RECENT ADVANCES IN ULTRASOUND DIAGNOSIS 2

RECENT ADVANCES IN ULTRASOUND DIAGNOSIS 2

Proceedings of the International Symposium on Recent Advances in Ultrasound Diagnosis, Dubrovnik, October 1-5, 1979

Editor: Asim Kurjak

1980
EXCERPTA MEDICA, Amsterdam - Oxford - Princeton

International Congress Series No. 498
ISBN Excerpta Medica 90 219 0427 6
ISBN Elsevier North-Holland 0 444 90125 6

Publisher:
Excerpta Medica
305 Keizersgracht
1000 BC Amsterdam
P.O. Box 1126

Sole Distributor for the USA and Canada:
Elsevier / North-Holland Inc.
52 Vanderbilt Avenue
New York, N.Y. 10017

Printed in The Netherlands by Groen, IJmuiden

CONTENTS

1. Introductory

2. Automatic and Computer-aided Sonography

3. Display Quantisation, Limitations and Testing

9. Recent Advances in Echocardiography

10. New Clinical Applications

11. Ultrasound Monitoring of Ovarian Stimulation

12. Ultrasound and the Radiologist

13. Invited Reviews

14. Free Communications

1. INTRODUCTORY

A. Kurjak
I.   Donald
G. Kossoff

WELCOME

This is the International Year of the Child. What occasion could be more fitting for such an event than this Third International Conference on the Recent Advances in Ultrasound Diagnosis--a meeting dedicated almost throughout to the welfare of humans from their earliest moments of embryonic life.

The participants in this meeting come from all over the world. Thirty-two countries are represented here, from as far apart as Australia and Japan to Europe and America. The Yugoslav Association of Societies for Ultrasound in Medicine and Biology and the city of Dubrovnik are proud indeed to be the host to so many men and women of international reputation. Among the many famous people here, I would like to distinguish two outstanding gentlemen, Professor Ian Donald, the father of diagnostic ultrasound in obstetrics and gynecology and Professor Inge Edler, the father of echocardiology.

At first, it may seem paradoxical that in a town as old as Dubrovnik, colleagues should gather to discuss ideas which project us all into the world of tomorrow, but perhaps Dubrovnik, by that enduring stability which comes with age, provides just the right environment for such an interchange. In a world where fortune now seems to change so rapidly, I believe we appreciate constancy more than ever before. But there is something else. Many of the delegates here also share a bond of friendship born of respect. Friendship has long been the thread which, in this old city, has woven together the past, the present and the future.

The word of friendship is "WELCOME". We have before us, for five days, not only the opportunity to work together but also, through our social program, to regenerate old friendships and create new ones.

Ladies and gentlemen, on behalf of the Organizing Committee, in the interest of science, and in the name of friendship, I bid you welcome.

A. Kurjak

MEDICAL SONAR - THE FIRST 25 YEARS

Ian Donald

Emeritus Professor, University of Glasgow
Consultant to EMI/Nuclear Enterprises Ltd,
Edinburgh, Scotland.

The first 25 years of medical sonar comes really as the finale in the much longer history of a subject whose origins go back into maritime history. What I have to say is no more than a personal account.

My often stated preference for the term "sonar" (which stands for "sound navigation and ranging") when referring to ultrasonic echography is based on my acknowledgement of this historical fact and our survival in the face of the German U-boat menace which, twice in my own lifetime, nearly defeated us in two world wars.

It was in about 1916/1917 that the French and British Admiralties formed a joint committee to counter the growing threat, the Anti-Submarine-Detection and Investigation Committee (ASDIC) and for whom the French physicist, Paul Langevin, (19) a one-time colleague of Marie Curie, conceived the principle of locating submarines in the ocean by using beams of sound waves of such high frequency as to be non-divergent and thus under directional control; and since the speed of sound, and therefore ultrasound in its passage through water is known, both the direction and distance of an object in the ocean could be determined.

As a schoolboy and student I knew of the application of the principle to depth sounding above the floor of the seabed from my enthusiastic attendance at engineering exhibitions at that time and, during my service with the RAF during the last war, I observed the fuller development of the technique of anti-U-boat warfare at closer and more sophisticated range. Little did I then think that I would one day apply it to the depiction of an early fetus in utero.

The miniaturisation of the technique came as a breakthrough in the USA during the last war by Firestone with his "reflectoscope" (14) for detecting flaws in metal structures, since the passage of a beam of ultrasound directly through a homogeneous metal was found to be interrupted in varying degree by cracks or flaws. This vital discovery was classified as a military secret and therefore not published until after the war but has since become standard metallurgical practice in engineering and affords a much simpler alternative to cumbersome high voltage X-ray examination.

By the 1950s my interest was thoroughly aroused. As medical usage was unexplored my own opportunity roughly synchronised with my translation to Glasgow, a city with heavy engineering as its principal industrial activity.

It was shortly before leaving London that I met Jack Wild whose early work with Reid in Minneapolis I had already read about (24). Wild's misfortune at the time was the premature hope that he would be able to differentiate between malignant and non-malignant tissue, a matter which, to my surgically-trained mind, must still remain with proper histology. Wild told me that he was even considering the possibility of diagnosing a carcinoma of the stomach from within its lumen - I thought then, and still do, an improbable feat. Nevertheless, I persuaded the late Professor Ian Aird to grant him the opportunity of giving a University of London lecture which my departure for Glasgow prevented me from attending, nor could I find a published account of it.

On arrival in Glasgow in 1954 I soon set about trying to learn something about the energy properties of ultrasound and managed to borrow from an engineering firm a powerful ultrasonic generator situated in a bath of carbon tetrachloride in which it created massive turbulence. I then suspended samples of unclotted blood in it for varying periods and then, by cell counting, determined the degree of haemolysis. The heating effect in the case of control specimens was found to be entirely respon-sible for this destructive phenomenon and at this early stage I recognised that power ultrasound was destructive in proportion with its heat generating capacity - a fact born out later by many subsequent experiments of other workers and very fully confirmed by a team of Professor Wagai and his colleagues in Japan who visited me in Glasgow some years later and showed me the negative results of their exhaustive experiments using diagnostic types of ultrasonic energy. This provides another reason for preferring the term "sonar" to "ultrasound" which, in the eyes of the public, may conjure up visions of dental drills, cooking and instrument cleansing apparatus!

One of my initial clinical frustrations on coming to Glasgow was the problem of the woman with the grossly-distended abdomen in which the tradi-tional methods of clinical diagnosis were simply in-adequate. Those were the days of massive tumours, both ovarian and uterine, of ascites whether cardiac, neoplastic or hepatic in origin and of obesity such as one seldom sees in the working classes of today.

One patient was so obese that she had been bedridden for years, lying like a turtle on her back with arms and legs waving about like flippers. It took four nurses all their strength to turn her over in bed to attend to her pressure sores. I could not believe such abdominal distension could be due simply to obesity and not to a pelvic tumour, yet neither I nor my colleagues could make the diagnosis and I even recklessly considered getting my hand in by laparotomy to be sure. It was a humiliating bafflement, and by no means an isolated case.

Thus it came about that I began to copy the techniques of my new Glasgow engineering friends and sought help from their contact A-scan method of probing metal structures and welds for cracks and flaws.

I began by thoroughly digesting Carlin's textbook on ultrasonic physics (2). Then, by good fortune, the wife of an eminent engineer at this time gratefully survived a hysterectomy at my hands and introduced me to her husband. Following a lunch party with their research directors a session was arranged in the research department of Messrs Babcock & Wilcox. I shall always remember that hot sunny afternoon of 21 July 1955 when we took to the factory some selections of the last few days operating, in the boots of two cars, large ovarian cysts and uterine fibroids, calcified and plain. The firm very thoughtfully provided a truly massive piece of prime steak as a control material.

All I wanted to know, and this was surely not asking too much, was whether a metal flaw detector could show me on A-scan, which was then all we had, the difference between a cyst and a myoma and so forth. To my surprise and delight the differences were exactly as my reading had led me to expect, the cyst showing clear margins without intervening echoes because of its fluid content and the fibroid progressively attenuating the returning echoes.

Photographic facilities were not at that time available and the factory artist was called in to sketch the blips on the cathode ray tube face. Furthermore, it was noted that the degree of penetration was inversely proportional to the frequency. The steak gave confusing and intermediate results which was rather a waste, especially since nobody would accept it to take home for cooking!

Armed with this knowledge and with borrowed apparatus, I returned to the clinical problem of the grossly-distended female abdomen - initially a gynaecological problem (6). The study of pregnancy came later.

I suspect that most engineers are doctors at heart. They like mending machines but people as well

6

if they could. The converse is unusual although I may be an exception. My personal role throughout this quarter of a century's research has been insignificant and no more than that of a catalyst or synthesiser of the fertile minds of my engineering friends.

Babcock & Wilcox referred me to Messrs Kelvin Hughes nearby who manufactured the apparatus and whose attitude was equally generous, both with advice, the loan of apparatus and with expertise. Their directors came to lunch with me at the hospital and promptly voted the princely sum of £500 towards helping my research. In particular, Mr W T Slater, the Managing Director, provided invaluable help. They put me in touch with Professor Mayneord of the then Royal Cancer Hospital in London who was having a discouraging time with their mark 2 flaw detector on the cranial vault - we now know why.

As a result, this hellish machine was passed on to us. As far as I remember, it had a 1 or $1\frac{1}{2}$ MHz quartz crystal and a paralysis time of 8 cms, i.e. nothing showed up within the first 8 cms of penetration.

This led us, inevitably, to devising water tanks with flexible latex bottoms which were applied with a film of grease to the protuberant female abdomen and into the surface of which our probes were cautiously dipped. Accidental spillages were frequent with such precarious balance and the resulting wet beds endeared me to neither patients nor nurses who had to clear up the mess!

Contraceptive condoms, blown up with water, seemed an obvious solution. Being rather well-known, by sight if not by repute, in a city like Glasgow I was naturally a little reticent in those days about being seen entering one of those shops for surgical rubber goods in West Nile Street - now long since swept away in a municipal slum clearance operation. My friend, the late Professor James Louw from Cape Town, was visiting me at the time and jumped out of the car offering to buy them for me. On being asked by the middle-aged blonde behind the counter whether he wanted teat-ended or plain he astonished her by saying that he would go out to the car and enquire! The puritanical nursing staff viewed the following experiments with even less enthusiasm, though less often inconvenienced.

Perhaps because of such failures, I developed a hearty dislike of tanks and stand-off mechanisms and from that time onwards have always favoured the direct contact approach as in engineering practice. I can remember arguing heatedly with George Kossoff, years later, in about 1960 when he visited me in my office, but I must admit that I had neither the

ingenuity nor the patience to go to the lengths which
he has to secure ultrasonograms of his very striking
quality.

Still limited to uni-dimensional A-scan, we got
hold of a much improved mark 4 Kelvin Hughes flaw
detector and tried to study the cranium with it, as
had Professor Mayneord. Our distinguished colleague,
Dr James Willocks, appeared to be the obvious subject
for experiment having a head which was both large
and bald. The fact that no intracranial echoes could
be discerned gave rise to a lot of frivolous and un-
charitable suggestions from all of us which were
without scientific basis.

Returning to the problematical female abdomen,
dramatic, life-saving success soon came our way. I
was invited to see a poor woman who had a grossly-
distended abdomen, believed due to massive ascites
as a result of malignant portal obstruction. A
barium meal X-ray had revealed a carcinoma of stomach
and her case was regarded as hopeless with progressive anaemia from incessant haematemeses and rapid
loss of weight. My own clinical examination of this
very tense abdomen fully supported the physicians'
diagnosis and I expected to find on A-scan examination a mass of bowel echoes in the central abdomen
due to the presence of contained gas - as I explained
to the surrounding throng of disbelieving medical
onlookers. To my dismay all I could demonstrate was
a clear space with, at great depth, a very strong
echo so that I began to doubt the validity of the
technique. My senior lecturer, John MacVicar, now
Professor in Leicester, insisted that if this was not
a large cyst then it ought to be. My own diffidence
vanished when the physicians admitted with commend-
able modesty that they could, of course, be wrong.
They agreed that, however hopeless, the patient
deserved a laparotomy so she was transferred to my
department. At operation I found a mammoth-sized
mucinous cystadenoma which was entirely benign. Her
recovery was immediate. Vomiting and haematemesis
ceased, the X-rays were declared to be an artefact,
she put on weight and remained well for many years
when I lost sight of her with the family's emigration
to New Zealand. This life-saving stroke of luck
abolished all thought of slackening our research
which had, up to then, been rather discouraging.

Soon I was being asked to do the impossible but
fortunately a brilliant young man, Tom Brown, who
was on the research staff of Kelvin Hughes, came on
the scene. I was later to learn that the girl he
subsequently married happened to be one of my staff
nurses. He was also expecting to find himself on
military draft as conscription still operated at that
time. He soon made himself indispensable by

borrowing all manner of equipment from his firm and later introducing me to polaroid photography of our results. Following a General Election, the usual exhortations from visiting politicians to reduce expenditure whatever the successful political party, prompted me to make a request that would cost the Exchequer nothing. The Under-Secretary of State, who had been haranguing us, looked at me with disbelief until I explained that I needed this young man to assist me and not at Government expense either. Brown was taken off military draft and our association, for many years to come, was most productive.

Our incursion into the study of pregnancy did not begin until ˌ1957 because my Obstetric Department at that time was situated at the other side of the town and it was difficult to transfer my apparatus from one hospital to another. The Queen Mother's Hospital was not in fact completed until seven years later. Nevertheless, we continued to attempt the impossible.

One striking and tragic case was that of a man who had recently undergone thoracotomy for the relief of mitral stenosis. The surgeon, however, had palpated a large mass within the left atrium which he opined was an atrial myxoma. He was, therefore, unwilling to proceed further without the establishment of cardio-pulmonary by-pass for which preparations had not been made. He accordingly closed the chest - to the fury of the physicians who reckoned that the lump was a well-organised intra-atrial clot which could have been turned out before proceeding to commissurotomy. They turned to me for a differential diagnosis with my new-fangled apparatus (remember this was in about 1957). The man, in pyjamas and dressing gown, was brought by ambulance to the maternity hospital where I put him to bed in the antenatal ward while I made ready to examine him. It was at this point that the ward sister from another department, who disapproved of me and all my works, suddenly took an interest in my research for the first and only time. She was eager to behold with her own eyes the sight of a male, no matter how sick, installed in a bed among highly pregnant females. She was not disappointed. Like Julius Caesar invading Britain she came, she saw and went away scandalised! The clarity of the echo picture which I got led me correctly to diagnose ˌa thrombus and not a myxoma but the poor man died in the course of his second thoracotomy a few days later.

In pregnancy the only echoes of which we could be reasonably sure at that time were those provided by the fetal head, a fact which enabled my staff nurse, Miss Marjorie Marr (later promoted to Matron at the new Queen Mother's Hospital), to be certain of the presentation in obese or difficult cases by the secret use of the apparatus in advance of our staff rounds on Friday mornings. It was this which led me to undertake a series of water tank experiments in which I learned to identify the biparietal diameter and, with later development, its accurate measurement.

Nevertheless, the limitations of A-scan technique were becoming all too obvious and the decision was made to adopt the PPI (plan position indication) system developed in wartime radar and thus to graduate from uni-dimensional to two-dimensional scanning. This involved transferring the echo signals from the vertical deflecting plates of the cathode ray oscilloscope to the grid or cathode, thereby influencing the energy of the cathode ray beam on its way to the phosphor screen, which now produced a series of dots of light, instead of blips, which coalesced to provide tissue outlines. The orientation of the time-base sweep was determined by X and Y linear potentiometers and its inclination by sine/cosine potentiometers, the latter giving us endless trouble in those early days.

The object was, of course, to position the echo dots geometrically in accordance with the attitude of the exploring crystal on the patients body surface and to relate them to their points of origin within the body. This all sounds remarkably obvious today but, believe me, we hardly knew at that time how or where to look and were like the blind leading the blind.

One of the difficulties with our makeshift apparatus (Figures 1, 2), made up largely of purloined ingredients, was that only echoes specularly reflected could be identified with any certainty and hence compound scanning was necessary in order to outline the shape of a viscus. Only by reference to frequency and power attenuation could we form any idea of the "transonicity" of different tissues. True tissue differentiation was only to come many years later, especially with the development of grey scaling. Nevertheless, we acquired a lot of experience and were able to give a demonstration on a patient to a meeting of the American College of Surgeons, which was held in Glasgow. At this time in 1958 we could differentiate with reasonable certainty between quite a variety of gynaecological tumours and ascites both benign and malignant (the latter having a characteristically bizarre appearance) and, of course, gross obesity. We could also demonstrate fetal echoes in utero, particularly the fetal head provided the uterus was enlarged above the level of the symphysis pubis.

We first went to press in The Lancet in 1958 (12)

and I still regard this as one of the most important papers I have ever written, noteworthy also because there has, so far, been no subsequent need to repeal anything I then wrote.

It was our attempts to diagnose hydatidiform mole which awakened us to the danger of being deceived by "electronic grass" if gain settings were set too high. Also, we recognised that we could cheat and make the diagnosis fit the clinical diagnosis by manipulating the controls and by the degree of deliberate overscanning. We were still operating literally in the dark as regards crystal frequency, pulse repetition frequency, amplification gain settings and duration of exposure so that results were often not reproducible. It was for this reason that we decided to resort to an automatic scanner which standardised as many of these variables as possible. This costly but necessary step was taken by Tom Brown and his research colleagues John Fleming and, presently, by Brian Fraser, at Kelvin Hughes and led to the ribald statement by a very senior gynaecologist, to an hilarious group of Edinburgh students, that in Glasgow we needed an apparatus costing more than £10,000 to diagnose a cyst which he could diagnose with a twopenny glove. This step led us into our first serious financial confrontation. The firm agreed to fulfil its promise and complete the automatic scanner but after that we could expect no more. In the next hectic ten days I managed to raise about £15,000, first from my University, then from Sir John Erskine (later Lord Erskine) Chairman of the Scottish Hospitals Endowment Research Trust, and finally from the National Research Development Corporation. (This latter body fully expected to recover its expenses in due course). Support from the Medical Research Council came much later.

It is pleasing to recall that many years later Lord Erskine, now well over eighty years old and with a most distinguished career behind him, came to visit me in Hammersmith Hospital while I was recovering from one of my cardiac valve replacement operations and told me that his decision to back me at this necessitous time gave him more satisfaction than any other achievement in his eventful life as a public figure, including governorship of Northern Ireland.

The automatic scanner was completed in 1960 and exhibited by Tom Brown at Olympia in London (Figs 3 & 4). We used a full-size adult doll from the nurses training school on which to demonstrate its automatic action. This was the first time I met the late Douglas Howry who was enraptured with our work. The results of his own genius, years earlier, with a circumferential B-scanner in a large water tank constructed from the gun turret of a Boeing bomber, should not be forgotten (17, 18) and his untimely death was a tragedy for our subject.

I think it was Lord Hailsham who observed the scanner rocking up and down over the length and breadth of the abdomen of our dummy doll and asked, frivolously, if we were trying to roll off some fat!

I have already mentioned our identification of the fetal biparietal diameter and my hopes of measuring it accurately (11). The glimpses which we obtained with a hand-held probe left insufficient time to measure the distance between the relevant blips from the parietal eminences on the cathode ray tube face. Accordingly, Tom Brown borrowed from his employers a two-channel gated flaw alarm unit which triggered a solenoid-operated polaroid camera from whose photographs measurements could be accurately made. This was an ingenious device with which it was hoped to simplify biparietal cephalometry in the course of random searching in the region of the anterior fetal parietal bone.

A physicist, hitherto engaged in rocketry and all its associated need for mathematical precision, now joined our team, namely Tom Duggan. He was initially horrified and sceptical of the concept of ultrasonic cephalometry. However, he introduced electronic cursors consisting of bright-up dots which could be placed by knob manipulation on the leading edges of the blips and provide a digital read-out of the distance between them. This proved even more accurate and saved money on photographic materials.

Meanwhile, Dr Willocks made a series of consecutive growth studies of fetal head enlargement (25, 26) which were later to be perfected by the more exact and exacting method of Stuart Campbell who later joined us and established a well-deserved international reputation (1).

Bertil Sunden from Sweden was our first distinguished foreign pupil to whom I taught all I then knew. He returned to Lund with his own apparatus and contributed greatly to the subject (23), mainly in the identification of twins by counting fetal heads and in recognising the characteristic features of hydramnios. I had the privilege, later, of examining him in Lund for his Docent degree in the course of a Saturday morning, in full academic regalia in a large public hall where the audience came and went as nature demanded, throughout a very lengthy morning. He defended his thesis so well that I was proud to recommend the award of his Docent.

Around this time I was emboldened to try to diagnose multiple pregnancy in animals. My veterinary colleagues were constantly impressing on me the need to differentiate between twin and singleton lambs since the feeding requirements differ and the matter was of considerable financial, though callous, importance. I felt that there was altogether too much wool about for contact scanning. In addition, others wanted to be able to tell what sort of bacon lay beneath the skin of a pig's backside. A large pig was brought into the factory in a very strong wooden box to restrain its movement. The danger of escape and running amok in such a sophisticated department was too awful to contemplate. The pig squealed and struggled uncontrollably and proved most unco-operative. It was quite clear that all the female secretaries were on the pig's side regardless of what might happen if he broke loose. Alas, he died, presumably of fright, while we suspended our investigations for a drink and lunch. The fact that he was destined for the slaughterhouse made little difference to the female sympathy which he evoked.

My other incursion into veterinary experiment was the interesting case of my youngest daughter's bitch who, after a series of unplanned indiscretions, showed all the signs of being pregnant, to her great delight. The animal was thus brought one evening to the hospital and placed on the examination couch to determine the number of puppies to be expected since my daughter had now reached the stage of promising them to her friends at school. She rigidly refused to allow me to shave the abdomen as she feared that I would damage what she called its "milkers". So, we did our best. Without cranial vaults to identify we were confused by the profusion of echoes and recklessly diagnosed triplets. Alas, term came and went and to this day no puppies have emerged. My child's regard for ultrasonic diagnosis is still one of withering contempt.

However, it was not always failure that greeted our efforts. Our experience grew in a number of directions, most notably of all perhaps in the rapid and easy diagnosis of hydatidiform mole (20). The vesicular pattern was found to be so gain sensitive that we have always recommended confirming the diagnosis at a second and higher frequency, e.g. 5MHz. It was from this principle that we sought to identify the placenta.

In 1961 Kelvin Hughes, who had done so much for us, were absorbed by Smith's Industrial Division from England whose more massive financial resources were better able to shoulder the considerable expense to which I was putting them, which dwarfed the contributions I had been able to raise. The team of workers, meanwhile, continued to work as before including John Fleming and Brian Fraser, the latter now in charge of ultrasonic production at Nuclear

Enterprises in Edinburgh. Throughout all these
worrying times of uncertainty the team always
managed to reform.

The late Managing Director of Smith's, who died
prematurely, came to see me and asked how long I
thought it would be before the project became commercially viable. I replied with almost prophetic
insight, fifteen years. He felt that this was a long
time to justify to shareholders, nevertheless I shall
always be grateful for their continuing help over the
next few years.

From 1962 onwards we had established contact
with Joe Holmes and his colleagues in Denver with
whom a very happy co-operation and association has
been maintained ever since. They followed us into
obstetrics and we all set about seeking to identify
the placenta, in our case as an extension of the
principles underlying the diagnosis of hydatidiform
mole. I was lucky to be able to import Usama Abdulla
from Baghdad specifically for the purpose of ultrasonic placentography, although he has since gone from
strength to strength. We worked in close liaison
with our Denver friends and published our findings in
the UK (10) shortly after their own publication in
America (15). Since that time sonar has come to
replace all other methods of placental localisation.

A really important breakthrough occurred in
1963 when a nervous patient presented herself for
examination with a full bladder. This at once made
possible the visualisation of the pelvic viscera,
even though not enlarged, since it had the effect of
displacing gas containing and therefore impenetrable
bowel out of the field and also provided a built-in
viewing tank without interfering with the ultrasonic
picture. Even the contents of a normal size uterus
could now be studied (3).

It was not long before I saw a very early
gestation sac in a woman who had a history of four
previous abortions and no living children and who,
at 6-7 weeks, did not even know that she was pregnant.
I delivered her myself at term and demonstrated my
early slides to the centenary meeting of the New York
Obstetric Society in Manhattan in 1964 (4), a society
older, I believe, than any similar society in the UK.

Early pregnancies, normal, abnormal, aborting
and continuing could now be studied serially in great
detail from the fifth week onwards and we soon
collected a mass of material. I published the
various appearances throughout prenatal development
in an article in the Journal of Pediatrics in 1969
(5). This was written under quite difficult circumstances since I was being treated in hospital at the
time for acute cardiac failure, just prior to my
first mitral valve replacement with a homograft. I

had a portable tape recorder hidden under the bed-
clothes and my secretary was allowed to visit me
briefly once a day. I was thus able to smuggle
photographs and tapes in and out. Later, as I was
recovering from this frightful operation, I wrote to
the editors in Chicago enquiring what had happened
to my article. They replied, reassuringly, that they
had corrected the proofs themselves, since they knew
I was sick, and they promised that it read like
excellent American. During the latter half of the
1960s things were going well and cases were being
referred to us from far and wide; also eminent
pupils from other countries came to us and each, in
his way, contributed. One of them, my friend Dr Lou
Hellman from New York, spent three weeks with us,
learning avidly and fast. He was rewarded on his
last day by correctly diagnosing a hydatidiform mole
and announced triumphantly, if a little unscientifi-
cally, "I may be wrong but I am not in doubt"!! In
actual fact, he missed the associated fetus which I
later discovered on rescanning, but no matter. He
set up his own department in Brooklyn and we later
produced a joint paper with Sunden in Sweden on the
safety of ultrasound in pregnancy (16).

What could have been a disaster struck, however,
in 1966 when Smith's, who had so generously helped
us, decided to pull out of Scotland and close the
Kelvin Hughes factory. I was desperate and could
foresee the dust-sheet phenomenon befalling my work.
In despair I turned to the University of Glasgow for
help and, to my astonished delight, was instructed to
form my own department of ultrasonic technology at
the Queen Mother's Hospital and to engage staff at
competitive rates of pay. Thus we acquired John
Fleming again and Angus Hall and some MRC help.
Meanwhile, Nuclear Enterprises Ltd in Edinburgh took
over the medical ultrasonics section, including the
aforementioned Brian Fraser with whom I have now
co-operated over a very large slice of our working
lives. In other words, the team again reformed and
the work continued.

By the early 1970s we began to recognise the
phenomenon of ovum blighting, which we now believe
to be common, and, with the now highly enthusiastic
radiologists in Glasgow, published our findings on
the subject in 1972 (13). Its frequency in early
pregnancy failure, if searched for, is not surprising
in terms of biology. That it should recur so often
in the same patient is a tragedy often associated
with abnormal karyotypes. All such cases should be
investigated by tissue culture and full genetic
assessment and not just dismissed as idiopathic early
abortions. Hugh Robinson came on the scene to
replace Stuart Campbell who had done so much to

import sonar to a backward city like London.
Robinson's most significant contributions, in
addition to all his other work, were the determination of the fetal crown/rump length and its accurate
relation to early gestational age and the positive
identification of early fetal heart movement by time
motion display (21, 22). These provide concrete
evidence of continuing fetal life long before ultrasonic Doppler studies become worthwhile.

Up to now our B-scanning technique (Figure
5), with varying degrees of compounding, had served
us well but true grey scaling was still far from our
grasp. In 1974, however, I was due to give the
Mackenzie Davidson Memorial Lecture at the British
Institute of Radiology and had already prepared my
script when Brian Fraser brought over to my ultrasonics department at the Queen Mother's Hospital a
scan converter and accessories which were then
linked up with my standard Diasonograph B-scanner.
This immediately made grey scaling possible. The
quality of the pictures as regards organ outline
remained as good as ever but also, by different
shades of grey, gave a far better indication of
tissue characterisation. In fact I scrapped my projected lecture and wrote another around the subject,
explaining the rationale of this new development
derived from radio technology and illustrating it
copiously with new illustrations (7). This facility
is now taken for granted but it has opened up a whole
new avenue of approach, especially in the study of
tissue parenchyma.

Finally, just before my retirement in 1976,
there came on the scene a whole crop of real-time
scanning machines whose different characteristics I
described two years ago in this hall and published in
Dr Kurjak's edited version of the proceedings of that
delightfully successful meeting (9).

Immediately following my retirement from my
clinical chair and being now free to undertake non-
university work I was invited by my colleagues of
long-standing in what is now the combined EMI/Nuclear
Enterprises group to join them as medical consultant,
so that my interest in the subject is not only sustained but positively heightened as I observe and try
out equipment of ever-increasing sophistication.

For me it has been a happy story with a happy
ending as I watch the subject of medical sonar going
from strength to strength in the hands of an ever-
widening circle of friends (8).

In conclusion, I can only reflect how different
was the sudden impact of X-rays upon medicine
compared with the long induction-delivery interval of
sonar. I would probably agree that the first twenty-
five years have been the worst. Nowadays one can

take for granted at least some sort of a result from
any functioning set of apparatus but I can remember
the days, twenty years ago, when we might spend three
weeks without being able to outline a simple cyst the
size of a baby's head.

I believe it was Louis Pasteur who talked of the
chance observation and the prepared mind. Certainly
I have had more than my share of chance observations.
Whether my mind has exploited them as fully as it
might have is more questionable.

REFERENCES

1.   Campbell, S. (1968): J. Obstet. Gynaec.
      Brit. Cwlth., 75, 568.
2.   Carlin, B. (1949): Ultrasonics. McGraw-Hill.
      New York - Toronto - London.
3.   Donald, I. (1963): Brit. Med. J. 2, 1154.
4.   Donald, I. (1965): Amer. J. Obstet. Gynec.,
      93, 935.
5.   Donald, I. (1969): J. Pediatr., 75, 326.
6.   Donald, I. (1974): Annals Roy. Coll. Surg. Eng.,
      54, 132.
7.   Donald, I. (1976): Brit. J. Radiol., 49, 306.
8.   Donald, I. (1976): J. Clin. Ultrasound, 4, 323.
9.   Donald, I. (1978): In: Recent Advances in Ultra-
      sound Diagnosis, pp5 - 21.
      Editor: A. Kurjak, Excerpta Medica, Amsterdam -
      Oxford.
10.   Donald, I. and Abdulla, A. (1968): J. Obstet.
      Gynaec. Brit. Cwlth., 75, 993.
11.   Donald, I. and Brown, T.G. (1961): Brit. J.
      Radiol., 34, 539.
12.   Donald, I., MacVicar, J. and Brown, T.G. (1958):
      Lancet, 1, 1188.
13.   Donald, I., Morley, P. and Barnett, E. (1972):
      J. Obstet. Gynaec. Brit. Cwlth., 79, 304.
14.   Firestone, F.A. (1945): Metal. Progr., 48, 505.
15.   Gottesfeld, K.R., Thompson, H.E., Holmes, J.H.
      and Taylor, E.S. (1966): Amer. J. Obstet.
      Gynec., 96, 538.
16.   Hellman, L.M., Duffus, G.M., Donald, I. and
      Sunden, B. (1970): Lancet 1, 1133.
17.   Holmes, J.H., Howry, D.H., Posakony, G.J. and
      Cushman, C.R. (1954): Trans. Amer. Clin. &
      Climatol, 66, 208.
18.   Howry, D.H. and Bliss, W.R. (1952): J. Lab &
      Clin. Med., 40, 579.
19.   Langevin, M.P. (1928): Revue général de
      l'électricité, 23, 626.
20.   MacVicar, J. and Donald, I. (1963): J. Obstet.
      Gynaec. Brit. Cwlth., 70, 387.
21.   Robinson, H.O. (1972): Brit. Med. J., 4, 466.
22.   Robinson, H.P. (1973): Brit. Med. J., 4, 28.

23. Sunden, B. (1964): Acta. Obstet. Gynec. Scand., 43, Suppl. 6.
24. Wild, J.J. and Reid, J.M. (1952): Science, 115, 226.
25. Willocks, J., Donald, I., Duggan, T.C. and Day, N. (1964): J. Obstet. Gynaec. Brit. Cwlth., 71, 11.
26. Willocks, J., Donald, I., Campbell, S. and Dunsmore, J.R. (1967): J. Obstet. Gynaec. Brit. Cwlth., 74, 639.

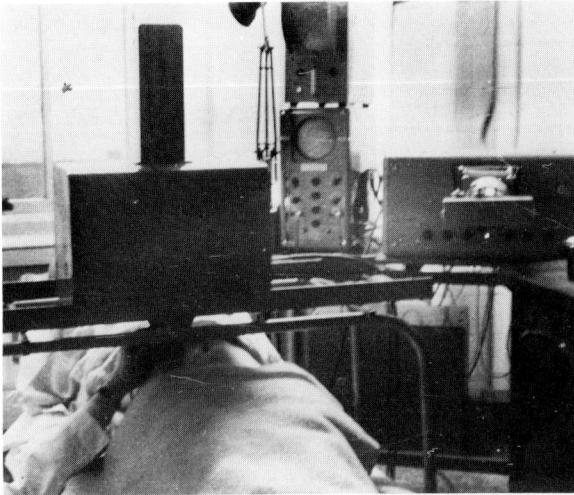

Figure 1 - 1957

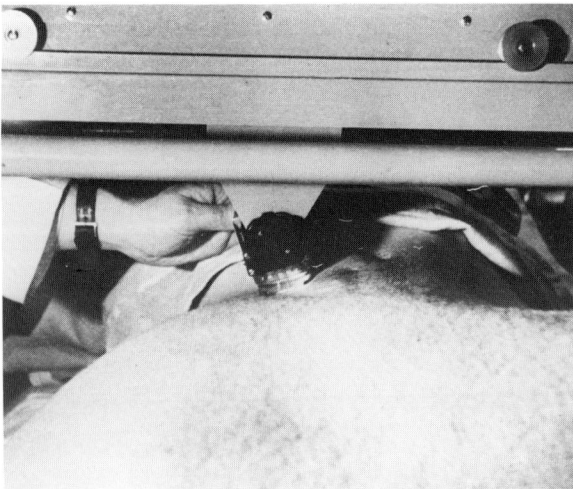

Figure 2 - 1957

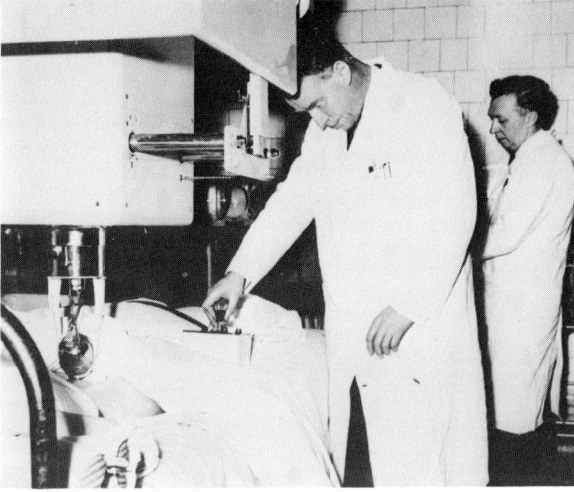

Figure 3 - 1960

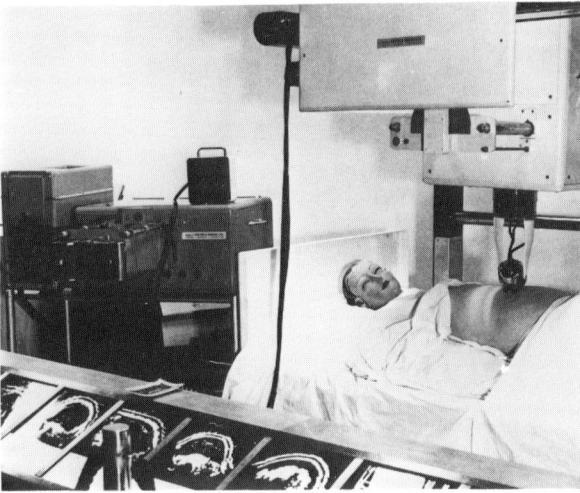

Figure 4 - 1960

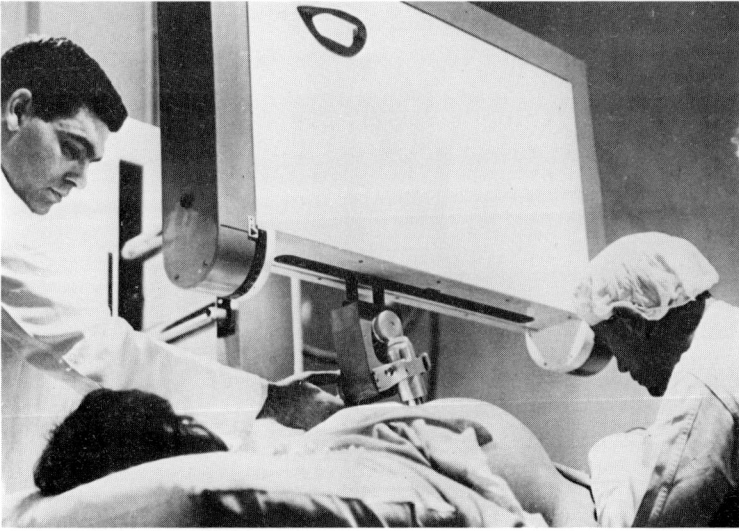

Figure 5 - 1965

LOOK INTO THE FUTURE OF DIAGNOSTIC ULTRASOUND

G. Kossoff

Ultrasonics Institute, Sydney, Australia

It is always an honour to be invited to present the opening address at a major international meeting and on this occasion I am particularly pleased to be able to share this address with Ian Donald. I must admit that invitations to speak on the future of diagnostic ultrasound give me some anxious moments. I do not consider myself a clairvoyant nor do I possess a magic crystal ball that lets me glimpse into the future. Thus in the past when I have given lectures on this subject I've made a number of predictions that have remained unrealised (1). Also I have not been astute enough to foresee some of the major innovations in their developing stages. I therefore advise that you take a sceptical view of my predictions and take into account that I will undoubtedly omit to mention important future innovations.

Diagnostic ultrasound first gained clinical acceptance in obstetrics and its major contributions have been in the assessment of fetal size and growth, the management of antepartum haemorrhage and threatened abortion and the diagnosis of fetal malformations.

Indeed, ultrasound has been so successful that some obstetricians feel that it has achieved all of its potential and there is little scope for any major new development. I do not share this opinion and believe that improvements will continue to be made to the resolution and grey scale sensitivity of conventional and real time equipment and these will allow us to view the whole conceptus in more detail. This improved performance for example will allow us to determine whether the umbilical cord is entwined around the fetal neck and reduce the risk of this cause of fetal demise.

In the future examinations based on morphological data will be complemented by studies concerned with the functional status of the fetus. An obvious example is the analysis of fetal breathing and limb movement made possible by real time equipment in the formulation of the biophysical profile to identify the fetus at risk for intrauterine compromise.

A recent study of the pattern of fetal breathing promises to become another example of the ultrasonic functional assessment of the fetus. This study has shown that prior to 32 weeks the fetal breath time is short and is characterised by an uneven period. The pattern changes between 32 and 36 weeks when breath is characterised by a long inspiratory phase with multiple augmenting movements. After 36

weeks the breath is more uniform and a definite periodicity
occurs in the last 2 weeks of pregnancy. In some pregnancies
in which the fetus has been subject to stress it achieves
the more developed breathing pattern at an earlier gestational
age suggesting that the method may be useful in the assessment
of functional maturity of fetal breathing (2).

Further advances will be achieved by the use of the
combined B-mode and pulsed Doppler technique. The former
allows the visualisation and measurement of the size and
orientation of deep lying vessels whilst the latter allows
the measurement of the mean velocity of the flow of blood in
the vessel. This information permits the quantitative
measurement of blood flow in the vessel and the technique is
being used to measure blood flow in the fetal umbilical vein.
Clinical studies on normal pregnancies from 20 weeks to term
have shown that the blood flow to the fetus increases prop-
prtionately with fetal growth, averaging 100 mls per minute
per kilogram weight of the foetus throughout pregnancy. The
flow decreases one or two weeks before term and appears to
coincide with the slow down or cessation of fetal growth.

A study of blood flow in growth retarded fetuses has
shown that the flow is reduced below the normal range.
Exceptions have been noted in cases of maternal hypertension,
placental dysfunction and other complications when the flow
per unit weight was found to be significantly higher (3).

Tissue characterisation studies have considerable
potential in obstetrics. In particular these should allow
the classification of placental function and fetal lung
development. If successful these would open up new areas
of application that would allow for instance, to dispense
with amniocentesis and the lecithin sphingomyelin ratio
test in the estimation of fetal lung maturity.

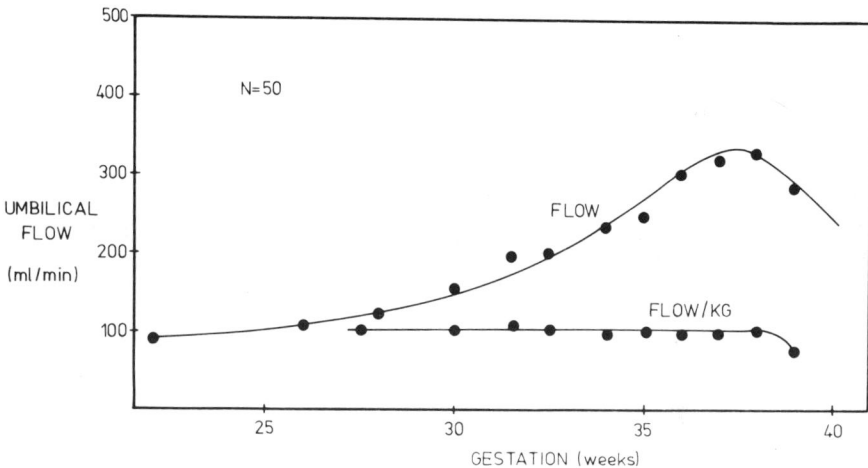

Umbilical vein flow in normal pregnancies.

Cardiology was the second specialty in which diagnostic ultrasound gained clinical acceptance. Indeed, if the level of acceptance of a technique may be judged by the degree of training provided at post-graduate level it is cardiology that has most fully integrated diagnostic ultrasound into its range of diagnostic procedures. It is estimated that well over half of the patients referred to specialist cardiology centres are examined by ultrasound and the M-mode technique has become as indispensable as an ECG examination for the total evaluation of the clinical condition of the patient.

I believe that the aggressive spirit of exploration that has characterised the development of echocardiography in the past will continue in the future. The identification of infarcted areas in the myocardium either by conventional techniques or by tissue characterisation is one example of advances that are likely to be achieved in the near future (4).

The development of different approaches to examine the heart should provide novel and valuable information. For instance, the cross-sectional examination of the heart by an oesophageal transducer is not impeded by overlying lung tissue and the technique may be used to examine a patient who cannot be examined by the conventional technique. This approach should also allow the visualisation of the structures near the oesophagus that are difficult to visualise by conventional methods.

Advances in Doppler technology will also undoubtedly take place and should ultimately allow the quantitative measurement of blood flow in all of the major vessels. We are currently attempting by the combined B-mode and pulsed Doppler method to measure the blood flow in the inferior and superior vena cava in paediatric patients. A number of centres throughout the world are also studying these applications and I'm sure that in the not too distant future all of our efforts will bear fruit and the quantitative measurement of blood flow will become a major application of diagnostic ultrasound.

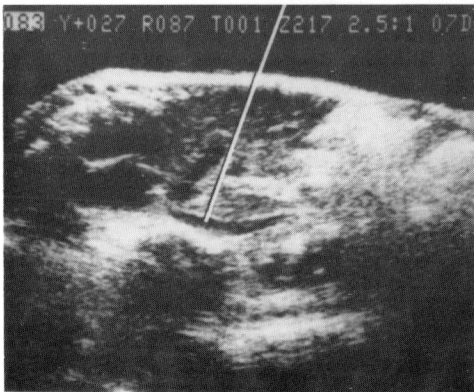

Flow = 360 mls/min
= 55 ml/kg min

Measurement of blood flow in inferior vena cava in 2 year old child.

Although ultrasound was first applied to examine the upper abdomen in the early 50's, it took 20 years for the technique to gain clinical acceptance. The two crucial factors that accelerated this acceptance were the development of grey scale and the application of this technique to the parasagittal scanning of the liver (5). These two developments allowed the reliable portrayal of the soft tissue texture of upper abdominal organs. Radiologists quickly recognised the clinical value of the procedure and developed it to its present stage of widespread acceptance.

The use of the liquid filled stomach with the patient examined in the prone position has been a major development in the examination of the upper abdomen (6). The liquid filled stomach and duodenum creates an acoustic window which acts as a landmark assisting the identification of neighbouring structures and allows the visualisation of posterior structures such as the body and tail of the pancreas. The stomach and duodenum wall may also be examined using this technique.

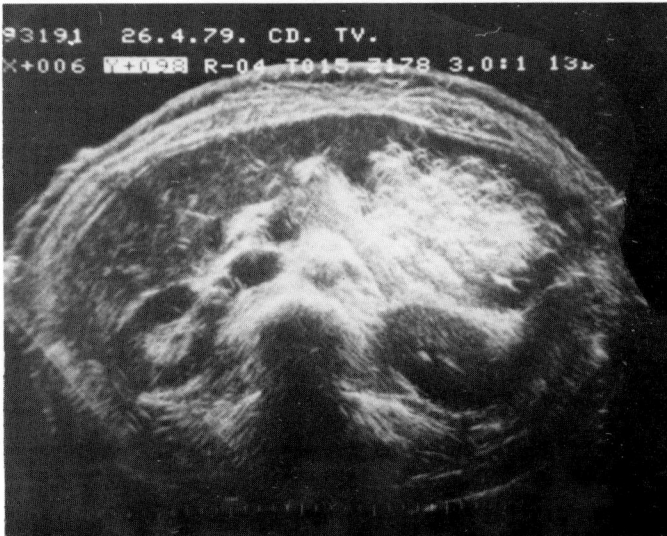

Upper abdominal scan in normal patient. Stomach filled with tomato juice. The pancreas and the left kidney are visualised.

Despite all the current advances one still frequently encounters patients who are difficult to examine and there is a tendency to blame the patient for the poor quality of images that are obtained. I believe that diagnostically useful information is resident in processes which degrade our images at present. In the future I'm sure that techniques will be developed that will allow the measurement of these processes and by reprocessing of the data, remove the degrading effects.

24

Digital signal processing is likely to play an important role in this development. One of the projects pursued at our Institute is the setting up of a computer interfaced with an Octoson which stores the whole A-mode data obtained during the scan (7). With this data in the computer it is possible to select the type of signal processing that optimises the display of selected anatomical detail without the need to rescan the patient. In the future it will be possible to also remove the degrading effects of superficial tissues and calculate the value of TGC that will portray the whole liver with uniform texture. The echogram may then be reconstructed with this value of TGC. The quantified value of this TGC setting could also be useful in the assessment of the degree of involvement by diffuse liver disease.

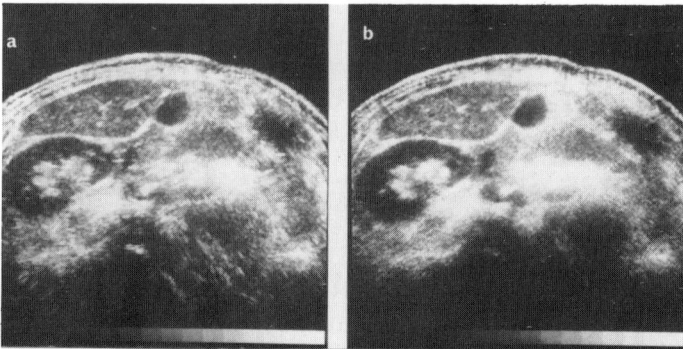

Computer reconstruction of data stored in line mode using peak and average detect.

Undoubtedly many new applications will also emerge in the future. One example is the use of the combined B-mode and pulsed Doppler technique for the measurement of blood flow in the portal and renal veins in patients with right heart failure and in renal hypertension.

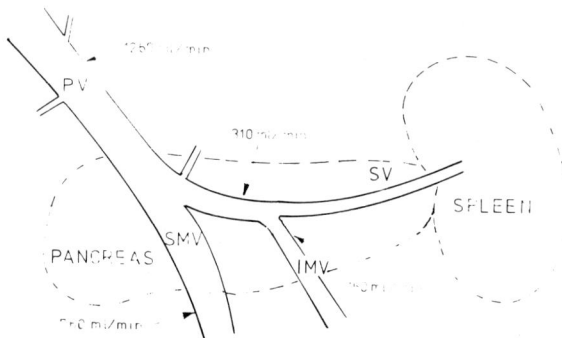

Blood flow in splanchnic system.

Paediatrics is a specialty in which ultrasound has made and will continue to make significant contributions. The safety of the technique is a particularly important feature in the examination of neonates and young children as it avoids unnecessary ionising radiation exposure to rapidly developing tissues. The simple and non-traumatic manner in which these examinations are performed without any requirement for anaesthesia are further advantages of the method in this application.

The less ossified skull in children does not impede the transmission of ultrasound as it does later in life. It has been shown that considerable intracranial detail may be demonstrated in children under the age of two years and that the size of the ventricular system may be reliably measured in children up to the age of four (8). In children with hydrocephalus the enlarged and presumably reduced thickness of the skull does not impede the visualisation to the same degree and satisfactory results may be obtained even in ten year olds. Correlation studies with CT have shown that ultrasound provides identical size data and in many centres the ultrasonic examination has considerably reduced the number of CT scans that are performed on young children, particularly in hydrocephaly where frequent repeat examinations are required to monitor the progress of disease or its response to treatment.

Similarly, the bony sternum and the ribs in infants do not impede to the same extent the passage of ultrasound and the cross-sectional examination of the heart and the mediastinum will provide unique diagnostic information in paediatrics

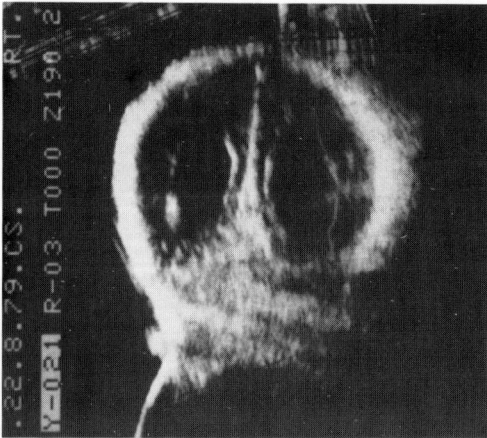

Coronal section in 2 day old infant showing enlarged lateral ventricles.

The breast was one of the first organs to be visualised by ultrasound but it is only in the last few years that this superficially lying organ, which from preliminary considerations could be thought to be ideally suited for ultrasonic visualisation, has finally become amenable to examination by ultrasound. The primary reason for this long latent period is the highly heterogeneous composition of the constituent tissues of the breast. This heterogeneous composition gives rise to a variable echo pattern and this complicates the detection and diagnosis of pathological changes.

The recent advent of water coupling equipment has shown that ultrasound may be employed to provide valuable information on patients with breast disease (9). In Australia patients with breast disease are managed by surgeons. Surgeons in Australia, as I am sure in other countries, are pragmatic in purpose and aggressive in treatment. For this reason patients who on physical examination have obvious signs of carcinoma or in whom a definite lesion may be palpated are seldom referred for an imaging investigation. Such patients are immediately referred to biopsy and are managed on the basis of this information. The majority of patients referred to imaging are patients with lumpy breasts where the referring physician is unable to make up his mind about the underlying pathology but is not sufficiently impressed by it to undertake biopsy. Alternatively, patients are referred when the physician feels that the biopsy of a lesion, which is probably benign, may lead to a "round robin" situation of repeated biopsies of little benefit to the patient. The safety of the method is an important advantage in these applications, particularly in younger women where it is desirable to avoid cumulative ionising radiation exposure.

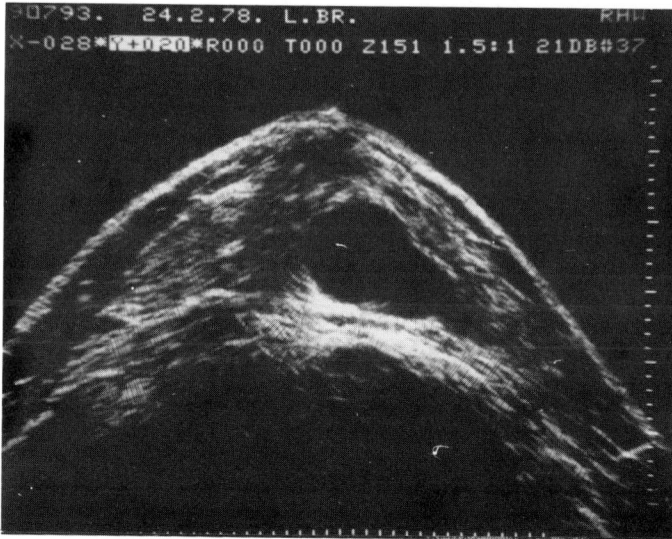

Fibrocystic breast disease.

We have recently completed a correlative study of ultrasound and xerography on the last 100 patients to whom a biopsy was also undertaken. Ultrasound was found to be the most accurate technique for the diagnosis of liquid filled lesions in the breast where it reliably identified cysts less than 5 mm in diameter and enlarged ducts 2 mm in diameter. In benign conditions it has been found to be more accurate than xeroradiography particularly in the younger, more dense breast. Finally, the two techniques were found to have approximately the same accuracy in the detection of malignant lesions greater than 1 cm in diameter. The method has limitations as it is unable to visualise small microcalcifications that form such an important part of diagnosis by xeroradiography. Difficulties are also encountered in accurately identifying fatty tissue and in patients with large breasts.

No. of Patients	Histology	Ultrasound			Mammography		
		Correct	?	Incorrect	Correct	?	Incorrect
56	Solid Dysplasia	46	6	4	33	15	8
13	Large Cyst(s)	13			3	6	5
8	Fibrocystic	8			4	3	1
4	Fibroadenoma	3		1		3	1
6	Duct Ectasia	4	1	1	2	2	2
1	Duct Papilloma	1			1		
2	Fat Lobule	2				1	1
7	Carcinoma	5		5	6		1
1	Lymph Node	1					1
2	Normal	2			1	1	

At the present stage of instrumentation development ultrasound is not suitable for screening examinations. It is likely that the method will be developed for this application where it could be made to identify high risk patients who would then be examined on a regular basis either by ultrasound or other methods such as xeroradiography or thermography. Potentially the method may also be developed to detect premalignant changes in the breast and this would open up a vast new area of application.
Studies on ultrasonic reconstruction techniques similar to those performed on x-ray computerised tomography equipment to determine the velocity and attenuation in breast tissue also hold considerable promise and will complement the information obtained by conventional B-mode techniques (10).

Recently it has been demonstrated that grey scale echography may be used to visualise the testes (11). The normal testis is displayed by homogeneous distribution of echoes and this facilitates the detection of lesions within the testis. Our experience to date shows that the referring physicians are considerably influenced by the information provided to them by ultrasound. In particular, a demonstration of a normal texture within the testis can avoid a biopsy or if abnormal echoes are obtained, guide the biopsy directly to affected areas. Biopsy of the testis frequently destroys the function of the testis particularly if the epididymis is pierced and the ultrasonic non-invasive visualisation will make an important contribution to the management of patients with scrotal enlargements.

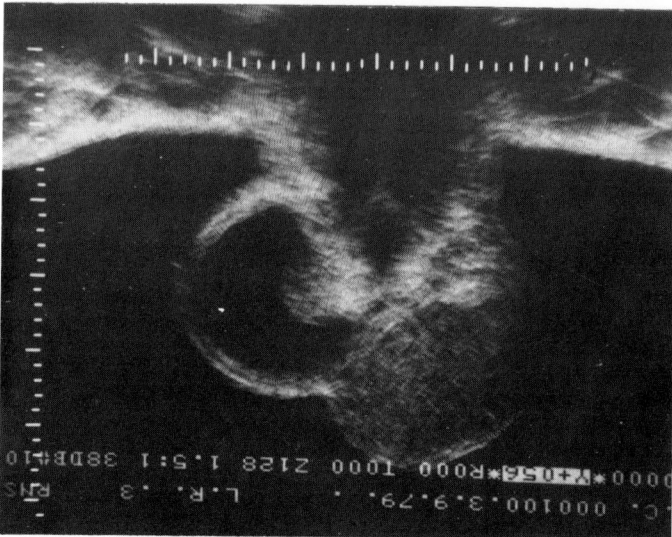

Post-surgical hydrocele following ligation of varicocele. There is some oedema in the right scrotal wall.

Internal devices such as used with transrectal and transurethral scanners are also likely to gain widespread clinical acceptance in the near future. This type of equipment has achieved a high level of performance particularly in the examination of the bladder and the prostate and will undoubtedly become commonly used by urologists. Many new instruments of this type are in the process of development. These include endoscope probes which contain small linear array transducers to provide real time viewing and ultrasonic catheters for measurement of biophysical parameters.

29

Erythrocytes in flowing blood return a signal which is Doppler frequency shifted proportional to their velocity. This information may be quantified and Doppler techniques will continue to make important contributions to our knowledge on haemodynamics and to vascular applications. Imaging techniques based on the visualisation of moving structures will also become used more frequently in the future. Such techniques are already being used to visualise vessels such as the carotid and to demonstrate internal occlusions, stenoses and plaques. This information combined with the measurement of flow by Doppler techniques has considerable potential in the detection and evaluation of patients with a variety of vascular disease and, for example, could significantly reduce the mortality associated with strokes by the early identification of patients at high risk to this disease.

No discussion on the future of diagnostic ultrasound would be complete without some mention on education. The Australian Society for Ultrasound in Medicine has held discussion on this matter with the representative bodies of cardiologists, nuclear medicine physicians, internists, radiologists and obstetricians and all agree that training should be provided at two levels of expertise, basic and advanced (12).

It seems reasonable that training at the basic level should be provided by the appropriate specialty. Just as an obstetrician and other clinicians are trained in the interpretation of aspects of radiology related to their specialty, so they should be trained in diagnostic ultrasound. The development of real time equipment which is finding a place in private practice, raises specific problems. Thus, it is important to detail not only the nature of training at the basic level, but just as important to list areas which should not be included so that the application and limitation of the simpler examinations are clearly understood.

The basic level of competence is different to the advanced level required of practitioners who see patients on a referral basis. Their training must be more comprehensive and they should have certified evidence of their competence. The Australian Society for Ultrasound in Medicine has set up such certification in the form of a Diploma of Diagnostic Ultrasound. The Diploma is granted by the Council of the Society on recommendation of the Board of Examiners to medical practitioners registered to practise in Australia and New Zealand. The examination is in two parts. Part I consists of a written paper on the physics of ultrasound. The questions are not too technical but require knowledge of instrumentation, biological effects and features of the subjects such as artifacts, which a specialist must be expected to understand thoroughly. The Part II examination is open to the candidates who have two years experience in ultrasound and consists of a written paper, an oral examination and a reporting test. The written paper has some choice and allows, for instance, the cardiologist to restrict himself to cardiological and vascular application but does not allow the imaging physician to avoid major areas of application of B-mode ultrasound. The oral and the reporting test are based on the evaluation of 12 sets of echograms and a test on anatomy.

The examination for the Diploma has now been conducted for over three years and currently 115 practitioners have been awarded the Diploma. Approximately half of them are radiologists, while 25% are obstetricians and cardiologists respectively. Currently there are also 50 practitioners who have completed Part I requirements.

The Diploma of Diagnostic Ultrasound is an attempt to establish a standard where none has previously existed. The Diploma is in no way exclusive and is open to other academic or professional bodies and indeed the Australasian College of Radiologists recognises the Diploma as appropriate qualification in diagnostic ultrasound as a sub-specialty in radiology.

As diagnostic ultrasound has made significant contribution across the whole spectrum of medical specialties, it is unlikely that ultrasound will be restricted to any one specialty but rather it will continue to be developed and practiced by those specialties interested in its application. It is even possible that once a sufficient number of specialists start practising ultrasound on a full-time basis, ultrasound could become accepted as a medical specialty in its own right.

In summary, it is clear that diagnostic ultrasound will continue to make a considerable impact on modern medical practice. In many ways it is an ideal form of energy to examine soft tissues. A wide variety of interactions take place when ultrasound propagates in tissue and we are still learning how to measure and utilise the information that is resident in these interactions. For instance, diagnostic ultrasound allows the measurement of six independent acoustic parameters of tissue, namely, acoustic impedance mismatch, attenuation, Doppler frequency shift, velocity, echo scattering cross section and impedance. By contrast, conventional x-ray and CT measure only one parameter of tissue, namely, the x-ray absorption by tissue. To date most of the ultrasonic applications measure only in a semi-quantitative way the first three parameters. I have no doubt that as more investigators enter the field and bring their imagination and expertise to the subject they will develop techniques which will measure quantitatively all of the six ultrasonic parameters and this will ensure the continuing growth of ultrasound in the foreseeable future.

REFERENCES

1. Kossoff, G. (1978): Diagnostic Ultrasound - The View from Down Under. J. Clin. Ultrasound, 6, 144-149.
2. Trudinger, B.J., Gordon, Y.B., Grudzinskas, J.G., Hill, M.G.R., Lewis T.J. and Arrans, Marie e Lozano. (1979): Fetal Breathing Movements and Other Tests of Fetal Wellbeing: A Comparative Evaluation. Brit. Med. J. (in press).
3. Gill, R.W.: Pulsed Doppler with B-mode Imaging for Quantitative Blood Flow Measurement. Ultrasound in Medicine and Biology (in press).
4. Gramiak, R., Waag, R.C., Schenk, E.A., Thomson, K. and Macintosh, P. (1979): Ultrasonic Imaging of Experimental Myocardial Infarcts. In: Echocardiology. Editor C.T. Lancee. Martinus Nyhoff Publishers, The Hague.
5. Taylor, K.J.W., Carpenter, D.A. and McCready, V.R. (1973): Grey Scale Echography in the Diagnosis of Intrehepatic Disease. J. Clin. Ultrasound, 1, 284-287.
6. Warren, P.S., Garrett, W.J. and Kossoff, G. (1978): The Liquid-Filled Stomach - An Ultrasonic Window to the Upper Abdomen. J. Clin. Ultrasound, 6, 315-320.
7. Robinson, D.E. and Kossoff, G. (1979): Computer Processing of Line Mode Echogram Data. In: Proc. 2nd Meeting of World Federation for Ultrasound in Med. & Biol., Miyazaki. Excerpta Medica (in press).
8. Garrett, W.J. and Kossoff, G. (1979): Grey Scale Examination of the Brain in Children. In: Ultrasound in Medicine, Vol. 3A, p. 821-828. Editor D. White and R. Brown. Plenum Press, New York.
9. Jellins, J., Kossoff, G., Barraclough, B.H. and Reeve, T.S. (1978): Comparative Study of Breast Imaging by Echography and Xerography. In: Recent Advances in Ultrasound Diagnosis. p. 299-304. Editor A. Kurjak, Excerpta Medica, Amsterdam.
10. Greenleaf, J.F., Johnson, S.A. and Lent, A.H. (1978): Measurement of Spatial Distribution of Refractive Index in Tissues by Ultrasonic Computer Assisted Tomography. Ultrasound in Med. and Biol., 3, 327-339.
11. Jellins, J. and Barraclough, V.H. (1978): Ultrasonic Imaging of the Scrotum. In: Ultrasound in Medicine, Vol. 4. p. 151-154. Editor D. White and T. Lyons. Plenum Press, New York.
12. Garrett, W.J. The Australian Diploma of Diagnostic Ultrasound. The Place of Real Time and Static B-Mode Scanning in Obstetric Practice. Ultrasound in Med. and Biol. (in press).

2. AUTOMATIC AND COMPUTER-AIDED SONOGRAPHY

N. Bom, Chairman

INTRODUCTION TO THE WORKSHOP ON AUTOMATIC AND COMPUTER-AIDED SONOGRAPHY.

N. Bom

Thoraxcenter, Erasmus University Rotterdam and
Interuniversity Cardiology Institute, the Netherlands.

Computers are being applied in a large number of applications to help facilitate the ultrasound methods. Applications range from optical image reconstruction techniques to the construction of sound velocity or sound attenuation images as used in breast scanning. In this session the topics will be focussed on recognition of tissue parameters, a line mode data acquisition and reconstruction method, recent advances in M-mode analysis and two-dimensional cardiac imaging and, finally, reconstruction of mitral valve motion combined with two-dimensional Doppler information in the same cross-sectional plane.

Many research laboratories are presently investigating the capabilities of differentiating tissues by careful study of stored and digitized echo information on "coarseness" of the acoustic structure or on irregularity in for instance echo peak distribution in the image. Promising use of computers to identify more than geometrical echo information will be extensively dealt with in this session. These methods are most likely the first practical applications to be used on a larger scale in future.

Some exciting examples of contour enhancement in two-dimensional cardiac real time imaging are presented. Since the analysis process is yet rather complicated, the contour enhancement and the two-dimensional real time blood velocity information obtained in the left ventricular sagittal plane will most likely be limited in the near future to cardiac research applications only.

Of course, the clinical result remains the ultimate judge as to whether the computer has really "aided" the echography. During this session therefore, the authors have tried to examplify their methods with clinical examples wherever possible.

An entirely different aspect of computer application to echography is the possibility to calculate beam patterns and thus establish transducer element configurations for optimal resolution. A less well known but logical step further is the use of such methods in combination with a water tank to simulate images during the design stage of an echo system. This topic will be discussed during the first lecture of this session on computer-aided sonography.

COMPUTER AND WATERTANK IN THE DESIGN OF AN ULTRASOUND SYSTEM

N. Bom, J. Vogel and L.F. van der Wal.

Thoraxcenter, Erasmus University, P.O.Box 1738, Rotterdam, the Netherlands and Interuniversity Cardiology Institute, Rotterdam, the Netherlands.

Description of a film presented in Dubrovnik, October 1979.

The transducer is considered a very important part of any ultrasound system. Not only the ultrasonic beam pattern, but also the transducer efficiency and band width must be optimal. New methods of multi-layer element structures whereby element dimensions have to be within narrow limits have been described.
Particularly in the design of multi-element transducers with extremely small individual elements the mode of resonance, the matching layer characteristics on both sides of the transducer, the individual element shape and inter element spacing are important.

Given element configuration and frequency the beam pattern may be calculated. Based on such calculations the theory may be confirmed with a similar prototype transducer when tested in a watertank experiment. These experiments have been carried out with a subset of individual elements from a large transducer array.

A programmable positioning mechanism allows registration of probe position. Together with echo information, it now is possible to simulate system performance when data are recorded and superimposed in the computer memory to produce the result of a fictive total transducer.

In a film this process was presented and an example of a cardiac image was shown. At the end of this lecture the clinical results of a dynamically focussed real time system were presented. The system was designed following the calculation methods as illustrated.

COMPUTER SIMULATION

A convenient method for evaluation of array performance is the use of a computer model of the array. In order to get a realistic representation of beam patterns a program has been developed which allows for the modelling of arbitrarily shaped two-dimensional transducers or transducer arrays. A continuous wave solution of the Huygens integral is derived for every point in the imaging field.

The resulting round trip sensitivity is displayed in shades of grey and provides an excellent insight into transducer performance. An example of a pattern output is shown in figure 1.

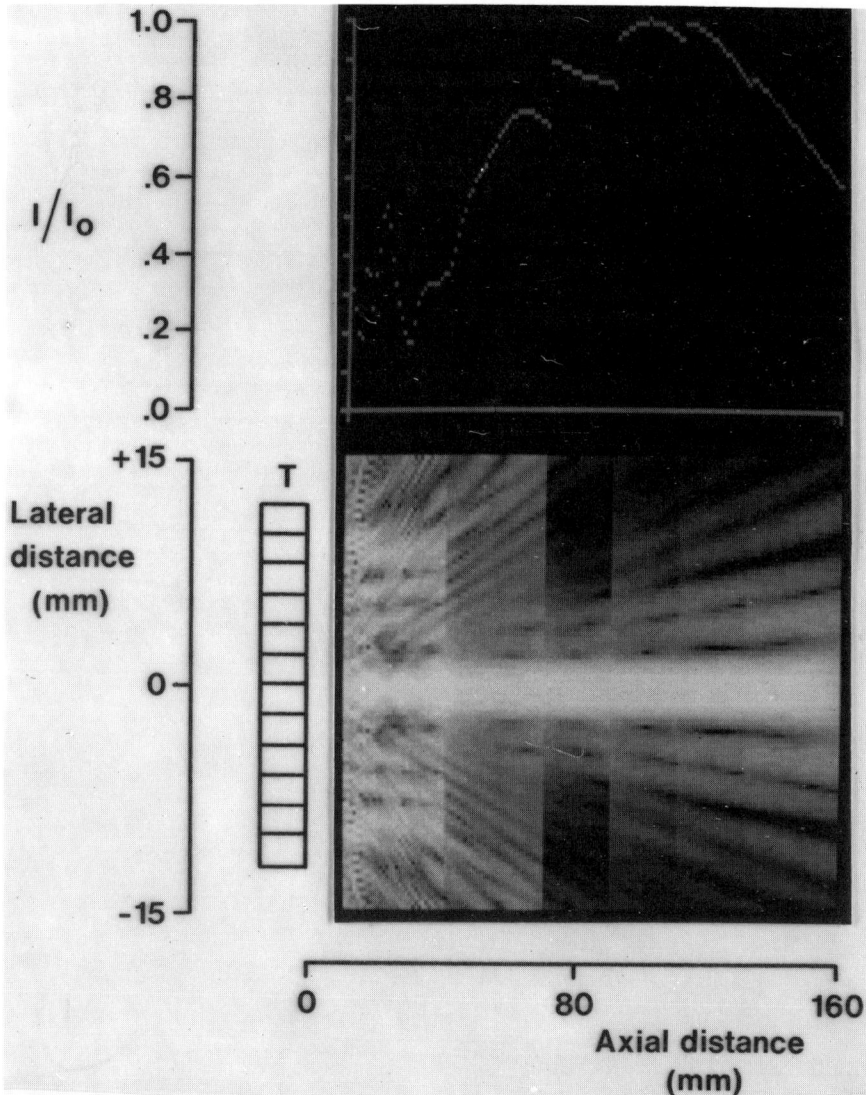

Figure 1: This figure illustrates the calculated round trip sensitivity distribution of a dynamically focussed linear array subgroup (12 elements, height 10 mm, element width 2 mm, f = 3.12 MHz).

The intensity variation as function of depth is shown at the top. This intensity level has been used to introduce a normalization for each line parallel to the transducer surface. At each line maximum sensitivity is indicated as 100% white. Stepsize: -3.75 dB, with 16 grey scale levels in total.

In figure 2 the entire computer configuration is shown.

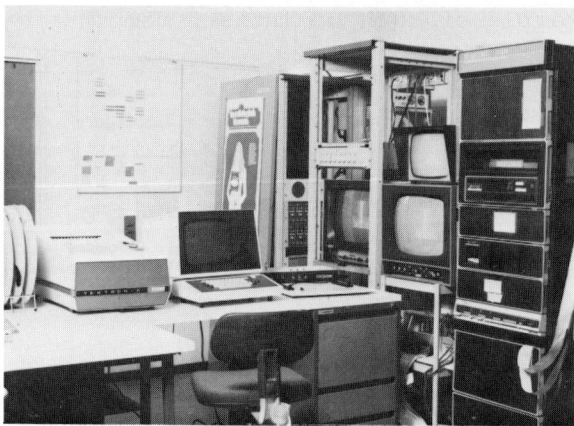

Figure 2: Computer configuration as used for calculation of beam patterns. This system is directly linked to the watertank.

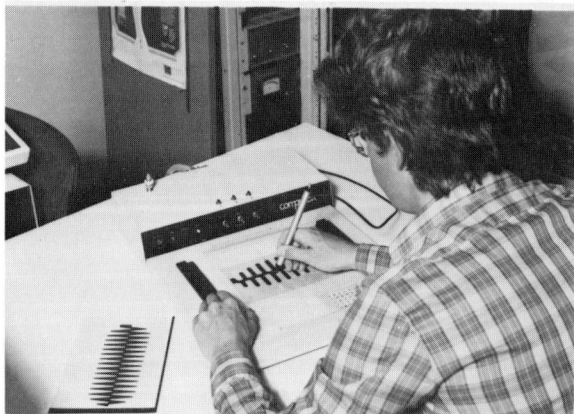

Figure 3: Amplitude weighing will occur when electrode material is not equally distributed over the transducer material. This effects the beam shape. With sometimes rather complicated element shapes also the grating lobe effects may be diminished by using anti-aliasing tech-

niques. This figure shows input of element geometry into the program for calculation of the beam pattern.

Input data such as number of elements, element spacing and frequency are fed into the system. Element shape is stored in the program through use of a digitizing tablet. It is well known that the regularity of parallel small rectangular individual elements may cause grating lobe effects. As a result image artefacts occur. A variety of element shapes has been tested in our laboratory to minimize grating lobe effects. The input of a complicated element shape for beam pattern calculation is shown in figure 3.

THE WATERTANK

The watertank as shown in figure 4 for ultrasound measurements has been constructed for a joint project with the technical university of Delft to allow very precise (10 micron steps) automatic positioning of a probe or object. The set-up has been completed by addition of an echo

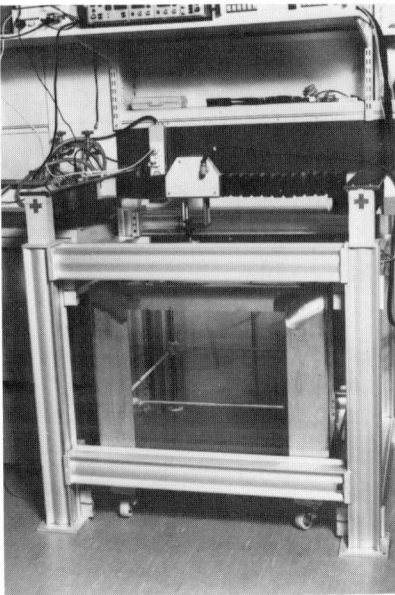

Figure 4: Watertank as used for simulation study.

data link with the computer through a biomation transient recorder. This allows full amplitude and phase information to be stored in memory for image reconstruction.

Many laboratories presently carry out research on instantaneous compound scanners where real time information in overlapping acoustic beams is used to form the image. A linear array with three or five sets of parallel beams, each set under a different beam axis angle, is a simple example of such an instant compound system.
A simulation of the complete echo image as obtained in the watertank with an in vitro heart is shown in figure 5.

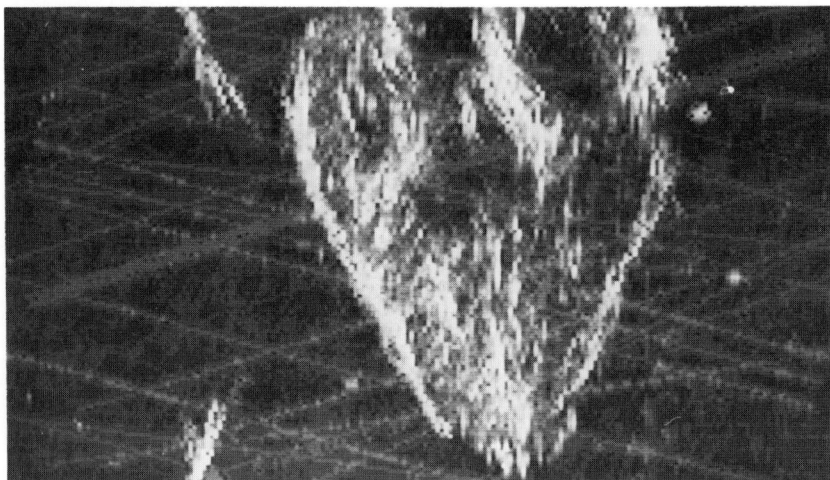

Figure 5: Simulation of system performance by echo data accumulation and computer image reconstruction of information from a variety of angles as obtained a few years ago on a heart, positioned in a watertank (courtesy J.Ridder).

CONCLUSION

In this paper it is shown that easy interaction with a computer and appropriate programs greatly facilitate insight in transducer behaviour. In watertank experiments image reconstruction programs may subsequently be used for simulation of system performance when a prototype transducer according to the calculated specifications has been built.

B-SCAN IMAGE QUANTITATION OF HUMAN HEPATIC TISSUE

D. Nicholas

Physics Department, Royal Marsden Hospital, Downs Road,
Sutton, Surrey, U.K.

Present day interpretation of clinical B-scan images
is entirely dependent upon a subjective evaluation of
their information content. Although much useful and
accurate diagnosis is achieved a preference must be for a
quantitative assessment of B-scans coupled with a rigorous
description (where possible) of related pathology. Our
attempt at this requirement has resulted in a system which
permits the retrospective analysis of the ultrasonic
information displayed in conventional B-scan images (1).
Recent diagnostic machines utilise scan-conversion
memories (both analogue and digital) as temporary storage
devices for the ultrasonic information. This makes it
possible to generate specific read out rasters and to
select portions of the image for digitisation (in the case
of analogue devices) and subsequent storage. The digitised pictures can then be analysed on a mini-computer by
a variety of mathematical techniques.
The majority of our examinations have been limited to
the liver where our past experience, at the Royal Marsden
Hospital, has led us to pose the following questions :
(1) can secondary focal deposits be classified with
respect to their primary type by either the intensity or
spatial distributions of the internal echo producing
structures ?
(2) Can tumour response to chemotherapy and/or
radiotherapy be monitored by an ultrasonic evaluation ?
(3) Can diffuse infiltrations of hepatic tissues be
characterised by quantifying the 'parenchymal' echoes ?
It will be shown that simple quantitative appraisal
of B-scan images is capable of providing useful diagnostic information to complement existing ultrasonic
investigations.

APPARATUS

As a preliminary pilot study a system was devised
which transferred data, on-line, from an analogue scan
conversion memory (associated with our existing diagnostic equipment) into a PDP 8/e mini computer. A line
selector enabled specific lines (corresponding to the 625
lines of video information fed to the standard monitor)

41

to be accessed for digitisation. This was accomplished
by reading the relevant line of information directly from
the scan-convertor into a 20 MHz 8-bit transient recorder
with 4k byte memory. Rejection of unwanted portions of
the digitised signal finally led to the storing of data in
the form of a 64 x 64 matrix corresponding to a small
region of the original B-scan image.

PRELIMINARY RESULTS

        In a preliminary survey, 62 independent B-scan images
were digitised and subsequently analysed. Two basic techniques which will be reported here involved an estimation
of echo peak separation and the general distribution of
echo amplitudes.
        Replotting the original data in the form of a histo-
gram of echo amplitude against frequency of occurrence
permits the extraction of simple first order statistics as
potential measures for characterising differing tissue
pathologies. Two of these parameters are summarised in
Table I (the mean echo amplitude is expressed in relation
to the general intensity level of the liver parenchyma
adjacent to the focal lesion under investigation). An
absolute value for the mean will not be meaningful until
the machine settings can be accurately calibrated and
patient variability accounted for.
        Two measures of echo peak separation are also listed
in Table I. The first is a simple measure of the number
of discrete peaks existing in the digitised region where a
peak is only accepted if its amplitude is significantly
higher than the surrounding picture elements. This
measure relates to the 'coarseness' of the acoustic structure but is incapable of assessing the presence of
regularity. For this latter purpose a second parameter
was calculated. A two-dimensionsal Fourier transform of
the data was performed and any regular structure extracted
from the resulting spectrum. This spectrum was then re-
converted to the spatial domain and is recorded in Table I
as the most predominant regularity.

DISCUSSION

        It is apparent that the number of discrete echo peaks
within a scan is a significant parameter, with most of the
focal neoplasms exhibiting significantly fewer echo peaks
per unit area than is usual for normal liver tissue. The
notable exception to date is the adenoma which produced
more echo peaks than normal tissue (though the limited
number of cases prevents the attachment of any significance to this result at present). Of the diffuse conditions the infiltrated liver (lymphomatous) indicated a
possible overall decrease in echo amplitude, whilst the
cirrhosis showed a distinct increase in the number of echo
peaks per unit area. Until an absolute measure can be

42

TABLE I. Quantitative analysis of 62 liver B-scans

Hepatic Condition	No.of scans	No.of peaks cm^{-2}	Regularity mm	Mean * dB	Coeff.of Variation
NORMAL	35	6±0.4	3.9±0.4		12 ±1.5
FOCAL LESIONS**					
Teratoma	8	4±0.2	4.8±0.2	+&-	11 ±0.5
Adenoma	3	8±0.2	3.3±0.2	O	9.5±0.2
Carcinoma	8	4±0.4	4.2±0.3	-2 ±1	12 ±0.5
Fibrosarcoma	3	4±0.2	-	-1.5±0.1	10.5±0.2
DIFFUSE INFILTRATIONS					
Lymphoma	2	6±0.1	-	-ve	14.5±0.1
Cirrhosis	3	7±0.2	3.6±0.1	+ve	12.5±1.0

*   expressed as a difference from the mean associated
     with normal liver parenchyma

**   where the hepatic lesions are secondary focal
     metastases they have been catalogued according to
     primary type.

placed upon the mean echo amplitude its use as a variable
for tissue differentiation is limited.   Similarly the
coefficient of variation (as a measure of dispersion) has
yet to show any marked significance as a measure of
abnormality.   Although only a few preliminary examinations have been reported the results suggest that
quantification has an important role in aiding clinical
diagnosis using ultrasound.

     The success of our pilot study has prompted the
development of an off-line data acquisition device which
can be attached to any ultrasonic diagnostic machine in
clinical use.   The data is now stored directly onto a
magnetic cartridge device which has a capacity of 34.5
million bits; in effect 400 images (of 64 x 64 elements)
can be stored on a single cartridge.   This frees the
computer for off-line analysis and provides a useful
store for the data.   This system is at present being
introduced into the clinic.

REFERENCES

1. Nicholas, D., Barrett, A., Chu, J.M.G., Cosgrove, D.O.
    Garbutt, P., Green, J., Pussell, S. and Hill, C.R.
    (1979) : In: Acoustical Holography, vol.8, Plenum
    Press, New York.

LINE MODE ECHOGRAM DATA ACQUISITION AND COMPUTER RECONSTRUCTION TECHNIQUES

D.E. Robinson and G. Kossoff

Ultrasonics Institute, Sydney, Australia

The grey scale ultrasonic pulse-echo imaging system relies on the use of appropriate signal processing techniques. In conventional systems these controls are manually set but in the recently released micro-processor based digital scan converter systems the signal processing options may be set up automatically by the microprocessor for a new scan. However, the use of a digital scan converter to store the signals still places limitations on the types of processing possible. This paper describes a computer based signal acquisition and processing system which stores the echogram signals line by line. This approach allows a range of different signal processing and image forming techniques to be applied without the need to rescan the patient.

In a digital scan converter system the signals are fed through a time-gain-control (TGC) amplifier, compressed, pulse shaped and combined to form an image. The values of intensity at each location in the cross-section are stored in a digital memory with up to 512 x 512 picture elements or pixels and a range of intensity of 16 or 32 shades of grey. This method of data storage is called Section Mode. Processing carried out after the image has been formed is referred to as post-processing and in the digital scan converter is limited by the restricted range of echo values stored in the memory. The image may be smoothed, filtered, amplitude histogrammed and amplitude windowed. For any change in signal processing and for some post-processing the patient must be rescanned.

The UI computer system is installed at the Royal Hospital for Women and interfaced with the UI Octoson. It consists of an Interdata Model 85 mini computer with dual 67 MByte disc drives for bulk storage and a Biomation 8100 Waveform recorder for signal input. The echoes from each ultrasonic line of sight are stored directly without being first formed into an image and are known as Line Mode Data. The system samples the video signals at 2 MHz. A total of 800 eight bit samples, corresponding to 400 us of data are recorded for each line. The acquisition cycle takes approximately 1.5 ms per line and a full eight transducer 5200 line compound scan containing 4.2 MBytes of data is stored on disc in approximately 8 seconds.

Because the recorded Line Mode data contains all the echo amplitude information with 8 bit resolution there is no need to rescan the patient for subsequent processing. The image is formed with 256 x 256 pixels within the computer in the reconstruction process. The reconstruction mode used in scan converters is peak detect (Figure 1a). Each pixel is assigned a value corresponding to the maximum signal received at that location. The point targets have the familiar star-shaped appearance due to the transducer beamwidth being displayed from different directions. Minimum detect (Figure 1b) stores the smallest signals from each location. It gives the best resolution for point targets as the echo only remains in the image if it is present within the pixel from all trans- ducers. The beamwidth effects are removed. Integrate mode (Figure 1c) sums all the echoes in each pixel. Because there is a denser scan line pattern at the top of the image there are more echo samples in each pixel and the echoes appear brighter. The resolution appears good since the maximum echoes all add up whereas the beamwidth echoes do not coincide. Average mode (Figure 1d) sums the echoes as in integrate mode but also keeps a count of the number of echoes summed into each location and divides the summed total echo by the number of bits for each picture point. Average has the same resol- ution as integrate, but the echo brightness is more uniform throughout the image.

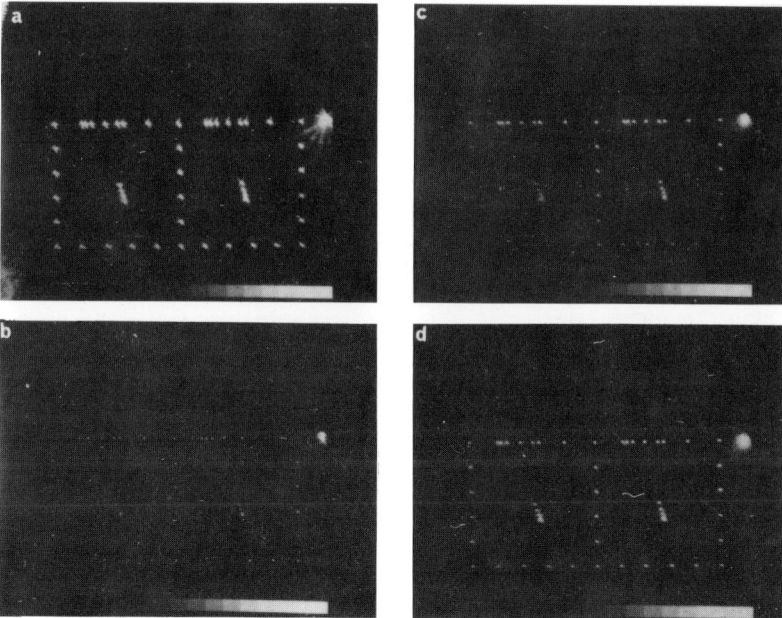

Figure 1. Reconstruction of test object using (a) peak detect, (b) minimum detect, (c) integrate and (d) average.

45

In tissue the appearances are somewhat different. When comparing the various reconstruction modes it is useful to process each image so that the histogram of the final result is the same. The differences observed are then due to the reconstruction effects rather than differences in visual perception due to brightness, contrast and dynamic range. The histogram found most suitable for these images was a constant up to half intensity and then a sine wave reducing to zero at maximum intensity. The peak detect mode (Figure 2a) gives the conventional echogram appearance. Minimum detect (Figure 2b) tends to enhance scattered echoes and suppress specular reflections. Thus, abdominal wall layers and out-line echoes are suppressed while scattered echoes are enhanced. However, a shadow on any single sector of the original data remains on the final image. Integrate mode (Figure 2c) displays an interference pattern due to the different number of samples of echoes added into each pixel. This effect is removed by the average mode (Figure 2d). The average mode retains the resolution improvement over the peak detect. It tends to enhance scattered reflectors and reduce specular highlights, resulting in a less attractive echogram appearance. This effect can be reduced while retaining the resolution improvement by reducing the amount of compression applied to the echoes before reconstruction. All other images shown in this paper are formed in peak detect mode. If the scale is expanded (Figure 3) the image reconstruction still uses 256 x 256 pixels and the resolution is limited only by the original ultrasound data.

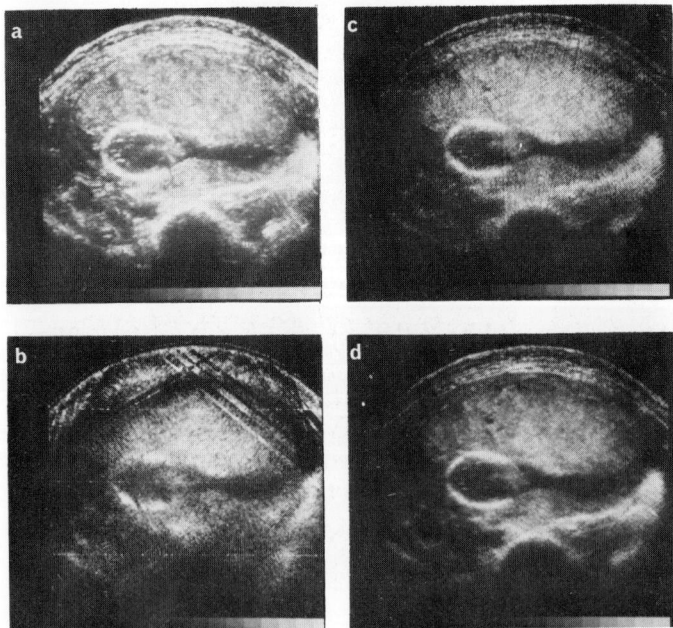

Figure 2. Reconstruction of patient data using (a) peak detect, (b) minimum detect, (c) integrate and (d) average.

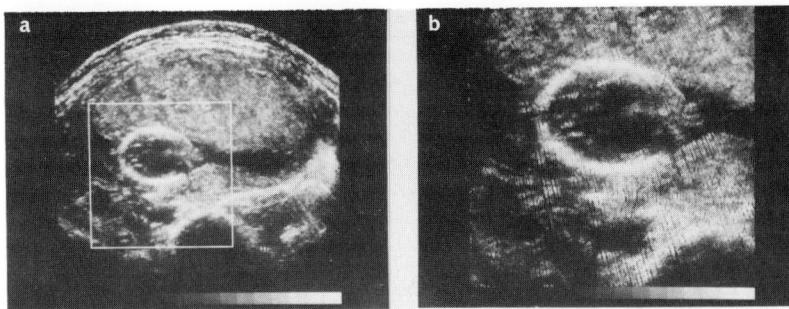

Figure 3. Reconstruction at (a) 2.5:1 and (b) 1.25:1 with
no increase in display pixel size.

　　　Processing which is carried out before image reconstruction
is called pre-processing. The preprocessing program applies
TGC, compression and pulse shaping functions to the Line Mode
data. To pre-process a typical eight transducer Octoson image
of 4.2 MBytes takes approximately 2½ minutes. Data acquired
with equipment settings not optimal to make the interpretation
can be reconstructed with corrected settings without any need
to rescan the patient. In Figure 4b the TGC was set with the
slope too steep, resulting in a bright band in the centre of
the image. This was removed by applying some negative TGC
in the pre-processing. For some data it is of advantage to
apply leading-edge enhancement by adding in a small proportion
of the differentiated signal. This accentuates small variations in texture and reduces long-lasting strong echoes
(Figure 4c).
　　　Computer processing of stored Line Mode data has been
shown to allow variation in reconstruction modes and signal
processing parameters to provide different and more informative images. This feature may well prove invaluable in the
future. The main application at present is in research into
ultrasonic visualisation techniques. It is now possible to
critically compare different processing and reconstruction
techniques using precisely the same input data, with no
variation due to differing scan patterns or patient movement.

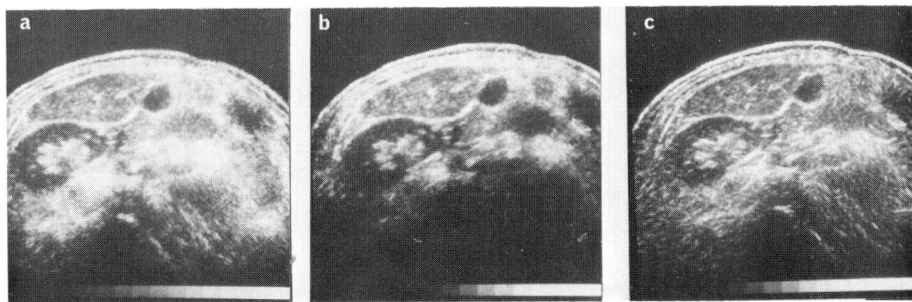

Figure 4. Effect of pre-processing with (a) as acquired,
(b) TGC reduced and (c) differentiate (leading-edge) processing,
before the image formation procedure.

M-MODE COMPUTATIONS AND TWO-DIMENSIONAL IMAGE RECONSTRUCTION

Jan A. Vogel, Olchert L. Bastiaans, Klaas Bom, Folkert J. ten Cate

Thoraxcentrum, Erasmus University, Rotterdam, The Netherlands.

INTRODUCTION

A number of methods have been developed for computer-based analysis of echocardiographic recordings. Two methods for analysis of this information can be distinguished:
1. off-line processing of time-motion recordings (M-modes) as obtained with the single element technique.
2. processing methods using more advanced techniques for the analysis of two-dimensional (2D) echocardiograms.
Recent progress in both fields will be discussed.

M-MODE ANALYSIS

To facilitate the use of a computer, the analysis of M-mode recordings is carried out in an interactive process. By responding to program messages and questions which are displayed on a TV-monitor, the operator can store the required patient data in the memory of the computer in a simple procedure. The data consist of general information like name, sex, age, weight etc, as well as the judgement of the operator on static and dynamic aspects of the cardiac structures. In the same procedure measurements of cardiac dimensions and tracing of motion-patterns can be carried out.

Computerized analysis of M-mode recordings is mainly based on digitization of positions of cardiac structures. With the aid of a digitizing tablet (1,2,3,4). In our experience however, this is a cumbersome procedure in studies on specific cardiac parameters for larger series of heartbeats. Digitization with the aid of a TV camera will be discussed as an alternative for the tablet tracing method. The camera method is based on our experience that normally the echocardiograms are pretraced with a leadpencil by the echocardiographer, who is responsible for the interpretation, whereas the actual digitization is performed by a technician. The new method employs a TV camera to read pretraced recordings directly into the computer; this overcomes the need to retrace the recordings on the tablet.

SYSTEM OPERATION

A pretraced recording is placed on a lightbox with
a constant illumination. Herewith, a good contrast is
obtained between pretraced pencil lines and background.
The transmitted light is converted into a video signal,
using a vidicon camera. After A/D conversion, the signal
is stored in a video scanned memory, as illustrated in
figure 1.

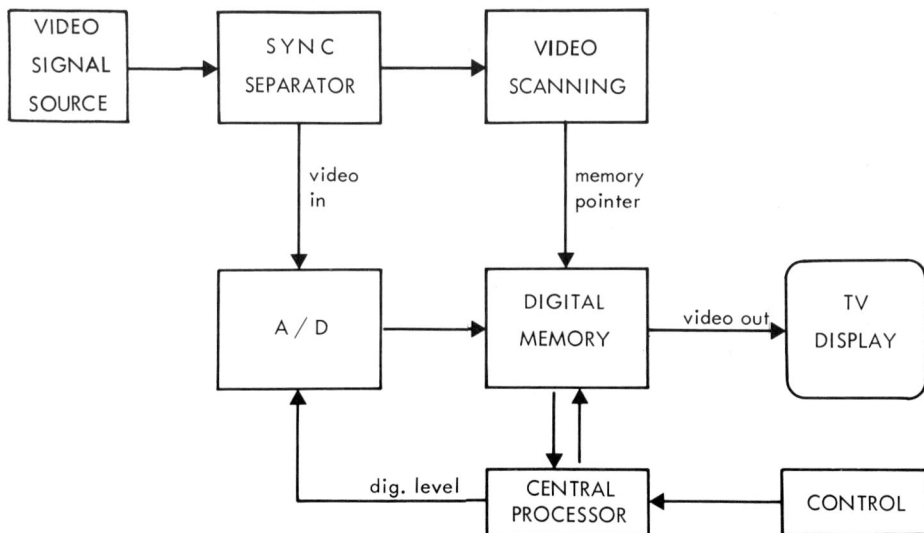

Fig. 1. Block diagram of a video digitizer. In M-mode
scanning the block "video signal source" is a camera
positioned above a light box. In 2D image analysis the
video recorder is represented by this block. The sync
separation unit allows correct video scanning for any
video signal.
Video images can be digitized with 256 greylevels, 256
video lines and 256 points per line. Digitized images
are displayed via a video scanned digital memory.

Under processor control an optimal threshold level is
selected out of 256 greylevels. Thresholding of the image
at this level results in a binary image showing the pencil
lines in black on a background that is displayed in white.
A line-search algorithme takes care of the translation

49

of the black traces into strings of co-ordinates. In
this way a pencil line can be digitized in less then
one second. The result of this tracing process is superimposed on the camera image for review of the digitization
procedure. After acceptance by the operator the string
of co-ordinates is stored on behalf of the calculations
that are carried out as soon as the digitization session
is finished. The discussed video tracing method has been
designed for the analysis of larger series of M-mode
recordings (5).
- In a research study for evaluation of ventricular performance during intensive training all 180 M-mode were
  processed in a total time of 150 minutes.
- For the analysis of atrial fibrillation 100 consecutive
  heartbeats of one patient are digitized in 20 mintues.
- A third field of application of this fast tracing method
  is the study of ischemia in the myocardium. This study
  is performed on young pigs with a small ultrasound
  transducer, sutured on the epicardium of the exposed
  heart. Changes in myocardial wall function are obtained
  in coronary artery occlusion, followed by reperfusion.
  Also in this study, where larger series of consecutive
  heartbeats are processed, processing time is largely
  reduced by the video tracing method. With this method
  the same resolution is obtained as by manual digitizing, using a tablet.

TWO-DIMENSIONAL IMAGE RECONSTRUCTION

    The video digitizing set-up, as illustrated in
fig. 1, is also used for processing of two-dimensional
cardiac images. Video tape recording is selected as the
general clinical practice; the required images for computer processing are selected from the complete video
recordings of a patient. A video digitizer is available
for A/D conversion of a still video frame and a video-
scanned memory for display of the final result. Images
are digitized with 200 points on each line and each point
contains 4 bit of image information. Data reduction is
accomplished by automatic rejection of all TV lines
without echo information. The method requires manual
positioning of the sequential video frames, therefore
the processing of a recording period of two seconds requires several minutes per patient.

ANALYSIS OF ECHOCARDIOGRAPHIC IMAGES

    In the analysis of the digitized 2D images attention
is directed to the registration of the motion of cardiac
structures. Structures in the images are recognized by
their motion in time. Time-motion, as an important help
in recognition, is not available in still video frames,
therefore quantitative analysis of the motional informa-

tion is carried out in a time-motion reconstruction
technique. Extraction of a selected video line from the
successive images and display of these lines along the
video screen results in a reconstructed time-motion (M-
mode) recording. Segmentation of the cardiac structures
is an interactive process, based on structure recognition in successively reconstructed M-modes from top to
bottom of the 2D images. This segmentation technique
is a semi-automatic procedure based on a matching algorithme (6). The first reconstructed M-mode from the top
of the cross-section is traced by the operator using
the pen of a graphic tablet. The information entered
with this pen is superimposed on the reconstructed M-
mode in order to trace the motion-patterns. Tracings
in the next M-modes are estimated by the computer. This
proces is interactive; after each estimated tracing by
the computer, the operator may accept, reject or correct
the tracing with the pen system. After segmentation of
all structures the data are rearranged into a lay-out
which is similar to that of the 2D images. A result of
this segmentation process is shown in fig. 2.

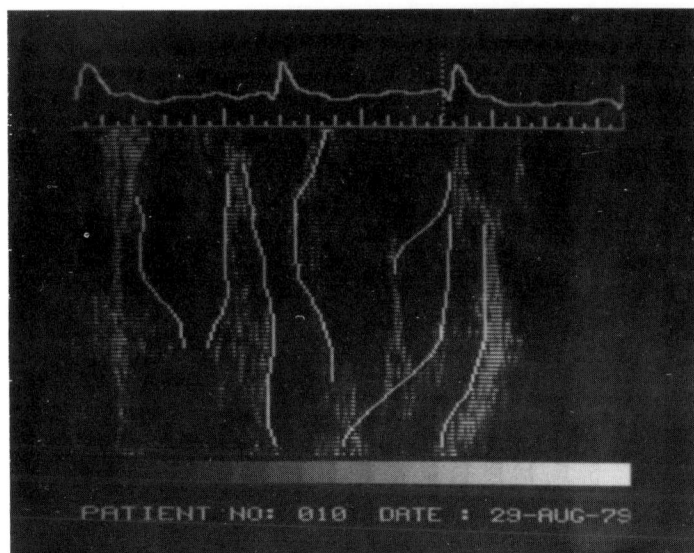

Fig. 2 An original cross-section with superposition
of detected data for several cardiac structures.

Two methods for display of the dynamics of cardiac structures are described here.

A three dimensional display technique allows for display of motional and structural information as available in the time series. In fig. 3 the endocardium of the left ventricular posterior wall is shown as a function of time.

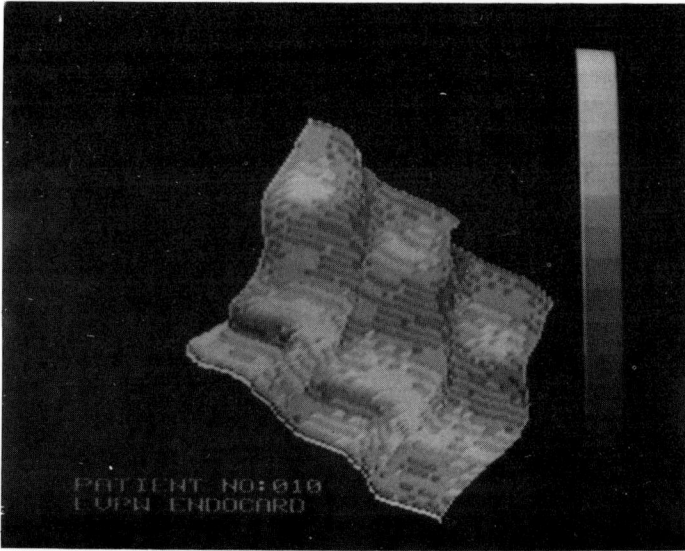

Fig. 3. The endocardium of the left ventricular posterior wall displayed as function of time (see text for details).

The right side of this image is a representation of the endocardium from the aortic region down to the apex. The structure is displayed from right to left as a func tion of time. Greyscale imaging is used as a simulation of the effect of a lightsource, that alluminates this object.

A direct quantitative impression of motion, thicke-ning or thickness of complete structures during the car-diac cycle is obtained in a so-called amplitude spectrum. In fig. 4 the thickening of the left ventricular posterior wall is shown as a function of time. Time is represented on the horizontal axis and the wall thickening is displayed on the vertical axis from the attachment of the anterior mitral valve down to the apex. Thickening is converted in greyscale. A separate greyscale indicator allows for direct conversion of greylevels into milli-meters.

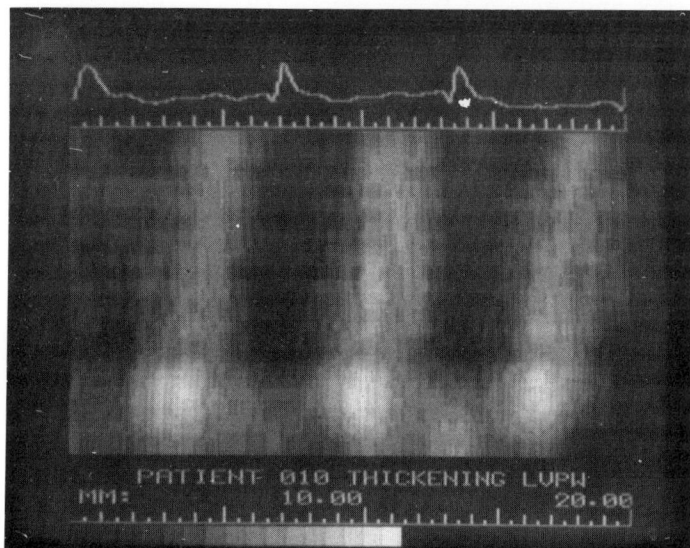

Fig. 4. Two-dimensional amplitude spectrum of thickening
of the left ventricular posterior wall for a recording
period of 2 seconds (see text for details).

DISCUSSION

     Two methods for extraction of data from echocardio-
graphic recordings have been discussed. Quantitative
extraction of data from conventional M-mode recordings
is already an established technique in several cardiac
centers. Usually the data are extracted with digitizing
pen systems.
     Analysis of larger series of M-modes is still time
consuming. The discussed video tracing technique reduces
the data aquisition time with at least a factor ten.
     On-line real-time digitizing of 2D images is beyond
us proposed by many other authors (7-15). However, the
most practical way for analysis of real-time 2D echograms
has proven to be the digitization from standard video
recordings. The segmentation procedure is based on tracing
in reconstructed M-modes, so advantage can be taken from
all knowledge in the field of M-mode tracing. The display
techniques developed in our laboratory allow for assessment of overall and regional cardiac function and the
measurement of dynamics of structures. This technique
seems to be a practical tool in clinical research and
will be evaluated for larger series of patients.

REFERENCES

1. Gibson, D.G. and Brown, D.J. (1976):Brit. Heart J. 38:8.
2. Decoodt, P.R., Mathey, D.G. and Swan, H.J.C. (1976): Computers and Biomed. Res. 9-549.
3. Teichholz, L.E., Caputo, G.R. Meller, J., Kashdan, N., LeBlanc, D. and Herman, M.V. (1977): Computers in cardiology IEEE Cat. no. 77CH 1254-C.
4. Van Zwieten, G., Vogel, J.A., Bom, A.H.A. and Rijsterborgh, H. (1977): Computers in Cardiology IEEE Cat. no. 77CH 1254-C.
5. Van Zwieten, G., Bastiaans, O.L., Honkoop, J. and Vogel, J.A. (1979): Charles T. Lancée (ed.) Echocardiology, 469-475.
6. Vogel, J.A., Bastiaans, O.L., Roelandt, J. and Honkoop, J. (1979): Charles T. Lancée (ed.) Echocardiology, 457-467.
7. Vogel, J.A., Ligtvoet, C.M., Bom, N., Van Zwieten, G. and Hugenholtz, P.G. (1975): Ultrasound in Med. Biol. Pergamon Press.
8. Vogel, J.A., Brower, R.W., Bom, N., Van Zwieten, G. and Roelandt, J. (1975): Computers in Cardiology.
9. Waag, R.C. and Gramiak, R. (1976): Ultrasound in Med. & Biol. 147-1:8.
10. Gramiak, R. and Waag, R.C. (1976): Am.J. Röntgenol. 127:91.
11. McSherry, D.H. (1974): IEEE Trans Sonic & Ultrasonics 21:91.
12. Matsumoto, M., Matsuo, H., Kitabatake, A., Inque, M., Hamanaka, Y., Tumara, S., Tanaka, K. and Abe, H. (1977): Ultrasound In Med. & Biol. 3:163.
13. Romic, C.A. and Hagan, A.D. (1974): Proc. San Diego Biomedical Symposium, 145.
14. Hirsch, M., Sanders, W.J., Popp, R.L. and Harrison, D.C. (1973) Comp. Bio-Med. Res. 6:336.
15. Robinson, E.P., Pryor, T.A., WIllard, S.J., Jones, D.S. and Ridges, J.D. (1976): Comp. Bio-Med. Res. 9:247.

MITRAL VALVE MOTION AND BLOOD FLOW VELOCITY IN THE LEFT VENTRICLE

BRUN P., LAPORTE J. P., ODDOU C.

Groupe de Recherche U 138 de l'I.N.S.E.R.M. Service d'Exploration Fonctionnelle. Hopital Henri Mondor. F 94000 Créteil (France)

The ultrasonic data, here referring to cardiac structures and intracardiac blood flow, contain quantitative informations which one can hardly extract if not computer-aided. Apart from large systems a place seems possible for small units, namely the micro-computer range. A physiological problem, the relations between a valve motion and the blood flow characteristics, is discussed here, documented exclusively on data derived from ultrasonic techniques. The suggested answers could contribute to a decisive understanding of the phenomena, despite their complexity. The graphic expression, as illustrated by blood velocity maps, appears as one of the most important features.

MATERIALS AND METHODS

Ultrasonic data about the walls of the left ventricle (LV), the left auricle (LA) and the anterior mitral leaflet (AML) were obtained with a multiscan system (Organon Technika). The specific usage of the multitransducer probe, the multi-TM technique, was described elsewhere (1,2). Information about blood velocity in the LV was obtained with a pulsed Doppler system (A.T.L.). a specific technique, referred to as the multi sector scan pulsed Doppler velocimetry, was described elsewhere (3).

In a first period, computations were made on a desk computer (Wang 2200). More recently a micro-computer (Apple II) was used, with floppy disk storage and high resolution video display. Programs included the computation of the AML instantaneous shape, derived from the multi-TM technique and the elaboration of blood velocity maps in the LV based on multi sector scan Doppler velocimetry (fig. 1 & 2).

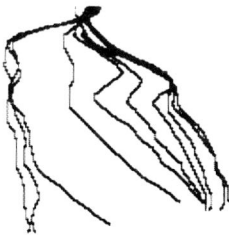

ANTERIOR MITRAL LEAFLET OPENING

Figure 1 - Video display of the successive instantaneous shapes of the AML during its opening motion.

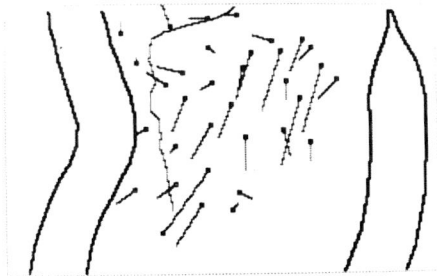

MAP N0 7

Figure 2 - Video display of the LV walls, the AML shape (peak E wave) and the instantaneous blood velocity field.

RESULTS AND DISCUSSION

Diastole - besides the isovolumic relaxation - is conceptually divided by the physiologist in three phases referred to a fast filling, slow filling and filling related to the atrial contraction. It is known from the cineangiographic measurements of LV internal volumes that such a scheme does take place in man. It is known from echography that the LV posterior wall has a backward motion during diastole and - if its subaortic region is excluded - the interventricular septum a forward motion. It is known, also from echography, that the AML presents an E and an A wave. Nothing is known either from cineangiography or echography about the LV blood flow during diastole, if one excepts the perception given by the non-opaque blood invading the LV in selective angiograms. Finally little is known about the interrelations between these different informations. Experimental results about cardiac valves as well as analogic or mathematical models give conflicting answers if are considered for instance the mechanisms involved in the mitral valve closure. Everyone agrees with the generation of a so called recirculation process during diastole, but there is a complete disagreement about its location and chronology - with correlated divergence about its relation with the valve closure. An alternate mechanism could be the breaking of a jet phenomenon which would act on the valve with a collapse effect.

The purposes of this paper which intended to resume and coordinate different works of the laboratory referring to the relation of LV wall and mitral valve motions (1), the shape of the AML (2), the instantaneous blood flow field in the LV (3), were to demonstrate thatusing exclusively ultrasonic techniques - with commercially available equipments - and computer facilities restricted to a desk computer or a micro-computer with their peripherals, it was possible to obtain a rather complete set of informations about the mechanical events occuring during diastole and give a coordinated description of the phenomena concerning LV flow, wall motion and mitral leaflets motion and shape. All informations were derived from conventionnal echography except flow which demanded the pulsed Doppler technique, though pulsed Doppler does not give proper informations for a flow field description : the velocity recorded is precisely oriented as the ultrasonic beam. In the technique used here, the bood velocity vector had to be composed after two velocity components, assuming the third component of negligeable value, which is certainly untrue if the whole cardiac cycle is considered.

The fast-filling period was arbitrarily divided in six subphases. Each description referred successively to 1) flow in the mitral region, 2) flow in other areas of the LV, 3) mitral leaflet motion, 4) LV wall motion and diameter rate of change. Peak E wave of the AML was used as time reference.

I. 60 ms before E wave. Slightly after the first early echographic signes of mitral valve opening, the situation could be resumed as follow : The signs of an apex-oriented flow, with low magnitude vectors, appeared in the inlet part of the LV - blood in the other regions of the ventricle was quiescent - The AML was uncompletly open : The

56

opening was obvious in the medial part of the valve, but near its free edge the motion seemed negligible. This asynchronism of opening conferred to a cross section of the leaflet a convexity toward the ventricle - There was no conspicuous change in the LV diameter, though both walls (posterior wall and septum) started slowly to move backward.

II. 20 ms before E wave.The zone affected by the apex-oriented flow presented a significant enlargement due to an increase of its anteroposterior diameter and length, and an increase of the magnitude of the velocity vectors. All vectors seemed roughly parallel - In other regions of the LV the blood was no more quiescent and one could notice small vortices formation at the tip of the AML and along its ventricular surface - The opening of the valve had widely increased, though the leaflet free edge remained late in its motion : There was a buckling motion of the valve, the leaflet being still convex toward the ventricle - The LV diameter increased steeply, at the exclusive expense of the posterior wall, as the septum still moved posteriorly.

III. E wave (peak).The maximal size of the zone affected by the apex-oriented flow was obtained here, with a peak value of the velocity vectors moduli. The flow had the structure of a jet, slightly diverging, structure which was already noticeable in the preceding stage. The inflow track of the LV extended now to nearly the entire area of the ventricle explored - The blood seemed quiescent in the small triangular area delimited by the AML and the septum - The maximal opening of the mitral valve was obtained : At last the AML was straightened, its free edge motion being no longer delayed (whipping motion) - Peak diameter rate of change took place here at the expense of the both the posterior wall (its peak motion rate of change was achieved between stage II and stage III), and the septum, initiating its anterior motion.

IV. 40 ms after E wave. Slightly after peak flow a zero velocity zone appeared in the inlet part of the LV : The apex-oriented flow was still present further down in the ventricle, but had considerably decreased in size and vector magnitude - In front of the AML an aorta-oriented flow pattern had appeared, with rather high velocity vector magnitude and a conspicuous extent. Under the tip of the valve a consistant flow, septum-oriented, was also present. These adjacent orientations highly suggested a recirculation process in contiguity with the AML - The AML was no longer in its fully-opened position though it had kept its straight shape. It must be stressed that the leaflet, parting an apex-oriented flow and an aorta-oriented flow, behaved differently as would have been expected from the simulations - The posterior wall ceased abruptly its steep posterior motion, though the LV diameter persisted to increase, due to the anterior displacement of the septum, now at full rate.

V. 80 ms after E wawe. In the inflow track of the ventricle, two opposite directions of flow could be observed 1) near the annulus the flow was oriented toward the LA, backward flow but not regurgitant flow, as 2) near the leaflet free edgen the flow was still apex-oriented. In between, zero flow was noted, and one could imagine a force exerted on the leaflets in that region,with a resulting collapse, effect, as observed in the breaking of a jet experience- In front of the AML, the recirculation flow orientation had changed and was now directed toward the LA, forming a straight angle with the leaflet surface. The AML continued its closing motion and became convex toward the LA. One can imagine that both actions 1) collapse, related to a breaking of a jet phenomenon and 2) recirculation did contribute to the valve closure - Though the valve was far from being entirely closed, the LV diameter no longer continued to increase and rather dicreased : The posterior wall had still a light posterior motion, but the motion of the septum had reversed and it was also moving backward with a slightly superior velocity.

VI. <u>160 ms after E wave</u>. Flow in the mitral area was negligible - Flow pattern in front of the AML did not receive a complete explanation, but probably resulted from a recirculation process moving out of the observation plane, as apex-oriented velocity vectors appeared unexpectedly in the sub-aortic area - The AML motion depicted the singular point F - The LV diameter rate of change was null, both walls still moving slightly backward in parallel motions.

The combination of factors involved in the mechanical events occuring during diastole is certainly not unique and we are well aware that the LV blood velocities here measured and the inertial effects, velocity-dependant, could have been of different magnitudes and lead to different descriptions. Nevertheless, the present description seems coherent, and illustrates how ultrasonic informations could be enhanced by the use of computer processing. The choice of a microcomputer solution resulted partly from financial considerations but the major argument was the versatility of the system, here entirely dedicated to echography. Another example was given by the elaboration of the small film, given as a comment or résumé of the above descriptions. A graphic terminal, computer monitored and filmed with a frame by frame camera, is a low price and low time consuming way to realise motion pictures, as the high resolution image, given by the microcomputer can be repeatedly edited with small and/or iterative changes. The solution here retained to suggest flow yelded only five basic shapes, oriented as the velocity vector angles, and alterning at a rate dependant of the vector magnitudes. These small light garlands simulated particles in the blood and the eye of the observer intended to be used as integrator to convert the velocity spatial and temporal information into flow information. The LV wall silhouette and mitral shape, derived from imaging and TM information, added borderlines to the flow patterns, contributed to their undestanding and to the avant-garde title of the film, Ultrasonic Cineangiography, presented here in a preliminary version.

REFERENCES.

1. BRUN P., ODDOU C., BERALDO E., KULAS A., LAURENT F., PHILIPPON A., VERNEJOUL F. Acta Med. Scand., Suppl. 627, 230.

2. BRUN P., ODDOU C., KULAS A., LAURENT F. Computers in Cardiology, p. 267. Editors IEEE.

3. BRUN P., LAPORTE J.P., DION M., LAURENT F., ODDOU C. Computers in Cardiology, p. 175. Editors IEEE.

3. DISPLAY QUANTISATION, LIMITATIONS AND TESTING

B. Breyer, Chairman

INTRODUCTION

There is no doubt that grey scale imaging is a helpful tool for the diagnostician, however, after the initial
enthusiasm one has to start asking questions about the limitations of the method.

The idea of the workshop on DISPLAY QUANTISATION,
LIMITATIONS AND TESTING was to survey the limits and problems in ultrasonic grey scaling, as well as to see how much
of the information readily available at the screen can be
extracted in quantitative terms by the eye and how much
must be left to computer processing.

For this purpose the workshop members have presented
their accounts on various aspects of such quantisation.
Differences between analogue and digital systems were considered in order to see whether digital technology brings
something in terms of image quality. Compound and real-
time systems were compared because new and more sophisticated real-time instruments can give a decent real-time
grey scale image. Attention has been drawn to interference
patterns in images which are often considered true (echo B
mode) structures of the parenchyma, while in fact these interference patterns are indirect descriptions of the tissue
texture. The limitations of the eye brain complex to perceive grey tones were considered since the examiner is an
integral part of the diagnostic system. Geometrical measurement problems and limitations have an important role
in the quantitative measurement of ultrasonic images. On
the other hand, the intensity profile and knowledge of
transmitting and reflected sound intensity should quantitatively be assessed if any numbers are to be attached to
grey tones. This aspect of the problem was also discussed.
A general conclusion which can be drawn from the papers and
discussions is that direct quantisation of perceived grey
tones is not as yet available. For this purpose, a combination of visual inspection of the image with digital computer analysis is probably indispensable.

B. Breyer

RESOLUTION AND IMAGING PROPERTIES OF REAL-TIME SCANNERS VERSUS CONVENTIONAL COMPOUND SCANNERS

M Halliwell and P N T Wells

Department of Medical Physics, Bristol General Hospital, Bristol BS1 6SY, UK

Summary

Resolution is conveniently specified in terms of the dimensions of the resolution cell. These dimensions depend on the effective duration of the ultrasonic pulse and the effective cross-section of the beam. Conventional scanners employing skin-contact single-element transducers give satisfactory performance with fixed focusing, but arrays can be dynamically focused on reception. The line density with conventional scanners is usually adequate, but some image information can be lost because of sparseness of lines with real-time systems. Digital image storage is free from drift, but the image may be degraded in real-time scanning by blank pixels and fringing. Electrical noise is more troublesome with real-time systems, which lack temporal and spatial averaging; likewise speckle and fluctuation noise, due to the random distribution of scatterers, can markedly degrade single frames from real-time sequences.

1.   Introduction

Conventional compound scanners use the same physical principles as real-time scanners but have the advantages of operating slowly so that the image line density is higher and of producing images with overlapping lines. These basic differences result in different characteristics which may be considered in terms of resolution, line density, ultrasonic beam effects, image storage, noise and speckle.

2.   Resolution

The resolution cell is the volume of material within which the inter-action providing the image datum takes place [1]. Its dimensions depend on the duration of the ultrasonic pulse and on the beam geometry [Fig. 1]. Typically the pulse duration is equivalent to two wavelengths, for a dynamic range of 10 dB, for all transducers; the beam geometry, however, depends on the kind of focusing employed. Single element, internally focused transducers can have 10 dB beam widths of 3 wavelengths at the focus (100 wavelengths range) increasing to about 6 at 40 wavelengths either side of the focus. The small aperture of these compound scanner transducers means that dynamic focusing systems do not significantly improve these figures [2].
    Dynamic focusing does improve the resolution of electronically switched linear arrays because apertures of over 30 wavelengths can be used [3]. The azimuth resolution can be about 8 wavelengths over the range 15-200 wavelengths [4]. The resolution in elevation cannot be controlled except by fixed lens focusing, which produces beam geometries similar to those of single element transducers.

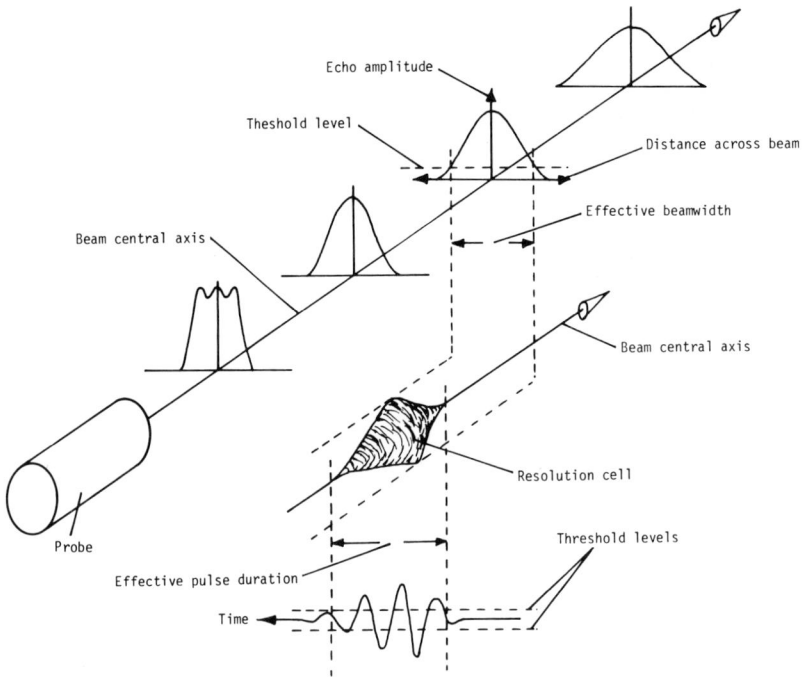

Figure 1 The resolution cell

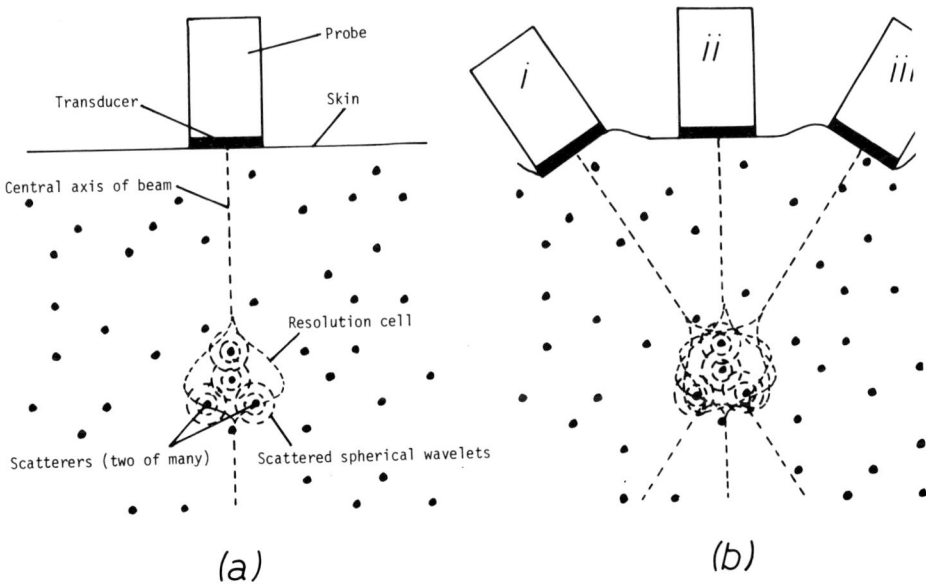

Figure 2 Speckle production (see text).

The apertures of electronically steered arrays (inaccurately termed "phased") are large enough to allow a useful degree of swept focusing [5], however as the beam angle increases the effective aperture is reduced causing degradation of the resolution. Typical 10 dB beam widths vary from 3 wavelengths (for a straight ahead beam at 40 wavelengths) to 5 at 200 wavelengths range.

3. Imaging Properties

3.1. Line density

Each pulse-echo wavetrain contributes one line to an image, the number of wavetrains per image (the line density) depends on the pulse repetition frequency and the scan time. The pulse repetition frequency is limited by the required penetration. For a penetration of 150 mm each pulse must be separated by 200 µs from the next and the P.R.F. cannot be greater than 5,000 s^{-1}.

Conventional scans take about 2 s and contain 10,000 lines with an average spacing of 0.02 mm. Real-time scans may contain 100 lines (because of the frame rate/P.R.F. limitations) with an average spacing of 2 mm. This reduction in spatial sampling frequency can result in a loss of image information. The aesthetic effects can be reduced by duplicating or interpolating lines [6], but these processes cannot retrieve uncollected data.

3.2. Ultrasonic Beam Effects

Single element transducers have well-defined main beams and low-amplitude side lobes, as do electronically switched linear arrays in which the beam is directed straight ahead from an adequate aperture. Unfortunately, however, when the main beam of an electronically steered array is deviated through an angle, the side-lobe amplitudes may be high enough to cause troublesome artifacts. The effect can be reduced by multiplicative processing [7] but evidence of it can be seen with most contemporary instruments.

3.3. Scan Conversion and Image Storage

Analogue scan converters perform adequately in terms of resolution and dynamic range but are prone to electronic drift. Digital scan converters (computer memories of 512 x 512 5-bit words) are free from drift but have slightly poorer resolution. The capability of post-image processing and flicker-free display of the 'last value' of the echo amplitude means that most modern scanners use them.

One important problem of digital storage may occur when the ultrasonic beam is not aligned with the storage matrix. Echo amplitude values must be assigned to pixels only partially intersected by the line-of-sight of the ultrasonic beam. This can result in blank pixels, jittering at the frame rate, and in Moiré fringing (particularly with real-time sector scanners).

3.4. Noise

(a) Electrical Noise

The dynamic range is ultimately limited by the echo amplitude falling below the electrical noise level. Electrical noise is stochastic, so that averaging improves the signal-to-noise ratio. Compound scans exhibit both temporal and spatial averaging. Real-time displays are temporally averaged, spatial averaging being introduced by slight movements of the image field around the object.

(b)   Speckle and Fluctuation Noise

Ultrasonic images are characterised by a granular structure, or 'speckle' [8]. This is not random as electrical noise is random and a particular fixed target situation will produce exactly the same granular image every time it is scanned, provided that the ultrasonic scanning conditions do not alter. Moreover, the granular image is independent of the scanning time (ie, line density) until the image lines become visually separable.

A realistic model considers the target issue to be composed of Rayleigh scatterers (Fig. 2). The spherical wavelets radiated by the scatterers within the resolution cell produce a high amplitude 'echo' if constructive interference predominates and a low amplitude one if the interference is destructive. The addition of the phasors is a random walk problem and the fluctuation of echo amplitude becomes smaller as the dimensions of the resolution cell are increased. Real soft tissues contain a multitude of scatterers, from sub-cellular components to complete organs, so that within the resolution cell it is the distribution of ultrasonic wavelengths - or the frequency spectrum - which determines the dimensions of those scatterers which are predominately detected. Bandpass filtering introduced by the intervening tissue, the receiving transducer and the electronics further affect this.

For stationary tissues (ie, motionless during at least the pulse transit time) the image forming process can be considered to be purely coherent and the granular structure of the image is determined by the physics of fluctuation scattering. In a compound scan, however, it can be seen, from Fig. 4, that each ensemble of scatterers within the target tissue is interrogated from several different directions. Each direction has a different set of phasors so that each A-scan is independent. The integration of these separate A-scan lines to form a two-dimensional B-scope image in which the average echo value is displayed is not subject to interference. Therefore this integration is an incoherent process. The result is that the granularity seen in simple or sector scans, which does not represent separately resolvable structures but is a distracting image artifact, is smoothed and reduced by compounding. The reduction is by a factor of $\sqrt{n}$, where n is the number of different directions of interrogation [8]. (Because of the detailed characterisation of 'maximum value' stores even B-scans produced with this processing show signal-to-noise ratio improvements only slightly less than with 'average value' storage.)

4.   Conclusions

The resolutions of conventional and real-time scanners are similar, except that arrays with swept focusing have the advantage. Single real-time images are inferior to conventional B-scans, but when viewed in real-time the artifacts due to speckle and electrical noise are significantly reduced.

References

[1]   Wells, P N T (1977) Biomedical Ultrasonics, pp 147-158. Academic Press, London.

[2]   Guibarra, E J, Wells, P N T, and Evans, K T (1976). A swept

focusing system for ultrasonic pulse-echo diagnosis. In Applications of Electronics in Medicine, pp 387-394. Institution of Electronic and Radio Engineers, London.

[3]   Whittingham, T A (1976). A hand-held electronically switched array for rapid ultrasonic scanning. Ultrasonics, 14, 29-33.

[4]   Ligtvoet, C M, Ridder, J, et al (1977). A dynamically focused multiscan system. In Echocardiology, ed N Bom, pp 313-323. Nijhoff, The Hague.

[5]   von Ramm, O T, Thurstone, F L and Kisslo, J (1975). Cardiovascular diagnosis with real-time ultrasound imaging. In Acoustical Holography, vol 6, ed N Booth, pp 91-102. Plenum Press.

[6]   Ligtvoet, C, Vogel, J, et al (1977). Direct conversion of real-time two-dimensional echocardiographic images. Ultrasonics, 15, 89-92.

[7]   Somer, J C, Oosterbaan, W A and Freund, H J (1973). Ultrasonic tomographic imaging of the brain with an electronic scanning system. In Ultrasonics Symposium Proceedings, 73 CHO 708-8SU, pp 43-48. Institute of Electrical and Electronics Engineers, New York.

[8]   Burckhardt, C B (1978). Speckle in ultrasound B-mode scans. I.E.E.E. Trans. Sonics Ultrason., SU-25, 1-6.

DIGITAL AND ANALOG SCAN CONVERTERS FOR ULTRASOUND IMAGING

D.A. Carpenter, D.E. Robinson and G. Kossoff

Ultrasonics Institute, Sydney, Australia

INTRODUCTION

In ultrasonic imaging the scan converter is used to change from the format produced by the scanning gantry to a television raster. It provides good grey scale image display and allows manipulation of the grey levels in the displayed image. Early models were analog units with the digital scan converter being introduced more recently. Table 1 shows the main performance characteristics of the two types.

CHARACTERISTICS	ANALOG S.C.	DIGITAL S.C.
Resolution	750,000 points	260,000 points
Grey Levels	Continuous ($\approx$50)	16 or 32
Processing	Limited	Extensive
Storage Time	< 30 minutes	Indefinite
Stability	Variable	Excellent
Aging	Degrades Performance	No Effect
Cost	$7,000	$15,000

ANALOG SCAN CONVERTER

In the analog scan converter the image is stored as charge levels on a storage surface. As the tube uses the same electron gun for writing and reading the image, these two operations cannot be done simultaneously. During the scanning process one can get a series of black bands across the image which represents the time that the tube is in the writing mode, commonly called the "venetian blind" effect. This can be overcome by reading and writing on alternate lines but with a loss in performance. The scan converter may be operated in the integration mode where the echo levels are summed for each point, or in the peak detection or equilibrium writing mode, in which the maximum value for each point is stored with no build-up on overlapping scans. This has proved of considerable advantage in the use of contact scanners as it reduces the critical requirement for even scanning. The analog scan converter offers excellent resolution with a wide grey scale range at a reasonable cost. Thus, up to nine images may be recorded on the storage surface,or part of a single image may be zoomed to greater magnification with adequate resolution. The wide range of stored echoes allows the grey scale levels to be expanded as the image is read onto a TV monitor (called post-processing) to emphasise a particular range of echoes within the scan. Lack of stability of operating characteristics at manufacture and during use has been a major problem with analog scan converters. Also, with the scan rates used for medical ultrasound the unit operates in a mode somewhere between peak detect and integrate. This means that it is still possible with poor scanning techniques to overwrite parts of the image. The image degrades with time and will start to lose contrast after a few minutes of storage.

DIGITAL SCAN CONVERTER

The digital scan converter stores the elements of the picture as number values in a digital memory. This generally means an image of 512 x 512 points with either 16 or 32 grey levels (1). If less points are used (say 256 x 256) the image has a coarse texture. Less grey levels (say 8) gives a contouring effect on the grey scale within the image. The present units do not have quite the resolution or grey scale capabilities of the best analog scan converters but offer considerable advantages in being able to read and write simultaneously and offering much greater versatility to process the image. They have no problems of stability and the image may be stored indefinitely with no degradation.

The unit can record a conventional M mode or a scrolling mode where the M mode image moves across the display screen as new information is added. The digital scan converter is particularly useful on a real time scanner to provide a freeze frame facility.

The digital storage technique allows much greater processing and measurement capability than is possible with an analog unit as shown in Table 2.

STORING MODE	POST-PROCESSING	MEASUREMENT
Integration Mode	Grey Scale Warping	Length
Peak Detect Mode	Grey Level Windowing	Area
Survey Mode	Bit Suppression	Echo Level at any Point
Exponential Mode	Level Slicing	Histogram of echo Levels
Subtraction Mode	Smoothing	in any areas
	Edge Enhancement	

Storing Mode

There are a number of different methods in which the signal at a point updates the value already in memory. The integrate and peak detect methods have already been described.

68

In the survey mode new data simply replaces the old so there
is a changeover from one scan to the next as the scan proceeds.
Alternatively there can be exponential build-up and decay of
the levels to give a gradual change from the old image into
the new one. The survey mode is particularly useful with an
automated scanner to maintain the overall image while rescanning and updating a small area of interest in a quasi real-time
mode. Figure 1 shows an overall longitudinal view of liver
with the central area rescanned rapidly to follow movement of
the I.V.C. and liver vessels.

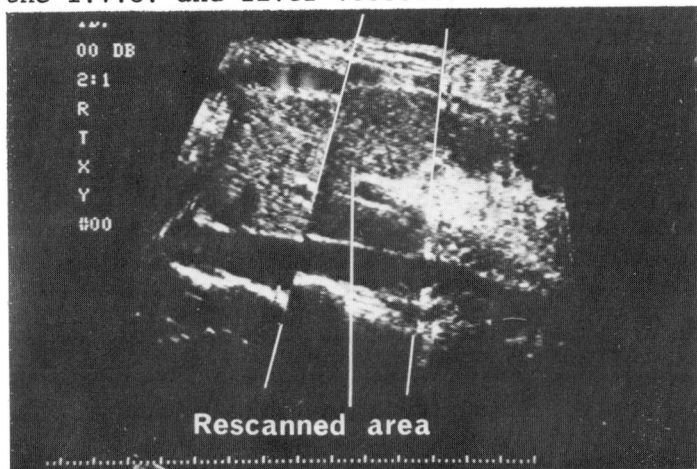

Post-Processing

Grey scale warping can be applied as the scan is read
out of memory, in a similar manner to the analog unit.
Figure 2 shows two examples where one is used to enhance
the low level echoes within structures and the other to show
well-defined boundaries.

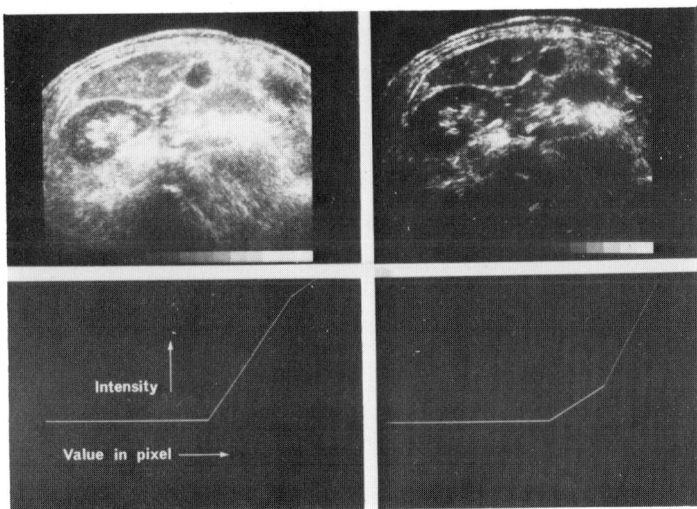

69

Grey scale windowing allows a selected group of grey levels to be expanded over the full range of the display while bit suppression and level slicing allows specific levels to be highlighted or suppressed. Filtering and differentiation techniques can be applied to give smoothing of the digital image and to enhance edges within the scan. Digital and analog scan converters normally supply both positive (white on black) and negative (black on white) video output signals.

Measurements

A considerable number of qualitative measurements can be taken from the scan converter. Calipers can define lengths or areas within the image which are then calculated and read out on the display. One can obtain a set of measurements of echo levels at a point or along any line of sight in the image and an area can be defined and the unit will produce a histogram or plot of relative frequency of occurrence of each echo level within the selected area.

CONCLUSION

The analog scan converter has been a major advance in ultrasound scanning as it offers excellent grey scale and resolution both for operator viewing and for recording of the image. It also offers the peak detection mode of operation which assists the scanning operation. The unit offers some grey scale processing capability and is available at a reasonable cost.

The digital scan converter has overcome the inherent stability and aging problems of the analog unit and gives simultaneous read-write capabilities with a greatly expanded versatility in processing of· the image but at a somewhat higher initial cost.

Recent research developments in this field are aimed at new processing techniques (2) for tissue characterisation.

REFERENCES

1. Ophir, J. and Maklad, N.F. (1979): Digital Scan Converters in Diagnostic Ultrasound Imaging. Proc. IEEE Vol. 67, No. 4.
2. Robinson, D.E. and Kossoff, G. (1979): Computer Processing of Line Mode Echogram Data. Proc. WFUM3 Meeting, Miyazaki, Japan. Excerpta Medica.

Analysis and Modelling of Grey Scale Images*

C. R. Hill, J. C. Bamber, R. J. Dickinson and D. Nicholas

Institute of Cancer Research, Royal Marsden Hospital, Sutton, Surrey, U.K.

ABSTRACT

This paper discusses the quantitative nature of the B-scan image from three related points of view. Conventional pattern recognition and image enhancement techniques have been applied to digitized B-scans and have been shown to aid both in distinguishing between the different diffuse parenchymal echo patterns characteristic of different disease conditions and also in differentiating small-scale local pathology from blood vessels or ducts. Such analysis raises the question of the precise relationship between small-scale anatomy and ultrasonic echo patterns, and computer modelling of the process of formation of a B-scan from a distributed scatterer model of tissue has demonstrated the interrelationship between anatomy and coherent wave speckle in the appearance of the resultant image. Finally, some consideration is given to the significance of coherent speckle as a form of image noise that may limit contrast resolution in a grey-scale image.

INTRODUCTION

The B-scan image has become a familiar tool in medical diagnosis and it is easy to forget that we know rather little about how it is formed and, therefore, about the precise nature of the information that it contains.

EMPIRICAL PATTERN RECOGNITION AND IMAGE ANALYSIS

A number of investigators have attempted to apply analytical techniques, developed for other branches of imaging such as aerial photography or sub-cellular biology, to the tasks of image enhancement and pattern recognition in B-scans (1-3). In a preliminary investigation (4) we have applied such techniques to liver B-scans

---

*
Paper for Conference on Recent Advances in Ultrasound Diagnosis, Dubrovnik, 1-5 October 1979.

with two practical objectives: (a) to characterize fine
scale parenchymal echo patterns in order either to
identify the presence and nature of pathology or to
monitor the response of an extended lesion to therapy,
and (b) to improve ability to identify or distinguish
discrete structures (e.g. tumours/vessels) on the basis
of their macroscopic shape.

Our techniques and preliminary results have been
reported in detail elsewhere (4) and some recent advances
are described in another paper in this volume (5). Of
particular relevance to the present discussion are the
results of attempts to quantitate B-scans in which, first,
a simple estimate was made of the spatial density of
echo peaks in particular regions of an image and, second,
Fourier methods were applied to search for periodicities
in the spatial frequency distribution of echo peaks. By
these means it appears to be possible to differentiate
in vivo between three categories: normal liver parenchyma
(intermediate spatial densities of echoes), cirrhosis
and possibly adenomata (relatively high spatial densities)
and other liver neoplasms (relatively low spatial
densities).

If findings of this sort can be substantiated in
more extensive and detailed clinical trials they will
represent a practical advance on the current approach
to differential diagnosis, which is based predominantly
on visual estimates of spatially integrated echo amplitude relative to a (supposed) normal tissue region.
Nonetheless they are "disappointing" in the sense that
the graduation of spatial density found in the images
seems to be markedly less than the variations in scale
and pattern of the corresponding histological structure.
It is therefore worth trying to investigate in detail the
manner in which the pulse echo process translates an
extended 3-dimensional tissue structure (in which much
of the ultrasonic interaction may take place with
structural elements comparable in size with an ultrasonic wavelength) into a 2-dimensional "B-scan image".

COMPUTER MODELLING OF THE B-SCAN PROCESS

The investigation suggested in the previous paragraph is at present impossible in an exact sense, because
the identity and nature of the tissue components responsible for ultrasonic scattering is not known. However,
recent developments in the theoretical description and
experimental observation of ultrasonic scattering by
tissues indicate that a useful first approach is to consider the acoustic scattering structure of tissue to be
an "inhomogeneous continuum", in which the density and
compressibility of tissues fluctuate in a continuous
manner from place to place, about their mean values (6,
7, 8). With such an assumption "tissues" of various types

and characteristics may be modelled mathematically. By then similarly modelling the features of an acoustic pulse, its scattering interaction with the chosen mathematical tissue model, and the subsequent process of signal reception and image formation, it is possible to explore the consequences for image structure of various combinations of machine settings and image parameters. This procedure has been described by some of us in a recent paper (9).

The results of this investigation are interesting in that they bear out and place in a quantitative framework the qualitative impressions, referred to above, of the limited extent of correlation between anatomical fine structure and the fine structure of the corresponding B-scan image. In particular they illustrate the importance, previously pointed out by Burckhardt(10), of wave coherence in the generation of image speckle. The modelling approach is quite general and appears to have very great potential. An example of its use is to compare the predicted B-scan appearances that result from scanning a tissue with two different pulses that are respectively short and long in relation to the "correlation length" (which can be thought of as a measure of coarseness of histological structure)of the tissue. The use of a "short" pulse, with non-linear signal processing, resolves the original object but gives the image an erroneously fine structure. A long pulse and/or a broad beam however leads to failure of anatomical resolution and an image appearance that is strongly dependent on pulse and beam parameters.

An important conclusion that can be drawn even at an early stage in this work is that attempts at image quantitation along the lines outlined in the previous section will need to take very careful account of the performance parameters of a scanner and that these may need to be chosen specifically in order to perform optimally in achieving a particular task of tissue differentiation.

IMPLICATIONS FOR IMAGE NOISE AND CONTRAST RESOLUTION

In this paper discussion hitherto has centred on the spatial characteristics of images. In diagnostic practice however it is probably true that the principal diagnostic criterion used in identifying and differentiating diffuse pathology is echo amplitude (or image brightness). There is a very important, although hitherto rather neglected, sense in which these two characteristics are related.

It is well known in other branches of imaging that contrast resolution (the difference in image brightness, compared with surrounding background, necessary for perception of an image region of given size) is very dependent on, among other factors, the level of image noise (see, e.g., Biberman, ref. 11).   In the absence of wave coherence noise is generally random in origin and nature (e.g., that due to the randomness of photon events in a radioisotope image).   Such noise is inevitably present in an ultrasound B-scan but may often be insignificant, in its influence on contrast resolution, in comparison with coherent speckle, which may, arguably, be considered as a special form of noise.   Means for controlling, or even eliminating, ultrasonic image speckle are therefore seen to be of considerable importance and this may well be the strongest scientific argument for the use of compounding techniques, where these can be applied without introduction of unacceptable movement and registration artefacts.

REFERENCES

1.   King, J. C. and Wong, A. K. C. (1972): Comput. Biomed. Res., 5, 190.
2.   Kay, M., Shimmins, J., Manson, G. and England, M. E. (1975): Ultrasonics, 13, 18.
3.   Waag, R. C., Gramiak, R., Lee, P. P. K. and Astheimer, J. (1976): I.E.E.E. Symp. Proceedings 76 CH 1120-55u, 163.
4.   Nicholas, D., Barrett, A., Chu, J. M. G., Cosgrove, D.O., Garbutt, P., Green, J., Pussell, S. and Hill, C. R. (1979): Acoustical Holography, 8, in press.
5.   Nicholas, D. (   ): B-scan image quantitation of human hepatic tissue (this volume).
6.   Chivers, R. C. (1977): Ultrasound Med. Biol., 3, 1.
7.   Gore, J. C. and Leeman, S. (1977): Phys. Med. Biol., 22, 317.
8.   Nicholas, D. (1977): In: Recent Advances in Ultrasound in Biomedicine, vol. 1, chap. 1. Editor: D. N. White.   Research Studies Press, Oregon.
9.   Bamber, J. C. and Dickinson, R. J. (   ): Ultrasonic B-scanning: a computer simulation.   Phys. Med. Biol. (in press).
10.   Burckhardt, C. B. (1978): I.E.E.E. Trans. Sonics and Ultrasonics, SU-25, 1.
11.   Biberman, L. A. (1973): Perception of displayed information, Plenum, New York and London.

PERCEPTION LIMITS OF GREY SCALE VISUALISATION

B. Breyer, B. Vojnovic and T. Viculin

Dept. of Obstetrics and Gynecology, University of Zagreb,
Rudjer Boskovic Institute, and Central Institute for Tumors
and Allied Diseases, Zagreb, Yugoslavia

ABSTRACT

Factors influencing grey scale visualisation are discussed. These include physical limits, such as random noise
or TV monitor limitations and physiological limits of the
eye that actually dictate the requirements on the instrumentation. One can show that random noise in the grey
scale image shifts the percepted average lightness and that
the eye's properties limit the useful dynamics to be shown
on the monitors for echography.

PERCEPTION LIMITATIONS

Human eye properties have developed during evolution in
such a way to optimally cope with necessities of perception
in normal life. Watching sonar images on a TV monitor is
in many respects different from everyday requirements.
Therefore, one should optimize the grey scale images in
such a way as to conform to the eye's properties and to recognize the limitations of such a straight forward diagnostic method.

The idea of grey scale imaging is simple and means only that different signals are being shown as different shades
of grey that are in some way proportional to the signal intensity.

The last word on how the eye brain complex perceives
an image still has not been said. Nevertheless there are
feasible, but partial explanations of the principles of the
integral image perception or at least some fair working
models. One of such theories relevant to image perception
on grey scale monitors is the Land's Retinex theory(1). It
explains how, on a black and white image, it is possible to
appreciate the lightness of an area even if the actual number of photons coming from that area does not conform to
our feeling. This property of visiion is useful because
we are normally interested in the reflectance of a surface,
rather than the actual lightness. A possible explanation
of this feature of our perception system is that we contin-
ually keep scanning the scene(2), and in fact recognize the
lightness boundaries that enable our brain to recalculate
the reflectances in the picture as if they were uniformly
illuminated. The fact that the eye scans the pictures makes

the impression dependent on the lightness boundaries and
their sharpness. If the lightness or reflectance boundary
is undefined, the scanning system is jammed and the number
of perceptible grey tones will be reduced (3). The sonar
images consist of dots and therefore on many occasions disturb our retinex system reducing the number of explicitly
definable grey shades to something between 5 and 8. This is
far less than one can occasionally find in literature (up
to over 30). Such an eye property reduces the possibility
and need for scan converters with a very high grey tone resolution if only whole images are to be shown on the screen.
In such cases, 3 or 4 bit digital scan converters would completely suffice. Obviously, the possibility of quantitative
analysis of the echoes, like amplitude analysis, has nothing to do with the eye's ability and in such a case the intensity resolution is not limited by the human eye. Compression of 60 dB or more of echo dynamics into the 20 dB
monitor dynamics may on occasion give images that are worse
for the diagnosis than it would be if not all echoes were
represented (4). A further limitation by the eye is the dependence of resolution on light intensity. It can be shown
(5) that the eye's ability to resolve adjacent structures
depends strongly (and proportionally) on the lightness and
contrast. Thus small echoes will be seen with a worse resolution. Increasing the lightness of the whole image will
brighten up small echoes, but will due to the other high level echoes induce a shrinking of the iris, thus counteract-
ing our efforts to see the small echoes better. This in fact
means that an intensity window for the monitor lightness
would help to perceive the low level echoes. We shall discuss a possibility for that in the last paragraph of this
paper.

SOME INSTRUMENTATION LIMITATIONS

     We shall try to briefly discuss the influence of ran-
dom noise on percepted lightness. Lightness perception characteristic is nonlinear, as shown in Figure 1. Random noise
will disturb a line spectrum in such a way as to produce a
whole (usually Gaussian) distribution of signals. This new
distribution will be transformed by the eye's characteristic into a nonsymmetrical actual perception distribution
that indicates the lightness feeling. Furthermore, a part
of the input signals will be cut off by the black level of
our eye. Owing to this and the nonlineariety, the net result will be a shift of the mean values of a noisy image as
opposed to a non-noisy one. This applies to fast renewing
pictures. Quantitatively, this is seen in Figure 2. The
perceived mean value of a noise disturbed line spectrum
(single lightness) changes with the additive noise in that
it first becomes smaller and then grows when the noise effects overcome the signal significance in the image. Noise
measurement methods have been studied in our previous investigations and they have shown that appreciable effects

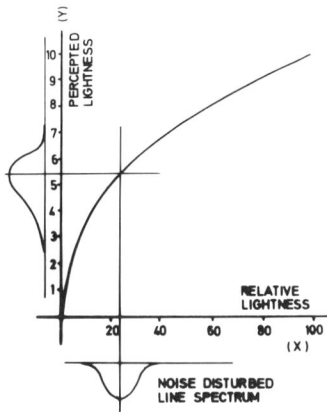

Fig. 1. Transformation of a noise disturbed line spectrum of light intensity.

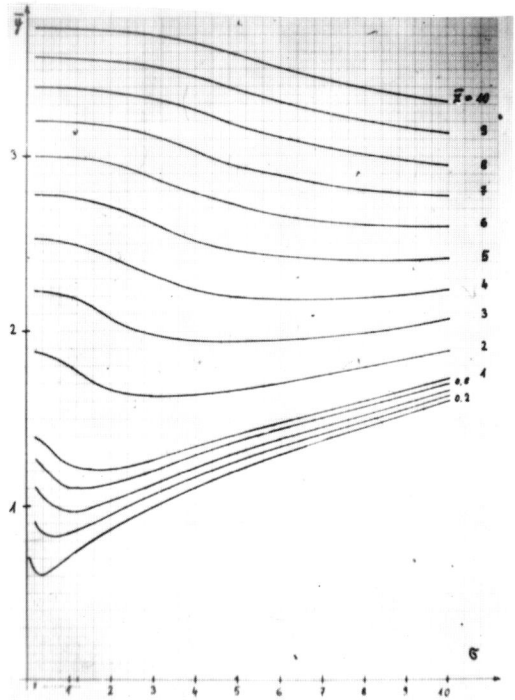

Fig. 2. Dependence of perceived mean value on noise SD. Ordinate-perceived mean value. Abscissa-noise SD. Parameter-physical lightness (7).

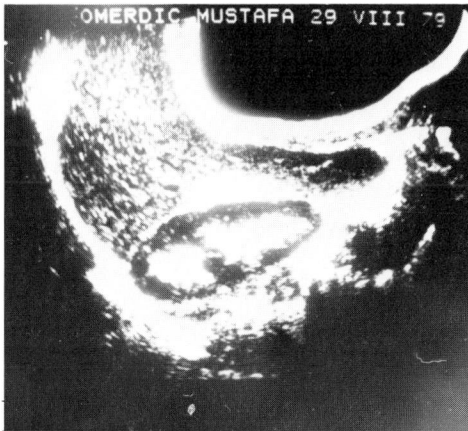

Fig. 3a. Normal display of liver and kidney

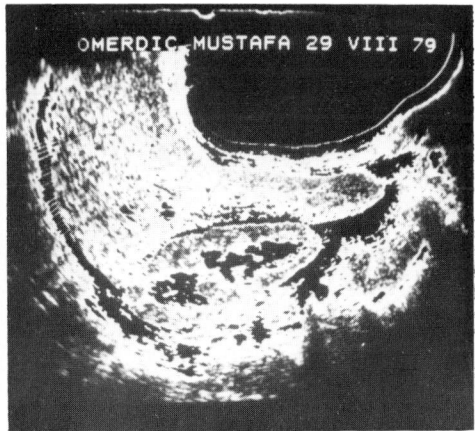

Fig. 3b. Window display of Fig. 3a. Kidney parenchyma can be seen better.

of noise can be demonstrated with good quality echoscopes at their highest sensitivities. Some authors quote useful echo dynamics of up to 120 dB and thus, if the ultrasound intensity is not to be increased, the noise disturbance will become a problem.

MONITOR LIGHTNESS WINDOW

Normally, the signals obtained from the transducer are being compressed in order to adapt them to the much narrower dynamics of TV monitors. This enables us to visualize all echoes in one image with different shades of grey. However, the nonlinearity of the eye combined with the compression characteristic degrades the differentiation of high grade echoes. On the other hand, small echoes are shown as very dark dots on the screen and thus they are not easy to detect in the presence of large signals. Brightening of all echoes does not help much because the eye and the monitor electronics counteract this action. A possibility for overcoming this problem in some particular cases is demonstrated in Figures 3a & b. The largest echoes are "blacked out", thus leaving only a window to be seen between the lowest and some maximum value. Dots that are brighter than a chosen value (level) are shown as dark areas and do not disturb the vision. The window thus excludes the brightest parts of the image and allows the darkness adapted eye to see only the low level part of the image. The brightness of the excluded parts can be adjusted to any desired level. Clearly, such image processing is only useful in those particular cases when in an overall bright image some darker areas are of special interest.

REFERENCES

1. Land, E.H., McCann, J.J. (1971): Lightness and retinex theory, J. Optical Society of America, 61, 1.
2. McCann, J.J., Benton, J.L. (1969): Interaction of long wave cones and the rods to produce color sensations. J. Optical Society of America, 59, 104.
3. Breyer, B., Kurjak, A., Latin, V. (1978): Subjektive Grauwer-schätzung. Perinatale Medizin (eds. E. Schmidt, J.W. Dudenhausen, E. Saling). Georg Thieme Verlag, Stuttgart, p. 454.
4. Robinson, D.E., Kossoff, G.(1974): The imaging properties of ultrasonic pulse echo visualisation systems. Proc. of the Society of Photo Optical Instrumentation Engineers Meeting, Kansas City, USA, Aug. 1-2, 47, 84.
5. Rose, A. (1973): Vision,Human and Electronic. Plenum Press, New York.
6. Breyer, B., Vojnovic, B. (1978): Noise measurement in ultrasonic pulse echo systems. In: Recent Advances in Ultrasound Diagnosis (ed. A. Kurjak), Excerpta Medica, Amsterdam, p. 48.
7. Breyer, B., Viculin, T., Vojnovic, B. (1980): Noise in ultrasonic imaging. To be published in Ultrasonics.

LIMITATIONS OF MEASUREMENTS FROM ULTRASOUND IMAGES

A.J. Hall

University of Glasgow Department of Midwifery, Queen
Mother's Hospital, Glasgow Scotland.

Various fetal dimensions are used, either singly or
severally, to monitor fetal growth. These include:
biparietal diameter, crown rump length, trunk area and
circumference, and head area and circumference. The
accuracy and reproducibility of the estimations are
influenced by image quality, equipment calibration
velocity, scale factor accuracy and display distortions.
Grey scale imaging by its nature produces images with
diffuse boundary regions thus causing uncertainty about
the exact dimensions to be measured. Exceptions are
the biparietal diameter and crown rump length where
the boundaries are relatively well defined. Diffuse
boundaries are more usual when measuring the area or
perimeter of a fetal trunk or head. The calibration
velocity selected affects the represented size of a
fetal cross section and measurement errors result from
variations with time or the use of the wrong velocity
with previously published data. For example if the
velocity 1524 msec^{-1} is used instead of 1540 msec^{-1}
the linear dimensions will change by 1%. The change in
area will depend on whether the image has been formed
using a compound scanner or a real time scanner and on
the type of scan. For a simple linear B scan or a real
time linear array scan there will be a change in one
axis only. If the image is formed by a sector scan
there will be change in the dimensions of both axes.
The size of the image also depends on the picture scaling
amplifiers and their design. For example if they are
fixed gain operational amplifiers with no presets using
1% tolerance resistors, a worst case gain error of ± 2%
is possible. However, if present, this linear error is
unlikely to change with time. This is not so for
television monitors which display the scan converter
output. These can introduce distortions which are
very dependent upon the settings of the brilliance and
contrast controls.

Measurement from Photographs - Area and perimeter
can be measured from either photographs or hard copy
output using a planimeter and a map measurer. Such an
approach is open to errors in picture scaling unless an
electronic reference graticule is used to allow for linear
scale errors. This graticule however cannot compensate
for the non-linearities in television monitors. Monitor
distortion can be avoided by using a hard copy unit which
accepts a video signal from the scan converter to modulate
a fibre optic CRT as a dry silver paper sheet moves past

it.

To investigate the errors likely in measurements obtained with a planimeter and a map measurer, two operators carried out multiple independent measurements on circles scribed with dividers on Polaroid film. The sizes of the circles varied from 10 mm diameter to 70 mm diameter. Typically the areas and perimeters were overestimated by 5% with coefficients of variation which ranged from 22% to 1%; the variation being worst for the smaller circles. Possibly the above errors could be reduced if a graphics analyser was used to digitise and compute the results but it is a method we have not explored.

Electronic Methods - An intrinsically better though technologically more complex solution to area and perimeter determination is electronic measurement - preferably "through the system" so that drift in picture size or other variations do not affect the measurement. By replacing the measuring frame X and Y voltages representing the transducer's position, with ones generated by a joystick connected to the measuring frame reference supply, the operator can place a marker dot anywhere within the X,Y space defined by the measuring frame dimensions. While the outline is being marked on the screen, the joystick voltages are fed to computing circuits which calculate area and perimeter or the distance between two points. The joystick can use either polar (RØ) or cartesian (X,Y) co-ordinate measurements for spot steering and computation. An R,Ø joystick uses two marker dots, one defines the measurement origin and must be placed inside the object to be outlined while the other is controlled by the joystick and defines the outline. Rotation is measured by an incremental angular digitiser (Ø) and radius (R) with a potentiometer. This approach allows the use of simple analogue computation: the equations used are - Area $\propto R^2 \emptyset$; Perimeter R Ø. A voltage to frequency converter is used to connect the radius voltage to a pulse train whose frequency is proportional to voltage. The pulse train is then gated so that each pulse represents 0.1 mm. The monostable controlling the gate is pulsed each time the angular digitiser moves through Ø. The pulse trains are summed to give perimeter in mm. Area is similarly computed but using an analogue multiplier to produce R^2 before voltage to frequency conversion, gating and storage. The computational process is halted electronically when the angular digitiser has moved through 360°. It can be shown that the computations of area and perimeter are independent of the value of Ø. The calculated area is independent of the origin location but perimeter is not and errors occur if the origin is far from the centre.

A cartesian co-ordinate system is electronically more complex but allows a single spot to be used for measurement. Additionally convoluted images can be

measured. Fig. 1 illustrates a system which uses a puck
or ring to steer the spot on the image.

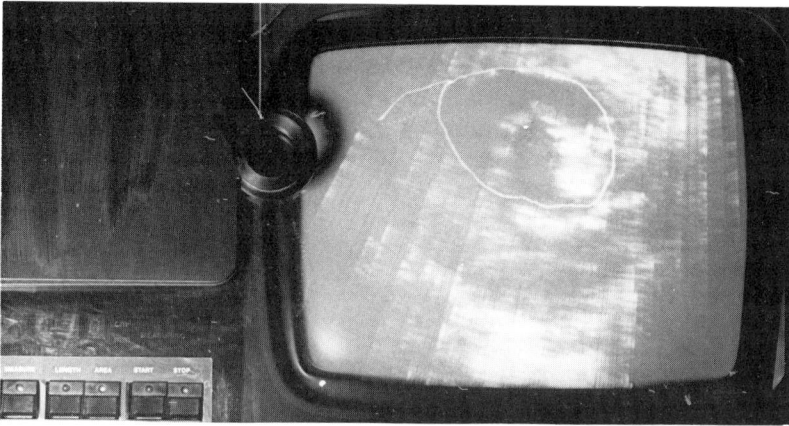

Figure 1   Close up view of cartesian co-ordinate
measuring system showing puck and typical
area outline.

This puck is connected to potentiometers and via scaling
and positioning amplifiers to the X and Y measuring
frame inputs of the ultrasound machine. Two 8 bit
analogue to digital converters digitise these voltages
and compute area and perimeter using hard wired logic
circuitry. The resolution of the analogue to digital
converters varys with picture size from 0.5 mm per bit
on life size to 2 mm per bit on 2/5 life size.
    The X axis position is measured by a tracking
analogue to digital converter which is unbalanced by
movement; each unbalance initiates a sample of the
current Y axis value. The circuitry calculates the area
under the curve; while the puck is moving from left to
right the X axis values are increasing and incremental
areas are added; decreasing values cause subtraction.
The net result is a calculation of the outlined area.
Perimeter is calculated from an algorithm based on the
differences between successive Y values. The measurement
is automatically terminated when the operator returns
the spot to within a specified distance of the start; an
essential feature if computational errors are to be
avoided.
    To quantify the accuracy and variability of measure-
ment due to the operator and the electronics, measurements
were performed on a variety of well defined electronically
generated circles - circular because most fetal structures
are circular or ellipsoid. The circles were drawn using
a test facility and the computational circuitry automatically calculated the areas and perimeters. The values
were found to be within -1% of the values calculated using

the usual formulae. Two operators were then required to trace 3 circles at various display scale factors and found that the coefficients of variation were within ± 1% for area and perimeter except for the smallest circle (30 mm diameter) where the variation in area reading was ± 2.2%. To test for overall accuracy including the effects of poor image definition, a water immersed target was used. It comprised a 77.2 mm diameter cylinder made of Melinex film, thickness 0.025 mm wrapped round a skeleton framework. Five scans were made and measured by each of three operators. The percentage difference between the mean of each group of five readings of area and perimeter are given in Table I along with the corresponding coefficients of variation.

Operator	AREA		PERIMETER	
	mean error %	coefficient of variation %	mean error %	coefficient of variation %
1	-1.8	2.7	-1.5	1.3
2	-3.3	1.5	-2.1	0.7
3	-2.4	1.5	-1.8	0.7

Table I. Errors in electronic measurements of area and perimeter of 77.2 mm diameter target in water bath.

The figures suggest that the overall accuracy likely when measuring ultrasonic images of this size is in the region of 2 to 3%. In considering the magnitude of these errors it should be noted that a two percent error in area would result from a one percent error in radius; for an 80 mm diameter circle this represents 0.4 mm which is less than the diameter of the marker spot used to outline the area.

OBTAINING QUANTITATIVE DATA FOR ULTRASONIC EQUIPMENT TESTING

K. Brendel and G. Ludwig

Physikalisch-Technische Bundesanstalt, Bundesallee 100,
3300 Braunschweig, Germany

A knowledge of the quantitative data of ultrasonic medical devices is necessary if optimal equipment for the various fields of application is to be chosen. It also enables the user to compare his results with those of other colleagues and to reduce avoidable risks to the patient. It is the objective of this paper to outline measurement methods for the various ultrasonic field parameters.

In table 1 the most important measurement methods, their approximate threshold sensitivities and their spatial and temporal resolutions are listed. Here, p is the sound pressure, ξ the particle displacement, v the particle velocity, P the acoustic power and I the sound intensity.

TABLE 1. Measurement methods for the various ultrasonic field parameters

Method	Measured Quantity	Resolution: Intensity W/cm^2	Power W	Space mm	Time s
Interferometry	ξ	10^{-6}		0,05	10^{-8}
Electrostatic Probe	ξ	10^{-4}		10	10^{-8}
Electrodynamic "	v	10^{-3}		10	3.10^{-8}
Float	P		10^{-2}	10	1
Balance	P		10^{-4}	10	1
Sphere	I	10^{-2}		1	1
Double Exposure Holography	I	10^{-3}		0,05	1
Piezoelectric Probe	p	10^{-10}		1	10^{-8}
Light Diffraction	p	10^{-3}		5	10^{-5}
Light Deflection	p	10^{-4}		0,1	10^{-8}
Calorimetry	P	10^{-3}		-	10

The table starts with three measurement procedures for the particle displacement and the particle velocity. A comparison of the characteristic data shows the advantages of interferometric methods, namely their high resolution in intensity, time and space. The quoted resolution in intensity can be still further increased, depending on the power of the laser used. By the use of sophisticated techniques such as the wiggler, or exploiting the two independent

orthogonal polarisations possible in a beam of light, a high
temporal stability at very high sensitivities is achieved (1). The
main value of this technique is that it allows the representation of
the pressure distribution over a cross-section of the radiated sound
field.

Electrostatic and electrodynamic probes are predominantly suited to
the measurement of particle displacement and velocity of short-
duration pulses, due to the problems with standing waves when
continuous waves are detected (2).

The following four measurement methods are based on the measurement
of the radiation force which is a direct result of the transport of
energy by the ultrasonic wave.

The float technique has been used since 1952 (4,5) for the determination of the total acoustic power radiated by therapeutic equipment. The float consists of a cone-shaped reflector with a stem
dipping into a liquid which is not miscible with water and which has
a density larger than 1, e.g tetracarbonchloride. The radiation
force displaces the float until its stem moves into the heavier
liquid far enough to develop an equal force. The main advantages of
this method are, first, that the calibration can be carried out very
easily by dropping weights on the float, and secondly, that the
float is self-centering. Unfortunately, this simple method originally
developed for the watt range, creates a lot of problems when power
measurements in the milliwatt range are performed, due to adhesive
and surface tension forces acting on the stem of the float. When
using Teflon-coated stems, the disturbing forces in the boundary
layer are diminished, as preliminary measurements in the milliwatt
range have shown (6).

Power measurements in the milliwatt range are usually performed
with a feed-back microbalance (7). The ultrasonic power is radiated
vertically upwards. The sound beam is intercepted by a target and
the mechanical force acting upon it is measured.
Performing measurements with modulated radiation pressure (8), the
lowest measurable power is of the order of 10^{-5} W, but this method is
restricted to transducer characterization. These measurement methods
reveal only the temporal and spatial average values of the sound
intensity.

The spatial intensity distribution can be determined performing
point-by-point measurements using a ball, the elongation of which is
measured. The double-exposure holography method is much more convenient, revealing a quantitative representation of the spatial
intensity distribution in a cross-section of an ultrasonic beam (9).
This method makes use of the fact that an ultrasonic beam striking
a liquid surface produces a surface relief caused by the radiation
pressure. Holographic interferometry makes this relief visible by
contour lines. The sound intensity is calculated by numerical
evaluation, taking into account the surface tension effect. Although
until now, this method has been tested in detail for continuous
waves, preliminary measurements with pulsed sound waves indicate

its applicability also to pulsed medical equipment (10).

Calibrated piezoelectric probes must be used for sound field measurements in absolute terms if a high resolution in both space and time domains is required, i.e. if the spatial and temporal peak pressure value must be determined. A probe for ultrasonic equipment testing should fulfil several fundamental specifications, i.e. it should be temporally stable, small relative to the wavelength, adequately sensitive, and broad-banded. At present these specifications cannot all be met simultanuously and special probes with restricted qualities have been recommended. One interesting proposal is the use of a thick piezoelectric disc for the measurement of the instantaneous pressure value of short ultrasonic pulses (11). This method is restricted to plane waves only. The sensitivity of the device is calculated from the piezoelectric data of the material used. The calibration of the piezoelectric probes is generally performed by measuring the output voltage with the instrument placed in an ultrasonic field of known intensity. As a calibration procedure for piezoelectric probes used in dosimetry, the competent IEC Working Group has recommended the reciprocity method using an auxiliary transducer (12). The receiving sensitivity can be calculated from the measured electric values of current and voltage. This measuring procedure has the advantage that the determination of the relevant acoustic quantities can be reduced to the measurement of electric quantities.

The acousto-optic methods have the principal advantage that there is no disturbance of the sound field by the placing of any measuring device into it. The diffraction method (Debye-Sears effect) is restricted to continuous waves or tone bursts. The calibration is performed by the measurement of the light intensity in the zeroth and first diffraction orders. The light deflection method has a high resolution in intensity, space, and time and is therefore suited to the investigation of short pulses. When using these acousto-optically investigated sound fields for the calibration of probe transducers, care should be taken that the light beam integrates over a volume of the sound beam (13).

The calorimetric techniques are based on the measurement of the temperature rise when ultrasonic energy is absorbed. This method requires that the thermal losses to the environment be kept at a minimum or, at least, determinable. These boundary conditions are not so easily met. Measuring devices for the intensity range of dosimetry must be regarded as laboratory instruments (14). Thermocouple probes yield a high spatial resolution, but their application is restricted to sound fields with intensities of about 1 W or more.

The measurement uncertainty is estimated to be of the order of $\pm$ 10% in most cases. Systematic errors are the main reason for this rather low accuracy, the elimination of which requires a great deal of effort. The essential source of error is that usually, the calibration facilities at megahertz frequencies are far from corresponding to the ideal boundary conditions assumed in theory. Further errors are caused by the medium itself. Gas content, wetting problems and non-linear properties all influence the results obtained.

References

1. Vilkomerson, D., Mezrich, R., and Etzold, K-F., An improved system for visualizing and measuring ultrasonic wavefronts, in Acoustical Holography. Vol. 7, Editor L.W. Kessler, Plenum Press, New York and London 1977
2. Filipczyński, L., Absolute measurements of particle velocity, displacement or intensity of ultrasonic pulses in liquids and solids. Acustica 21(1969) pp. 173-180
3. O'Brien W.D.,Jr., Ultrasonic dosimetry, in Ultrasound: Its Applications in Medicine and Biology, Editor Fry, F.J. Elsevier, Scientific Publishing Company 1978
4. Oberst, H. and Rieckmann, P., Das Verfahren der Physikalisch-Technischen Bundesanstalt bei der Bauartprüfung medizinischer Ultraschallgeräte, Amtsblatt der PTB Nr. 3 (1952), 106
5. IEC-Publication 150, Testing and calibration of ultrasonic therapeutic equipment, 1963
6. Swamy, K.M., Ultrasonic power measurements in milliwatt-region by the float method, Unpublished report (1978)
7. Rooney, J.A., Determination of acoustic power outputs in the microwatt-milliwatt range, Ultrasound Med. Biol. 1 (1973) 13-16
8. Greenspan, M., Breckenridge, F.R. and Tschiegg, C.E. Ultrasonic transducer power output by modulated radiation pressure J. Acoust. Soc. Amer., Vol 63, (1978) 1031-1038
9. Reibold, R., Applicaton of holographic interferometry for the investigation of ultrasonic fields, Acustica 38, (1977) 253-257
10. Reibold, R., Recent advances in the holographic liquid-surface inspection of ultrasonic fields. Publication details to come
11. Baboux, J.C.; Lakestani, F. and Perdrix, M., Measurement of the ultrasonic energy radiated by transducers used in echography, Ultrasound Med. Biol. 5 (1979) 75-82
12. Brendel, K. and Ludwig, G., Calibration of ultrasonic standard probe transducers, Acustica 36 (1976), 203-208
13. Erikson, K.R., Calibration of standard ultrasonic probe transducers using light diffraction, in Interaction of Ultrasound and Biological Tissues, Editors Reid, J.M. and Sikov, M.R., DHEW Publication (FDA) 73-8008, 1972
14. Zapf, T.L., Harvey, M.E., Larsen, N.T. and Stoltenberg, R.E., Ultrasonic calorimeter for beam power measurements, NBS Technical note 686, 1976

CHARACTERIZATION OF ULTRASONIC TRANSDUCERS USING CHOLESTERIC
LIQUID CRYSTALS

R. Denis

E.E.C., N.D.T. Laborities, J.R.C., Ispra, Italy

ABSTRACT

This paper relates to two methods for characterisation
of ultrasonic transducers by means of a visualisation technique which exploits the particular properties of cholesteric liquid crystals. Examples illustrating these methods are
used to demonstrate the results obtained whilst maintaining
the advantages of a simple and economic technique. The methods do not require special qualifications for the operators.

INTRODUCTION

In order to provide the users and manufacturers of ultrasonic transducers with a simple and cheap means for controlling their apparatus, we have experimented with a technique, calling upon the particular properties of cholesteric
liquid crystals. Two methods were developed and made it
possible to obtain a considerable amount of information.

DIRECT METHOD

The first,known as the direct method, consists of observing a layer of liquid crystals deposited on the lens of
the transducer to be characterized. Any thermal phenomenon
occurring on the transducer surface of the lens is translat-
ed into a coloured image of the temperature distribution on
the surface.
The thermal phenomena observed during the characterisation of a transducer can have three origins:
1. The passage of a thermal flux from the body of the transducer towards the atmosphere through the lens, when the
   transducer is not powered.
2. Localized heat sources due to contact resistance.
3. Transformation of acoustic energy into thermal energy due
   to absorption of the acoustic wave.
In order to illustrate this method, we describe the successive phases in the characterisation of a medical transducer. After cleaning the surface of the lens, a coat of
black paint is applied in order to absorb the non-reflected
part of the incident light spectrum. Water soluble paint is
used, easily removable by a simple wash with water, once the

measurements are finished. The layer of liquid crystals is applied and then covered with a sheet of mylar that is used for homogenisation of the liquid crystal layer and for protection against atmospheric contamination, which might react with the liquid crystals. The cholesteric mixture is prepared so as to present its own mesophase at a temperature only slightly exceeding room temperature. When the transducer is held by hand, it heats up sufficiently for the liquid crystal coloration to appear. One can then observe the contour of the crystal, the housing and the heterogeneous areas of the lens as well as the unglued areas of the latter. This preliminary examination will remove doubts about the interpretation of thermal phenomena of acoustical origin. The transducer is then powered by a continuous wave generator and the frequency is varied until coloration appears on the surface. A contact resistance (defective velding of a connection, for example) will produce a very characteristic local heating. By means of the absorption of the acoustic wave, one can determine:

1. The energy peaks emitted by the transducer in function of the frequency (frequency spectrum).
2. Defects in parallelism between the two faces of the lens, its thickness and its adaptation to the central frequency of the crystal.
3. Several structural defects will be pin-pointed and defined on the basis of the information obtained before powering. (Figure 1)

TOMOGRAPHY METHOD

The second method, known as the tomography method, is based on the thermotropic properties of the cholesteric liquid crystals. It consists of visualisation of cross sections of the beam of the transducer to be characterized. The liquid crystals are sandwiched between an optical glass and an absorbant layer which transforms acoustic waves into heat. Figure 2 shows the optical device which is used for transducer characterisation. A movable screen with a 1 mm slit is placed in front of the printing frame. The slit can be positioned at the height of the plane of the desired longitudinal section. A photograph of a longitudinal section of the beam is obtained (Figure 3) by a succession of automatized sequences: -- vertical movement of the transducer
                                    -- positioning of the printing frame
                                    -- camer shutter release.

CONCLUSION

In conclusion, one can say that the technique becomes increasingly valid because it supplies a great deal of information at a very low operational cost. It has an additional advantage of not requiring any particular qualification for the operator, except of being familiar with liquid crystal manipulation.

REFERENCE

1. R. Denis (1978): Characterisation of ultrasonic trans-
    ducers using cholesteric liquid crystals (Part 1), Ul-
    trasonics, EUR 5710e.

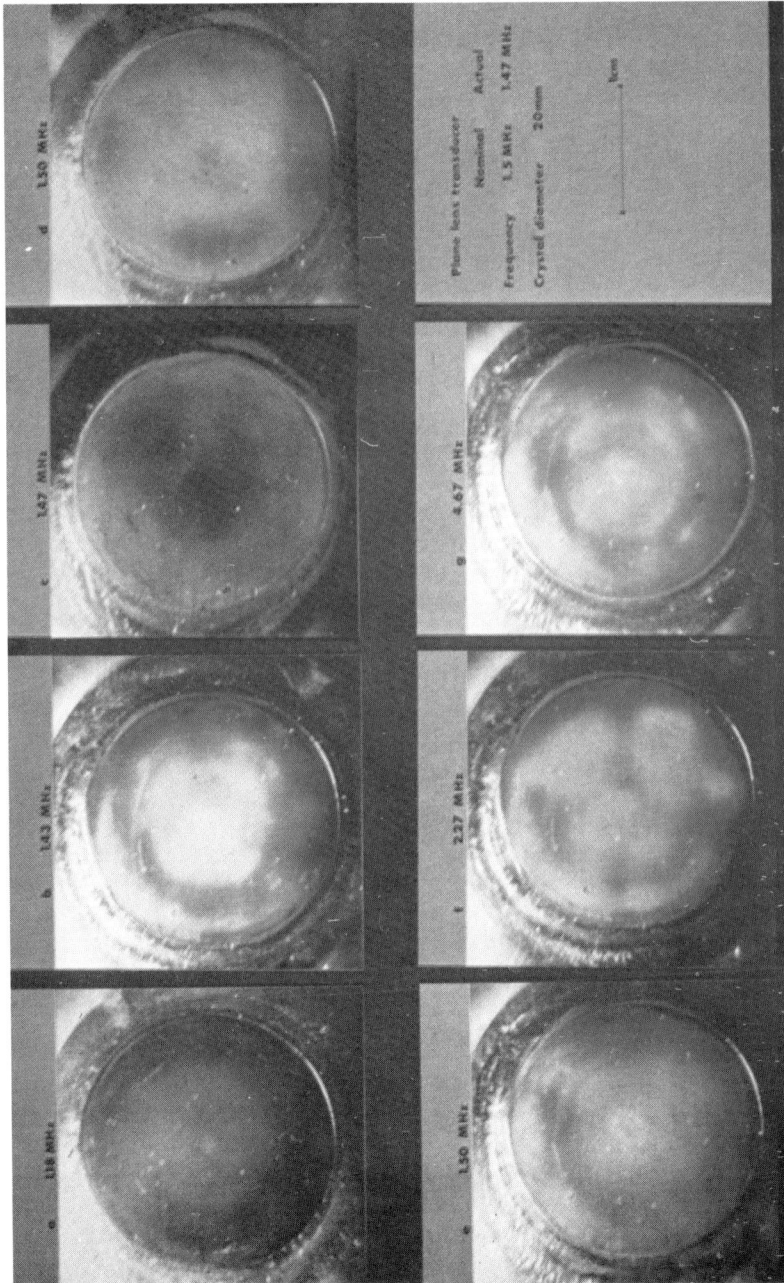

Fig. 1. The direct method.

89

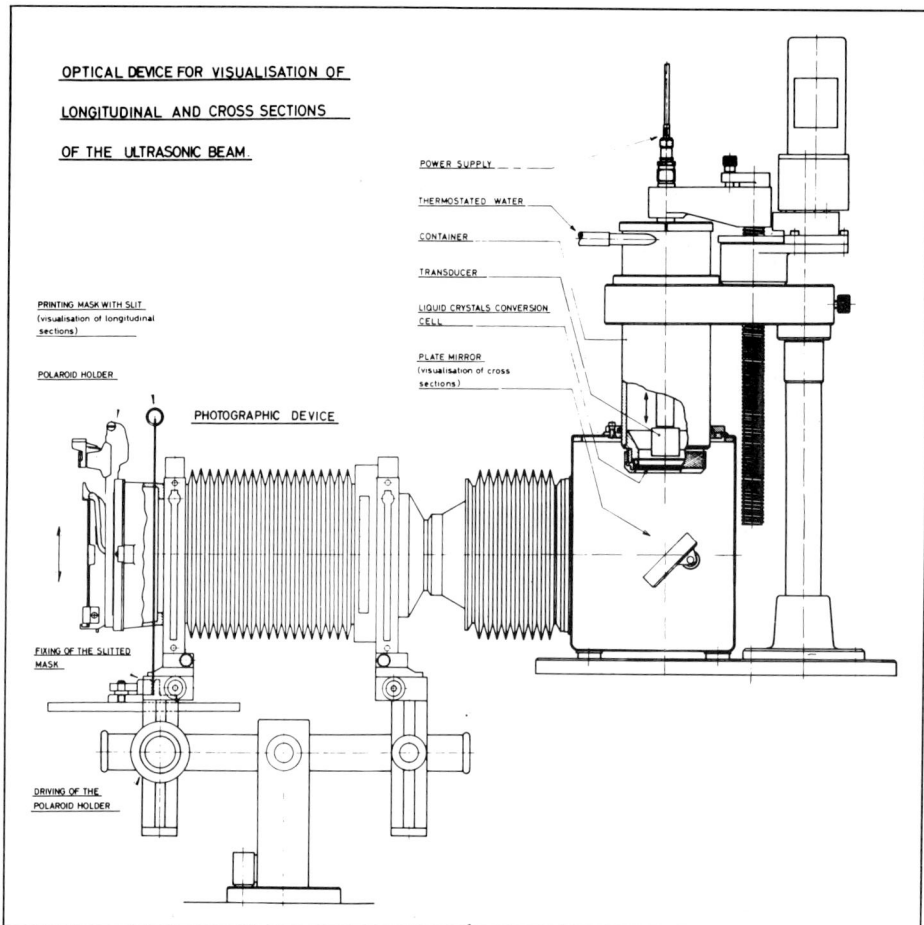

Fig. 2. Optical device for visualisation of longitudinal and cross sections of the ultrasonic beam.

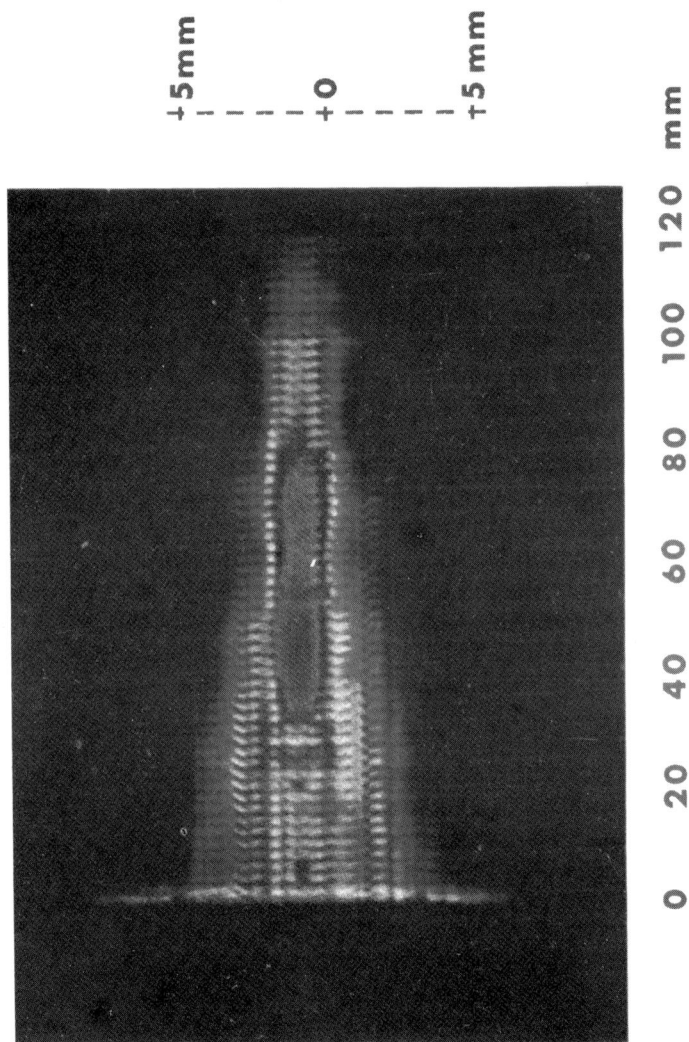

Fig. 3. The tomography method.

4. BIOLOGICAL ACTION OF ULTRASOUND IN RELATION TO THE RADIATION SAFETY QUESTION

C. R. Hill, Chairman

Ultrasonic Radiation Safety: Is There a Problem?

C. R. Hill.

Institute of Cancer Research, Royal Marsden Hospital,
Sutton, Surrey. U.K.

Over the past ten years the diagnostic use of ultrasound has grown very fast, to the point where some investigative procedures, particularly in obstetrics, are used on a large fraction of the population in many countries. In addition, therapeutic uses of ultrasound have been in quite widespread use for the past 30 years or more. In all this experience there has been no clearly established report of damage to a patient, other than from occasional fairly minor therepeutic over-exposures.

However, scientific caution and professional ethics make it necessary to question whether such rather uncertain evidence is adequate to provide a basis for guiding the continued and widespread use of ultrasound in medicine. This question is underlined by the inevitable comparison that is made between ultrasound and X-ray techniques and by the evidence that has been claimed for the genetic and carcinogenic actions of diagnostic doses of ionizing radiations.

A considerable body of research has been carried out into this question of the safety of ultrasonic radiation. This has been the subject of a major review that was recently commissioned by the World Health Organization(1). Work published since the WHO review was prepared is summarized in the first of what is intended to be a series of updating review articles (2). It is not immediately obvious what lines of research are most necessary and relevant to providing answers to this question and the purpose of the following group of papers is to discuss the value and relevance of the main lines of work that have seemed to be appropriate.

High on any list of relevance must be any systematic evidence that can be derived from studying statistically the consequences of human exposure: epidemiology. This however is a difficult and potentially expensive field of study, and one in which answers can only come after many years of study. One thus turns to laboratory studies and, particularly in the light of experience in radiobiology and other branches of toxicology, searches for genetic, cytogenetic and teratogenic changes seen to be relevant here. In addition, and particularly because of the potential of ultrasound for inducing mechanical changes in fragile structures, it seems sensible to look for evidence of damage at the cellular and ultrastructural level.

In all this it is important to bear in mind that ultrasound is known to be able to induce biological damage by a variety of mechanisms, amongst which that of "cavitation" in particular seems to be particularly sensitive to specific environmental conditions, in such a way that care needs to be taken in extrapolating from in vitro laboratory conditions to the situation of intact living tissues.

Finally a very valuable line of evidence must come from studies of the therapeutic use of ultrasound. Until recently practice in this field has been empirical and, some would say, unscientific, but some good research evidence is now starting to accumulate.

REFERENCES

1.   Hill, C. R. (-): Chapter on Ultrasound in "WHO Manual on Health Effects of Non-Ionizing Radiation" World Health Organization (in press since mid 1977 but single copies available free from Dr M. J. Suess, WHO Europe, Scherfigsvej 8, Copenhagen, Denmark).
2.   ter Haar, G. R. (-): Safety of Medical Ultrasound. In: Progress in Medical Ultrasound. Editor: A. Kurjak. Excerpta Medica, Amsterdam (in press).

Strategy For Safety Studies And The Place Of Epidemiology

Jens Bang

Department of Diagnostic Ultrasound, Rigshospitalet, University Hospital, Copenhagen, Denmark.

In the last 5o. years ultrasonics has been used in continious in creasing extent. Many of the applications involves exposure to humans neither occasionally or as in the medical application of ultrasonics as an essentiel part of the procedure. The existens of those applications involves of course the question about possible corresponding harmful effects for the individual influenced by the exposition.

Hill (2) has asked the question about the biological effects of ultrasound in a very good survey as early as 1968 specially concerning the medical application of ultrasound but it must be recognized until now here is no complete answer of the problem. In considering the exposure possibilities generally it needs to be born in mind that ultrasound propagates rather poorly through air and that liquid-air or solid-air interfaces constitute major differences in impedance and thus effective barriers to transmission in the frequences used in medical diagnostics. This means that the sonoghraphe will not receive any kind of ultrasound.

In relation to the very great and even stil growing number of patients exposed to ultrasonic diagnostics and here not the least important in gynecology and obstetrics where fetuses are exposed even very early in pregnancy, it may be of great importance to support the impression that there is no harmful effects and it is of great importance to encourage this problems examined both by experimental and e-pidemiological work.

AIUM had issued in 1976 a communication on "Mammation In Vivo Ultrasonic Biological Effects". It was started by the AIUM that in any application of the statement to safety decisions, consideration should be given to the following.

a. most of the data applied to mammals, other than man, and it is not always clear how to relate these to the human situation.
b. most experiments have not been repeated by independent investigators.
c. data are scarce on exposures both with repeated short pulses and with long exposure times at low intensities.
d. exposure levels for which bio-effects have been reported are not necessarily minimum levels (if, indeed, definite minima exist).

WHO had a working group in London 1976 with the purpose to make a chapter on ultrasound in a manual on health aspects of exposure to non-ionizing radiation. After the meeting Hill( ) made a very good chapter on ultrasound and we hope this manual will be avaible soon. In the manuscript there is a list over litterature concerning ultra-sounds biological effects published until now.

The working group has made a general recommendation.
1. A primary (traceable) standard for ultrasound exposure parameters should be developed along with procedures for the measurement of these ultrasound exposure parameters.
2. Encouragement should be given to the developement of improved measurement equipment including portable devices to determine exposure parameters for biological and biomedical research and for the determination of equipment performance.
3. Research with bio-effects should be encouraged on suitable chosen test systems to quantify better potential risks to human associated with exposure to ultrasound.
4. Encouragement should be given to the training of operators og medical ultrasound equipment.
5. Evaluation and improvment of the diagnostic capability of ultrasound should be encouraged.
6. Guidlines for the safe use of ultrasound in medicine in relation to current data on its bio-effects should be developed.
7. Epidemiological studies should be encouraged in populations exposed to diagnostic and therapeutic ultrasound.
8. Test phantom should be developed for use in both equipment performance evaluations and operator training.
9. When stating ultrasound exposure parameters, experimenters are recommended to indicate whether they are reporting spatial peak or spatial average values of intensity (a destination which may be specially important in the case af those experiments involving focused transducers).
1o. The investigation should be encouraged of possible hazards to the operators of all forms of ultrasound equipment and where necessary appropriate protection procedures should be developed.
11. Finally hope was expressed for a workshop in Bologna in 1978.

As experimental research progress and more sensitive endpoints are investigated in the laboratory, and increasing number of biological effects are reported at diagnostic intensities. These effects include delayed neuromuscular developement in rats, congenital anomalies in mice evoked electro-encephalografic responses in primates and immunuglobulin depression in mice. (1,3,5,6,).
Additional considerations that heighten concern about intrauterine exposure to ultrasonic energy are the increasing use of ultrasound during pregnancy and the recognized susceptibility of the fetus to environmental influences.

The initial step of a strategy to assess possible effects of ultrasound is to examine avaiable information either from litterature or unpublished data from existing studies. This informations could provide suggestions or clues to possible effects within the immediate future. Such an opportunity was given recently by the National Institut of Child Health and Human Development's amniocentesis registry (4) The population consisted of 3o3 amniocentesis patients exposed to ultrasound, 679 amniocentesis patients not exposed to ultrasound and for additional comparision 97o women receiving neither amniocentesis nor ultrasound. In the study no association was demonstrated between second trimester ultrasound exposure and abnormalities in the neonatalperiod or at 1 years of age.

However, as with other of these studies sample size and design of the study limit the interpretation of this data and only the possibility of rather common effects can be excluded. Of course, no inference can be made about possible effects associated with ultrasound exposure during the first or third trimesters or about possible effects becomming apparently after 1 year of age. Answers to questions of infrequent or delayed effects must await investigation using longer follow up periods and larger study populations. To definitively assess the benefits and possible effects of ultrasound exposure, experimentel human study (controlled clinical trial) is clearly the most powerful method. For the past several years British Medical Research Council has been planning a clinical trial of obstetric ultrasound. This study proposed to randomly 2o.ooo pregnant women to receive ultrasound examination for the determination of fetal maturity or alternative to complete the pregnancy without ultrasound examination. Comparison of the groups for the subsequent management of pregnancy would indicate benefite from the examination. Comparison for the frequency of abnormalities of the fetus or child could establish whether there are important hazards attributed to ultrasonic examination.Unfortunately, because of financial stringency this entire project has been abandoned.

Under prof. Horace E.Thompson and with a contract with Bureau of Radiological Health there is a epidemiological study planned in USA. The goal of this study is to determine whether children at 8-1o years of age who were exposed to ultrasound in utero are different with respect to general health, growth, physical development,intellectual development and neurological function when compared to an unexposed but otherwise similar group of children. Indeed, clinical trials are expensive and time consuming. A randomised clinical trial of adequate size requires at least 5 years before results would be available.

Is it justificated to use such extensive commitment of resources.? The routine use of ultrasound has been recommanded to monitor normal pregnancies to locate the placenta when performing amniocentesis and to continuously monitor the fetus during delivery. The routine exposure of most pregnancies could, if hazardous effects exist, create great harm. This necessitates that safety be assured with a high degree of security. Since improved outcome of pregnancy from routine ultrasonic monitoring of uncomplicated pregnancies or deliveries has not to my knowledge been demonstrated, nor has the possibility of adverse effects been adequately investigated, clinical trials in my opinion is not only ethically justified but a necessity. Futher more it is an urgent matter because in very few years it will be impossible to find a control group because of the increasing use of ultrasonic diagnostics.

REFERENCES
1. Anderson,D.W. and Barret,J.T.(1977)Presented at the meeting of the American Association of immunologist, Chicago.
2. Hill,D.R. (1968): Br.J.Radiol. 41:561-569.
3. Hu,J.H. and Ulrich,W.D.(1976):Aviat space environment 46:64o.
4. The NICHD National Registry for amniocentesis for prenatal diagnosis (1976) JAMA 236:1467.
5. Shohi,R.E. Shuriza, T. and Matsuta,S.: Teratology 6:119.
6. Sikow,M.R., Hildebrand,B.P.and Stearns,J.D.:Postnatal sequelae of ultrasound exposure at fifteen days of gestation in the rat. (1976)3rd World Congress of Ultrasonics in medicine.

GENETIC AND CYTOGENETIC EVIDENCE AND ITS RELEVANCE

Hans-Dieter Rott

Institute for Human Genetics and Anthropology, University
of Erlangen-Nürnberg, 8520 Erlangen, F.R.G.

Discussing mutagenic effects, there are generally to distinguish two fundamentally different types of mutations
with different methods necessary to prove them.
Gene mutations (point mutations) are changes in the base
sequence of DNA and cannot be seen by microscope. They
can only be proved by a missing or a pathological gene
product of a biochemical or morphological kind, for instance.
Chromosomal aberrations in contrast are changes of the
genetic constitution, which can be revealed by microscopic techniques. One has to distinguish between numerical
aberrations, which are caused primarily by lesions of the
spindle, and structural aberrations due to a preceding DNA
lesion. Most of the mutagenic agents known to us produce
both gene and chromosomal mutations.

Gene mutations

Investigations into a possible gene mutation producing
effect of US have been made with different experimental
sets and different test objects. Especially in bacterio-
logical investigations US intensities have been used with
the primary aim of killing the bacteria and getting sterility. In spite of these high intensities mutations have
not been found to be increased under the surviving individuals. In contrast , test with insects gave contradictory results: KATO (6) found gene mutations increased after US application to Drosophila, but he did not communicate the US intensity used and possibly the effects were
merely thermic. GRUBBS and CONNER (4), too, found a higher
mutation rate in the wasp MORMONIELLA after exposure to US
at intensities up to 1 W cm^{-2} at 20 kHz. Although temperature rose in some experiments by 20° C, the authors believe the mutations not to be caused by the heating effect.
In contrast to that, THACKER and BAKER (9) carefully investigated successive generations of flies having survived
irradiations. They found no increase in the frequency of
mutations and chromosomal non-disjunction, even under exposure conditions (2 W cm^{-2} at 1 MHz) sufficient to kill
a substantial proportion of the animals. Investigations
with mammals as mice, rats, and rabbits all gave negative
results.

Chromosomal aberrations

Investigations into a possible chromosome damaging effect

of US are numerous. It may have been the stimulating effect of the positive results of MACINTOSH and DAVEY, which motivated different groups to these experiments. The authors named above found increasing rates of chromatidal and chromosomal breaks after insonication of lymphocyte cultures with US intensities of 8 and 80 mW cm^{-2} at 2 MHz, but they were unable to reproduce their findings three years later together with COAKLEY. Altogether, there are now 23 papers in the literature referring to chromosomal investigations after US application to mammalian cells in vitro or in vivo with higher than diagnostic intensities. Only two authors found an increase of chromosomal aberration rates: BUGNON et al. (1) saw gaps and breaks increased after US application of 10 mW cm^{-2} at 2,25 MHz. FISHMAN et al. (3) registered the same effect after application of US above 20 W cm^{-2}. Here the effect was probably thermic. All other authers were unable to show any chromosome damaging effect although in some experiments much higher than diagnostic or therapeutic intensities have been used. In vivo studies in man gave all negative results. Due to these findings there are no hints for a mutagenic effect of US independent of heating or cavitation.

Comutagenic effect

An enhancement of ionizing radiation effects by US has been repeatedly reported. These synergistic effects have been quite variable and have included cell death, reduction of ionizing radiation dose to achieve tumour remission, decrease in plant growth ect. (Review by BURR et al. (2). But there are only three recent investigations on chromosome aberration rates in mammalian cells after US and ionizing radiation combined. KUNZE-MÜHL (7) treated human lymphocytes with X-rays and US (3 W cm^{-2} at 810 kHz) BURR et al. (2) used CO-60 and US (2 W cm^{-2} at 1 MHz) for treatment of human lymphocytes, and HARKANYI et al. (5) irradiated mice with X-rays and US (0,1 to 1 W cm^{-2} at 0,8 MHz). These authors found unanimously an increase of chromosomal aberration rates after simultaneous US application. In addition, KUNZE-MÜHL and BURR et al. proved that US alone and US treatment before ionizing radiation had no harmful effect, while sonication up to two hours after sonication increased chromosomal aberration rates. BURR et al. discuss three possible mechanisms of these effects:
1. US causes the chromosomes to move about, thereby increasing the probability of misrepair.
2. US which is not capable to fracture double strand DNA may be able to fracture single strand DNA. Since ionizing radiation causes many more single strand DNA fractures, there would be many single strands available for US action.
3. US may cause some as yet undetermined change in the kinetics and/or chemical nature of the repair mechanisms.

From chromosomal aberration patterns no decision can be made whether one or more of these possibilities prove to be right.
In this context a new and exciting method is the visualisation of Sister Chromatid Exchanges (SCE's). By incorporation of Bromedesoxyuridine (BUdR) instead of thymidine into DNA the two chromatides of metaphase chromosomes can differently be stained and thus sister chromatid exchange can be seen. These exchanges are believed to be comparable to meiotic crossing overs and are interpreted as the effect of at least one type of repair. The normal SCE rate in man is about 8 to 12 exchanges per metaphase. The usual chemical and physical mutagens are able to increase the rates yet with the chemical mutagens for unknown reasons being much more effective than ionizing radiation. For US, there are only two investigations performed, both by LIEBESKIND et al. (8). This group found SCE's increased after US application at intensity of 4 mW cm^{-2} for 30 min. on human lymphocyte cultures.. In contrast to this, their experiments with HeLa cells gave negative results. Studies with the combination of US and ionizing radiation and following evaluation of SCE rates were not yet performed.
Whether US has an effect on SCE's will be cleared up in future. How SCE's are to be interpreted biologically and whether increased rates can prove a weak mutagenic or comutagenic effect is being discussed and cannot be judged definitely at the moment.
Summarizing a comutagenic effect of US is neither stated with sufficient probability nor is it refuted. Whether such a probable effect is due to a thermal property or has a mechanical component, is not known. Further research in this direction will probably give new aspects of intracellular effects of US to DNA and repairing enzymes.
At last, investigations into a possible comutagenic effect of US using chemical mutagens are lacking totally.

REFERENCES

1. Bugnon, C., Cottin, Y., Kraehenbuhl, J., Weill,F(1972): J. Radiol. Electrol. Med. Nucl. 53,750
2. Burr, J.G., Wald, N., Pan, S.,Preston, K.(1978):p 120 In: Mutagen induced damage in man. Editors: Evans, J. Lloyd, D.C., Edinburgh Univ. Press, Edinburgh 1918
3. Fishman,H.K., Coleman, D.J., Lizzi, F.L. (1972): J. Cell Biol. 55, 74a
4. Grubbs, S.C., Conner, G.W.(1976) J. Heredity 67,191
5. Harkanyi, Z., Szollar, J., Vigvari, Z. (1978): Brit. J. Radiol. 51, 46
6. Kato, M. (1966): Bull. Osaka Med. School 12,102
7. Kunze-Mühl,E.(1975)p 3 in:Proceedings,II. Europ.Congr. on Ultrasonics in Medicine. Excerpt. Med. 1975
8. Liebeskind et al.(1979): Radiology 131,177
9. Thacker, J., Baker,N.N.(1976): Brit.J.Radiol.46,367

CELLULAR EFFECTS AND THEIR RELEVANCE

Alun R. Williams

Department of Medical Biophysics, University of Manchester, Manchester, England, U.K.

A large proportion of the literature concerned with the interactions between ultrasound and living material is devoted to its interaction with cells in suspension. The rationale behind this approach is that any modality which alters the behaviour or function of living cells in vitro may exert a similar effect in vivo with potentially serious consequences for the complete organism. The use of a uniform population of cells in suspension is particularly attractive to experimentalists because one can look in exquisite detail at subtle aspects of cellular function and thereby detect small changes which would be undetectable in vivo.

There are many other practical advantages to be gained by irradiating cells in suspension. For example, the investigator is free to devise the most near ideal exposure conditions unfettered by the restrictions which plague most in vivo situations. In practice this means that one usually chooses to expose a small volume of cell suspension contained in a vessel whose walls are permeable to ultrasound. This vessel is usually placed at a specific point within a well-characterised beam of ultrasound which traverses a tank of water before being absorbed or reflected. Thus, the ultrasonic exposure conditions are almost completely under the control of the investigator.

Unfortunately, far less care and attention has usually been paid to the choice of the biological material to be irradiated. This has apparently been gleaned from some adjacent colleague who happens to use a suitable cell suspension for other research work. This serendipitous approach has been eminently successful in demonstrating the biological hazard resulting from exposure to ionizing radiation. However, the mechanisms of the interactions of ionizing radiation with living tissue to produce "sub-lethal" damage are essentially the same whether those cells are free in suspension or constrained within a block of tissue. This is not necessarily true for ultrasound.

There is general agreement that exposure of aerated cell suspensions to intensities of c.w. ultrasound in excess of about one Watt/cm^2 (s.a.t.a.) usually results in the production of some form of vapour/gas bubble activity commonly referred to as acoustic cavitation. Hydrodynamic shear stresses and shock waves associated with this phenomenon may disrupt cells, or at least subject them to mechanical trauma which may result in some form of "sublethal" damage.

At any given frequency, the "threshold" intensity needed to initiate some form of cavitation-like activity depends upon a number of other variables. Foremost amongst these are the presence of stable minute pockets of gas called micronuclei. These are apparently produced whenever a medium containing dissolved proteins is aerated or transferred from vessel to vessel, or when a liquid medium bathes a dry solid material which may have minute cavities or irregularities on its surface. Proteins tend to be orientated and denatured at a gas/liquid interface and form a "skin" which helps to stabilise each micronucleus. Thus, the procedures employed while preparing the biological samples for irradiation and their introduction into a suitable exposure chamber tend to increase the number of available micronuclei.

Consequently, the role of acoustically-induced cavitation as the physical agent responsible for any observed biological effect will almost certainly be enhanced whenever cells are irradiated in suspension in vitro. The degree of enhancement will be a function of the number of micronuclei or gas bodies which have been introduced. For example, ultrasonic intensities in excess of 1 Watt/cm^2 at 0.75 MHz were required to disrupt human erythrocytes in vitro when the blood had been carefully withdrawn into a syringe containing degassed anticoagulant and stringent precautions were taken to avoid turbulence or exposure to air or dry surfaces. A portion of this same blood sample was aerated by inverting the syringe and it was found that the "threshold" for lysis was reduced to about 0.8 Watts/cm^2 under the same exposure conditions. This "threshold" was reduced still further by deliberately introducing microscopic gas bodies which were stabilised against diffusion within the 4 μm diameter pores of hydrophobic nucleopore membranes. Under these extreme conditions erythrocytes were disrupted at s.a. intensities of the order of 30 mW/cm^2 at frequencies of 1 and 1.6 MHz.

Thus, irradiation of cell suspensions in vitro provides an excellent model system for investigating the effects of acoustically-induced cavitation on living tissues. However, it is difficult to extrapolate the results of these studies directly to the in vivo situation because the conditions necessary for the initiation and growth of cavitation sites will almost certainly be different.

104

SAFETY OF DIAGNOSTIC ULTRASOUND -
EVIDENCE FROM THERAPY STUDIES

Gail ter Haar

Physics Division, Institute of Cancer Research, Sutton,
Surrey, U.K.

Ultrasound is used extensively as a therapeutic
agent in physical medicine. The aim in this case is to
produce beneficial biological effects. In considering
the safety of diagnostic ultrasound, it may, therefore,
be informative to look at the changes brought about by
therapeutic ultrasonic intensities (0.25-3.0 Wcm^{-2};
0.75-5MHz) and to determine intensity thresholds for their
occurrence.
    This paper will consider some aspects of the inter-
action of therapeutic ultrasound with biological tissue
and its constituents. Effects on blood flow and blood
vessel ultrastructure will be considered in detail.

EFFECT OF THERAPEUTIC ULTRASOUND ON CELLULAR COMPONENTS

A considerable amount of work has been done to
investigate the effect of ultrasound on intracellular
components. Evidence exists for membrane changes. These
include alteration of permeability to potassium ions
(1), surface charge effects (2), and ultrastructural
changes (3). Electron microscope studies of organelles
have revealed mitochondrial changes (3,4) and lysosomal
disruption (5,6). The nucleus seems in most cases to be
undamaged (3) although disruption of the nuclear membrane
has been seen (7).

EFFECT OF THERAPEUTIC ULTRASOUND ON INTERCELLULAR
MATERIALS

Almost all ultrasonic treatment involves irradiation
of collagen. Harvey et al. (8) have shown an increase in
collagen synthesis _in vitro_ resulting from ultrasonic
irradiation. This has also been demonstrated _in vivo_.

EFFECT OF THERAPEUTIC ULTRASOUND ON TISSUES AND ORGANS

Much work has gone into the study of the effects of
ultrasonic therapy on organ function and structure. The
work to be described here will deal only with effects on
the circulation.

Effect of therapeutic ultrasound on blood flow:
Dyson et al. (9) have shown that irradiation of blood
vessels in a standing wave field may lead to modification
of blood flow. At intensities above 0.5 Wcm^{-2} at 3MHz,
the red cells in embryonic chick blood vessels clumped
together to form bands at half wavelength intervals.
This is shown in Fig. 1. The effect is usually revers-
ible.

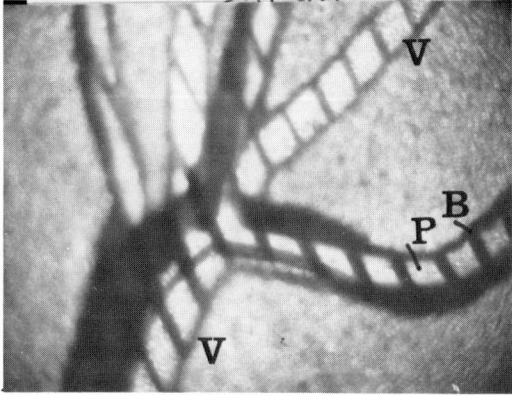

Fig. 1.   Red blood cell banding in vessels of the area
vasculosa of a 3½ day chick embryo. B: red cell band;
P: blood plasma; V: blood vessel. (10).

The same effect has also been seen in the blood
vessels of the mouse uterus at intensities above 1.2 Wcm^{-2}
(3MHz)(10). Electron micrographs of mouse uteri in
which stasis has been induced show red cell packing,
extravasated erythrocytes, and damage to the luminal
aspect of the plasma membrane (3).

MECHANISMS FOR THERAPEUTIC ACTION OF ULTRASOUND

The way in which therapeutic ultrasound interacts
with tissue to produce changes is not fully understood.
Energy is deposited within the tissue and this leads to
heating.   Non-thermal, mechanical effects such as acoustic
streaming, also take place, and these may be instrumental
in producing some of the changes seen at cell membranes.
The existence of cavitation effects in solid tissue has
still not been proven.

106

CONCLUSIONS

Therapeutic ultrasound can undoubtedly give rise to changes in biological tissue. The Bio-effects Committee of the AIUM have reviewed the existing bio-effects literature and have come to the conclusion that there have been "no demonstrated significant biological effects in mammalian tissues exposed to intensities below 100 mW cm^{-2}", and that for total irradiation times between 1 and 500 seconds no such effects have been shown at higher intensities where the product of intensity and exposure time is less than 50 J cm^{-2} (11). The intensity quoted is the spatial peak, temporal average intensity.

For effective therapeutic ultrasound usage, treatments lie in the region I.t $>$ 50 J cm^{-2}. Although this is the case, no reports of adverse "side" effects have appeared, despite extensive use of the technique.

REFERENCES

1. Chapman, I. V. (1974): Brit. J. Radiol., 47, 411.
2. Joshi, G. P., Hill, C. R., Forrester, J. A. (1973): Ultrasound in Med. and Biol., 1, 45.
3. ter Haar, G. R., Dyson, M., Smith, S.: Ultrasound in Med. and Biol. in press.
4. Hrazdira, I. (1970): In: Ultrasonographia Medica, p.457-463. Editors: J. Bock et al. Academy of Medicine, Vienna.
5. Taylor, K. J. W., Pond, J. B. (1972): In: Interaction of Ultrasound and biological tissues, p.87-92. Editors: J. M. Reid and M. R. Sikov. DHEW Publication (FDA) 73-8008.
6. Dvorak, M., Hrazdira, I. (1966): Zeitschrift Mikrosk. anat. Forsch., 4, 451.
7. Watmough, D. J., Dendy, P. P., Eastwood, L. H., Gregory, D. W., Gordon, F. C. H., Wheatley, D. N. (1977): Ultrasound in Med. and Biol., 3, 205.
8. Harvey, W., Dyson, M., Pond, J. B., Grahame, R. (1975): In: Proceedings 2nd European Congress on Ultrasonics in Medicine. p.10-21. Excerpta Medica Int. Congress Series no. 363.
9. Dyson, M., Pond, J. B., Woodward, B., Broadbent, J. (1974): Ultrasound in Med. and Biol., 1, 133.
10. ter Haar, G. R. (1977): In: The effect of ultrasonic standing wave fields on the flow of particles, with special reference to biological media. PhD Thesis, University of London.
11. AIUM Bio-effects Committee (1976): Ultrasound in Med. and Biol., 2, 351.

ULTRASTRUCTURAL CHANGES CAUSED BY ULTRASOUND

I. Hrazdira

Department of Biophysics, Faculty of Medicine, Purkyně
University Brno, Czechoslovakia

Last time in the connection with the expansion of
ultrasonic diagnostic methods in all branches of medicine, the studies of cell ultrastructure supply valuable
data for appreciation of safety criteria of ultrasonic
applications.

Living cells exposed to direct action of ultrasound
show a large scale of ultrastructural changes from slight
anomalies of single organelles up to the complete
disintegration of cell structures, often accompanied with
the vacuolation of the cytoplasm (3,4,1,11). The deepness
of observed changes is a function of ultrasonic intensity.
The different degree of damage in the same experimental
sample may be explained by the interfering character of
the ultrasonic field.

Ultrasonically induced changes appear in all cell
structures, i.e. in the cell membrane, in the nucleus
and in the cytoplasmic structures. The membrane structures react especially sensitively. (Fig.1). The first
in detail studied organelle was mitochondria (1,2).
The mean reason of this fact was the importance of
mitochondria as chemical energy transformators in the
cell metabolism. Ultrasonic action leads to changes in
the shape of mitochondria as well as in their internal
structure. The mitochondria swell and their shape become
round. Cristae mitochondriales disappear and their rests
enlarge. The general appearence of the altered mitochondria resembles the picture of multivesicular bodies.
The terminal phase of mitochondria disintegration is the
alteration of the double-layer structure of mitochondrial membrane. All basic functions of mitochondria -
Krebs´cycle, oxidative phosphorylation and electron-
transfer - are affected by ultrasonic action.

It was proved, however, that mitochondria react by
similar alteration of their structure and function also
to the action of other physical and chemical factors
(8). Thus the observed changes of mitochondria are not
typical for ultrasound. There is only an unspecific
sign of altered vital state of the sonicated cell.

The changes of another membrane structure - the
granular endoplasmic reticulum seem to be more specific

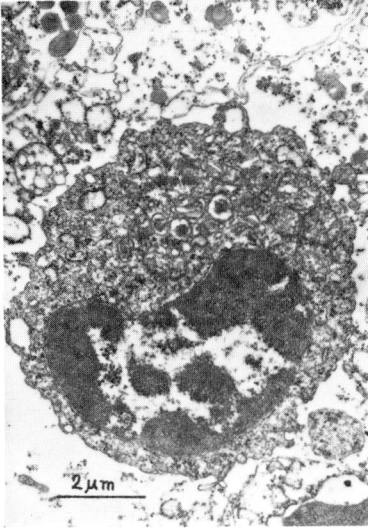

Figure 1

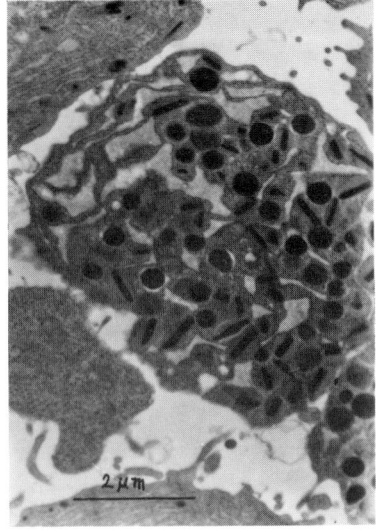

Figure 2

Fig. 1. Myelocyte grossly damaged by ultrasonic action
at therapeutic intensity. Alteration of all
cell structures.

Fig. 2. Eosinophilic myelocyte after ultrasonic treatment at low intensity. Enlargement of the rough
endoplasmic reticulum only.

for ultrasound. Under ultrasonic action their membranes
enlarge into vesicles or sacs (5,10). The spatial
distribution of ribosomes on the membranes is irregular. The changes of endoplasmic reticulum must be evaluated also from the functional point of view. By the
high content of RNA and connection to the protein
synthesis, endoplasmic reticulum seems to be one of the
most important cell organelles. The changes of endoplasmic reticulum may be considered therefore as the morphological basis of ultrasonically altered protein synthesis (stimulated or inhibited).

    The partial enlargement of endoplasmic reticulum
was also found in sensitive cells treated by diagnostic
intensities in vitro (Fig.2).

    The changes in the nucleus are always characte-
ristic even in the cases where the overall damage of
the cell is not too advanced. The chromatin granules
are strongly concentrated into extensive granular-like
areas. Among these areas, empty spaces with roughly
granulated intensely osmiophilic corpuscles appear in
the electron micrographs.

The changes of some cell structures show the signs of mechanical impairment. This is especially so of cell membrane, which as the largest continuous phase boundary is exposed to the greatest mechanical effect of ultrasonic waves. Other changes are mainly of colloidal-osmotical character. The enlargement of membrane surrounding spaces may be attributed to the increased permeability.'

The analogous changes were also proved in the ultrastructure of sonicated plant cells (6,7).

In spite of limitation of the morphological point of view, the published electron microscope studies proved all vital cell centres may be affected by direct and indirect ultrasonic action at therapeutic intensities. During the procedures of ultrasonic diagnostics there is no risk of mechanical damage of the cells. However, inexpressive but repeatedly established changes of endoplasmic reticulum must be taken into consideration as a warning sign in the evaluation of biologically effective ultrasonic intensity.

REFERENCES

1. Borovyagin, V.L., Elpiner, I.E. (1964): Biofizika, 9,312.
2. Dmitrieva, N.P. (1964): Biofizika, 9, 571.
3. Dvořák, M., Hrazdira, I. (1966): Zeitschr. mikr.-anat. Forsch., 75, 451.
4. Dyson, M., Pond, J.B., Woodward, B., Broadbent, J. (1974): Ultrasound Med. Biol., 1, 133.
5. Hrazdira, I. (1969): Ultrasonographia Medica. Proc. 1st World Congress on Ultrasonic Diagnostic in Medicine, p. 457. Editors: J.Böck, K. Ossoining. Verlag der Medizinischen Akademie Wien.
6. Hrazdira, I., Havelková, M. (1966): Naturwissenschaften, 53, 206.
7. Miller, D.L. (1977): Ultrasound Med. Biol., 3, 221.
8. Tairbekov, M.G. (1966): Biofizika, 11, 80.
9. Taylor, K.J.W., Pond, J.B. (1972): In: Interaction of Ultrasound and Biological Tissues, p. 87.Editors: J.M. Reid, M.R.Sikov. DHEW Publication 73-8008, Washington.
10. Webster, D.F., Pond, J.B., Dyson, M., Harvey, W. (1978): Ultrasound Med.Biol., 4, 343.
11. Williams, A.R., Sykes, S.M., O'Brien, W.D., Jr. (1976): Ultrasound Med. Biol., 2, 311.

5. THE VALUE OF ULTRASOUND IN PERINATAL MEDICINE FROM THE CLINICIAN'S POINT OF VIEW

J. M. Beazley, Chairman

ULTRASOUND AND CLINICAL DIAGNOSIS

John M. Beazley

Department of Obstetrics and Gynaecology, University of Liverpool, England.

In any medical discipline, good patient management requires the doctor to grapple with three fundamental issues. These are:-

Firstly, an understanding of the basic problem.

Next, recognition of that problem whenever it recurs;

And thirdly, treating the patient appropriately.

From the view-point of therapy, it is clear that, as yet, ultrasound has no application in perinatal medicine. In this speciality the value of ultrasound lies entirely in its capacity to enlarge our understanding and improve our diagnoses. Nor is it overstating the fact to say that in these two activities, ultrasound has changed the thinking of our age. The magnitude of this step alone is incalculable. But, what we can say is that ultrasound, more than any other modern technique, has made manifest that the fetus is an individual virtually from conception.

CLINICAL DIAGNOSIS

With regard to the place of ultrasound in reaching a clinical diagnosis, I should like to offer one word of caution.

Slide 1. (An Elephant)

I know that this is an elephant - not because I understand about elephants, (coming from Liverpool), but, because having seen one before, when I observe another I can recognise it for what it is. (I feel much the same about many congenital malformations).

Slide 2. (A Rolls Royce motor car)

I know this to be a motor car. But not just any motor car. It is a Rolls Royce. The bonnet is pathognomonic of a Rolls Royce. Yet having identified and labelled this fine machine, I freely admit that I understand little of how it functions. (I feel much the same about hypertension, oedema and proteinuria as signs of pre-eclampsia, or a small-for-dates baby as a sign of placental insufficiency).

In perinatal medicine, to observe and recognise, to identify and label, is not to understand. Nor is it to make a clinical diagnosis. A clinical diagnosis requires attention to at least six factors.

113

Slide 3.
Dis-ease/Dis-order

1. The Principle Site?
2. The Direction of the Unusual Deviation ?
3. The Extent of this Deviation?
4. "Who is Guilty"?
5. "Who is Responsible"?
6. The Clinical Implications?

Whether faced with "disease" or "disorder" the clinician is first required to determine the principle site of the problem. This is not always as obvious as it seems.

The direction of the deviation is usually "too much", or, "too little" of one of the pathogenic processes, which we classify as "congenital" or "acquired", "inflammatory", "degenerative", "neoplastic", "vascular", etc.

The extent of the pathogenic process usually has to be measured specifically, if it is to be graded correctly.

Precipitating aetiological factors, and the predisposing background, often require separate consideration. The precipitating factor in intra-uterine syphilis, for example, is usually obvious. The background factors predisposing to the problem, for example, social deprivation or promiscuity, may be less apparent.

The clinical implications of pathology always require careful and humanitarian consideration. For example, amniocentesis under ultrasound control, to detect mongolism in a sub-fertile woman of 40, is pointless if she is not interested in pregnancy termination anyway.

Translating the diagnostic concept into the practical discipline of ordering investigations, our junior staff in Liverpool are permitted to order what tests they wish so long as a) they can justify the test in terms of one of the six headings shown here and b) they are not simply confirming something that they know already from physical examination.

Under this discipline our general findings have been that precipitating aetiological factors are more readily determined by bacteriologists and geneticists than by ultrasound. Background aetiology is more relevant to sociologists and environmentalists than to ultrasound. The clinical implications of the condition, including the patient's wishes, her needs or anxieties, are determined more by compassionate clinicians than by ultrasound.

By contrast, ultrasound is often of considerable clinical value in detecting the chief site of disorder, especially if this is a gross malformation of the fetus, like anencephaly or hydrocephaly. (Soft tissue disorders are, as yet, less readily detectable, though this situation is improving steadily). The direction of the deviation, for example the appearance or disappearance of pregnancy, or, of more than one pregnancy, or, the development of a hydatidiform mole, or, the degenerative process of fetal starvation, these are all clearly demonstrable by ultrasound, as indeed is the extent to which these problems have progressed.

DIAGNOSTIC UNIT

PATIENT'S NAME ....

Diagnostic Investigations ordered; and their purpose

A) **Investigations to determine the principle site of disorder**

1.   6.
2.   7.
3.   8.
4.   9.
5.   10.

B) **Investigations to determine the direction of the deviation**

1.   6.
2.   7.
3.   8.
4.   9.
5.   10.

C) **Investigations to determine the extent of the deviation**

1.   6.
2.   7.
3.   8.
4.   9.
5.   10.

D) **Investigations to determine the precipitating cause(s) of the problem**

1.   6.
2.   7.
3.   8.
4.   9.
5.   10.

E) **Investigations to reveal factors which are probably responsible for the precipitating cause(s)**

1.   6.
2.   7.
3.   8.
4.   9.
5.   10.

F) **Investigations to assess the chief clinical effects or implications of the disorder**

1.   6.
2.   7.
3.   8.
4.   9.
5.   10.

115

CONCLUSION:-

My note of caution is simple. For the clinician, ultrasound technology, however wonderful, is never an end in itself. Thus, in our enthusiasm for observation by ultrasound, let us not forget that observation and recognition, even identification and labelling, do not by themselves comprise understanding. Nor do these four processes constitute a clinical diagnosis. Ultrasound may be the most useful tool we have in perinatal medicine. Nevertheless, as clinicians, let us keep its value in perspective, and continue to use it wisely.

ULTRASOUND IN ANTEPARTUM HAEMORRHAGE-PLACENTAL LOCALISATION

Maher Mahran

Ain Shams Ultrasound Unit, Ain Shams University, Cairo, Egypt

The introduction of ultrasound in clinical obstetrics made placental localisation available to the treating doctor. It is no more a matter of guess. Ultrasound revolutionzed our knowledge about the placenta, its development, migration and clinical disorders.

MATERIAL

During the period of twelve months starting the first of September 1978, 828 pregnant women 20 weeks or more were examined in our Ultrasound Unit. This material was used to assess the incidence of placenta praevia and its relation to antepartum haemorrhage. At the same time the sonographic information was used in the clinical management of these patients.

METHODS

Every patient had a complete ultrasound examination. The placental site was identified carefully to see whether it was:
1. anterior or posterior;
2. in the upper or the lower uterine segment;
3. its relation to the internal os if it encroached on the lower uterine segment--
    Grade 1: near the internal os.
    Grade 2: reaching but not covering the internal os.
    Grade 3: covering the internal os completely.
The fetal factors which might affect the management were also assessed, such as fetal maturity, presentation, twin pregnancy or fetal abnormality.

RESULTS

Out of the 828 patients, 60 presented clinically as cases of antepartum haemorrhage (7.2%). One case proved to be not pregnant and another was a case of degenerated bleeding fibroid. Out of the remaining 58 patients, 19(33%) had a normally situated placenta (accidental haemorrhage). The remaining 39 cases (67%) had placenta praevia. Cases of placenta praevia were 69% grade 1, 9% grade 2 and 8% grade 3.
Out of the 828 cases, there were 51 cases asymptomatic,

discovered accidentally during scanning (6%). There were
45% in grade 1, 23% in grade 2 and 32% in grade 3.

DISCUSSION

Ultrasound is a great help to the obstetrician in making decisions in the management of high risk pregnancies. Its availability improves perinatal mortality and morbidity. The practice of obstetrics in the management of antepartum haemorrhage varies from one place to another depending on such availability. With the help of ultrasound, it is possible for the first time to indicate the incidence of placenta praevia in any group of patients. In this study, there were 109 cases of placenta praevia out of 828 pregnant women (13%). The symytomatic cases were 58 (55%), while the asymptomatic cases were 51 (45%).

Faced with a case of antepartum haemorrhage, it is very important for the obstetrician to exclude placenta praevia. Placental localisation by ultrasound is a single technique and can answer very important clinical questions. A full bladder avoiding overdistension is important so that the lower segment can be easily visualized. The placenta is identified by the chorionic plate on the fetal side and by the characteristic internal echoes (speckling). However, if the whole uterus is not scanned, placenta praevia can be missed. Due to the longer distance between the transducer and a posterior placenta and interference of the in between structures, such as the head or trunk, its diagnosis might be difficult for a beginner. The separation of the fetal head by a distance from the bladder or the posterior uterine wall is suggestive of placental presence. The presence of some liquor amnii is a great help for identifying the chorionic plate. Pushing the head manually upwards or putting the patient in Trendelenburg's position allows more liquor to occupy the lower uterine segment and hence better visualization of placenta praevia and its chorionic plate (Kobayashi, 1974).

The degree of placental separation can be delineated by the echo free area between the placenta and the uterine wall. This can be clearly and usefully demonstrated in cases of concealed and mixed accidental haemorrhage with retroplacental haematoma. From the prognostic point of view it is also important for the clinician to know whether a placenta praevia is anteriorly or posteriorly located. Fetal information regarding the presentation, twin pregnancy and fetal abnormality can be immediately provided by ultrasound. The availability of the biparietal diameter measurement will enable the estimation of the gestational age. This information is essential as termination of pregnancy is always a possibility and particularly in a community where the date of the last menstrual period is usually forgotten and where the pill is a common method for contraception. The value of placental localization in relation to amniocentesis for LS ratio estimation in these patients cannot be ignored.

118

There is no doubt that an obstetrician who is supplied with this information will be in a better position to manage his patient. How far can he carry conservative treatment and its chance of success can be evaluated by ultrasound data. This is particularly important when the obstetrician thinks that the uterine milieu is better than the outside world. This is the situation in many countries where neonatal intensive care units are not always available.

The use of ultrasound has completely changed the way we manage cases of antepartum haemorrhage:

1. Radiological methods of investigation are no longer practiced. Ultrasound is safer, quicker and more accurate in placental localisation. Radiological methods carry a definite risk of irradiation to the fetus and is time consuming.

2. A quick and sure differentiation between placenta praevia and accidental haemorrhage is available. There is no longer need to examine patients under general anaesthesia. If the placenta is normally located inside the uterus it can be safely examined vaginally and induced by amniotomy without the use of general anaesthesia.

3. A quick decision about whether to keep the patient in the hospital or to allow her to go home, and whether to be in bed or ambulatory, is easy to make following the diagnosis of placenta praevia and its degree by ultrasound.

4. A decision can be taken about the place of delivery according to whether intensive care service is expected to be needed or not.

Asymptomatic cases discovered accidentally during the second trimester should be followed up every 4 weeks without any clinical restriction. Patients should be reassured that 90% will have no complications. Cases during the third trimester must have their activities restricted. They must be followed up. The decision to hospitalize or to restrict the patient to bed should be based on clinical data and ultrasound findings.

One word of warning is necessary regarding the translation of sonographic findings to clinical diagnosis and decision making. We should be aware of the phenomenon of placental migration. It is quite common to find a placenta covering the internal os completely during the second trimester which will be far away from the internal os in the third trimester (King, 1973; Young, 1978). Under no circumstances should the diagnosis of placenta praevia made more than two weeks prior to the time of delivery be used as an indication for elective Caesarean section (Winsberg,1974).

REFERENCES

1. King, D.L.(1973): Radiology, 109, 167.
2. Kobayashi and Mitsunao(1974): In: Illustrated Manual of Ultrasonography in Obstetrics and Gynecology. p.228.
3. Winsberg, F.(1974): In: Ultrasonography in Obstetrics and Gynecology.p.215. Ed. R.C.Sanders & A.E. James, Appleton-Century-Grafts, N.Y.
4. Young, G.B.(1978): Radiology, 128, 183.

FETAL GROWING - ABSTRACT

Bruno Salvadori

Istituto di Clinica Ostetrica e Ginecologica, University of Parma, Parma, Italy

The principle of fetal growing, followed during pregnancy by clinical or ultrasound procedures, is contrasted with that of growth estimated by weight at birth. Fetal growth is abstract and we need a concrete expression for it; usually weight at birth is adopted but for many years the habit of considering the birth weight as the "growth index" has been criticized by broad minded obstetricians and pediatricians. In our experience the frequency of chest circumference reduction in 1400 randomized newborns appear usually to be higher than that of weight. This was more evident in those born to gestotic mothers; 14.6% of such babies despite their appropriate weight presented a reduced chest circumference.

Clinical and biophysical procedures have made it possible to evaluate the fetal growth pattern. This is the real fetal growing assessment which gives us the possibility to detect the growth defect at the moment it occurs.

Some time ago we suggested the use of three Fetal Poor Growing (FPG) patterns: i.e., Primary, Secondary and Transitory, whatever the parameter chosen, and then we gave a practical confirmation using clinical (Symphysis-Fundus Length) and ultrasonic (BPD) criteria.

Now we are able to calculate the frequency and outcome of the three types of FPG. Using SFL measurements (Table 1) the Primary FPG is the most frequent, followed by the Transitory and the Secondary. Perinatal mortality is very high in the Primary form, whereas it is 0% in the Secondary one. Birth weight defects appear equally distributed. The Transitory FPG shows a frequent (35%) reduction of chest circumference and a perinatal mortality of 15%.

If we use BPD assessment (Table 2) the figures are very different: the most frequent appears to be the Primary and Transitory. Perinatal mortality is severe in Primary but is the highest in the Secondary FPG.

The variety of figures obtained from different criteria contributes to the opinion that fetal growth is more a series of increments than a homogeneous process.

Furthermore, fetal growing assessment enables us to foresee the outcome of pregnancy; in fact, the recognition of FPG in a clinically normal pregnancy is often followed, sooner or later, by severe clinical features, and mostly placenta separation.

Fetal growing assessment has made it possible to question the rigid but shaky concept of SGAI. The reality of
fetal development cannot be regarded as a unique process,
but rather as a series of increments, as a set of several
growth patterns--almost as a combination of many growths,
each running a different course during fetal life. Weight
can indicate one of these growth patterns but it is a mistake to consider weight as a sum of the patterns. On the
other hand, it is practically impossible to assess weight
exactly and directly in utero.

Birth weight was indicated as the first pillar supporting the concept of SGAI; the second pillar--gestational
age calculated from the last menstrual period--has proved
to be as uncertain as the first, and perhaps even more so.

We will be able to rubricate different types of FPG
(such as Primary, Secondary and Transitory) for each of the
different parameters considered during fetal life. Part of
the categories will also record low birth weight values,
but not necessarily.

Nevertheless, our conclusions will remain uncertain until pediatricians verify the early and late outcome of the
various types. Only then will we be able to realize the
full clinical meaning of a single deviation from the theoretically normal fetal growth and to decide on a practical
obstetrical strategy.

TABLE 1. Frequency, perinatal mortality and weight at birth
in Primary, Secondary and Transitory FPG assessed by SFL
measurement.

DIFFERENT TYPES OF FPG	FREQUENCY %	PERINATAL MORTALITY	WEIGHT AT BIRTH SGA%	AGA%
Primary	38.75	19.35	74.29	25.80
Secondary	27.50	0.00	77.28	22.72
Transitory	33.75	14.81	0.00	100.00

TABLE 2. Frequency, perinatal mortality and weight at birth
in Primary, Secondary and Transitory FPG assessed by BPD
measurment

DIFFERENT TYPES OF FPG	FREQUENCY %	PERINATAL MORTALITY	WEIGHT AT BIRTH SGA%	AGA%
Primary	43.58	17.64	70.58	29.41
Secondary	15.38	50.00	50.00	50.00
Transitory	41.02	0.00	31.25	68.75

THE APPLICATION OF ULTRASOUND IN PREVENTION OF PERINATAL MORTALITY IN ČSSR.

Z. Štembera

Research Institute for the Care of Mother and Child, Prague-Podolí, Czechoslovakia.

The obstetric ultrasound diagnostic has been used for many years in numerous institutions in ČSSR. The favourable results help us to further decrease perinatal mortality. At present it is on the first place prematurity with 6.1%o, on the second intrauterine hypoxia and placental insufficiency with 5.1%o and on the third malformations with 2.1%o that contribute most to the country-wide total perinatal mortality. Consequently the ultrasound diagnostics is focussed predominantly to those areas.

In an attempt to decrease the prematurity rate, ultrasound is used above all for an early detection of several risk factors leading to prematurity as e.g. placenta praevia, multiple pregnancy and uterine myoma. This makes it possible to take pertinent early measures (preventive hospitalization, administration of beta-mimetics etc.). It is also used for localization of the placenta before amniocenthesis performed in cases where the L/S ratio is to be measured.

The second area involves all cases of fetal jeopardy by hypoxia. Here ultrasound helps us first to diagnose SFD by repeated examinations of the biparietal/chest diameter and by comparison of the obtained data with the pertinent growth courves and second to register breathing movements either spontaneous or after stimulation, which is one of the methods for early detection of fetal hypoxia. In this area ultrasound is also used for localization of the placenta before amniocenthesis performed in cases of a suspect fetal isoimmunisation for measurement of bilirubinoids in the amniotic fluid.

In the third area dealing with an early detection of fetal malformation again the localization of placenta is performed before amniocenthesis for analysis of chromosomes, enzymes and different metabolites in the amniotic fluid. A positvie result has for consequence legal abortion because of genetic reasons. A direct ultrasound diagnosis of a severe fetal malformation before the 22nd week of pregnancy is an objective basis for legal abortion. If the diagnosis is made in the third trimester, then it prevents a needless caesarean section in cases where the malformed fetus exhibits at the end of pregnancy or in the course of labour signs of distress.

The results obtained during ultrasound examination can be divided into three groups:

In the first of them they can be considered a final diagnosis as e.g. in cases of severe fetal malformations, uterine myoma etc. In the second group the results complement the diagnosis in combination with other methods, biochemical, cytological or cardiotocographic as e.g. in cases of fetal hypoxia, small-for-dates fetuses etc. In the third group the results represent only an auxiliary basis for another diagnostic procedure. This is e.g. localization of the placenta preceding amniocenthesis.

Since the ultrasound technique equipped besides the basic B scan also by the grey scale and by real time is rather expensive and must be imported, it is necessary to organize an optimal distribution of these apparatuses from the economic point of view. Therefore they allocated in ČSSR primarily to the eight regional centers ensuring both the outpatient and institutional care for the most serious cases of high risk pregnancies (diabetes mellitus, cardiopathies, Rh-isoimmunisations, severe EPH gestoses, genetic complications etc.) from an area of some 1-1.5 mil. of inhabitants. In the second phase the equipment of selected 32 district centers taking care of some 250.000 inhabitants and concentrating the other high risk pregnancies was started. We plan to equip in the third stage another 100 centers covering each an area with some 100.000 inhabitants that would ensure a screening of high risk pregnancies, especially of those cases that have the greatest share in perinatal mortality. Together with the instrumental equipment also qualified training of the workers from the quoted centers is being centrally organized by the Institute for Postgraduate Training. Those theoretical and practical courses of instruction are ensured by selected experts having several years practice in our Institute and in some clinical workplaces. The ultrasound technique is one of the methods that helped to decrease the perinatal mortality rate in our Institute in the last years to 11‰.

THE VALUE OF ULTRASOUND IN PERINATAL MEDICINE FROM THE CLINICIAN'S POINT OF VIEW

D.M. Serr, Y. Itzchak, J. Shalev and S. Mashiach

Division of Obstetrics and Gynecology and the Section of Diagnostic Ultrasound, The Sheba Medical Center, Tel-Aviv University Medical School, Israel

Todays' science of ultrasonography can be approached in various ways and we have at this meeting studies of the most advanced nature and observations from those with the broadest experience. In this contribution I would like to try to put into words what the general obstetrician in practice feels as he compares life as an obstetrician before and after the advent of the use of ultrasound in our profession. The generation before us see this perhaps as a change in attitude to all the old principles and problems. The generation growing up in training today can barely visualize the thought of obstetrics without the use of ultrasound - and this can be verified by asking the average medical student to answer a typical examination question and qualifying the question by saying - "you do not have ultrasonic diagnostic aids available to you".

It is quite obvious that a major revolution has quietly - and I may say bloodlessly - taken over our profession. The contributors are many and through this presentation I will be referring in general to those who have given us so much in basic scientific and clinical observations such as Ian Donald, Asim Kurjak, Stuart Campbell, Kratochwill, Kossoff and their co-workers as well as many others who have devoted time and energy to the progress of perinatology.

I would like to step down for the present observations from the status of departmental and professional rank to the position as I sit at my obstetrician's desk and compare my observations, diagnoses, prognoses, way of thought in the pre-ultrasonic era to the present day.

I think most of us will agree that bleeding in early pregnancy is one of the most frequent conditions which we are faced in our daily practice. 12-15% of pregnancies terminate in spontaneous abortion. 20% of pregnancy women bleed in the first trimester. Our approach years ago varied from doing nothing but wait for the inevitable - either abortion or continued pregnancy having little idea of what was going on. During the pregnancy itself some would believe in bed-rest others not, but this is not really the core of the issue. The advent of ultrasound has given us the position of being able to have far more idea of diagnosis and prognosis of the condition of threatened abortion than before, and we have been upgraded from more or less unknowledgeable bystanders to professionals with sound physical diagnosis. When compared to our armementarium of 15 years ago, we could examine physically and that was and is important. We could have a quantitive hormonal pregnancy test performed, which in those days took some time to receive an answer. Not always did the result when it arrived from the laboratory reflect the state of the pregnancy at the present moment.

The following pictures demonstrate well known conditions which todays' obstetrician and gynecologist faced with bleeding in early pregnancy can firmly confirm or ruleout, or be prepared to follow-up some diagnostic suspicion which would have either escaped him or been impossible in the pre-ultrasonic era.

Blighted ovum
Twins - Multiple pregnancy
Hydatidiform Mole
Threatened Abortion
Missed Abortion
Uterus Bicornis
Ectopic Pregnancy
Pregnancy with IUD's
Gestational Age
Tumors in Pregnancy
(+ ovary, cysts and hyperstimulation)

From as early as in the 6th week of pregnancy a diagnosis of the gestational sac can be made. From 8 weeks a disc-like shape of the gestation sac and fetal movements can be seen. By the 9th week activity can be noted and the fetal heart beat can be demonstrated on real-time equipment. Beyond 12 weeks there is no difficulty in fetal heart detection and measuring the fetal heart. These possibilities enable the obstetrician to compile data concerning the state and prognosis of the pregnancy problem in question that not only enables him to come to much more rapid and decisive conclusions but to be more confident in answering his patient's questions. Thus the image of the clinician in the eyes of his patient is enhanced this being another by-product of not insignificant importance of the ultrasonic age.

THE SAFETY OF ULTRASOUND

One of the questions which our patients ask quite frequently concerns the safety of "taking a picture of the baby during pregnancy". This is also a pertinent question and one which we asked ourselves just as ultrasound was beginning to be applied in standard equipment form for Doppler effects, Doppler monitoring equipment and A- and B- Scan instruments. Our experiments were divided into two series animal and human, and I mention them only briefly here since it is from the results that we can reassure our patients and not the studies themselves which have been published previously.

The studies show that although ultrasound at an intensity of greater that 0.5 Watts/Cm2 can cause thermal damage - the damage to rat fetuses being the same as if the animals had been heated to a similar degree as the heat produced by insonation. However, there were no chromosomal or cavitational effects up to this intensity which is higher than that compiled by modern diagnostic equipment at present in use. Some experimental attempts to produce holographic ultrasonograms suggested that under certain conditions to achieve this might involve the use of higher intensities. I will avoid here the detail of frequency and duration of the pulses used in ultrasound apparatus but sum up the situation by saying that although no chromosomal or other damage in present day equipment has been definitely demonstrated, the rapid advances in technique and introduction of new devices based on ultrasound must keep us aware that reassessment of the safety factor must be kept constantly in mind.

GESTATIONAL AGE AND ANTE-PARTUM BLEEDING AND FETAL SIZE AND POSITION

Other members of the panel will be detailing these specific problems. However as the perinatologist follows-up his patient during the course of the pregnancy, these will be among his main concerns. In the generation of a decade ago, besides the palpation and manual estimation, clinical astuteness, care in handling painless ante-partum haemorrhage and such like conditions, the physician would often resort to the use of X-Rays to confirm doubtful assessment of these conditions. He was naturally limited in the amount of X-Ray films he could or should take since it was already shown at that time by the geneticists that there may be long-term effects on the developing fetus, X-Ray pelvimetry was popular and often involved many films. The changing attitude to caesarean sections today, the rapidly disappearing contracted pelvis and other changes in obstetric conditions have altered the demand for much of the pelvimetry that was performed. Following the publications in the literature that the possibility existed of a connection between leukemia and X-Ray pelvimetry, it fell further into disuse. Ultrasound today can almost eradicate the need for the use of roentgen films although here and there there may still be necessity for a specific diagnostic procedure such as amniography. Ultrasound can also be used to diagnose post-partum products of conception.

AMNIOCENTESIS

It is the practice of this procedure that the clinician has come to realize both in early and late pregnancy the joys of ultrasound, real-time and scans. I think that although until recently there was a race in some units between what was to become the most used daily procedure - amniocentesis or ultrasonic scanning, I think that today it should be considered that no amniocentesis should be performed prior to ultrasonic screening. The figure shows the growth of this procedure in our unit. For the physicians in practice once again he can reassure his patient who is being referred for amniocentesis that with the aid of ultrasound the procedure is even safer than before.

Fetoscopy is yet another offshoot of this approach, and as a procedure still in its infancy, just one real-time picture will suffice to show how essential it is to have such equipment in the operating room in use throughout the procedure.

CONGENITAL ANOMALIES

A case is presented here in which a huge cystic mass adjacent to the outline of a 29-week fetus was identified by ultrasonography. After delivery this was proven to be a common cloaca in a fetus with multiple congenital anomalies.

To the best of our knowledge such an ultrasonographic finding has not previously been reported. The possible teratogenic mechanisms of this anomaly are discussed.

To sum up this clinical observation series, I think that one of the most serious discussions a physician can have with his patient is during a pregnancy in a woman who has delivered a previous child with congenital anomalies. The possibilities here of ultrasound diagnosis are not unlimited but they certainly add so much to the assurance and diagnostic assistance to be considered a revolution in itself.

This is why I think that thinking and acting as a practising obstetrician and gynecologist I can say that ultrasound has revolutionized our times and the profession deserves to be proud that the greatest contributors to the introduction of ultrasound medicine have been physicians of our profession.

FETAL ASSESSMENT FROM CONCEPTION TO BIRTH

John M. Beazley

Department of Obstetrics and Gynaecology, University of Liverpool, England.

The Ancients believed that in each ovum or sperm there was a complete but tiny adult whose body and soul simultaneously came into existence at the time of fertilization.

The Theologians next introduced the idea that, in utero we exist firstly in a pre-human form and only later, i.e. after entrance of the soul, develop into the human fetus with which most people are familiar.

In a truly chauvenistic manner Hippocrates suggested that the soul entered a male fetus on the 30th day of intra-uterine life; and into a female on the 40th day.

With the development of embryological science, the notion that life in utero was divided into a pre-human and human era, remained unconfirmed. After fertilization there was only a continuum.

Generations of poets have led us to believe that life in utero, is a haven of peace and quiet, our birth equivalent to "paradise lost". The modern invasion of fetal privacy has substantially altered this notion.

The uterus is not a sound-proof box. The beating of the maternal heart and the reverberations of the maternal gut produce as much sound as a busy high street.

Nor is the uterus completely dark. Though the developing baby may not see objects clearly, transillumination allows some light to enter the uterus.

It is clear also that the baby can taste its surrounding liquor. If the liquor is made bitter by chemicals the child swallows less. If sweetened with saccharin the child swallows more.

It is evident that at an early stage of intra-uterine existence, we develop a remarkable individuality. Unfortunately this wonderful integration of events is subject to the malevolence of disease and chance just as much as in life after birth. In fact, because of our vulnerability in utero, after pregnancy and delivery we are not again subject to such risks of mortality until our old age. Hence there is a logical demand for perinatal medicine and with it comes a need for fetal assessment from conception to birth.

ADEQUACY OF THE PLACENTA

The vitality of the fetus, i.e. its capacity to sustain life, and to perform its functions in utero, must be served at all times by an adequate placenta. That placenta is perfectly matched to its fetus with respect to age. Nevertheless, the placenta's functional capacity spans a time-scale which is significantly reduced and which, under abnormal circumstances, may even be dangerously brief.

The adequacy of placental function is not measurable yet in all its components. Indeed our ability to assess its overall capacity remains both indirect and crude.

The most widely used index of placental sufficiency has been the maternal 24-hour urinary excretion of total estrogens. Where feasible, this test now has been superceded by measurement of either the oestrogen/creatinine ratio in an early morning sample of urine, or the assay of oestrogens in maternal plasma. Human placental lactogen, regrettably, has failed to fulfil its early promise as a more reliable index of placental function.

What obstetricians now require is a more detailed, more direct and more refined measurement of each major component of placental function. Some of these requirements may be met by thermographic studies of the placenta, which now are possible, or from the use of a computer linked gamma camera to measure patterns of isotope uptake during placentography. We also await with interest the further development of those ultrasound techniques which permit location of the umbilical cord and measurement of blood velocity in the umbilical vessels.

FETAL MATURITY

Given placental adequacy, the vitality of the fetus next depends on its maturity. Fetal maturity is a product of both age and development. By "development" I mean fetal organisation at both the cellular and organ level, plus an increase in fetal dimensions and weight.

ASSESSMENT OF FETAL AGE

In obstetric practice, probably no single assessment will ever be more important than determining fetal age. Traditionally this is calculated by Naegale's rule, which still suffices for all but 22% of patients whose menstrual history is unreliable. The use of obstetric milestones to assess fetal age, for example the fundal height, uterine size, quickening, engagement or cervical ripening have been shown to be too inaccurate for modern practice. Of the ancillary tests available the accuracy of ultrasonic techniques surpasses that of older methods, like the cellular and chemical analysis of liquor, or the radiological examination of epiphyseal centres. Not only are these former techniques invasive, they can be misleading when most required to help.

ASSESSMENT OF FETAL GROWTH OR DEVELOPMENT

When considering fetal growth it is probably fair to state that every senior obstetrician has suffered the embarrassment of delivering undiagnosed twins, the reported incidence of which varies from 20 - 49% - a serious indictment of abdominal palpation. Inasmuch as Swedish authors have shown that the incidence of detection before 25 weeks gestation, can be increased to 95% by the routine use of ultrasonic screening, little justification remains for relying upon outmoded clinical methods.

ASSESSMENT OF FETAL WEIGHT

Clinical attempts by experienced attendants, to assess fetal weight, also results in inaccuracies of ± 500 grams in about 75 - 80 per cent of patients. The error is greater in the remaining women, or when junior attendants make the assessment, or when a baby weighs as little as 2kg or as much as 4.5 kg. Fetal weight can be assessed by rather complicated ultrasonic techniques or by special Xray fetograms necessitating the prior injection of intra-amniotic oil. Regrettably, neither of these methods are widely available at present.

ASSESSMENT OF FETAL DIMENSION

The intra-uterine assessment of fetal dimensions, especially by ultrasound, has proved particularly valuable in the recognition of dysmaturity. Whereas in the past, clinicians were reliant upon such crude signs as poor maternal weight gain, oligohydramnios, or reduced uterine size to detect small babies, now ultrasonic measurements enables sudden growth retardation to be distinguished from low growth potential and symmetrically small babies to be distinguished from those with the asymmetrical growth caused by intra-uterine starvation.

ASSESSMENT OF FETAL ORGANISATION

i   Fetal organisation of the cellular level is evaluated by the geneticist or biochemist. Amniocentesis regularly facilitates the detection of mongolism, sex-linked disorders or inborn errors of metabolism. Increased alpha-feto protein is widely used as an index of defective neural tube development; Lecithin Sphingo-myelin ratios are measured routinely to assess the maturity of the fetal lung.

ii   The development of fetal organs, especially their gross anatomy and function now may be assessed to a limited degree by fetoscopy. This permits not only a direct study of the fetal limbs and body, but also facilitates direct blood sampling from early fetal blood vessels. Ultrasonic evaluation of fetal renal function, or of filling and emptying of the fetal bladder, helps to distinguish mature babies from dysmature and normal infants from those with Potter's Syndrome.

Fetal breathing movements have always aroused great interest. References to babies crying within the uterus may be found in the ancient writings of the Hindus, the Babylonians, the Assyrians, the Greeks and the Romans. St. Bartholomew and Mahommed are both reputed to have cried in utero.

In the middle ages, the physicians were loath to report such an occurence because of religious persecution. Midwives who claimed to have heard crying before birth were accused of witchcraft. Yet crying in utero is hardly surprising. All that is required is air within the uterus and an appropriate fetal stimulus. Both these conditions might be fulfilled readily with the introduction of modern endoscopes or needles.

Professor Dawes has clarified that breathing movements are detectable from 11 weeks of intra-uterine life. By 36 weeks, the chest of the normal child moves regularly, as in life after birth. Within the forseeable future, fetal breathing movements may provide an index of impending fetal death as reliable as cardiotocography. For the present however, non-stressed ante-natal cardiotocography still provides the best assessment of when to deliver a baby.

In his play "Love's Labour Lost", Shakespeare described early fetal movements by writing, "she is two months on her way. She is quick. The child brags in her belly". Less romantically modern classifications now recognise 4 different categories of fetal movement. Despite this advance, our life in utero continues to follow a circadian rhythm, periods of wakefulness being followed by periods of sleep. The maternal evaluation of this normal pattern is bedevilled, quite naturally, by an anxiety that when the baby is quiet, it may be dead. To overcome this fear a simple screening device has been used in Liverpool, known as a fetal "kick chart". Each day, from the thirtieth week of gestation, the mother records on this chart the time of which she receives the tenth kick from her baby. Should she not receive 10 kicks within 12 hours she is admitted immediately for further assessment.

FETAL ASSESSMENT IN LIVERPOOL

In Liverpool, my Department has been studying some clinical implications which arise from the routine application of the current technology I have mentioned.

Our approach has involved four major principles. Firstly, the statistical data relating to Britain has been evaluated so that it may be used according to its general predictive value. This provides an index of potential risk. Secondly, we have separated all maternal from fetal data, thus creating two case sheets from the beginning. Thirdly, in both maternal and fetal case records all quantitative data has been separated from qualitative data. Thereby, we extract all technical measurements from the equally important but qualitative records of patients complaints, medical compassion and fetal misfortunes. Lastly, all quantitative measures are grouped into an order which offers the best prediction of individual risk. Trend values are clearly distinguished from data which is either directive or permissive.

CONCLUSION

With these comments upon fetal assessment from conception to birth, I have tried to emphasise an increasing clinical demand for sophisticated technology, and a need to study dynamic data rather than static information.

THE VALUE OF ULTRASOUND IN PERINATAL MEDICINE FROM THE CLINICIAN'S POINT OF VIEW

A. Cretti, Z. Czajkowski, J. Bajorek, A. Nienartowicz

Department for Pathology of Pregnancy and Labour, Medical Academy, Szczecin, Poland

The relation of the ultrasound diagnostics to the obstetrical practice in my corner of the world is, generally speaking similar as in other regions of the world. The ultrasound equipment is localized in the obstetrical departments despite some few trials to make central ultrasound departments, connected with the X-ray departments.

However, there is a number of small hospitals which have no ultrasonography. Consequently, there are a number of gravidas, in whom the size and the growth of the fetus are not checked up by the ultrasound. In these cases the fetal growth is observed with the use of external measurements of uterine height (4, 6) and the fetal weight is estimated with the method of Johnson.

Of course the ultrasound method is more reliable than the palpation method by Johnson, but it seemed interesting how big is the error of this method in comparison with ultrasonography. This comparison was made in our department by Czajkowski and co-workers in 1976 (2). 198 hospitalized patients in third trimenon of pregnancy were examined with Johnson's method and with ultrasound; the biparietal and thoracic diameters were measured and the nomogram of Hansman-Voit was used. Results of both methods were compared with the postnatal weight of the newborns'. Statistical analysis consisted of the test 'u' and of the method of minimal quadrats.

The results are presented in Figure 1. It can be seen that: (a) the difference between the ultrasonically estimated weight and the real weight is in general smaller than the difference between the weight estimated by Johnson's method and the real weight. These values are statistically significant; (b) the Johnson's method gave values lower than the real ones in the sector below 3500 grams and higher than the real in the sector above 3500 grams.

To improve the accuracy of the Johnson's method a modification was elaborated in our department by Nienartowicz and co-worker in 1979 (5). The modification consists of the introduction of the factor 140 for 31st - 35th weeks of pregnancy and factor 150 for the 36th and 37th weeks of pregnancy; in the original method the factor 155 is used for the whole third trimenon. As we see in

Figure 2 our modification gave better results than the original method.

For some years we use the newborns maturity index by Dubowitz (3) which contains also the evaluation of neurological state. In the previous investigations made in our department, Bajorek and Czajkowski in 1976 (1) found that in poor intrauterine fetal growth there is no correlation between the BPD on one side and the birth-weight or duration of pregnancy on the other side (Fig. 3, Fig. 4), in contrast to the normally developing feti. It seemed interesting to see if there is a correlation between the BPD and the maturity index. As we see in Figure 5 it seems that there is such correlation, but it needs confirmation on a more numerous material.

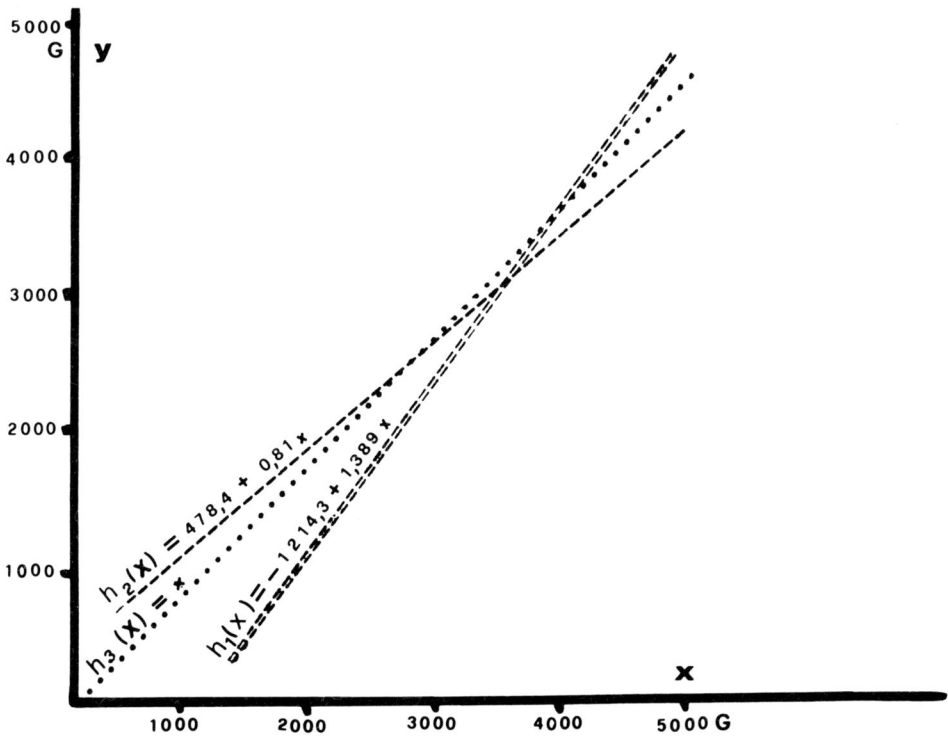

Figure 1. Diagram of the correlation between the fetal weight estimated with Johnson's method - h_1/x/, with ultrasonography - h_2/x/, and the real weight - h_3/x/.

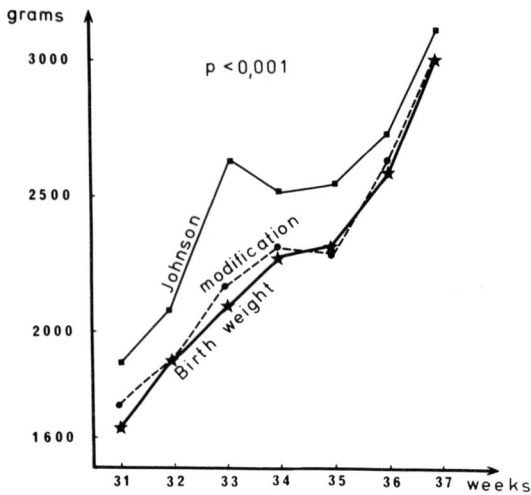

Figure 2. The differences between the fetal weight estimated with Johnson's method and the real weight, and the differences between the fetal weight estimated with our modification and the real weight.

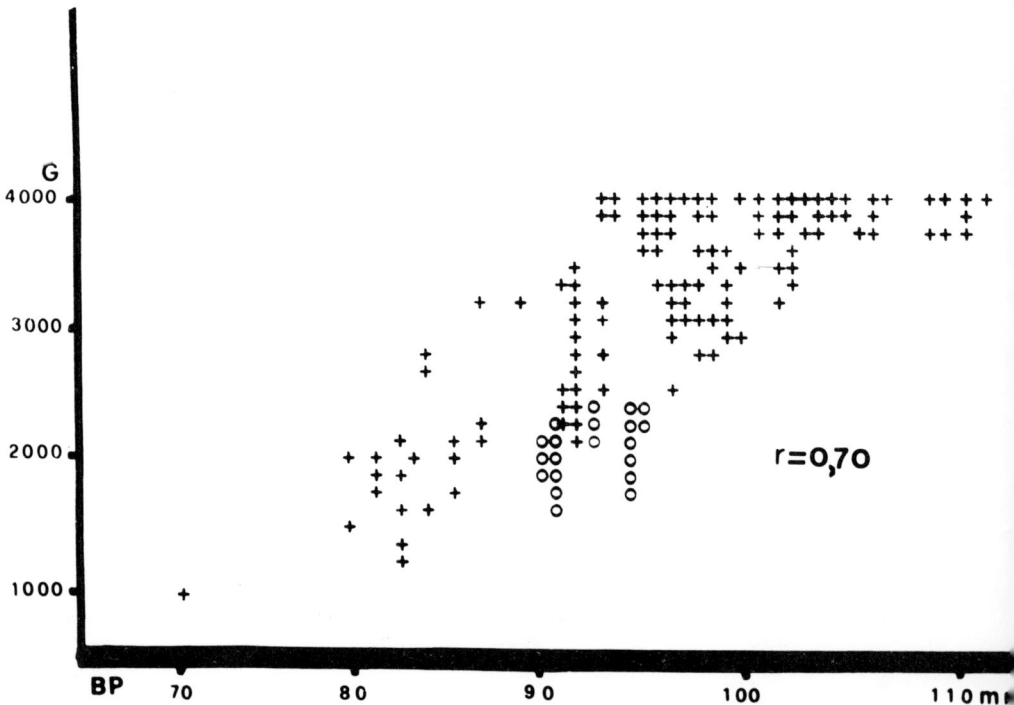

Figure 3. Diagram of the correlation between the biparietal diameter (BP) and the neonatal weight (G) in the feti with normal development (+) and in the cases with the poor intrauterine growth (O).

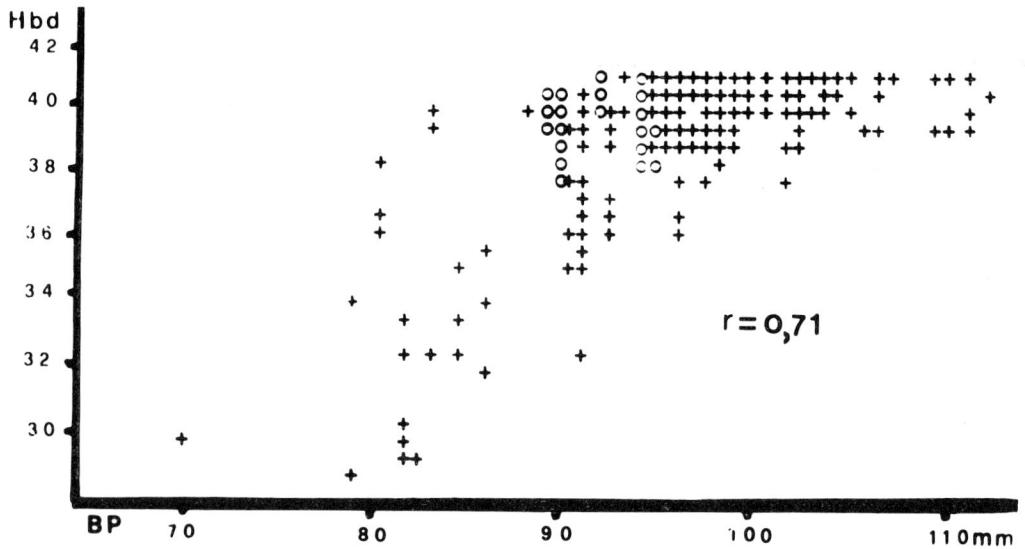

Figure 4. Diagram of the correlation between the biparietal diameter (BP) and the duration of the pregnancy in
weeks (Hbd) in the feti with normal development (+) and in
the cases of poor intrauterine fetal growth (0).

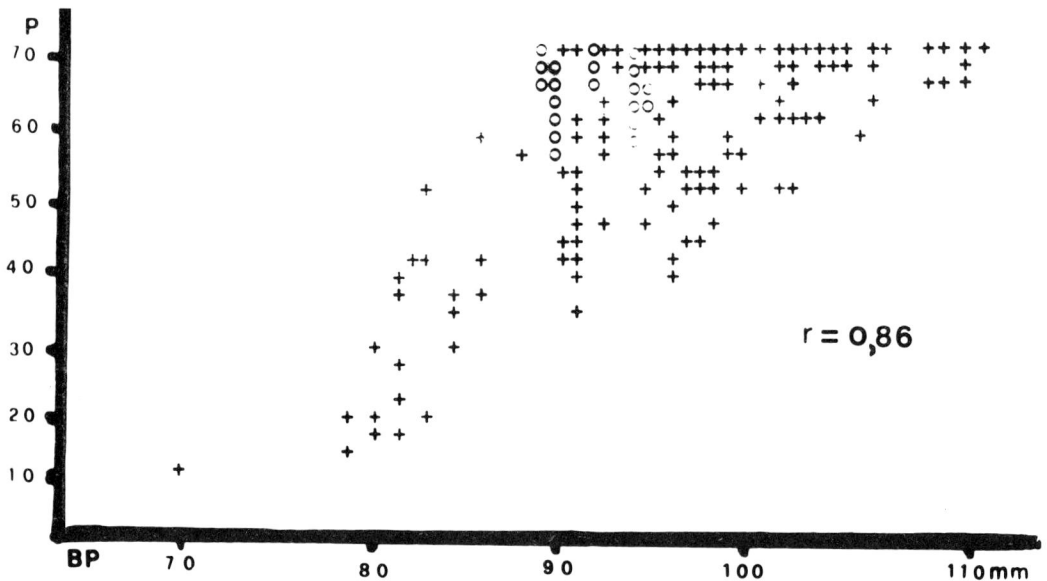

Figure 5. Diagram of the correlation between the biparietal diameter (BP) and the neonatal maturity score (P) in
the feti with normal development (+) and in the cases of
poor intrauterine fetal growth (0).

REFERENCES

1. Bajorek, J., Czajkowski, Z. (1976): Materialy Naukowe IV Ogőlopolskiego Sympozjum Neonatologieznego, Katowice, 5.
2. Czajkowski, Z. et al. (1976): Materialy Naukowe IV Ogőlnopolskiego Sympozjum Neonatologieznego, Katowice 14.
3. Dubowitz, L. et al. (1970): J.Ped., 70, 9.
4. Leroy B. et al. (1973): Rev. franc. Gynec., 68, 83.
5. Nienartowicz, A., Sych, Z. (1979): Ginekologia Polska, 50, 487.
6. Westin, B. (1977): Acta Obstet. Gynecol. Scand, 56, 273.

6. THE INFLUENCE OF DIAGNOSTIC ULTRASOUND IN PERINATAL MEDICINE

A. Kurjak, Chairman

REAL-TIME ULTRASONIC EVALUATION OF BLEEDING IN EARLY PREGNANCY

Asim Kurjak, Pertti Kirkinen, Ivo Banovic and Brigita Rukavina

Ultrasonic Center, Dept. of Obstetrics and Gynecology, University of Zagreb, Zagreb, Yugoslavia

The most common pathologic symptom in early pregnancy is bleeding. It has been established that 40 to 50% of those patients have an unfavourable outcome(1,2). The main problems in the management of these patients are diagnostic; after an accurate diagnosis has been made, the selection of possible therapeutic measures is easier. At this moment ultrasonography is considered to be the best diagnostic method for early pregnancy complications (2-4). With the real-time unit, it is now possible to obtain very reliable information on the actual state of the pregnancy and to predict with adequate certainty the later course of pregnancy at the time of a threatened abortion. Data on the reliability of this equipment compared to the conventional B-scanners are also increasing (5-8).

The intention of this study was to investigate the role of the real-time machine in the diagnosis and assessment of bleeding in early pregnancy in a busy department under everyday routine conditions.

PATIENTS

This series consisted of 1263 patients, who were sent for an ultrasonic examination because of clinical findings of bleeding in the first trimester. The examination was repeated once in 300 cases and twice in 169, mainly because of uncertain gestational age or for confirming an initially negative finding (Table 1). The gestational age was predicted by measurements of the crown-rump length.

METHOD

Aloca and ADR real-time equipment were used and the examinations were made by three experienced persons under routine conditions. For evaluating the ultrasonic findings, the criterion of a normal and abnormal situation presented by Robinson (1975) was used. The presence of fetal heart activity and movements and the number of amniotic sacs in utero were also recorded.

RESULTS

In the first examination, an intact pregnancy

139

with fetal life signs was verified in 1024 cases (80.5%).
In these patients the course of pregnancy was uncomplicated
to the end of the first trimester.

The final ultrasonic diagnosis of the 239 cases (19.5%)
in whom no fetal life was seen at the first ultrasonic examination is presented in table 2. Missed abortions and
blighted ovas constituted nearly 60% of these cases. The
first ultrasonic examination did not reveal fetal life in
15% of this group because of a very early pregnancy. However, the exact diagnosis of a living, normal pregnancy
could be verified in each of these cases at the next ultrasonic examination within one or two weeks. In 5.8% of the
cases in this group, the bleeding was caused by some non-
gestational reason, and in these cases the repeated ultrasonic examination did not reveal any finding of a normal or
pathologic pregnancy.

TABLE 1. OUR MATERIAL

No. of patients with 1 real-time scan	794	=	794
No. of patients with 2 real-time scans	300	=	600
No. of patients with 3 real-time scans	169	=	507
Total no. of patients	1263		
Total no. of scans			1901

Only 14 of these 239 cases (5.8%),in whom the first
ultrasonic examination did not reveal a normal pregnancy,
included an examiner's error in the interpretation of the
ultrasonic finding at this first examination. The succeeding examinations revealed in these cases the existence of
a normal pregnancy without any discrepancy between menstrual
delay and ultrasonically estimated gestational age, i.e. the
first finding was a human error.

TABLE 2. PATIENTS WITH NO SIGNS OF FETAL LIFE AT FIRST
ULTRASONIC EXAMINATION

Ultrasonic diagnosis	No.	%
Missed abortion	79	34.0
Blighted ovum	59	24.5
Retained product of conception	18	7.5
Very early pregnancy	37	15.0
Ectopic pregnancy	15	5.8
No pregnancy	14	5.8
Hydatid mole	3	1.2
Error	14	5.8
Total	239	100.0

Of those cases with early pregnancy failure (N=159),
the ultrasonic diagnosis was correct in the first examination in 76% and the second examination was needed after one
week in 24%. In each case the ultrasonic diagnosis could
be made after two examinations. Blighted ovum was most
difficult to diagnose at the first examination (Table 3).

TABLE 3. ACCURACY OF REAL-TIME DIAGNOSIS OF EARLY PREGNANCY
FAILURE

N=159

| | Number | | % | |
DIAGNOSIS	1st exam	2nd exam	1st exam	2nd exam
Missed abortion N = 79	65	14	82	18
Blighted ovum N = 59	39	20	66	34
Retained product of conception N = 18	17	1	95	5
Hydatid mole N = 3	2	1	66.5	33.5
Total	123	36	76	24

MULTIPLE PREGNANCIES

The material contained also 22 twin pregnancies, in
whom the ultrasonic finding was normal in 9 cases for both
of the twins. The findings of the remaining 13 cases are
presented in table 4. The most frequent abnormality was a
combination between blighted ova and coexisting normal pregnancy (9).

TABLE 4. ABNORMALITIES IN TWIN PREGNANCIES

Blighted ovum/Normal pregnancy	11
Missed abortion/Missed abortion	1
Blighted ovum/Blighted ovum	1
Total	13

DISCUSSION

Bleeding in the first trimester constitutes one of the most frequent diagnostic problems in the antenatal period. Having such a patient in his consulting room, any obstetrician should like to know several important facts which can radically alter the management. These are: Is the patient pregnant? Is the pregnancy single or multiple? Is the fetus alive or dead? What is the gestational age? Are there any signs that the pregnancy may abort? Is there any evidence to suggest that the pregnancy is extrauterine? In the event of an abortion, is it complete or incomplete? Is there an associated pelvic mass? Only after this differentiation can the controlling and possible therapeutic measures be applied to the cases in whom a normal outcome of the pregnancy can be expected.

The recent introduction of real-time ultrasound units has added a whole new parameter to obstetric practice. These inexpensive, portable machines are very suitable for use by the obstetrician in the consulting room and may be regarded as providing a logical extension of the classical methods of inspection, palpation and auscultation. The clinician can now look inside the uterus, see the fetus and placenta, note the presentation, position, fetal movements and multiple pregnancy. He may also do biometrical measurements.

The results of this material showed that with the real-time machine it is possible in the large majority of pregnancies with bleeding in the first trimester to make a correct diagnosis at the first examination. If the fetal life signs are seen, the reliability of the ultrasonic diagnosis is good. The good prognosis after confirming fetal life in these cases was also reported by Levine and Filly in 1978 (5), Jouppila in 1978 (4). In a series reported by Anderson in 1978 (10), there was a good outcome in 88% of the cases of threatened abortion after seeing fetal life with ultrasonography. Important is the fact that our series did not contain any false positive findings of fetal life in ultrasonography.

Also in the patients in whom no fetal life was demonstrated at the first examination, it was still possible to make a correct diagnosis at the same time. Fifteen percent of these cases had incorrectly estimated gestational age, which is further evidence for stressing the importance of a repeated ultrasonic examination. The diagnosis of blighted ova by clinical and biochemical methods is often very indefinite. Recent findings of the relation of this condition with a succeeding molar pregnancy stress the important value of a reliable and quick diagnosis in blighted ova pregnancies (11). This material reveals that with real-time ultrasonography, the diagnosis of blighted ovas is in 100% possible at two examinations with a one week interval. The improvement of the equipment will surely add to the percentage of correct diagnoses at the first examination,

when better resolution of the equipment will make it possible to see fetal anatomy and life earlier and better than
now.
 The most prominent practical finding at the ultrasonic
examination is the prognostic significance of fetal life
detection for the later course of pregnancy. In this series,92% delivered as diagnosed. This high prognostic predictive value gives ultrasonic examinations a primary role
in the diagnostic evaluation of problems in early pregnancy.
The interpretation of fetal life findings is simple enough
and the results are immediately available for use.

REFERENCES

1. Johansen, A. (1970): Acta Obstet. Gynecol. Scand. 49:89.
2. Jouppila, P. (1979): Br.J.Obstet.Gynecol. 86:343.
3. Robinson, H.P. (1975): Br.J.Obstet.Gynecol., 2:849.
4. Jouppila, P. (1978): Recent advances in ultrasound diag-
    nosis. Ed. A. Kurjak, Excerpta Medica, Amsterdam, p.175.
5. Levine, S. and Filly, R. (1978): Obstet. Gynecol. 51:
    170.
6. Adam, A., Robinson, H., Fleming, J. and Hall, A.(1978):
    Br.J.Obstet.Gynecol., 85:487.
7. Balfour, R. (1978): Br.J.Obstet.Gynecol., 85:492.
8. Davies, P. and Richardson, R. (1979): Br.J. Obstet.
    Gynecol., 86:765.
9. Kurjak, A. and Latin, V. (1979): Acta Obstet. Gynecol.
    Scand., 58:153.
10. Anderson, S. (1978): Obstet. Gynecol., 51:284.
11. Kurjak, A. and Jouppila, P. (1980): Ultrasonic, hormon-
    al and histopathological diagnosis and assessments of
    blighted ovum.Ultras.Med. Biol.; accepted for publica-
    tion.

ULTRASONIC AND BIOCHEMICAL ASSESSMENT OF FETAL BEHAVIOUR
IN RELATION TO MATERNAL MEALS IN NORMAL AND INSULIN-
DEPENDENT PREGNANCY

J.W. Wladimiroff, P. Roodenburg, J. Laar and G. Kroesen

Department of Obstetrics and Gynaecology, Academic
Hospital Rotterdam Dijkzigt, Erasmus University Rotterdam,
Rotterdam, The Netherlands

Fetal respiratory (FRM) and body movements (FBM) are
receiving great interest both in animal experimental work
(1,2) and in clinical Perinatology (3 - 8).
This paper presents preliminary data on FRM and FBM
relative to maternal meals in normal and insulin-dependent
diabetic pregnancies in the third trimester of pregnancy.

PATIENTS AND METHODS

A total of 8 normal and 8 insulin-dependent pregnancies was studied. In the former group pregnancy duration
varied between 31 and 40 weeks (median; 35 weeks) in the
latter group between 28 and 37 weeks (median; 34 weeks).
FRM and FBM were studied by real-time ultrasound on a
transverse cross-section of the fetal upper-abdomen and
plotted on a magnetic tape using an event marker. The
percentage incidence of FRM and FBM were subsequently
calculated over 15 minute periods on a computer..
In normal pregnancy FRM´and FTM were recorded 30
minutes before the beginning of a meal and 90 minutes
following the end of a meal. The meal itself started at
8.00 a.m., 12.00 p.m. and 5.00 p.m. and lasted 15 minutes
during which no recording was made. Maternal blood glucose
levels were measured 30 minutes before and 45, 75 and 105
minutes following the commencement of each meal (Fig. 1).
In diabetic pregnancy the same procedure was followed,
except for breakfast and dinner which was preceded by a
60-minute recording period, since insulin was administered
at 7.30 a.m. and 4.30 p.m., i.e. 30 minutes before the meal
(Fig. 1).
All patients were studied in the semi-recumbent
position.

Normal   (n = 8) : 31 - 40 weeks

Diabetes (n = 8) : 28 - 37 weeks

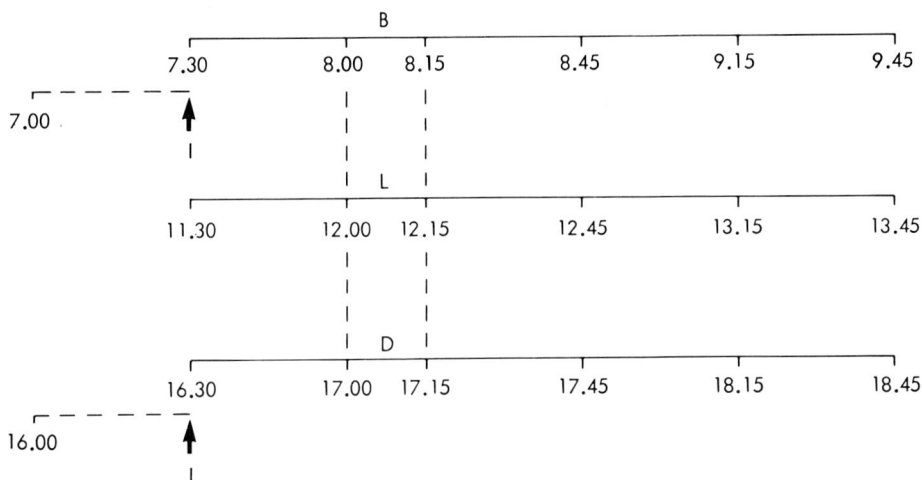

```
                        B
     ┌─────────┬────────┬─────────────┬───────────┬────────────┐
     7.30      8.00    8.15          8.45        9.15         9.45
┌ ─ ─ ─ ─ ─ ┐
7.00         ↑          |             |
             |          |             |
             |          |             |
             |          |  L          |
     ┌─────────┬────────┬─────────────┬───────────┬────────────┐
     11.30     12.00   12.15         12.45       13.15        13.45
                        |             |
                        |             |
                        |             |
                        |  D          |
     ┌─────────┬────────┬─────────────┬───────────┬────────────┐
     16.30     17.00   17.15         17.45       18.15        18.45
┌ ─ ─ ─ ─ ─ ┐
16.00        ↑
             |
```

Figure 1. Set-up of the fetal respiratory and body movements study relative to breakfast (B), lunch (L) and
dinner (D). I=insulin.

RESULTS

     Figures 2 and 3 present the mean values and standard
error of the mean for the percentage incidence of FRM
and FBM for each 15 minute period (continuous line) and
the maternal blood glucose levels for each 30 minute
period (dotted line) before and after breakfast, lunch and
dinner in normal pregnancy. Before meals the incidence of
FRM varies between 24 and 30%. Following breakfast a
steady increase from 14 to 57% can be observed. The study
period following lunch and dinner is characterized by an
initial rise and subsequent fall in percentage incidence
of FRM,although the post-lunch data is rather inconclusive.
Maternal blood glucose levels show a statistically
significant (p < 0.01) increase following meals.
     The preprandial percentage incidence of FBM varies
from 10 to 16%. The post-breakfast and post-lunch values
do not significantly differ from the preprandial values,

145

apart from an unexplained dip, 60 minutes following lunch.
An increase, however, can be observed up to 23%, 10-75
minutes following dinner coinciding with a maximum blood
glucose level of 5.4 mmol per liter.

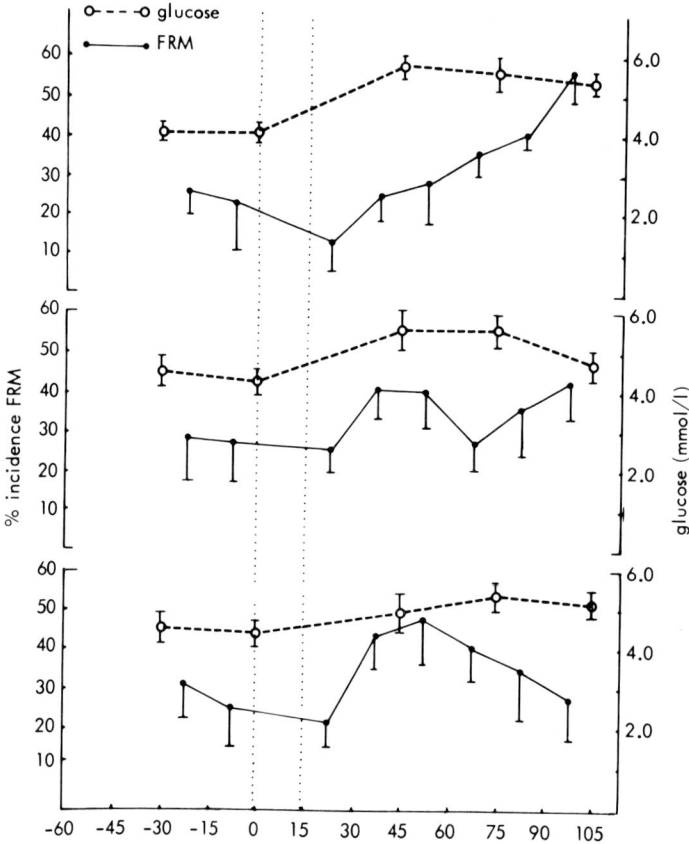

Figure 2.

Figures 4 and 5 demonstrate the mean values and
standard error of the mean for the percentage incidence of
FRM and FBM and maternal blood glucose levels relative to
breakfast, lunch and dinner in diabetic pregnancy   There
is an increase in FRM incidence from 15 to 31% before
breakfast and a slight fall before lunch. The pre-dinner
levels are inconsistent. The FRM pattern immediately
around the three meals very much resembles the maternal
blood glucose pattern. During the remainder of the study
period an impressive increase in FRM incidence and maternal blood glucose levels can be observed, particularly
following breakfast and lunch.

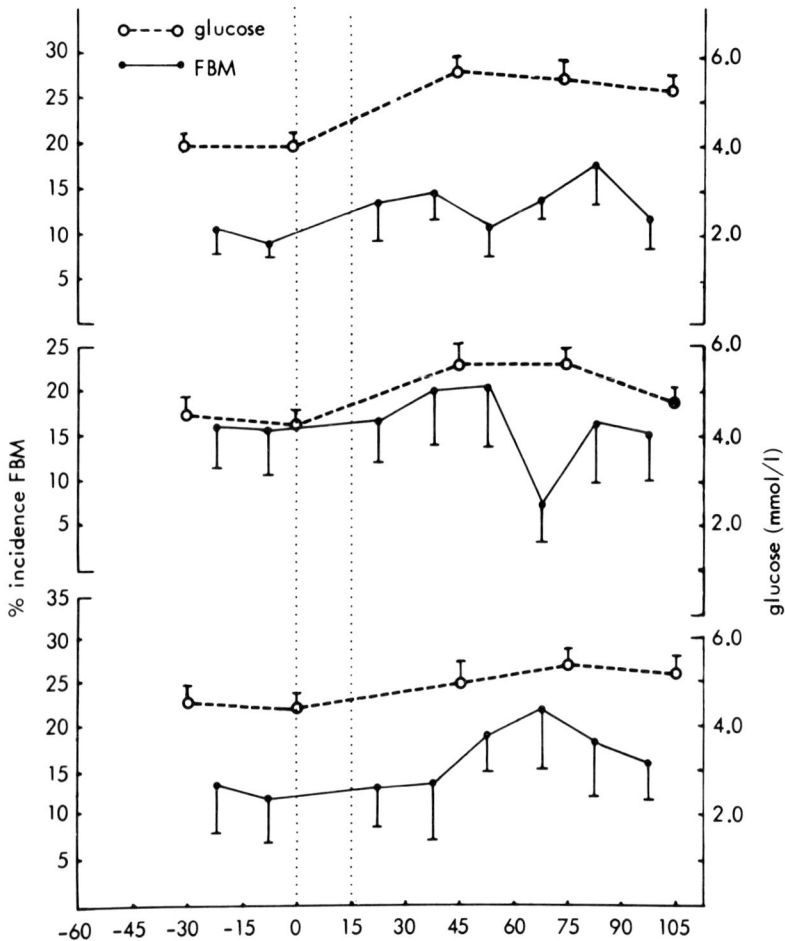

Figures 2 and 3. Mean values and S.E. for fetal respiratory (FRM; Fig. 2) and body movement incidence (FBM; Fig.3) and maternal blood glucose levels relative to breakfast (B), lunch (L) and dinner (D) in normal pregnancy.

The FBM incidence ranges from 10 to 20% before breakfast and from 12 to 22% before dinner. The post-breakfast and post-lunch values do not significantly differ from the preprandial values. There is, however, a marked rise up to 33%, 60-75 minutes following dinner. This increase is not related to the maternal blood glucose levels.

Comparing normal (dotted line) and diabetic (continuous line) pregnancy (Fig. 6),in the latter group the postprandial FRM incidence is higher after breakfast (8 against 31%) and lower after lunch (26 against 7%) and dinner (23 against 16%). During the remainder of the post-meal period, the rise in FRM incidence is more marked in

147

diabetic than in normal pregnancy, particularly after breakfast and lunch. A similar pattern could be observed in the maternal blood glucose levels following breakfast and to a lesser extent following lunch.

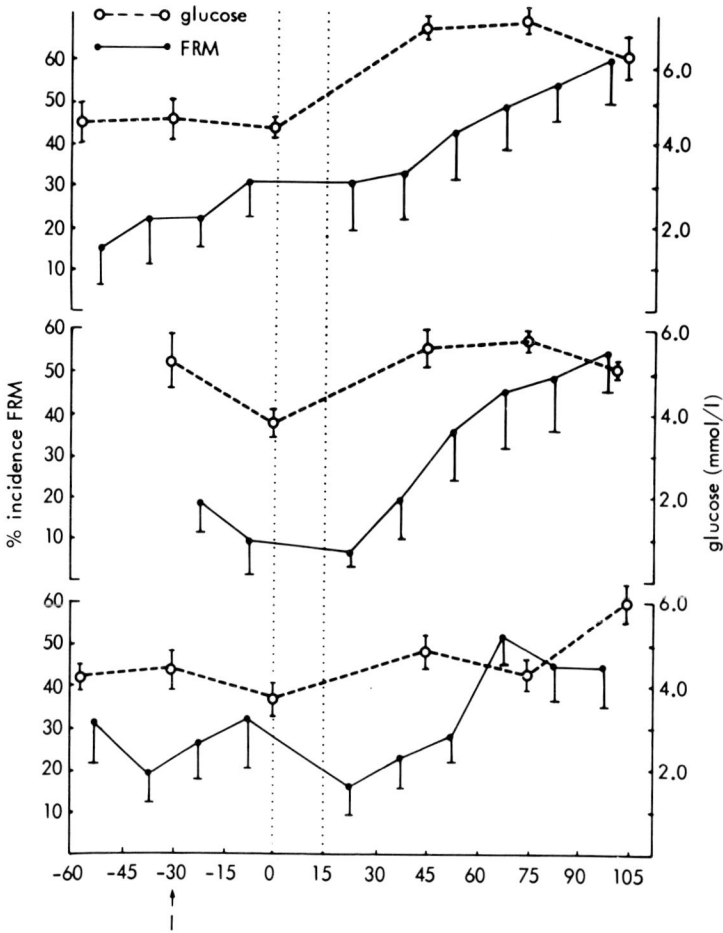

Figure 4.

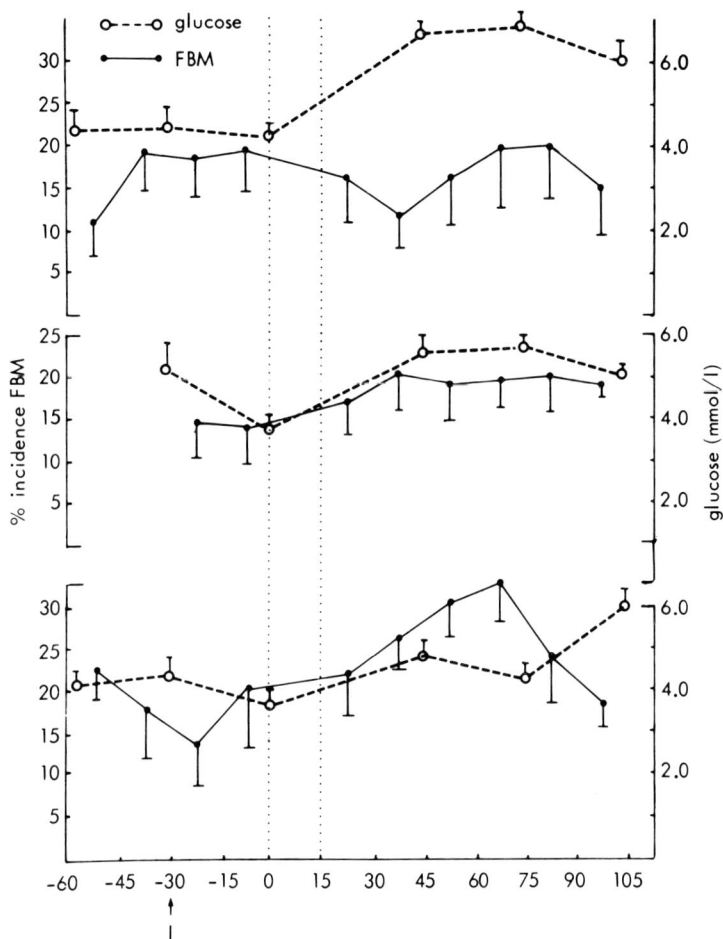

Figures 4 and 5. Mean values and S.E. for fetal respiratory (FRM; Fig. 4) and body movement incidence (FBM; Fig. 5)
and maternal blood glucose levels relative to breakfast
(B), lunch (L) and dinner (D) in diabetic pregnancy.
I=insulin.

Apart from pre-lunch and immediate post-breakfast and
post-lunch values, FBM incidence is generally higher in
diabetic than in normal pregnancy (Fig. 7).

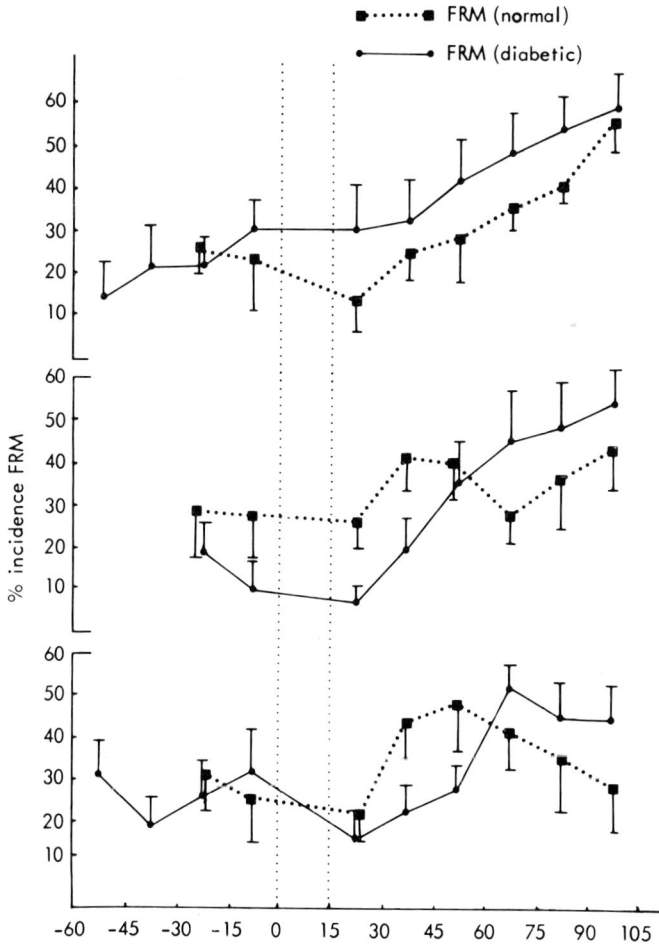

Figure 6. Mean values and S.E. for fetal respiratory movements (FRM) relative to breakfast (B),lunch (L) and dinner (D) in normal and diabetic pregnancy.

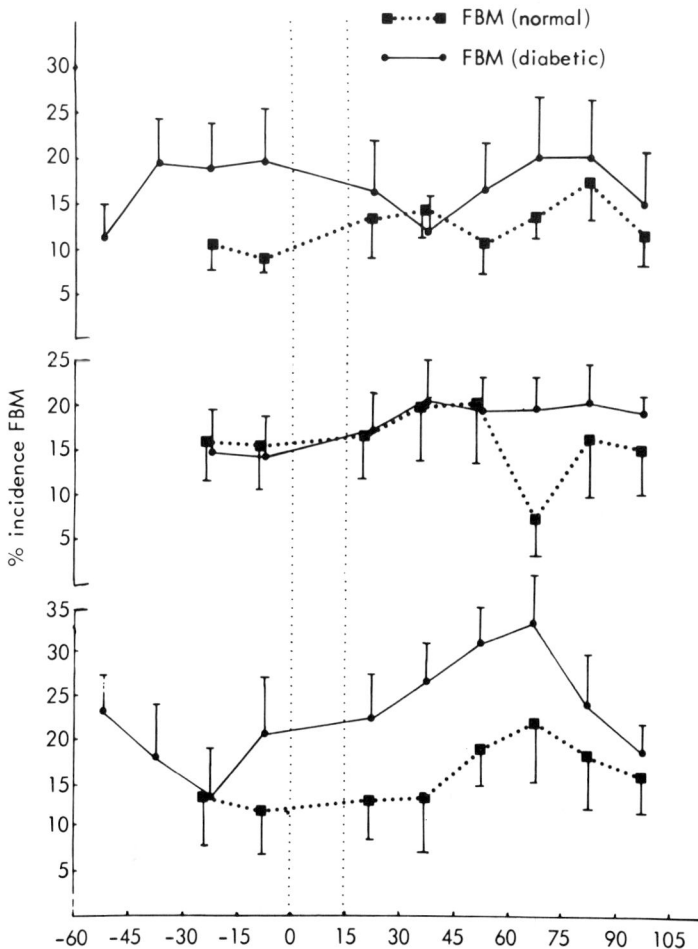

Figure 7. Mean values and S.E. for fetal body movements (FBM) relative to breakfast (B), lunch (L) and dinner (D) in normal and diabetic pregnancy.

Figure 8 represents total fetal activity as expressed by the sum of FRM and FBM incidence. Around breakfast time there is a significantly higher fetal activity in diabetic pregnancy. The lunch period is characterized by a significantly lower fetal activity before and during the first 45 minutes after lunch. The last 60 minutes of the study period starts off with a very pronounced rise in total fetal activity in diabetic pregnancy, resulting in activity levels well above those in normal pregnancy. Immediately around dinner there is not much difference in total fetal activity in normal and diabetic pregnancies. The activity patterns during the last 60 minutes of the study period very closely resemble those observed during the same period after lunch.

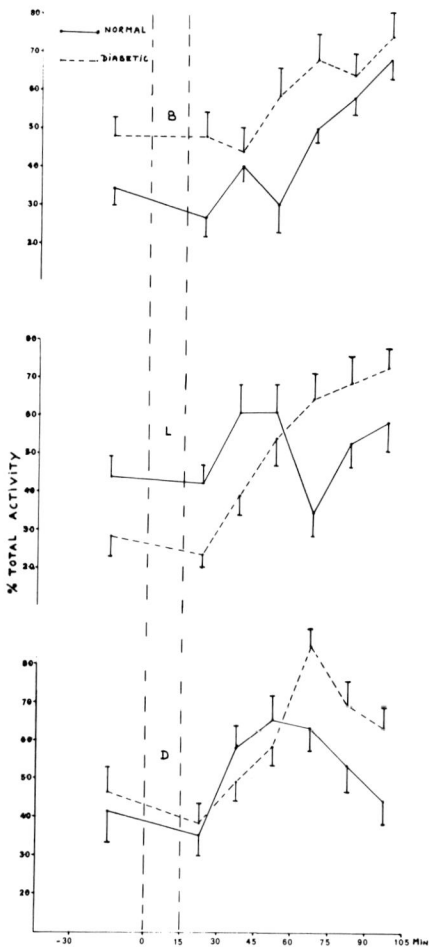

Figure 8. Mean values and S.E. for total fetal activity relative to breakfast (B), lunch (L) and dinner (D) in normal and diabetic pregnancy.

SUMMARY

1. In normal pregnancy a significant increase in FRM is observed within 45-60 minutes following each meal, particularly after breakfast. In diabetics a higher incidence of FRM is found following breakfast. Significantly lower levels are observed immediately following lunch and dinner, they are followed by a more marked and sustained increase during the remainder of the study period. This data seems to be glucose dependent.

152

2. In normal pregnancy, the post-dinner period is characterized by a steady increase in FBM. In diabetic pregnancy the incidence of FBM is significantly higher following lunch and dinner as compared with normal pregnancy.

3. Total fetal activity is generally slightly more pronounced in diabetics during the breakfast study period. Total fetal activity is significantly lower in diabetics immediately before and following lunch and dinner, but shows a very marked rise during the last 60 minutes of the study period.

REFERENCES

1. Dawes, G.S., Fox, H.E., Leduc, B.M., Liggins, G.C. and Richards, R.T. (1972): J. Physiol. 220:119.

2. Chapman, R.L.K., Dawes, G.S., Rurak, D.W. and Wilds, P.L. (1978): Am. J. Obstet. Gynecol. 131:894.

3. Gennser, G., Marsal, K. and Brantmark, K. (1975): Am. J. Obstet. Gynecol. 123 : 861.

4. Wladimiroff, J.W., Ligtvoet, C.M. and Spermon, J.A. (1976): Br. Med. J. 2:975.

5. Manning, F.A., Platt, L.D. and Lemay, M. (1977): Br. Med. J. 4 : 1582.

6. Patrick, J., Natale, R. and Richardson, B. (1978): Am. J. Obstet. Gynecol. 132 507.

7. Lewis, P.J., Trudinger, B.J. and Mangez, J. (1978): Br. J. Obstet. Gynaecol. 85 : 86.

8. Wladimiroff, J.W., Roodenburg, P. and Bovenlander, J. (1979): Br. J. Obstet. Gynaecol., in press.

RECENT ADVANCES IN ULTRASONOGRAPHY OF THE PLACENTA

K. Vandenberghe, P. Goddeeris* and F. De Wolf

Departments of Obstetrics-Gynecology, and of Pathology I*,
Academic Hospital Sint-Rafaël , University of Leuven,
Leuven, Belgium.

The direct object of placental ultrasonography is the
in vivo placenta, which is about 60 percent larger in surface, thickness and volume than the delivered placenta,
and which can be studied repeatedly at different stages in
its deveolopment. Moreover it appears as a dynamic organ
because of uterine contractility and flexibility, fetal positioning and movements, and circulation conditions.

VISUALIZATION

The technical capabilities of the present day gray
scale compound and real time systems have enabled to make
the information already contented in the A-scan data - a
large range of echo amplitudes and real time information -
more readily accessible.
The typical sickle or dome shape of the placenta can
be visualized from eight-ten weeks on, the period of differentiation between chorion frondosum and chorion leave.
The placenta appears as a soft tissue mass (Fig. 1) with a
homogeneous medium-strong echo pattern, delineated by the
dense echo line of the chorionic plate and the less echogenic zone of the decidualized uterine wall. The umbilical cord with its two arteries and one vein can often be
visualized, sometimes also its insertion into the placenta;
membranes between twins can be identified. An accessory
lobe or a bilobate placenta is mostly diagnosed but these
images are to be differentiated from local uterine contractions; placenta membranacea has been reported (15), and
large hemangiomas of the placenta can be diagnosed.

LOCALISATION

Placental localisation proved to be one of the first
valuable clinical applications of obstetric echography (8).
Because of the factors of uterine movability, flexibility
and contractility, it is important to stress the necessity
to use uterine and not maternal points of reference to indicate the exact placental location (Fig. 2 and 3). The
differential growth of the uterine wall with progressive
elongation of the lower, isthmic segment, suffices to explain the increasing distance between the lower placental
margin and the internal cervical os, in the follow-up of
early low placental implantation. There seems to be no
need for a hypothesis of dynamic placental migration (7),
and there is certainly no scientific proof for the validity

of such hypothesis.

MEASUREMENTS

Apart from thickness measurements,which are linear, other placental mensurations such as volume and implanta-

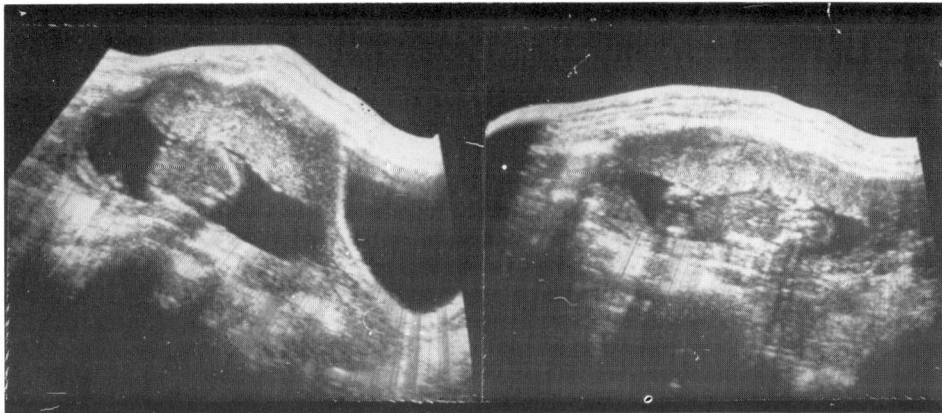

Figure 1. Placenta anterior. Longitudinal and transverse tomograms; pregnancy of 17 weeks duration.

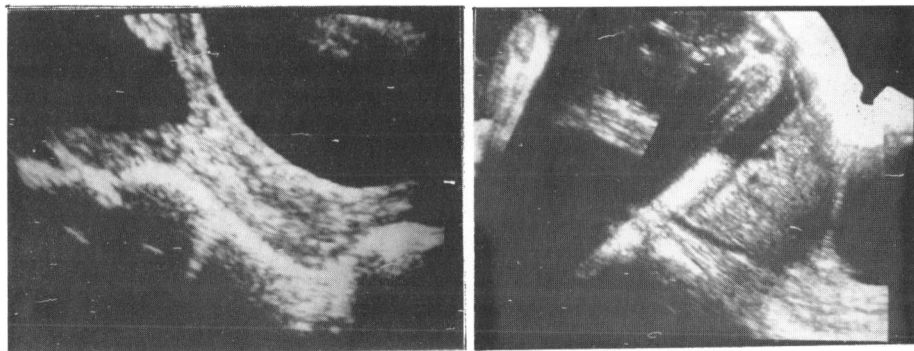

Figure 2. Uterine cervix. Longitudinal tomogram showing lower uterine segment and cervix with internal os and cervical canal.

Figure 3. Total placenta previa. Longitudinal tomogram in 37 weeks pregnancy with transverse lie of the fetus and placenta previa.

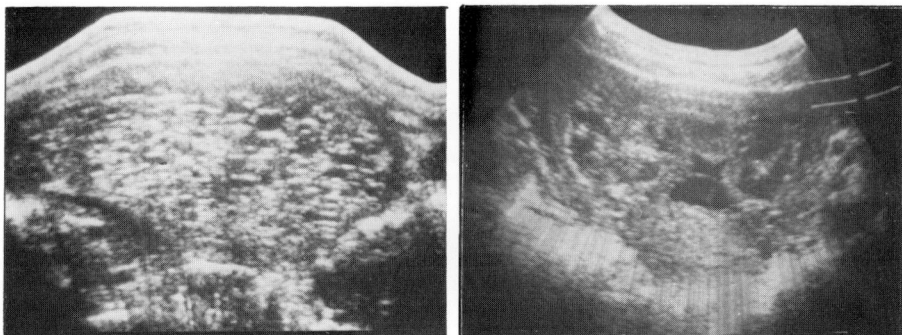

Figure 4. Mola hydatiformis.   Transverse tomogram; amenorrhea of 14 weeks.

Figure 5. Hydropic changes in longstanding missed abortion
(or blighted ovum).   Amenorrhea of 14 weeks; no fetus was
recognized either at the echography or at the curettage.
Transverse tomogram.

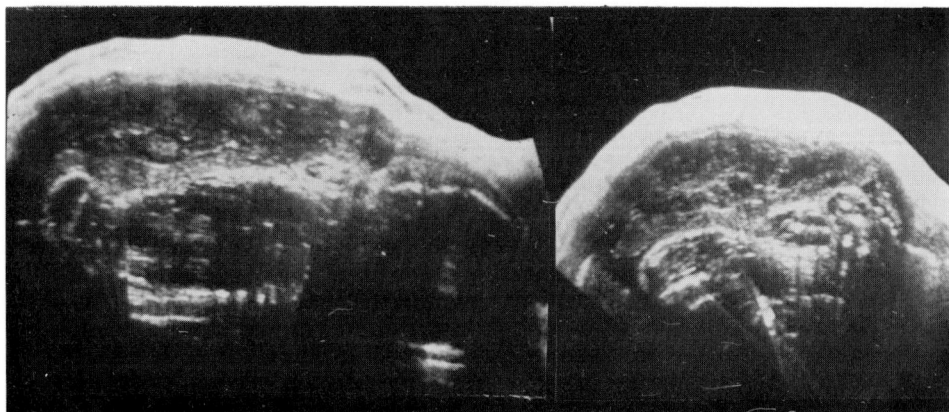

Figure 6. Total placental abruption.   Longitudinal and
transverse tomogram in a pregnancy of 39 weeks with a dead
fetus, showing a total cleavage of the anterior placenta
from the uterine wall by retained blood clots and serum.

tion area, suppose tridimensional estimations. Of the two appropriate methods, namely integration of serial tomograms (1,11), and calculations with approximative formulae (5,12), the first one is definitely the most accurate. Recent technical facilities, such as light pen and digital computer programs, will enable to apply the integration method in more large scale research projects and in routine clinical situations.

TISSUE CHARACTERISTICS

The normal developmental stages of the placenta can be recognised from the trophoblastic shell and the chorion frondosum until the term and postterm placenta. Some already clinically accepted applications of tissue typing and pattern recognition in related conditions should be mentioned : abruption of the placenta (Fig. 6), intramural and submucous myomata, local uterine contractions, hydatiform mole (Fig. 4), hydropic changes in blighted ova and missed aboration (Fig. 5), and choriocarcinoma invasion in the uterine wall. With present systems the small grapelike cysts of hydatiform mole can be demonstrated (Fig. 4) in a more realistic way than in the bistable snowstorm image.

With better gray scaling and real time, optimally focused transducers, and higher frequencies, tissue characterisation within the placenta itself has become feasible (2,10,14). It is to be realized that the placenta consists of many different tissues : the placental parenchym is delineated at the fetal side by the chorionic plate from which the fetal stem vessels branch, and at the maternal side by the basal plate with its septa protruding into the parenchym. The parenchym itself consists of the villous trees, grouped in cotyledons, immersed within the intervillous space. Most of the placental changes currently visualised by echography, are not to be situated in the villous trees, but in the other placental structures. There is however evidence from histopathological studies that the villous changes are more closely related to the fetal condition, than the changes in the other placental tissues (3).

One should bear in mind that the present ultrasonographic pulse echo reflection methods produce cross-sectional tomographic views with possible effects of posterior enhancement and shadowing. The maximal axial resolution is function of the wavelength, which is in the order of the resolution capabilities of the human eye - i.e. macroscopic -. The ultrasonographic information is a function of differences in acoustical impedance, while visual information is a function of differences in electromagnetic impedance.

Project on placental tissue typing with ultrasonographic and histological correlations.

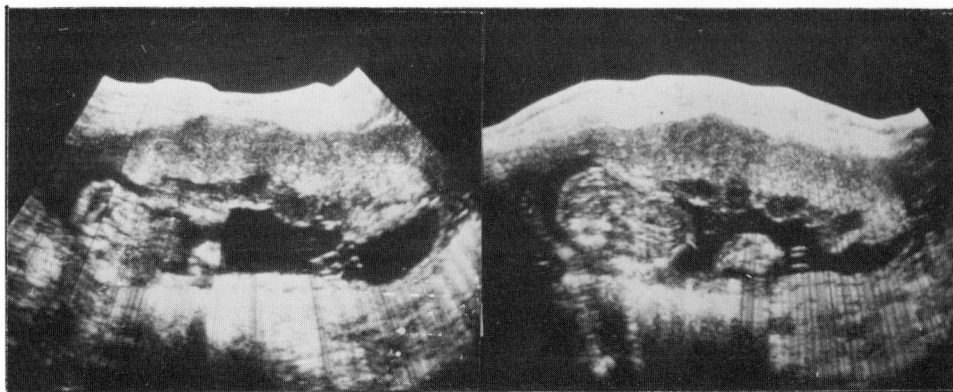

Figure 7. Placenta with subchorionic transsonic area. Longitudinal and transverse tomogram in a pregnancy of 23 weeks; at delivery a large subchorionic fibrin plaque was noted, and confirmed by histology.

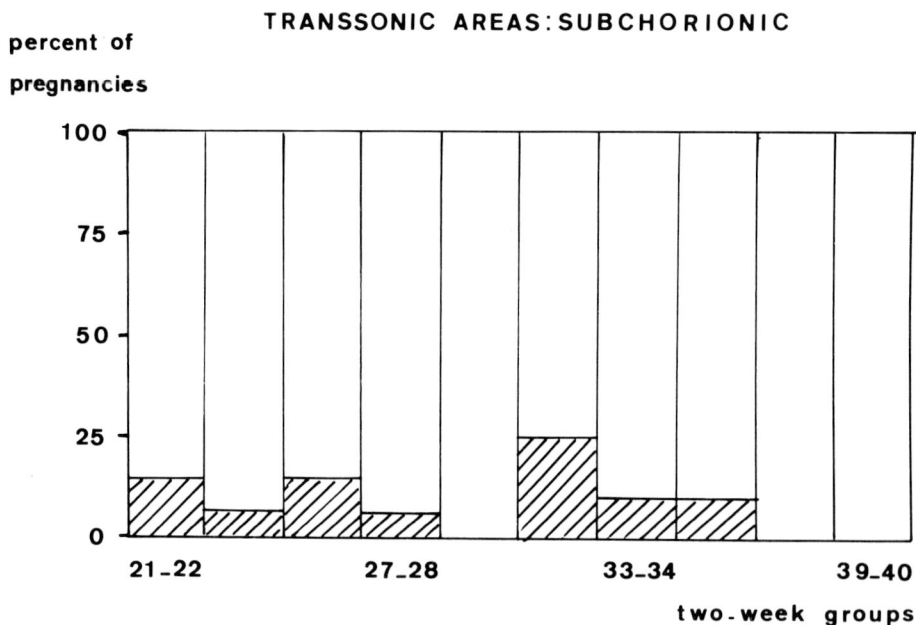

Figure 8. Incidence of subchorionic transsonic areas in the placenta, in a cross-sectional study of 204 normal single pregnancies between 21 and 40 weeks.

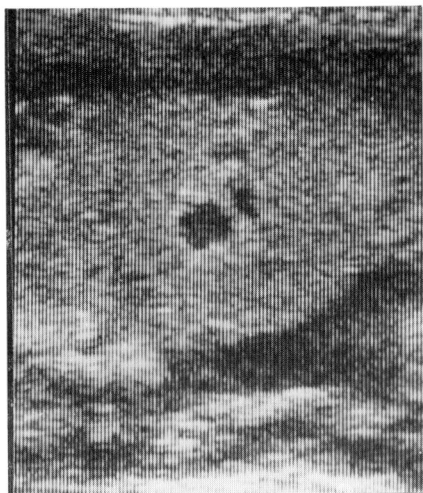
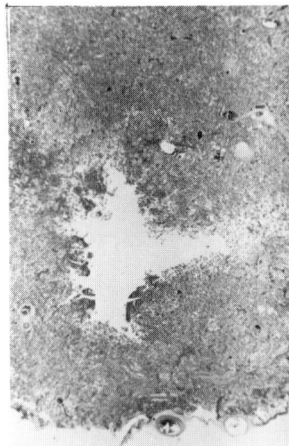

Figure 9. Transsonic areas in the placental parenchym.
Transverse tomogram; pregnancy of 37 weeks.

Figure 10. Histology (hematoxylin-eosin staining) of one of
the transsonic areas in the placenta from Fig. 9, showing
an open intervillous space, surrounded by normal villi.

The aim of a current project is to evaluate the incidence of ultrasonographic changes in placental tissue
characteristics in the second half of normal pregnancy,
and to identify and type some tissue changes - mainly sonodensifications and transsonic areas - by prospective follow-
up, waterbath scanning, and histology of selected areas.

Material and methods.

A cross-sectional study was performed in 204 normal
single pregnancies between 21 and 40 weeks. In each subject two to four tomograms of the placenta were performed
with a compoundB-scanner, Diasonograph NE 4102 - Emisonic -
with PEP 500 scanconverter, with a 3.5 MHz transducer, and/
or with a real time system, Toshiba Sonolayergraph SAL 10,
with a linear electronically focused multielement transducer of 3.5 MHz. Most tomograms were made crossing the
central part of the placenta; when only a real time examination was performed, one tomogram was also made in the
lateral part of the placenta. Since most of the echographic
changes that at present can be visualized, are to be situated in the non-villous compartments, the villous tissue

159

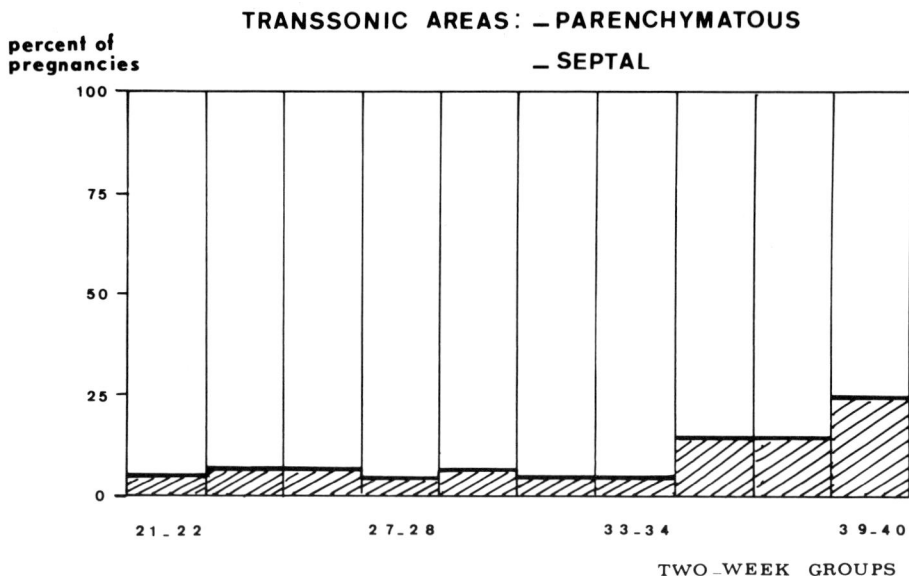

TRANSSONIC AREAS: —PARENCHYMATOUS
— SEPTAL

Figure 11. Incidence of parenchymatous transsonic areas in the placenta, in a cross-sectional study of 204 normal single pregnancies between 21 and 40 weeks.

pattern was used as an internal standard reference medium; the system settings were adapted visually, subjectively, to present always about the same level of medium strong echoes from the villous parenchym. ·

Results

The observations are grouped into three parts, following the geographical distribution and the ultrasonographic appearance : subchorionic transsonic areas, intraplacental transsonic areas, and basal plate and septal sonodensifications.

1) Subchorionic transsonic areas are seen incidentally in about 10 % of normal pregnancies, over the whole second half of pregnancy (Fig. 8). These areas generally correspond with massive subchorial thrombosis or fibrin plaques (Fig. 7). On two occasions, but not in this series a cytotrophoblastic cyst was found. Large blood vessels can be seen frequently in the chorionic plate; a subamniotic hemorrhage should sometimes be considered.

2) Intraplacental transsonic areas are occasionally found, in about 5 % of pregnancy, between 21 and 34 weeks; they are observed more frequently in the last six weeks of pregnancy (Fig. 9), the frequency going up to 25 % by term

160

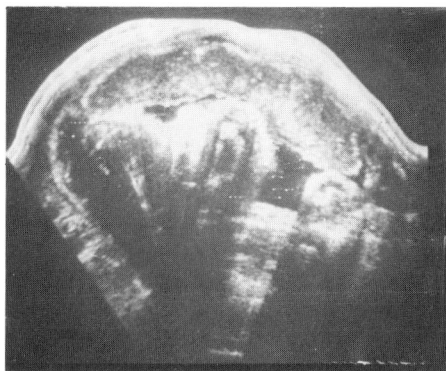

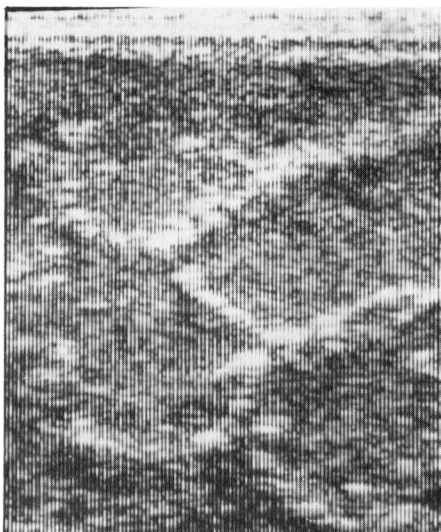

Figure 12. Sonodensifications in the placental basal plate.
Pregnancy of 39 weeks; transverse tomogram of anterior
placenta.

Figure 13. Sonodensification of the placental basal plate
and septa. Pregnancy of 37 weeks; transverse tomogram
through a fundal placenta, showing a honey comb-like structure of the intercotyledonary septa.

(Fig. 11); they also tend to become larger; the diameter
can amount up to two cm., so that they are identified more
readily. Histologically (Fig. 10) there is some evidence
that the transsonic areas correspond with small avillous
lakes within the intervillous space, known as "cavernes" and
"plazentar Hohlräume" (13,9); the real time signals are
suggestive of blood flow in these areas. No histological
evidence was found until now that these areas correspond
with fresh intervillous thrombosis or Kline's hemorrhage
(4). The possibilities of septal cysts, and of fresh perivillous fibrin deposition should also be envisaged.
    3)Sonodensifications in the basal plate and septa
(Fig. 12,13,15). In the second trimester of pregnancy it is
often difficult to identify exactly the basal plate because
there is a gradual transition between the stronger villous
echoes and the weaker echoes from the decidualised uterine
wall (Fig. 1). Sonodensifications of the basal plate appear
for the first time at 25 weeks, in 3 % of the subjects;
the incidence and degree gradually increase until 40 weeks
(Fig. 14). Those densifications occurring only marginally

161

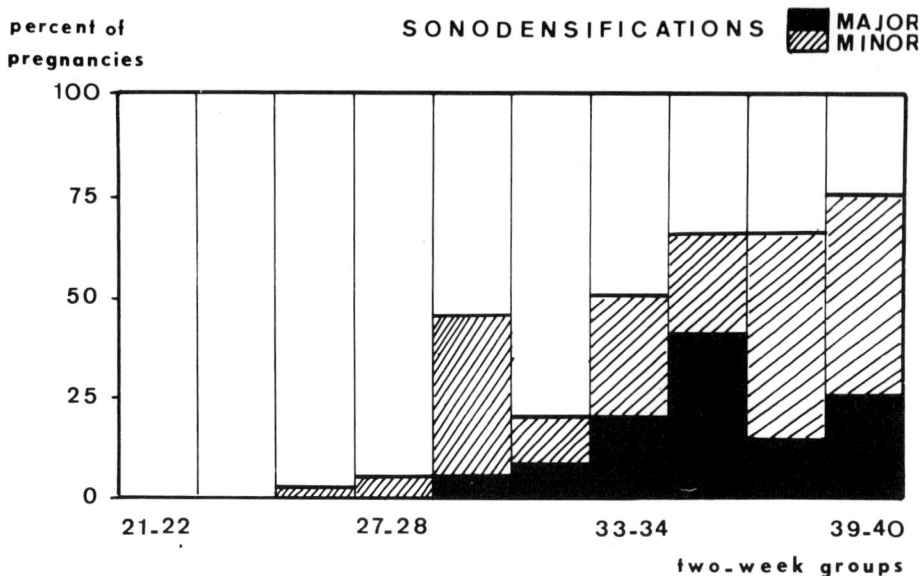

Figure 14. Incidence of sonodensifications in the placental basal plate and septa, in a cross-sectional study of 204 normal single pregnancies between 21 and 40 weeks.

or locally in the basal plate are called minor; those involving the whole basal plate and also very often the septa are called major sonodensifications. Near term major densifications were found in about 25 % of subjects, and minor ones in about 50 %.

Histologically (Fig. 16) the sonodensifications in the basal plate and in the septa correspond to fibrinoid deposits mixed with decidual tissue; they can mostly be differentiated from calcifications which produce shadowing.

In this series no infarctions, large fresh thrombosis, or massive perivillous fibrin deposition were identified prospectively. Some gross lesions were recognised in the delivered placentas, and subsequently scanned in a waterbath with 3.5 and 5.0 MHz transducers. Old infarctions appear slightly less echogenic than normal villous tissue (Fig. 17); fresh red thrombi appear as large sharply delineated transsonic lesions (Fig. 18).

DISCUSSION

The clinical feasibility of tissue typing in the placenta, with current systems, has been demonstrated. The clinical importance of ultrasonic pattern recognition in placental abruption, molar pregnancy and some related con-

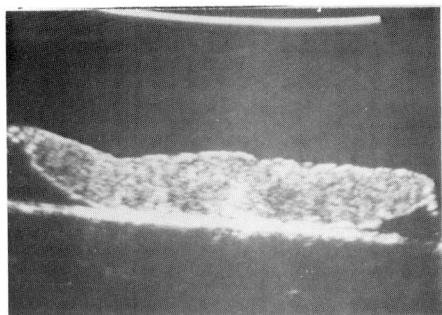

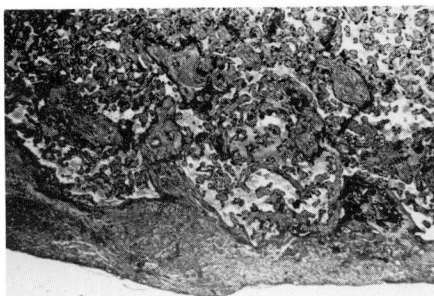

Figure 15. Waterbath scanning of a placenta which - in utero - was showing a sonodensification of the basal plate at
echography, as documented in Fig. 12. The thin sonodense
line at the maternal side (down) represents the basal plate.

Figure 16. Histology (hematoxylin-eosin staining) of a
biopsy from the maternal side of the same placenta as in
Fig. 15, demonstrating the basal plate layer containing
fibrinoid and decidua, as seen at higher magnification.

ditions is already well established.
    Most of the ultrasonic changes observed in the cross-
sectional study, namely in the subchorionic region, intra-
placentally and in the basal plate and septa, are mainly
to be located in the non-villous placental structures; the
significance of these changes is not yet well established.
There is a correlation between some of these changes and
gestational age as demonstrated in this study ; some alter-
rations have been correlated to fetal lung maturation by
the Yale group (5). However in a certain percentage of normal pregnancies without apparent differences in course or
 outcome, these echographic alterations are not observed;
before the correlation with placental function and fetal
condition is clearly demonstrated, it seems preferable not
to employ terms such as "aging" and "maturation" in this
context with too much emphasis.
    The villous tissue changes, which are more closely
linked to the fetal condition (3) are certainly much more
subtle than the ones described here. A major problem in
the assessment of these alterations is the lack of an internal reference standard. Moreover it is apparent that
even with digital computer programs such as histograms,
one will have to differentiate strictly between villous and
non-villous compartments. The in vivo recognition of perivil-

163

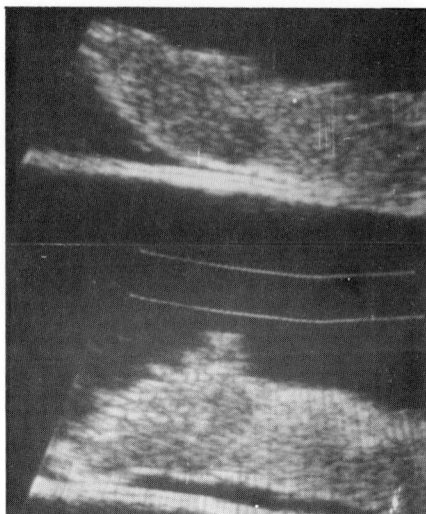

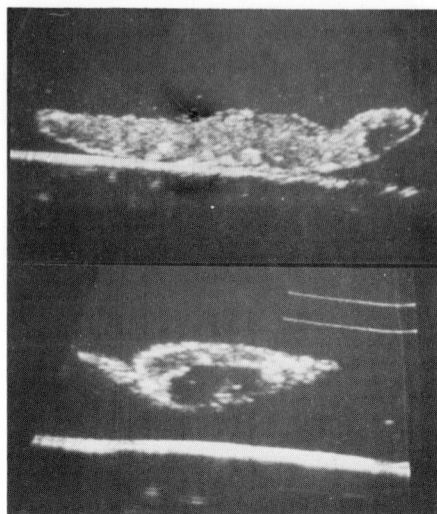

Figure 17. Waterbath scanning of a placenta with an old marginal infarction. Frequency : 5.0 MHz.; the upper scan with chorionic plate up, the lower with chorionic plate down. A slightly less echogenic lesion is shown.

Figure 18. Waterbath scanning of a placenta with a marginal fresh red thrombus. A longitudinal and transverse tomogram with 3,5 MHZ, demonstrate an anechoic, transsonic lesion.

lous fibrin deposition and placental infarctions seems a next important step in placental tissue characterisation.

REFERENCES

1. Bleker, O.P., Kloosterman, G.J., et al. (1977) : Am. J. Ob. Gyn., 127, 657.
2. Fisher, C.C., Garrett, W., Kossoff, G. (1976) : Am. J. Ob. Gyn., 124, 483.
3. Fox, H. (1975) : In : The Placenta and Its Maternal Supply Line, p. 217. Editor : P. Gruenwald, MTP, Lancaster.
4. Fox, H. (1978) : Pathology of the Placenta, p. 129, Saunders, London.
5. Grannum, P.A.T., Berkowitz, R.L., Hobbins, J.C. (1979) Am. J. Ob. Gyn. , 133, 915.
6. Hellman, L.M., Kobayashi, M. et al. (1970) : Am. J. Obst. Gyn., 108, 740.
7. King, D.L., (1973) : Radiology, 109, 167.

8. Kratochwil, A. (1978) : In : Handbook of Clinical Ultrasound, p. 175. Editors : M. De Vlieger, et al., Wiley Medical, New York.
9. Spanner, R. (1935) : Zeitschr. Entwickl., 105, 163.
10. Spirt, B.A., Kagan, E.H., Rozanski, R.M. (1978) : Am. J. Roentg., 131, 961.
11. Terinde, R., Bender, H.G., et al. (1978) : In : Ultraschalldiagnostik, p. 85. Editors : A. Kratochwil, E. Reinold, Thieme Stuttgart.
12. Vandenberghe,K.(1979):In :Proceedings of the 1st. International Berlin Meeting of Perinatal Medicine, In press.
13. Wilkin, P. (1965) : Pathologie du Placenta, p. 16, Masson, Paris.
14. Winsberg, F. (1973) : J. Clin. Ultras., 1, 52.
15. Wladimiroff, J.W., Wallenburg, H.C.S. et et. (1976) : Arch. für Gyn., 221, 167.

ULTRASOUND DIAGNOSIS OF MAJOR FETAL ABNORMALITIES.

Pat Farrant

X-Ray Department, Northwick Park Hospital, Harrow, Middx, U.K.

This paper is a review of our results over the past two years in the ultrasonic diagnosis of major fetal abnormalities. During the period of the study there were 6665 deliveries with an incidence of 11.5 per 1000 major malformations including congenital heart disease and Downs syndrome. Ultrasound was performed on about 4000 of these patients, and in this sub group there were 28 major malformations which ultrasound is theoretically able to detect. We correctly identified 25 of these.

	CORRECTLY DIAGNOSED	MISSED
ANENCEPHALY	7	
HYDROCEPHALY	2	
HYDRANENCEPHALY	1	1
ENCEPHALOCOELE	1	
SPINA BIFIDA	4	
URINARY TRACT OBSTRUCTION	5	
POTTER'S SYNDROME	1	
GASTRO INTESTINAL OBSTRUCTION	2	2
OSTEOPATHIA STRIATA	1	

The ultrasonic appearances of anencephaly and hydrocephaly are now well known (1,3) and I shall mention these cases no further. However, I would like to briefly discuss our technique for scanning the spinal column. It has previously been stated that transverse scans should be performed along the whole length of the spinal canal in order to check its integrity (2), but we now favour longitudinal scans as our routine procedure for visualising the spine. Occasionally the whole spine may be visualised on one single sweep (Figure 1), but it is more usual to have to perform two or three scans along the length of the spine to allow for fetal flexion. All our patients have the spine routinely scanned, and we have found this method reliable and quick. It has been our

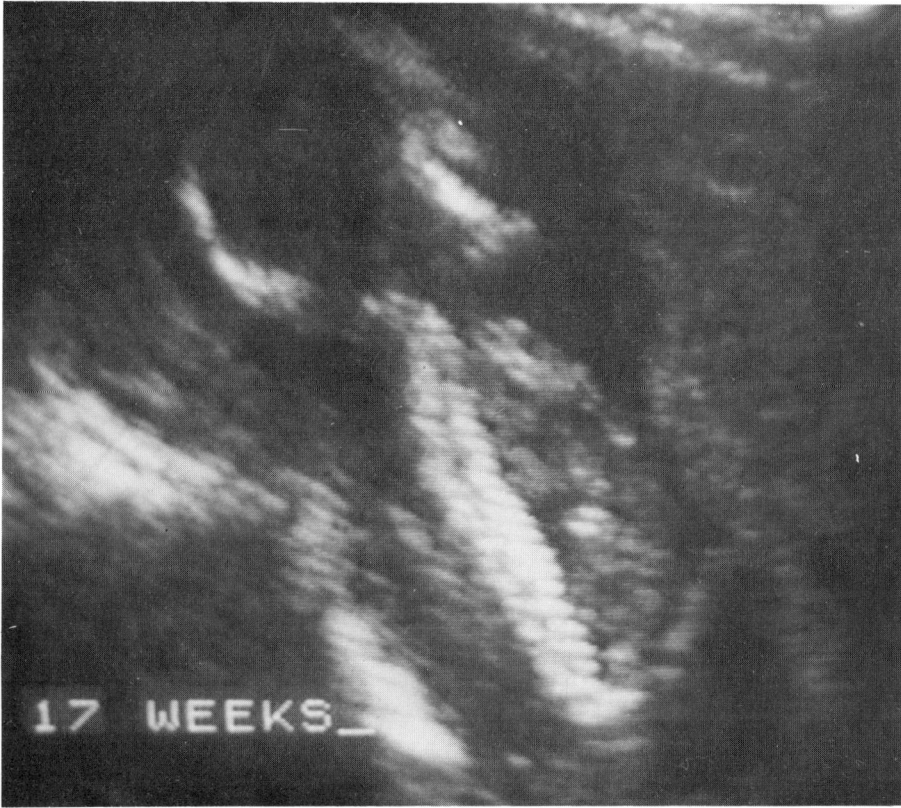

Figure 1 - Longitudinal scan of a normal 17 week fetal spine.

experience that spinal abnormalities are well demonstrated on longitudinal scans. Figure 2 shows a normal thoracic spine with a sudden angulation in the upper lumbar region and absence of the lumbar neural arches, both of which are abnormal findings. An amniocentesis was performed on this patient at the same time as the ultrasound, and the alfa feto protein level was found to be normal. The pregnancy was terminated on ultrasound findings alone, and the aborted fetus exhibited a lumbar spinal defect with an intact meningocoele.

Our first case of hydranencephaly remained undiagnosed by ultrasound as at that time I was unaware of the existence of such a condition, and also inadequate views of the fetal head were obtained as it persistently lay very low in the maternal pelvis.

167

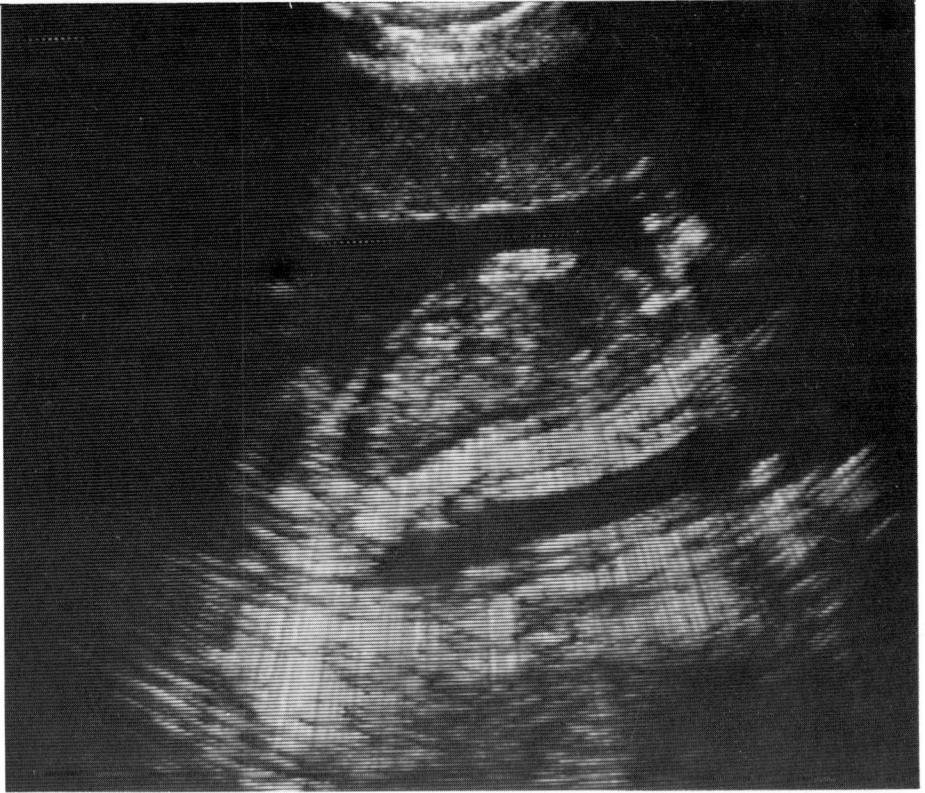

Figure 2 - Longitudinal scan of 19 week fetal spine demonstrating spina bifida.

Figure 3 shows the typical appearance we now associate with this malformation. The fetal skull contains only a small remnant of brain tissue in the middle, the rest of the skull being filled with fluid. The BPD measurements obtained were normal, and a midline echo was observed because the falx is present. The baby was scanned neonatally, and exactly the same appearances were demonstrated as in utero. Since this condition is invariably fatal, it is important to make the diagnosis prenatally as this may help the obstetrician in management of labour.

Ultrasound diagnosis of fetal urinary obstruction has previously been reported (4), and in the last 2 years we have had 5 such patients, 2 with bladder neck obstructions and 3 with obstructed kidneys. Figure 4 is a midline scan showing a breech

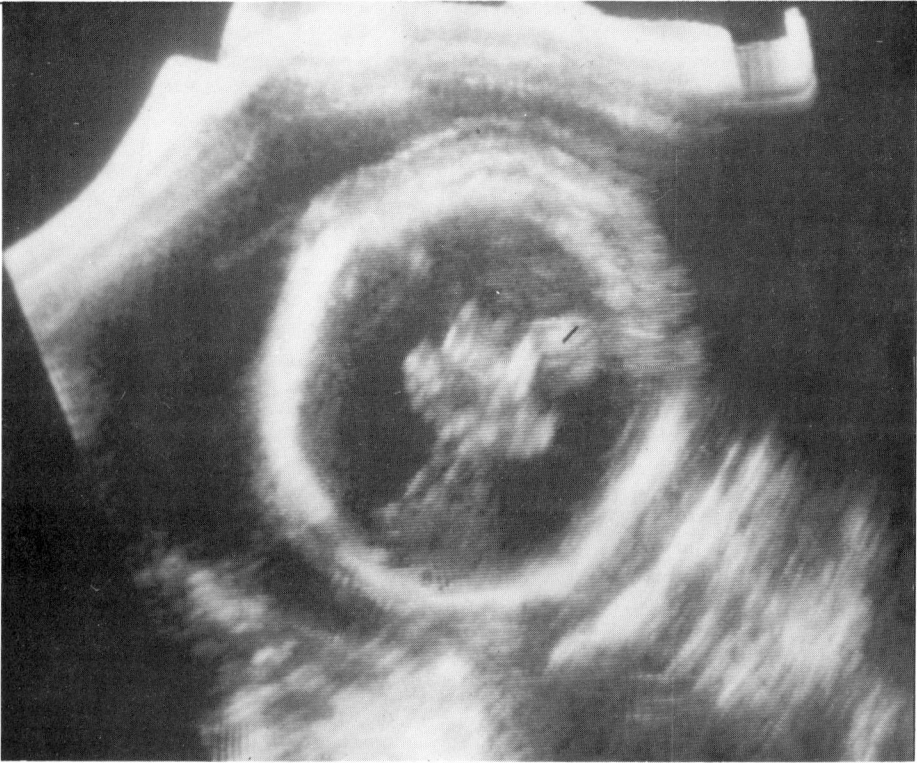

Figure 3 - Transverse scan of fetal head showing hydranencephaly.

fetus with a large cyst in its abdomen and no liquor around it. Our first such case was routinely scanned at 17 weeks and it was thought that the cystic structure might possibly represent an obstructed fetal bladder. The obstetrician in charge of the case decided to perform paracentesis under ultrasound control to obtain some of the fluid for analysis. 40 mls of fluid were drained from the cyst and 2 days later a repeat scan showed that the cyst was smaller and obviously arose from the fetal pelvis. The fetus, however, had developed ascites, and some liquor was also present. A paediatric pathologist was consulted as to the possible outcome of such a case, and the probability of pulmonary hypoplasia was raised. After consultation with the parents it was decided to terminate the pregnancy and the post mortem findings demonstrated a total bladder neck obstruction with associated pulmonary hypoplasia. Our second case was found on a slightly more advanced fetus. The patient was referred at 23 weeks gestational age because of poor weight gain and small uterine size. Figure 4 shows the ultrasound appearance. A dilated ureter was visualised and the kidneys appeared moderately hydronephrotic. Again the cystic structure was catheterised, and a follow up scan two days later showed a smaller cyst, and a minimal quantity of liquor. This pregnancy was allowed to continue, but the patient went into premature labour at 34 weeks, delivering a live baby which subsequently died (20 minutes later) because of pulmonary hypoplasia. Post mortem examination confirmed the presence of bladder neck obstruction and dilated ureters, but the kidneys were shown to be polycystic and not hydronephrotic. Both our patients with complete bladder neck obstruction diagnosed early in pregnancy were confirmed to have severe pulmonary hypoplasia. We therefore consider it reasonable to offer

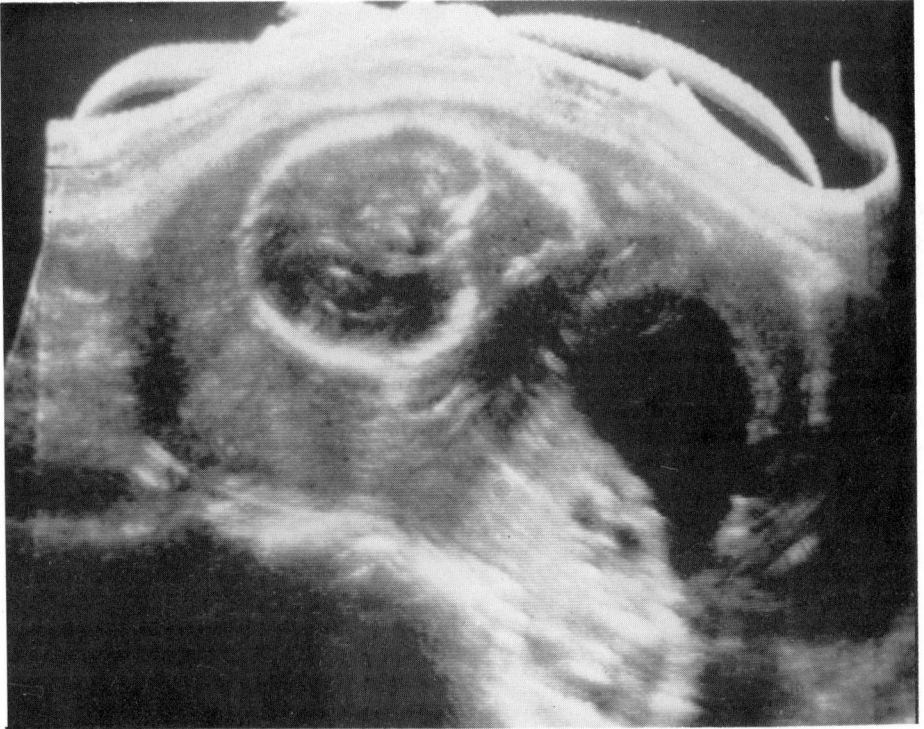

Figure 4 - Midline scan of 23 week fetus with bladder neck obstruction.

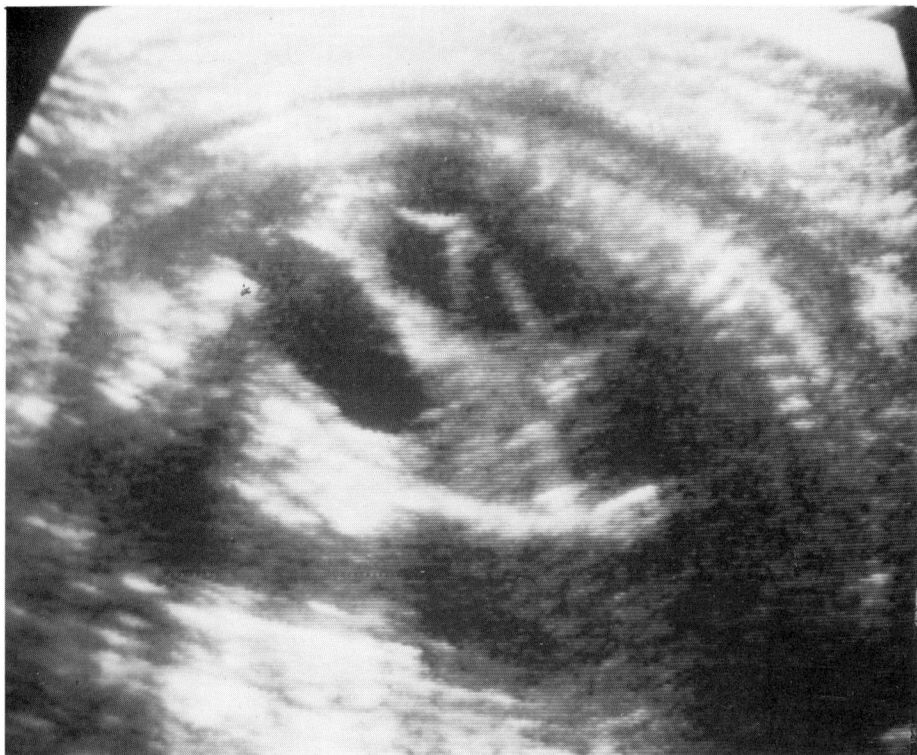

Figure 5 - Longitudinal scan of 34 week fetus with hydronephrosis.

termination of pregnancy to any patients diagnosed as having this condition in future.

Figure 5 shows a longitudinal scan of a 34 week fetus with bilateral hydronephrosis and a dilated bladder. The kidney was catheterised under ultrasound control and an indwelling catheter left in situ to drain the kidney. Follow up scans showed that the kidneys remained slightly hydronephrotic, but the catheter continued draining for the 3 weeks until delivery. The baby had an early post natal operation to relieve a partial bladder neck obstruction, and is now alive and well.

One of our other cases of obstructed kidneys had no post natal follow up as the fetus exhibited only mild hydronephrosis in utero, but our last case with moderate hydronephrosis was scanned post natally, on the day it was born, and subsequently 2 weeks later. The baby had no clinical signs of urinary tract obstruction whatsoever, but the scans showed bilateral hydronephrosis with a dilated bladder on both occasions, and the baby was referred to a paediatric hospital for an intravenous urogram and probable bladder neck surgery.

It is important to make the diagnosis of partial bladder neck obstruction before delivery, to allow corrective surgery before further renal impairment occurs.

Over the past 2 years we have had 4 cases of gastrointestinal obstruction, 2 of which we did not detect. These were both cases of oesophageal atresia and they both had tracheo oesophageal fistulae, a finding which occurs in about 90% of cases of oesophageal atresia

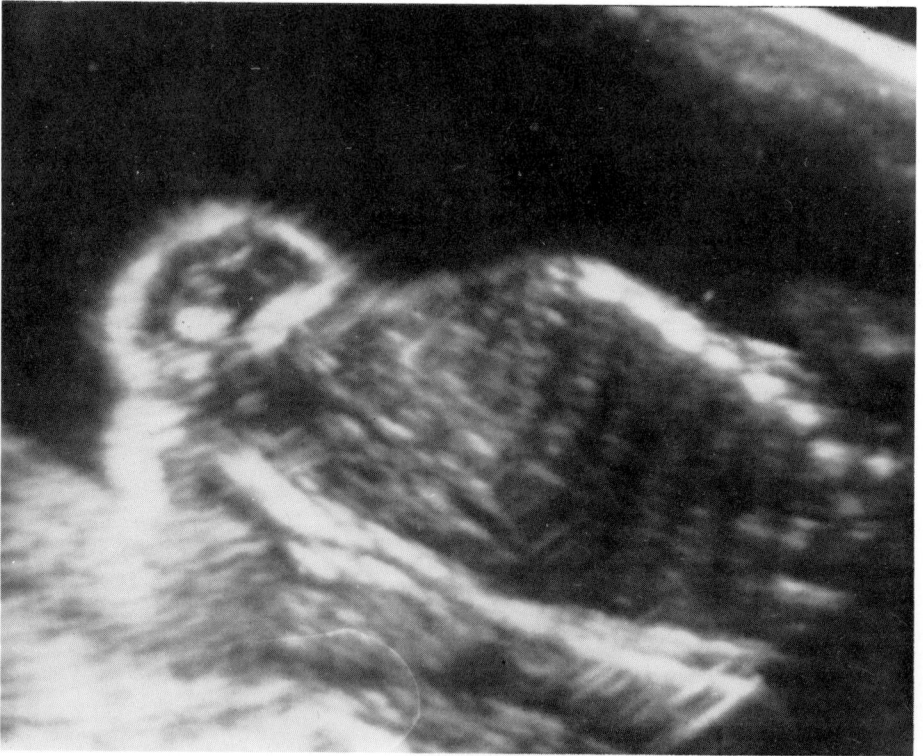

Figure 6 - Longitudinal scan of 27 week fetus with oesophageal and tracheal atresia.

(6). Fluid is therefore able to pass into the fetal stomach and a
normal ultrasonic appearance is obtained. However, in the other 10%
of these cases there is no fistula present and fluid cannot reach the
fetal stomach. We have had one such case recently in a patient
referred because of hydramnios at 27 weeks gestational age, and she
had started to go into spontaneous labour. The fetal spine and head
appeared normal, and Figure 6 shows a longitudinal section of the
fetus in the region of the fetal stomach (which is not visible). We
routinely visualise the fetal stomach as we use it as a land mark for
fetal abdominal circumference measurements, and when no stomach could
be visualised, the diagnosis of oesophageal atresia was made. Labour
continued and a stillborn fetus was delivered which at post mortem
was confirmed to have oesophageal and tracheal atresia.

Our last gastro intestinal obstruction is a case of duodenal
atresia, which clearly shows the "double bubble" sign (5). (Figure 7)
We do not have confirmation of this diagnosis as the patient

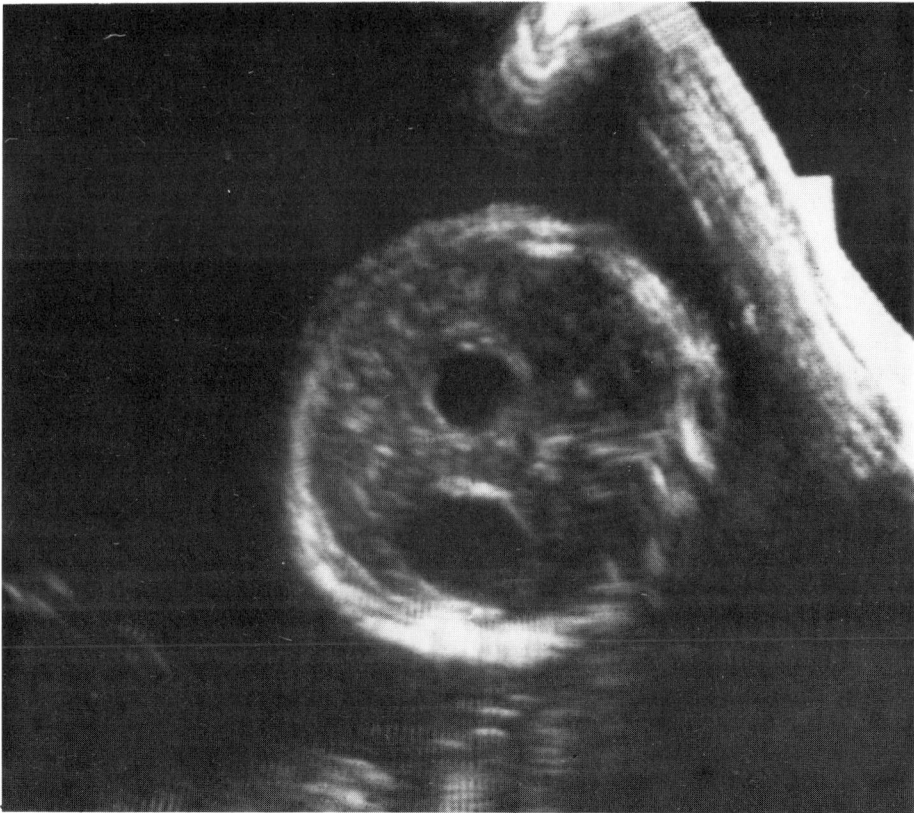

Figure 7 - Transverse scan of 31 week fetus showing duodenal atresia.

has not yet delivered, but the connection between the 2 "bubbles" was demonstrated on oblique scans. Fortunately this condition is able to be surgically corrected and with the prior warning, this may now be performed as soon after birth as is practical.

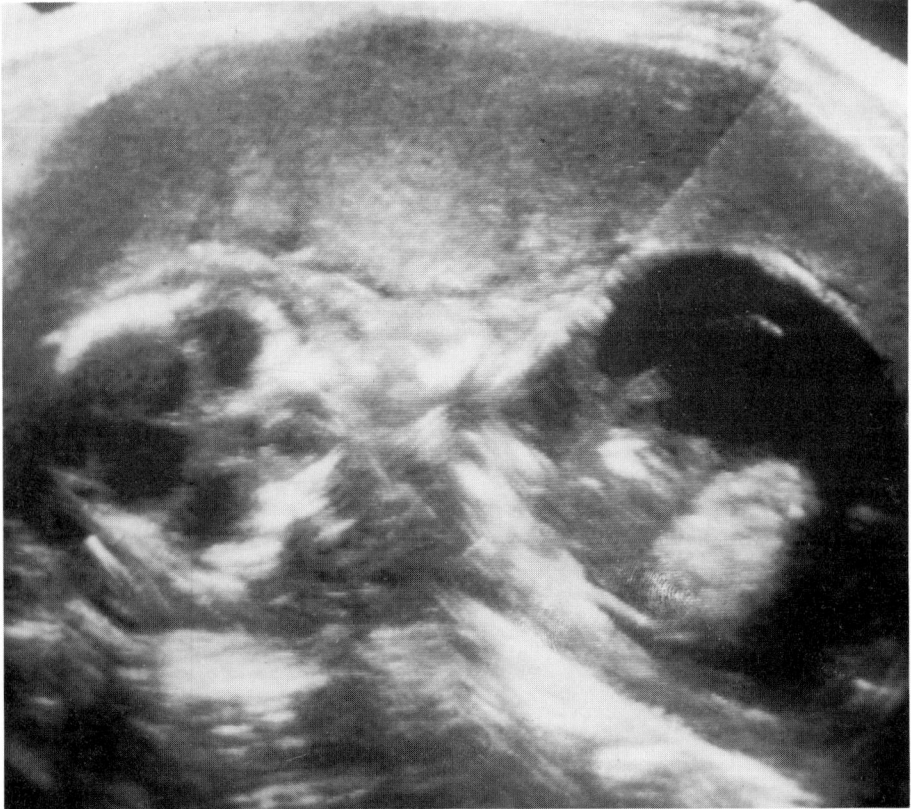

Figure 8 - Longitudinal scan of 31 week fetus with multiple abnormalities.

The last picture (Figure 8) shows a longitudinal scan of a grossly abnormal fetus of 31 weeks gestational age exhibiting multiple congenital abnormalities. It is microcephalic with gross ascites, and the placenta was enormous and very oedematous. We can be of little help in cases such as these as the fetus was too grossly malformed to survive, but it is nevertheless important to make the diagnosis prenatally, as this will help the obstetrician in his management of labour.

We have found that by careful, systematic scanning we have been able to detect 96% of the ultrasonically detectable major fetal abnormalities.

REFERENCES

1. Campbell, S., Holt, E.M., Johnstone, F.D. and May, P. (1972):
   Lancet 2; 1226-7.

2. Campbell, S., Pryse-Davies,J. Cottart, T.M., Seller, M.J. and Singer, J.D. (1975):
   Lancet 2; 1065-1068.

3. Garrett, W.J., Fisher, C.C. and Kossoff, G. (1975):
   Med. J. Aust. 2; 587-9.

4. Garrett, W.J., Kossof, G. and Osborn, R.A. (1975):
   Brit. J. Obst. & Gynae. 82; 115-120.

5. Loveday, B.J., Barr, J.A. and Aitken, J. (1975):
   Brit. J. Radiol. 48; 1031-2.

6. Waterston, D.J., Bonham Carter, R.E. and Aberdeen, E. (1962):
   Lancet 1; 819-822.

FETOSCOPY AND ULTRASOUND SCANNING IN THE PRENATAL DIAGNOSIS OF FETAL LIMB DEFORMITIES

R. Rauskolb and V. Jovanovic

Universitäts-Frauenklinik, Giessen, West Germany

Fetoscopy has been applied diagnostically for 3 years now in the few centres where it is practised and so it could be said to have progressed beyond the experimental stage(3). The technique offers us a clinically valuable method for the early detection or exclusion of outwardly visible fetal malformations not accompanied by chromosomal defects.

Fetoscopy is generally indicated wherever there is a risk of fetal deformations severe enough to justify termination of the pregnancy (1,2). On the other hand, it is performed often enough with the aim of preventing an abortion already planned on the basis of a calculated risk, dispelling the parents' doubts and giving them new hope in a future with children.

INDICATIONS FOR FETAL EXAMINATION

The indications which have so far given us occasion to apply fetoscopy diagnostically are shown in Table 1.

TABLE 1. DIAGNOSTIC INDICATIONS FOR FETAL VISUALIZATION

Indication	No. of Fetoscopies
Limb deformities	13
Congenital syndromes	9
Cleft lip and palate	7
Neural tube defects	6
Others	3
Total	38

First of all there are 13 cases with increased risk of extremital deformation. Examples of what one could call "classical" indications are severe congenital syndromes, especially those obligatorily accompanied by clearly visible anomalies, in themselves apparently harmless. The remaining indications involved risk of recurrence of cleft lip and palate, whereby the particular circumstances surrounding each case and the personal situation of the parents were major considerations. For the prenatal diagnosis of neural tube defects fetoscopy was only applied in individual cases, where borderline AFP-levels made interpretation

somewhat difficult (2 cases to date) or where it is important to obtain final confirmation of a suspected anencephaly
without the time-loss involved in determining the AFP-con-
centration in the amniotic fluid (4 cases to date).

RESULTS WITH FETOSCOPY

Small-scale limb deformities

The limb deformities in question were in 7 out of 13
cases small-scale disturbances in the formation of hands
and feet, such as pero-, poly- and syndactyly or lobster
deformations present in the family (Table 2).

TABLE 2. SMALL-SCALE LIMB DEFORMITIES

Sort of Malformation	No. of Fetoscopies
Pero-. Poly- Syndactyly	5
Lobster deformations (hands and feet)	2
Total	7

These smaller-scale extremital malformations are mostly
disturbances with increased risk of recurrence but in themselves not too debilitating. In 5 out of a total of 7 cases
we could exclude the possibility of morphological anomalies
by means of fetoscopy. All of these children were born healthy with no sign of abnormality. Once the fetoscopy revealed bilateral syndactyly of the toes, where a 50% probability of lobster hands and feet had been calculated on the
grounds of this being present in the natural father and the
first-born child. The pregnancy ended with a premature birth
in the 31st week of gestation and the observed syndactyly was
fully confirmed. In the 4th diagnostic fetoscopy we ever performed, we failed to detect a syndactyly of the hand (1)- the
3rd and 4th fingers of one hand are cutaneously connected -
because the palmar side of both hands could only be judged
endoscopically with the fingers bent.

Large-scale limb deformities

We hoped to be able to exclude large-scale limb deformities by fetoscopy in 6 cases. The individual malformations in
question are shown in Table 3. Two of these were special cases
in which it was theoretically possible that indefinable disturbances in the development of the fetal extremities had resulted from outside influences. One of these special cases involved a young patient whose pregnancy continued in spite of
a curretage in the first weeks. Here the patient's fears culminated in the belief that a leg or arm had been damaged as a
result of the intervention. Sadly, it did then come to an
abortion following a premature rupture of the membrane in the
25th week, 8 weeks after the fetoscopy. In the other case,
abortion occurred 4 weeks after the intervention, the patient
having taken high doses of oestrogen in the form of a "morn-

ing-after pill" in early pregnancy.

In such cases of possible large-scale limb deformities the parents fear are often quite disproportionate to the usually low risk of recurrence. The very thought of a dysmelia becomes a nightmare for them. Such was the case, for example, with the parents of a child with an aplasia of the right arm (1,2) or with a family in which the father himself had a marked foreshortening of the lower (Fig 1) and left upper extremities due to a femur-fibula-ulna complex. With the exception of the 2 abortions already mentioned, the remaining 4 cases have all culminated in the birth of a healthy child.

Congenital syndromes

Seven of a total of 9 syndromes for which we performed fetoscopy also included specific limb deformities which served as important indicators for diagnosis. Five of these were small-scale disturbances in the formation of a hand or foot, such as the poly(syn)dactyly belonging to the Ellis van Creveld, Laurence-Moon-Biedl-Bardet, Meckel-Gruber and Mohr syndrome. The typical deformations arising out of the Holt-Oram or the Hanhart syndrome, on the other hand, already belong to the large-scale limb deformities. Five children have so far been born healthy.

TABLE 3.   LARGE-SCALE LIMB DEFORMITIES

Sort of Malformation	No. of Fetoscopies
Amelia, Peromelia	3
Femur-Fibula-Ulna-Complex	1
Limb deformities caused by	
- curettage in early pregnancy?	1
- high dosage of oestrogen?	1
Total	6

RESULTS WITH ULTRASOUND-SCANNING

The very success of fetoscopy in the prenatal diagnosis of large-scale limb deformities led us to start using the ultrasound diagnosis which was anyway an integral part of the fetoscopic technique (2,4,) as a less troublesome diagnostic alternative in its own right. Since we began seriously trying to judge fetal extremities in all ultrasound examinations carried out between the 15th and 20th week of pregnancy, we have been surprised to find how often this has been possible. On the basis of this experience, we have since been able in 4 cases (Table 4) to dispense altogether with the fetoscopy originally planned, after a careful ultrasound exploration had revealed diagnostically satisfactory results. In all cases the feared fetal limb deformities could be ruled out.

Twice it was a question of a peromelia, which in one case was recurrent in the family and in the other had appeared in the first child of a couple who are incidently colleagues of ours. Finally, in the 3rd and 4th cases, the first child had a bilateral micromelia and   foreshortening of the left lower leg.

TABLE 4. INDICATIONS FOR ULTRASOUND-SCANNING

Sort of Malformation	No. of cases
Peromelia, unilateral (arm)	2
Micromelia, bilateral (arm)	1
Dysmelia, unilateral (leg)	1
Total	4

In principle, we always aim at performing a first ultrasound exploration between 14 and 16 weeks' gestation with at least one follow-up a week or two later. The ultrasound inspection is first of all carried out by 2 examiners separately, whereby the whole procedure should, if possible, be recorded on videotape so that it can be interpreted jointly afterwards. It is in any case beneficial if a Compound- and a Real-time Scanner can be used in combination. In the 4 cases just mentioned, pregnancy is still in progress.

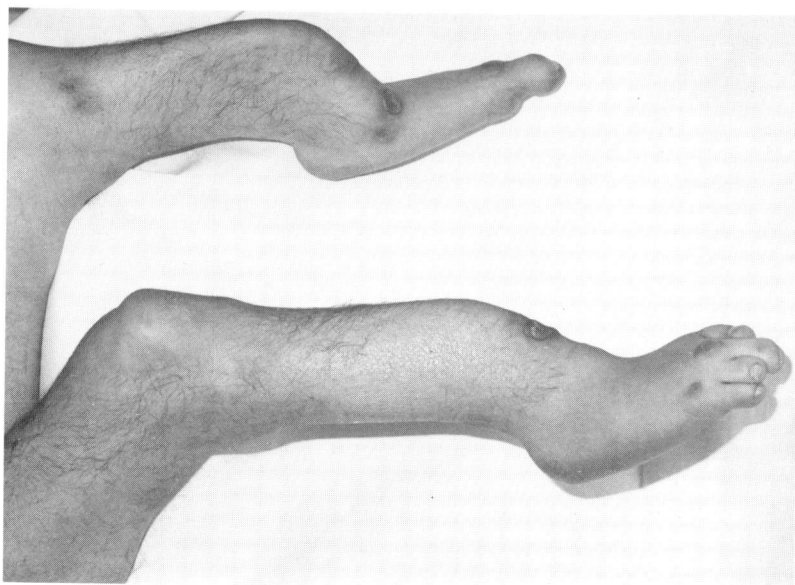

Fig. 1. Limb deformities of the natural father. Foreshortening of the lower extremities combined with a reduction deformity of the left arm (Femurfibula-ulna comples). Photo: Genetische Beratungsstelle Mainz.

179

DISCUSSION

Looking back on the 6 fetoscopies described earlier in the section on large-scale limb deformities, we would today have tried to replace at least two with an ultrasound diagnosis aimed specifically at ruling out the deformations in question, in both cases an aplasia of one arm. Two other cases may be seen as borderline cases, especially the limb deformity in the natural father already mentioned (Fig.1). Paradoxical as it sounds, the particularly serious femur-fibula complex is not striking enough to be identified with certainty in an ultrasound diagnosis. The legs are clearly foreshortened, but as this applies equally to both sides, the reduction deformity and indeed the completely crippled legs are hardly or not at all distinguishable in an ultrasound inspection. Such was the case here, where our preliminary attempt at ultrasound diagnosis produced unsatisfactory results and we decided to go ahead with the fetoscopy as planned. The child in question was born healthy and came for a follow-up examination only a few weeks ago.

The use of modern ultrasound equipment is gaining in clinical relevance also for the prenatal diagnosis of large-scale limb deformities (aplasia). It remains to be seen in the course of many more applications to what extent inspection of the fetus by ultrasound is in a position to replace a fetoscopy or to supplement the incomplete diagnosis of a fetoscopy impeded by turbid or bloodstained amniotic fluid. Small-scale disturbances in the formation of hands or feet, particularly where these are expected as indicators of a syndrome, should,however, still be inspected with the fetoscope.

REFERENCES

1. Fuhrman, W.(1979): In: J.D. Murken, S. Stengel-Rutkowski, E. Schwinger (Eds.) Prenatal Diagnosis. Proceedings of the 3rd European Conference on Prenatal Diagnosis of Genetic Disorders. Enke, Stuttgart, 205.
2. Rauskolb, R., W. Fuhrmann (1978): Die Fetoskopie (Übersicht). Z. Geburtsh. Perinat. 182, 243.
3. Rauskolb, R.(1979): Regoscopy in Western Europe-- A short preliminary survey (Group report). In: J.D. Murken, S. Stengel-Rutkowski, E. Schwinger (Eds.). Prenatal Diagnosis. Proceedings of the 3rd European Conference on Prenatal Diagnosis of Genetic Disorders. Enke, Stuttgart, 193.
4. Rauskolb, R. (1979): Fetoscopy-A new endoscopic approac Endoscopy, 2, 107.

ULTRASONIC ASSESSMENT OF POLYHYDRAMNIOS

P.Kirkinen

Department of Obstetrics and Gynaecology, University of Oulu,
Finland

Polyhydramnios is associated with very well known perinatal
hazards. (1,2,3,4,5). Therefore early antenatal diagnosis and
follow-up is important. A qualitative ultrasonic and clinical
diagnosis of this condition is easy in unambiguous cases, but
the quantification is still much more difficult.

The purpose of this work was to quantify the ultrasonic findings in polyhydramnios-pregnancies, to ascertain their prognostic significance and to evaluate the ultrasonic parameters
suitable for follow-up of these pregnancies.

Patients

The material consisted of 31 patients, in whom polyhydramnios
was suspected clinically during the last one and a half years.
The diagnosis of polyhydramnios was verified in 18 patients
at the delivery, in whom the amount of amniotic fluid measured
immediately after discision or rupture of the fetal membranes
was over 2 liters (polyhydramnios-group). In 13 cases the
amount of amniotic fluid measured upon delivery was greater
than normal, but exact measurement either was not done because of gradual discharge of the fluid or yielded a result
of 1 - 2 liters (borderline-group). A series of 74 normal
pregnancies was used as a control series. Multiple pregnancies
and pregnancies with unknown gestational age were excluded.

The average time of entering the follow-up shedule was the
31,4th gestational week in the polyhydramnios-group and the
32,6th week in the borderline-group.

The clinical data of the different series are presented in the
table 1.

Method

An ultrasonic examination was performed weekly. The following
parameters were evaluated: fetal position, fetal structure
with successive transverse scans, biparietal diameter,anterior-

posterior and transverse diameter of the fetal body at the
vena umbilicalis level, length of the uterine cavity, its mid-
point breadth and its mid-point height (anterior-posterior
diameter of uterine cavity). The placenta was measured for its
mid-point thickness and the length and breadth of the chorioi-
dal plate. Uterine volume was calculated by means of ellipsoid
approximation and placental volume by means of the equation for
the volume of planoconvex object. The ratio between the uterine
volume and the mean of fetal body anterior-posterior and transverse diameter was calculated (cm3/cm). The values obtained for
the normal pregnancies on the corresponding weeks were used as
the reference.

Results

Dimensions and fetal position in the last measurement

Biparietal diameter was below - 2 SD level or could not be
measured because of anomalies or abnormal head positions in
27,8% of the polyhydramnios-group and in 15,4% of the borderline-cases. The mean of the fetal body diameters was above
+ 2 SD level in 22,2% of the polyhydramnios-cases and in 30,8%
of the borderline-group. The uterine volume was in 94,4% of
the polyhydramnios-group above the + 2 SD, as it was in 53,8%
of the borderline-cases. Placental volume was between the normal mean + 2 SD in 88,9% and 92,3%, respectively.

The uterine dimension, which differed most from the normal was
uterine anterior-posterior diameter, which was on average 37,7%
greater in the polyhydramnios-group than the control group. The
similar difference was found in uterine length, on average
15,5%, and in uterine breadth 14,1%. The borderline-group showed the same tendency. Breech or transverse positions were
noted in 44,4% of the polyhydramnios-group and in 15,4% of the
borderline-group.

Growth of ultrasonic parameters and alteration of fetal
position

The growth of the uterine volume varied greatly in the polyhydramnios-group being on average 765 cm3/week (table 2). In
one case the calculated volume even transiently declined during
the follow-up. The increase in the biparietal diameter was on
average greater, but in the body diameters smaller in the polyhydramnios-group compired with normal, while in the borderline-
group the body dimension on average increased more rapidly than
normal. Individual variations were great. During the follow-up
examinations the fetal presentation changed in 22,2% of the
polyhydramnios-cases, compared to 13,5% normally during the
whole third trimester of pregnancy.

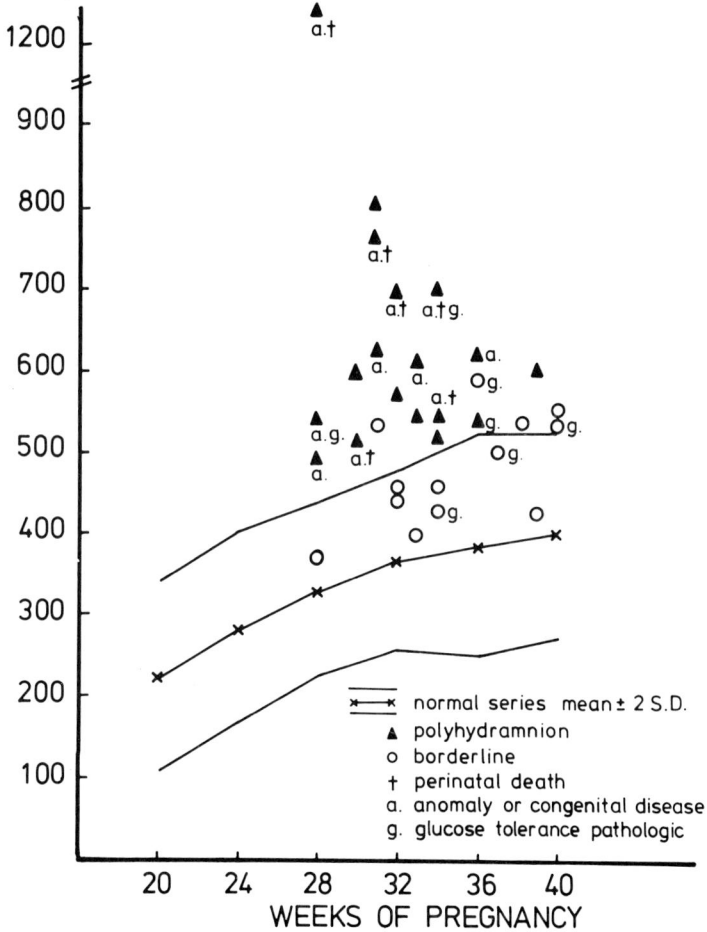

Figure 1. The ratio between uterine volume and fetal body diameter (the mean of fetal body anterior-posterior and transverse diameters at vena umbilicalis level).

Fetal anomalies

The ultrasonic examination revealed the cranial anomalies, the duodenal atresy and the sacrococcygeal teratoma in the material. The fetus with chloride diarrhoea was ultrasonically found to have distented loops of the bowel and large, apparently fluid-filled areas in the abdominal cavity. The fetus with Rhesus-incompatibility was found to have ascites, and ascites was noted in one case with cardiac anomaly.

Ratio between uterine volume and fetal body dimension

The figure 1 shows the ratios between uterine volume and the mean of fetal body diameters in the polyhydramnios- and border-line-groups during the last measurement. The cases with a great ratio frequently involved perinatal death. The cases with anomalies or congenital diseases were quite evenly distributed over the + 2 SD curve of the normal material. The cases with pathologic glucose tolerance were either in the normal range or slightly above it.

Discussion and conclusions

Our results confirmed that polyhydramnios is both ultrasonically and clinically a marked heterogenous condition. This was expected, when we know how various is the etiology of this complication. (1,5). Out of the uterine dimensions, the anterior -posterior diameter increased most clearly, and obviously among the single parameters it reveals this condition best. Uterine volume and fetal dimensions are indicative of fetal risks, high values being associated with perinatal death. The fetal anomalies, however, are not necessarily associated with a finding of an exceptionally great uterine volume, and apparently do not correlate directly with the amount of amniotic fluid. It is evident that the ratio of uterine volume to fetal body dimension appears suitable and sufficiently simple parameter for routine-like follow-up of women with suspected polyhydramnios, provided that placental hypertrophy, which is a rare condition, is excluded.

Table 1. The clinical data of the different series. Mean ± SD.

	Polyhydramnios	Borderline	Control series
N	18	13	74
Maternal age (years)	25,4 ± 10,5	29,8 ± 5,9	27,2 ± 6,4
Parity	2,9 ± 2,3	2,5 ± 1,7	2,2 ± 1,5
Week of delivery	34,3 ± 3,2	37,8 ± 1,7	39,9 ± 1,2
Weight of baby (g)	2389 ± 924	3433 ± 640	3604 ± 421
Weight of placenta (g)	679 ± 254	680 ± 229	655 ± 95
Apgar score (1 min)	4,1 ± 3,5	9,1 ± 0,9	8,6 ± 1,3
Perinatal mortality (	33,3	0	0
Fetal anomalies (%)	44,4	0	0
Pathologic glucose tolerence (%)	16,7	30,8	0

Table 2. Weekly growth of the most important ultrasonic parameters (mean ± SD) and the alteration in the fetal position during the follow-up.

Measured parameter	Polyhydramnios	Borderline	Control series (Mean of the last trimester values)
Uterine volume (cm^3/week)	765 ± 906	290 ± 198	174 ± 25
Biparietal diameter (cm/week)	0,21 ± 0,15	0,14 ± 0,08	0,18 ± 0,05
Body mean diameter (cm/week)	0,24 ± 0,23	0,39 ± 0,12	0,34 ± 0,07
Alteration in the fetal position (%)	22,2	15,3	13,5

References

1) Kirkinen P., Jouppila P.: Polyhydramnion. A clinical study. Ann. Chirurg. Gynaecol. 67: 117, 1978

2) Kirkinen P.: Estimation of the severity of polyhydramnion by ultrasonic examination. 6th Nordiska Kongressen for Perinatal Medicin. Abst.No 30, Oulun Yliopiston monistuskeskus, Oulu 1977

3) Kurjak A.: Direct ultrasonic diagnosis of fetal malformations and abnormalities. In: Recent advances in ultrasound diagnosis. (ed. Kurjak A.) International congress series 436:209. Excerpta Medica, 1978.

4) Kirkinen P.: Intrauterine growth followed ultrasonically in normal and some complicated pregnancies. Ann.Chirurg. Gynaecol. 68: suppl.194, 1979

5) Wallenburg H.C.S., Wladimiroff J.W.: The amniotic fluid. II Polyhydramnios and oligohydramnios. J.Perinat. Med. 6:233, 1977

7. ULTRASONIC ASSESSMENT OF FETAL CARDIO-VASCULAR FUNCTIONS. PHYSIOLOGY AND CLINIC

G. Gennser, Chairman

ULTRASONIC ASSESSMENT OF FETAL CARDIOVASCULAR FUNCTIONS.
PHYSIOLOGY AND CLINIC —— INTRODUCTION

G. Gennser

Department of Obstetrics and Gynecology, University
Hospital, Malmö, Sweden

> Without the special apparatus
> that is constructed mainly
> for anticipated functions,
> the results that lead ulti-
> mately to novelty could not
> occur.
>
> Thomas S. Kuhn: The Structure
> of Scientific Revolutions
> (1962)

In view of the present rapid development of methods
for antenatal investigations, it is appropriate to re-
collect that the human fetus and its cardiovascular system
have very long been beyond reach of our diagnostic capacity. In 1651, William Harvey, in his "Exercitationes de
Generatione Animalium", posed the since-famous question:
how does the fetus survive in utero during the last months
of gestation without obvious respiration? (1). Only 100
years ago (1876), the experiments performed by the young
Swiss obstetrician Paul Zweifel unequivocally demonstrated
that the fetus respires via the placenta and that it con-
sumes the oxygen carried to its tissues (2). The Harvey
Question and its answer have been said to open up the
modern study of fetal physiology, and they also pointed to
the problem of transportation and distribution of respiratory gases within the fetus. The cardiovascular function
before birth was touched upon in 1670 by Boyle, who reported the longer survival in asphyxia of kittens compared
with adult animals (3). Much later, it was shown that one
factor pertinent to the extraordinary ability of the fetus
and the newborn to withstand oxygen deprivation was the
glycogen content of the fetal heart (4). Thus, Boyle's
report, very early indicating an important feature of the
fetal heart, anticipated by several hundred years the
current interest in the fetal cardio-vascular field. The
time relation of the fetal heart beats has been an information available on human cardiac dynamics, since de
Kergaradec initiated in the early 19th century the auscultation of the fetal heart tones (5). However, until
recently, the fetal heart rate, in prenatal care, has

served mainly as an unspecific parameter of fetal well-being or compromise.

Studies on animals, such as the classic angiographic investigations of Barclay, Franklin and Prichard in ex-teriorized fetal lambs (7) clarified the specific features of fetal blood flow in the major vascular channels. The relative inaccessibility of the human fetus and ethical considerations have previously restricted studies on the human fetus to static observations on structures or to occasional investigations on a living previable fetus.

Our ability to evaluate the fetus in its intrauterine environment has significantly increased during the past few decades. Ultrasound was introduced as a method for investigating cardiac dynamics by Edler and Hertz in 1954 (6), and later this technique was applied to infants and, recently, to fetuses. The use of diagnostic ultrasound in examinations of the fetus was facilitated by its non-invasive character and by the absence of reported adverse effects on the fetus. Moreover, physical factors make the fetus, surrounded by amniotic fluid and lacking air in its lungs, a favourable ultrasound target with a large "window" for approach. Doppler ultrasound technique in diagnostic cardiotocography is one example of the rapid utilization of ultrasound in antenatal clinical work.

An increasing number of methods for studying fetal circulatory dynamics now include ultrasound. This section reports three recently developed applications.

Fetal echocardiography visualizes and quantifies the dynamic behaviour of the heart walls and valves. The two investigations on this subject both use multi-element scanners to orientate and pin-point details of the target in a cross-sectional image of the heart. The cardiac structures are then recorded by a single ultrasound beam and a TM-mode presentation.

Apart from giving the physiological range of fetal cardiodynamics, one paper reports the transitional changes at birth and estimates the myocardial contractility. In-formation on the contractile state of the fetal heart is also gained, in the third study, by measuring some of the electromechanical intervals from simultaneously recorded fetal ECG and Doppler scanning of the heart.

The second part of this section deals with blood flow measurements in the large fetal vessels. During recent years, flow velocity in superficial vessels has been measured by continuous Doppler devices. The calculation of flow is dependent on a thorough knowledge of the geometry of the particular vessel, which fact has long prevented the utilization of this method in deeper structures, such as the fetus in utero. The combination of a B-mode scan-ning with a pulsed Doppler technique makes it possible to localize a fetal vessel and, by measuring its diameter and the flow velocity, to estimate the blood flow. The last two reports give an account of the very recent data, which have been obtained by different solutions of this measuring problem. Both groups of authors report their results of recording the flow in the umbilical vein. The Norwegian equipment, including a contact scanner, allows quantification also of the higher flow velocities occurring in the fetal aorta: this has not been possible by the Australian water-bath scanner, whose transmission distance of the ultrasound beam is longer which physically limits the detection of Doppler shift frequencies.

The technological accent of this section presenting application of new electronic techniques should not conceal the fact that the following presentations are produced in the true spirit of pioneers in cardiovascular physiology.

REFERENCES

1. Harvey, W. (1651): Exercitationes de Generatione Animalium, London.
2. Zweifel, P. (1876): Arch. Gynaek., 9, 291.
3. Boyle, R. (1670): Phil. Trans. R. Soc., 5, 2011.
4. Dawes, G.S., Mott, J.C. and Shelley, H.J. (1959): J. Physiol., 146, 516.
5. De Kergaradec, L.: Mémoire sur L'auscultation Appliquée à L'étude de la Grossesse.
6. Edler, I. and Hertz, C.H. (1954): Kungl. Fysiogr. Sällsk. Lund Förhandl., 5, 1.
7. Barclay, A.E., Franklin, K.J. and Prichard, M.M.L. (1944): The Foetal Circulation and Cardiovascular System and the Changes That They Undergo at Birth. Blackwell, Oxford.

NEW CONCEPTS IN HUMAN FETAL AND NEONATAL CARDIAC GEOMETRY AND FUNCTION

J.W. Wladimiroff, R.P.L. Vosters, L. Vrij and
J.H.M. Wondergem

Department of Obstetrics and Gynaecology, Academic
Hospital Rotterdam Dijkzigt, Erasmus University Rotterdam,
Rotterdam, The Netherlands

Initially A-mode and later B and M-mode pulsed echo
systems (1-3) were used to establish fetal heart activity,
particularly in early pregnancy. Today, more detailed
information on fetal cardiac geometry and function can be
obtained by means of combined use of real-time scanners
and single beam ultrasonic transducers (4).
The objectives of our study were as follows:

- Development of a technique of obtaining an M-mode
  recording of a transverse cross-section of the fetal
  and neonatal heart which is at right angles to the intra-
  ventricular septum at the level of the mitral valve
  leaflets (Fig. 1).
- Assessment of ventricular geometry and function from
  measurements at this particular level.

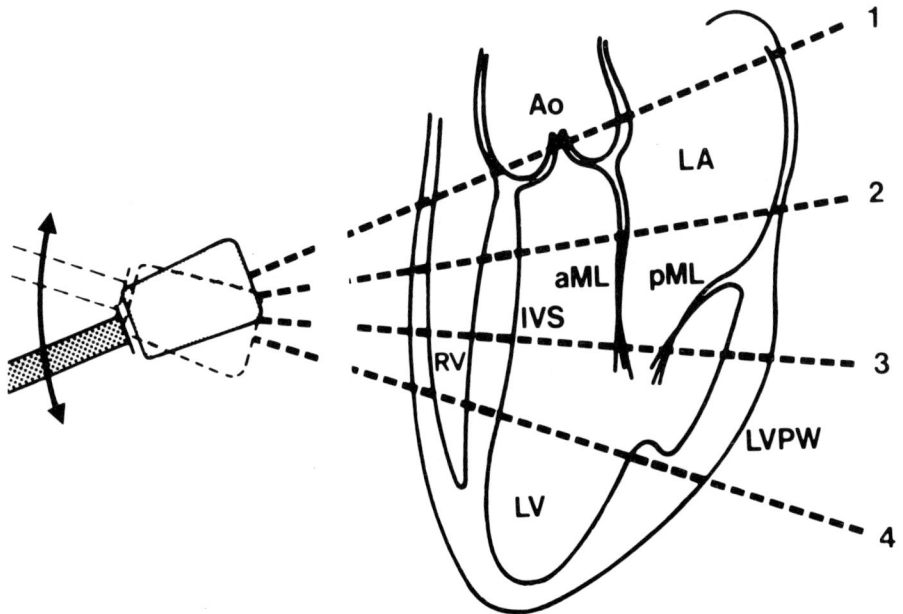

Figure 1. Schematic picture of plane of investigation in a
neonatal heart. Ao=aorta; LA=left atrium; aML and pML=

anterior and posterior mitral leaflets; IVS=intraventricular septum; LV and RV=left and right ventricle; LVPW=left ventricular posterior wall.

RECORDING TECHNIQUE

The antenatal recording technique is two-phased: First a two-dimensional cross-section of the fetal chest at the level of the heart is obtained by means of a dynamically focussing linear array real-time scanner (5) (Fig. 2). In the next step an annular array, dynamically focussing single-beam transducer (6) (Fig. 3) is positioned at an angle of 45° to the antero-posterior diameter of the fetal chest in order to be at right angles to the intra-ventricular septum at the level of the mitral valve leaflets (Figs. 4 and 5). In neonatal studies only the single beam transducer is needed. A fetal and neonatal M-mode recording of the plane of investigation is shown in Figs. 6 and 7.

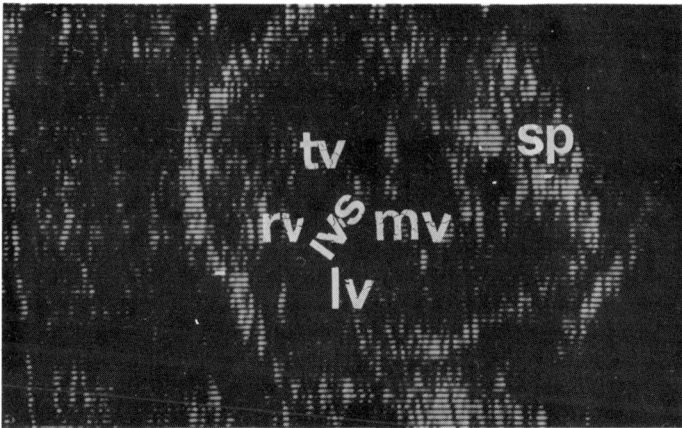

Figure 2. Real-time two-dimensional oblique cross-section of fetal chest at 39 weeks showing left and right ventricle (LV and RV), intraventricular septum (IVS) and mitral and tricuspid valves (MV and TV), SP is fetal spine.

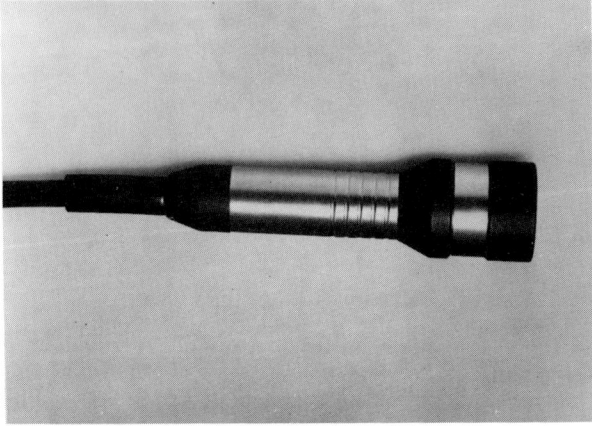

Figure 3. Annular array, dynamically focussing single beam transducer consisting of six concentric rings (diameter 24 mm).

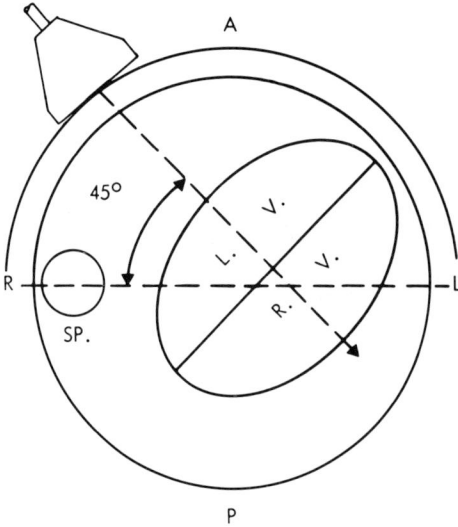

Figure 4.

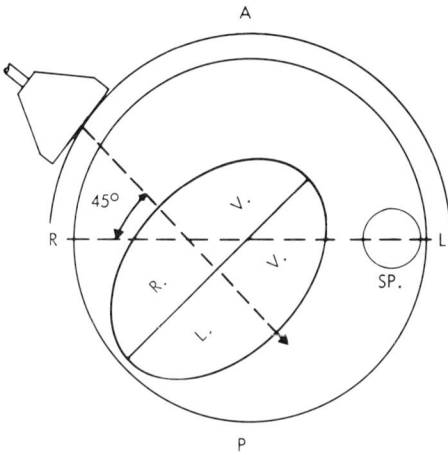

Figure 5.

Figures 4 and 5. Positioning of the single beam transducer relative to the fetal chest and heart. A=anterior; P=posterior; R=right; L=left; SP=spine; LV and RV= left and right ventricle.

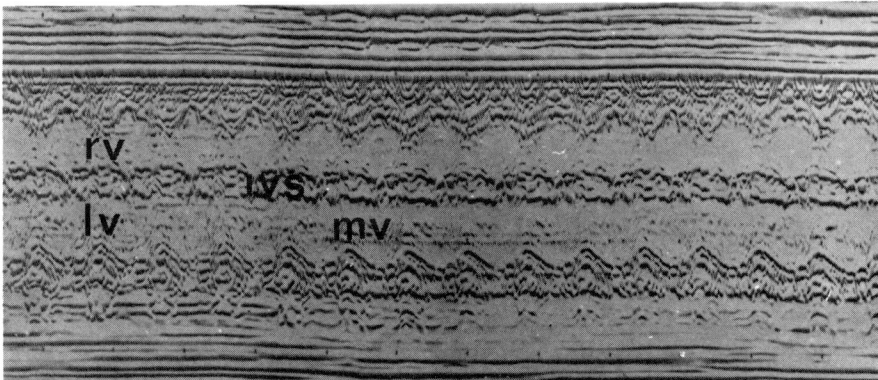

Figure 6.

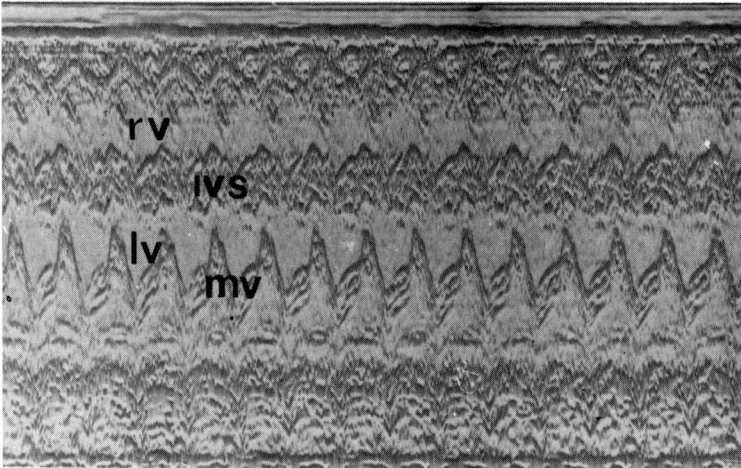

Figure 7.

Figures 6 and 7. M-mode recording of fetal heart at 38 weeks and neonatal heart at 2 days, showing LV (left ventricle), RV (right ventricle), IVS (intraventricular septum) and MV (mitral valve leaflets).

PATIENTS AND MEASUREMENTS

So far a total of 46 normal pregnancies has been studied. Pregnancy duration varied from 28 - 42 weeks. In 34 patients one antenatal M-mode recording was produced between 28 and 39 weeks. In the remaining 12 patients M-mode recordings were made between 39 and 42 weeks and within 10 minutes, 4 hours, 24 hours and 48 hours following delivery. From each M-mode recording about 10 cardiac cycles were included in the following measurements:

- Left and right ventricular transverse diameter in the end-diastolic (ED) and end-systolic (ES) position in mm.
- Intra-ventricular septum thickness in the end-diastolic and end-systolic position in mm.
- Left and right ventricular ejection time (ET) in msec as determined by the time interval between end-diastole and end-systole.

From these measurements the following calculations were made:

- The right-to-left ventricular ratio in the end-diastolic and end-systolic position.
- Two parameters expressing myocardial contractility of the ventricles:

  - The fractional shortening of ventricular dimension; this is the total shortening of ventricular dimension

196

expressed as a proportion of the end-diastolic dimension:

$$FS\ (\%) = \frac{ED - ES\ dimension}{ES\ dimension} \times 100$$

- The mean velocity of fractional shortening of ventricular dimension. In addition to the extent of shortening this parameter takes into account the velocity of ventricular wall motion.

$$VCF\ (sec^{-1}) = \frac{ED - ES\ dimension}{ES\ dimension \times ET}$$

RESULTS

Figure 8 shows the mean values and standard error for the left ventricular transverse diameter between 28 and 42 weeks and first 48 hours following delivery. A gradual increase in left ventricular diameter upto about 36 weeks can be observed. This increase is from 12.4 to 16.1 mm 32%) in the end-diastolic position and from 9.3 to 12.4 mm (31%) in the end-systolic position. After 36 weeks and in the neonatal period there seems to be a slight increase in left ventricular size in the end-diastolic and virtually no change in the end-systolic position.

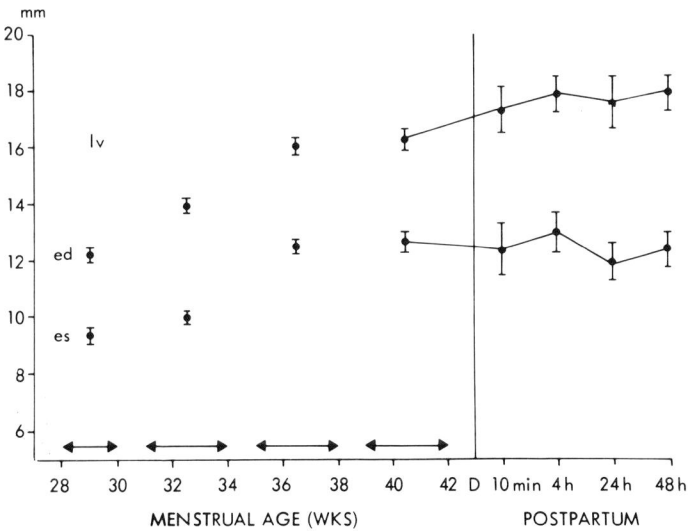

Figure 8.

The right ventricular transverse diameter in the antenatal period shows a pattern which is very similar to that of the left ventricle (Fig. 9). The percentage increase is 37% in the end-diastolic and 48% in the end-systolic position. Immediately following delivery, however, a marked drop in right ventricular diameter of 57% in the end-diastolic and of 41% in the end-systolic position can be observed. The remainder of the 48 hours study period is characterized by comparatively small changes in this particular diameter.

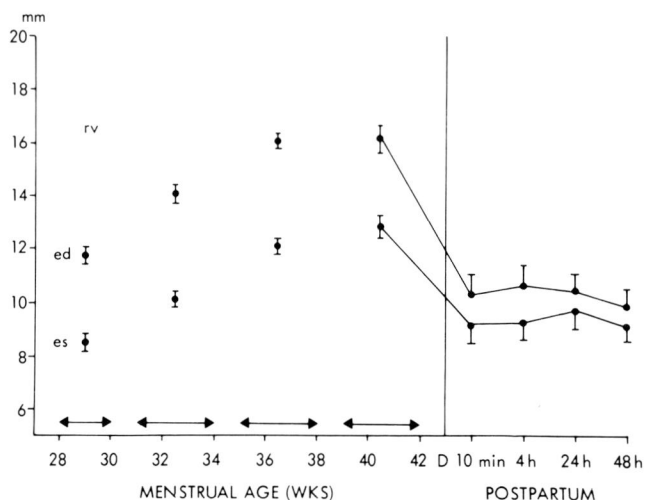

Figure 9.

Figures 8 and 9. Mean values + standard error for left (Fig. 8) and right ventricular transverse diameter (Fig. 9) between 28 and 42 weeks and first 48 hours following delivery. D=delivery; ED=end-diastolic; ES=end-systolic position.

The right-to-left ventricular ratio (Fig. 10) varies from 0.9 to 1.0 between 28 and 31 weeks and from 1.0 to 1.05 between 39 and 42 weeks, indicating a more or less equal ventricular size in the antenatal study period Within 10 minutes following delivery a pronounced drop in ratio of 71% in the end-diastolic and of 36% in the end-systolic position is demonstrated.

The thickness of the intra-ventricular septum (Fig.11) shows a gradual increase of just over 2 mm between 28 and 31 weeks to just over 3 mm in the last weeks of pregnancy. End-diastolic and end-systolic values do not significantly differ from each other. Immediately following delivery an impressive increase in septal thickness in the end-systolic position as opposed to the end-diastolic position can be demonstrated.

Figure 12 gives the data for right and left ventricular fractional shortening. Right ventricular fractional shortening shows a downward trend from 28% between 28 and 31 weeks to 25% between 39 and 42 weeks. These values are lower than the values for the left ventricular fractional shortening which are 36 and 29% respectively. Following delivery a further marked reduction in right ventricular fractional shortening occurs to values of 11-16% whereas left ventricular fractional shortening stays at a level of 30-35%.

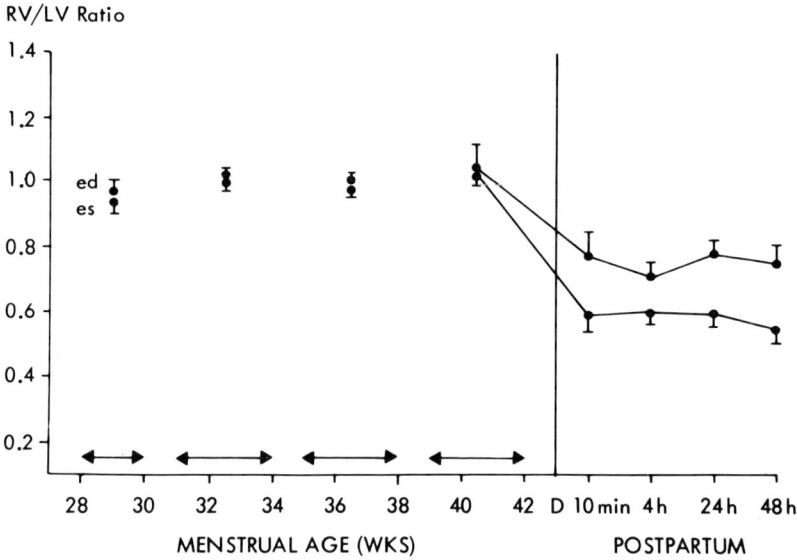

Figure 10. Right-to-left ventricular ratio

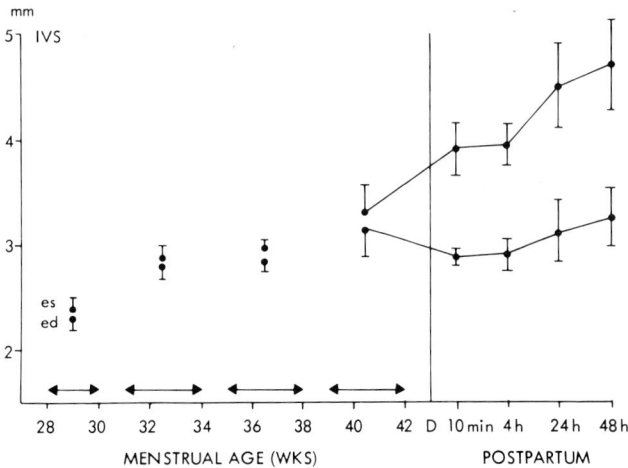

Figure 11. Intraventricular septum thickness (IVS)

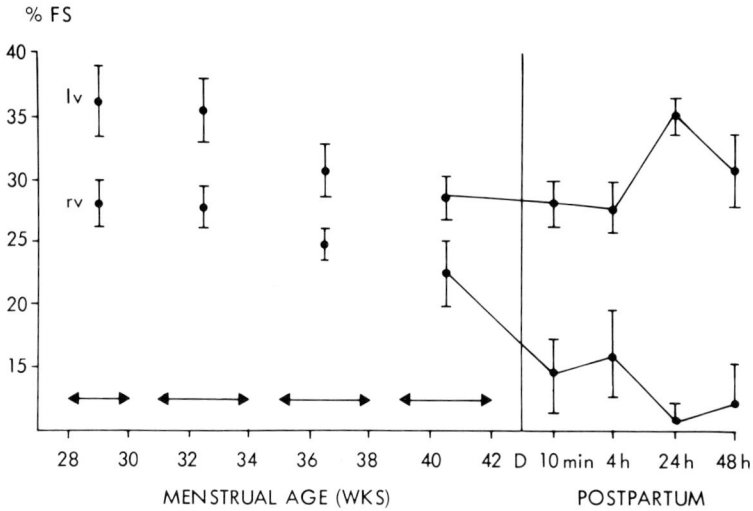

Figure 12. Left and right ventricular fractional shortening (FS).

The antenatal values for the mean velocity of fractional shortening (Fig. 13) range from 1.4 to 1.8 for the left ventricle and from 1.1 to 1.3 for the right ventricle. Postnatally, the left ventricular velocity of fractional shortening is always situated above 1.3,whereas the values for the right ventricle fall below the level of 0.8. Ideally, the mean velocity of fractional shortening should be corrected for fetal heart rate, however, a correction factor has not yet been established.

Antenatally, left and right ventricular ejection time (Fig. 14) ranges from 200 - 215 msec. There is a marked increase up to 250 msec for the right ventricle and a dip followed by an increase up to only 220 msec for the left ventricle 4 hours following delivery.

In the antenatal study period (Fig. 15) a gradual increase in beat-to-beat interval from 418 to 445 msec can be demonstrated. Postnatally there are marked changes in beat-to-beat variation which very much resemble the changes in ventricular ejection time.

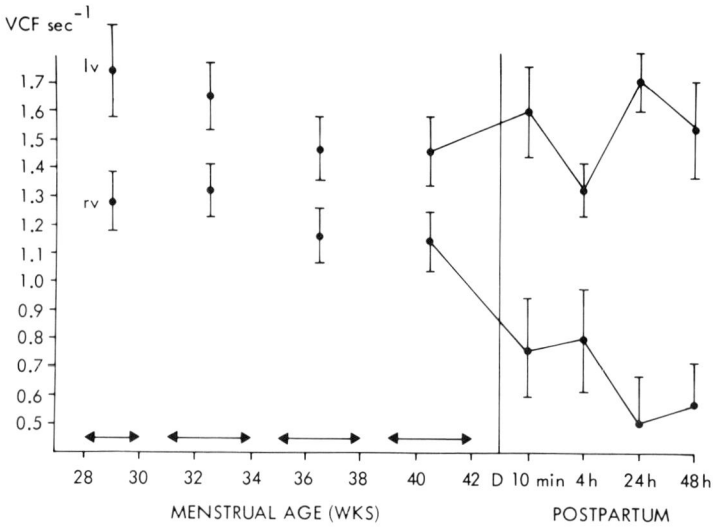

Figure 13. Mean velocity of left and right ventricular fractional shortening (VCF).

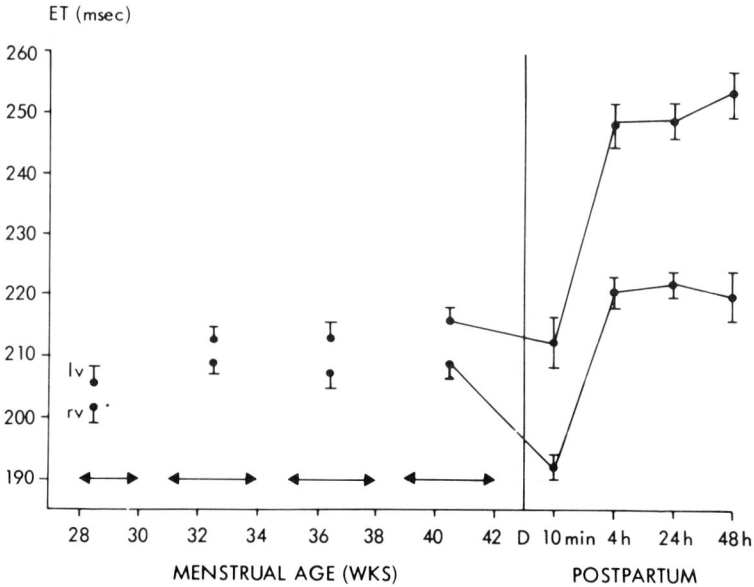

Figure 14. Left and right ventricular ejection time (ET) in msec.

BEAT-TO-BEAT INTERVAL (msec)

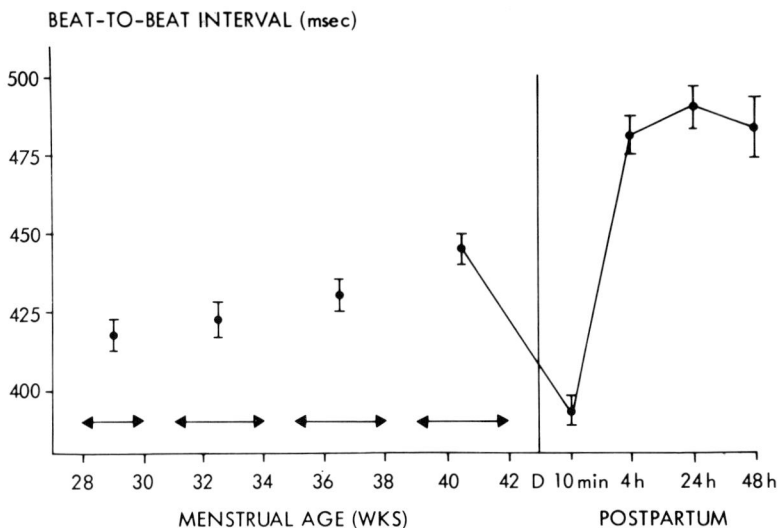

Figure 15. Beat-to-beat interval in msec.

DISCUSSION

In the antenatal period the right-to-left ventricular ratio is about 1 which underlines the fact that both ventricles of the fetal heart work in parallel and eject blood against the same pressure.

Following delivery marked circulatory changes take place: there is an arrest of the umbilical circulation, increase of pulmonary flow on ventilation of the lungs, closure of the foramen ovale and constriction of the ductus arteriosus. The marked drop in righ-to-left ventricular ratio immediately following delivery is mainly determined by a pronounced reduction in right ventricular size.

The nearly identical end-diastolic and end-systolic values for intra-ventricular septal thickness indicate a very limited involvement of the septum in ventricular activity in the antenatal period. If slight septal movement is observed, it is nearly always non-paradoxal, i.e. the septum moves toward the left ventricular posterior wall during systole. Following delivery, however, clear involvement of the septum in cardiac activity can be demonstrated through a marked increase in septal thickness in the end-systolic position.

The finding of slightly lower fractional shortening values for the right ventricle as compared with the left ventricle is rather puzzling since both ventricles eject blood against the same pressure. The gradual decrease in left and right ventricular fractional shortening during the course of pregnancy seems to be determined by the increase in left and right ventricular transverse diameter. Following delivery the marked drop in right ventricular

202

fractional shortening is probably entirely determined by the changes in right ventricular geometry. The same accounts for the mean velocity of fractional shortening values. Both data on left and right ventricular fractional shortening and mean velocity of fractional shortening are similar to those found during infancy and adult life.

The highly significant increase in neonatal right ventricular ejection time as compared with the antenatal values may be explained on a more functional basis, i.e. the reduction in pulmonary vascular resistance and subsequent reduction in pressure in the right ventricular outflow tract. The neonatal changes in both left and right ventricular ejection time resemble the changes in beat-to-beat variation indicating a positive relationship between those parameters.

More studies are underway, particularly in relation to the effect of fetal breathing movements, maternal drug administration and fetal hypoxia on the various cardiac parameters here presented. We are now able to accurately display the opening and closure of the aortic valve leaflets on M-mode tracings. This will provide a possibility of calculating Pre-ejection Period (P.E.P.) in simultaneous fetal E.C.G. and M-mode recordings.

REFERENCES

1. Kratochwil, A. and Eisenhut, L. (1967):
    In: Intrauterine Dangers to the Fetus, p. 258,
    Editors: H. Horsky and Z.K. Stembera. Excerpta
    Medica, Amsterdam

2. Robinson, H.P. (1972):
    Br. Med. J. 4 :466.

3. Piiroinen, O. (1975):
    M.D. Thesis, University of Turkey

4. Wladimiroff, J.W., Vosters, R. and Vletter, W. (1979):
    Contr. Gynecol. Obstet. 6:109.

5. Ligtvoet, C.M., Ridder, J., Hagemeijer, F. and
    Wladimiroff, J.W. (1977):
    In: Ultrasonics International 1977, p. 111, Editor:
    Z. Novak, IPC Science and Technology Press, Guildford,
    England.

6. Wal, van der L. (1978):
    Focussing systems, M.D. Thesis, Technical High School
    Delft, The Netherlands

CURRENT STATUS IN FETAL ECHOCARDIOGRAPHY

A. Ianniruberto

Department of Obstetrics and Gynecology, City Hospital
"M.Sarcone", 70038 Terlizzi (Bari), Italy.

Sonar is a noninvasive and harmless technique widely
employed in obstetrics for the identification of many
fetal internal structures. It has been used also in study
of the fetal heart, but technical difficulties have been
encountered when a single crystal transducer of a B-mode
or TM-mode scanner is used (6,7,8,11). Recently the fetal
heart structures and activity have been studied more extensively by using a real-time ultrasound apparatus associated with a TM-mode registration (5).

MATERIAL AND METHODS

Fetal heart activity has been evaluated in 90 pregnant patients from 34th - 41st week of pregnancy by using
an Aloka Echo Camera SSD-200 ultrasonic apparatus[*], which
allows a contemporaneous display in real-time gray-scale
B-mode and in TM-mode. With the 2.5 MHz linear array
multicrystal transducer of the equipment it is possible to
visualize and study the fetal heart structures and their
reciprocal relationship, after having located the fetal
back and head. The transducer is moved in different directions and inclinations in order to obtain satisfactory
images of the fetal heart in longitudinal and transverse
sections. The best pictures are obtained when the ultrasonic beam is directed perpendicularly to the fetal chest,
either anteriorly or posteriorly. The cardiac structures
are subsequently selected by means of a single ultrasonic
beam and recorded on a TM-mode oscilloscope.

Also assessment of the fetal cardiac dynamics has
been attempted by measuring the diastolic and systolic
diameters of both ventricles. The cardiac output (CO) of a
single ventricle is calculated according to the formula
$CO = SV \times HR$, where SV is the stroke volume and HR the
heart rate. The stroke volume is estimated by calculating
during 5 cardiac cycles the average difference between the
end-diastolic and the end-systolic volumes of each ventricle separately according to the formula $SV = Dd^3 - Ds^3$,
where Dd is the ventricular end-diastolic diameter and Ds

[*] Aloka Co., Ltd., Tokyo, Japan.

the end-systolic diameter (2). It should be emphasized
that the formulas above reported do not yield the true
ventricular volumes, because it is virtually impossible to
calculate a true volume of a complex object such as the
ventricle with a single dimension. However, several
studies have shown a good statistical relationship between
the echocardiographic dimensions and the angiographic ventricular volumes (1).

Since fetal circulation is not a series circuit, as
in the adult, but the two ventricles tend to function in
parallel (8), the fetal cardiac output is expressed as
the combined left and right ventricular outputs.

The ventricular diameters used for the calculations
above are perpendicular to the interventricular septum and
located close to the level of the chordae tendineae of the
mitral valve. An incorrect inclination of the transducer
gives wrong echocardiographic tracings (Fig. 1).

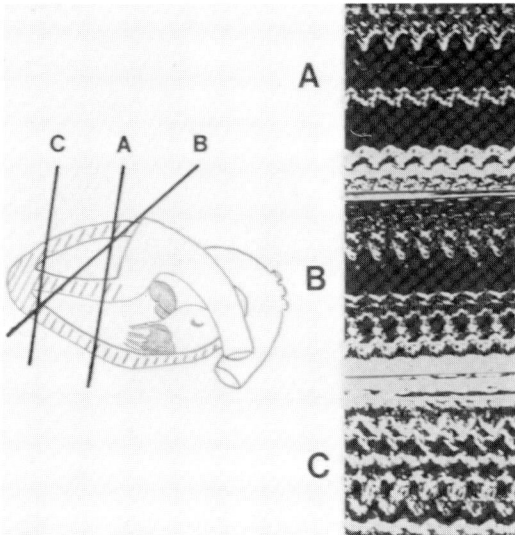

Figure 1. According to the direction and the inclination
of the ultrasonic beam to the fetal heart, it is possible
to obtain different echocardiographic tracings.
In A, the two ventricular sizes are almost equal.
In B, the right ventricle seems larger than the left one.
In C, both ventricles are considerably smaller because of
the tracing obtained at the level of the apex of the
heart.

For explaining the implication of the values reported
in the Results, it seems opportune to emphasize that
during ventricular diastole the leaflets of the mitral

valve fly apart as blood is rapidly dumped from the left
atrium into the left ventricle. If diastole is sufficiently long, there may occur a mid-diastolic flow of
blood with reopening of the leaflets. If the heart rate is
faster and diastole shorter, as during fetal life, then
the diastolic reopening of the valve does not occur. The
diastolic closing velocity is measured as the echocardiographic E-F slope, according to the original lettering
given to the mitral valve leaflets by Edler (1).

    Difficulties are encountered for the measurements of
the fetal heart if the fetus is too mobile, in case of
presence of fetal breathing movements and in case of
interposition of fetal small parts between the transducer
and the heart structures.

    In 40 % of the present cases it has been necessary to
repeat the ultrasonographic scanning after 24-48 hours in
order to obtain a satisfactory tracing of the TM-mode
recording, because of failure at the initial attempt to
visualize the structures of the fetal heart.

RESULTS

    The anterior leaflet of the mitral valve has been
visualized in all cases (Fig. 2). At term of pregnancy the
slope velocity E-F was almost equal to those of newborn
infants, being 60-120 mm/sec. The excursion movement
measured between the points D and E has been 0.8 cm in
average. The posterior leaflet has been registered in TM-
mode only in 22 cases.

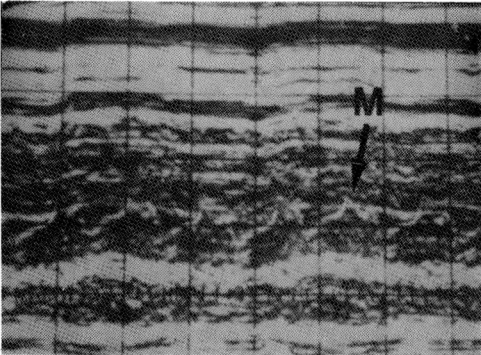

Figure 2. The anterior leaflet of the mitral valve (M)
registered by a TM-mode scanning in a fetus at term.

The tricuspid valve has been visualized in 37 % of the cases (Figg. 3 and 4) and its E-F slope velocity at term of normal pregnancy has been 70-110 mm/sec, with values very close to those of the anterior leaflet of the mitral valve.

The movements of the aortic root have been registered in 100 % of the cases (Figg. 3 and 4), but more difficult was the registration of the aortic leaflets, which have been visualized in 15 % of the cases. The diameter of the aortic root at term of normal pregnancy was 8-10 mm. It has always been possible to record the continuity from the aortic root to the anterior leaflet of the mitral valve by moving the transducer caudally a few millimeters.

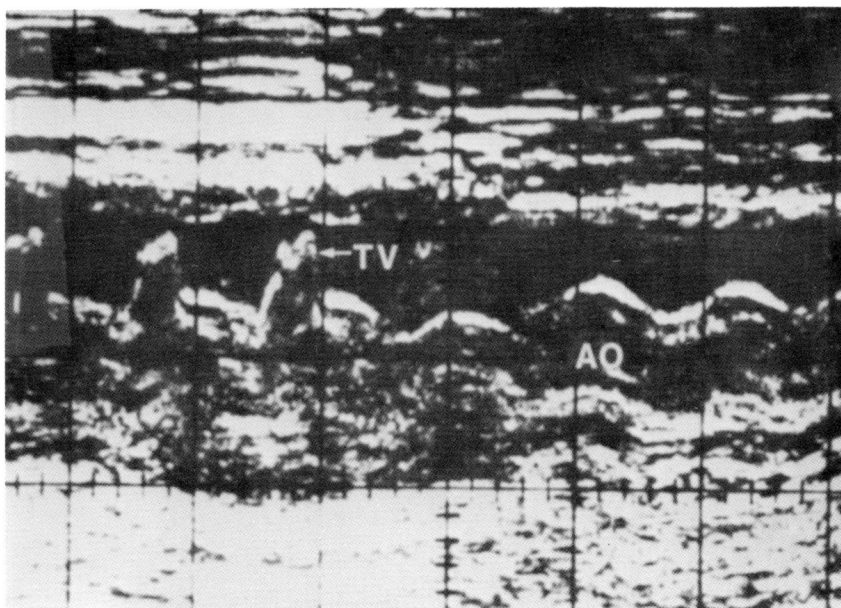

Figure 3. Registration of the tricuspid valve (TV), anteriorly to the aortic root (AO).

The pulmonary artery has been visualized in 40 % of the cases, anteriorly to the aortic root. When registered simultaneously, the pulmonary artery was usually larger than the aorta, having a diameter of 10-11 mm at term of pregnancy.

The posterior wall of the left ventricle, the anterior wall of the right ventricle and the interventricular septum have been visualized in 55 cases by using real-time scanning. However, a satisfactory contempor-

aneous tracing in TM-mode, mandatory for stroke volume
calculation, has been obtained only in ten fetuses at
term of normal pregnancy, from 38 - 41 weeks of gestational age. In the human fetus at term the internal dimensions of the left and right ventricles are almost equal
with a very small predominance of the left one. In the ten
fetuses at term the range of the end-diastolic and the end
-systolic diameters have been respectively 1.6-2 cm and
1.0-1.4 cm in the left ventricle and 1.2-1.8 cm and 0.8-
1.2 cm in the right ventricle.

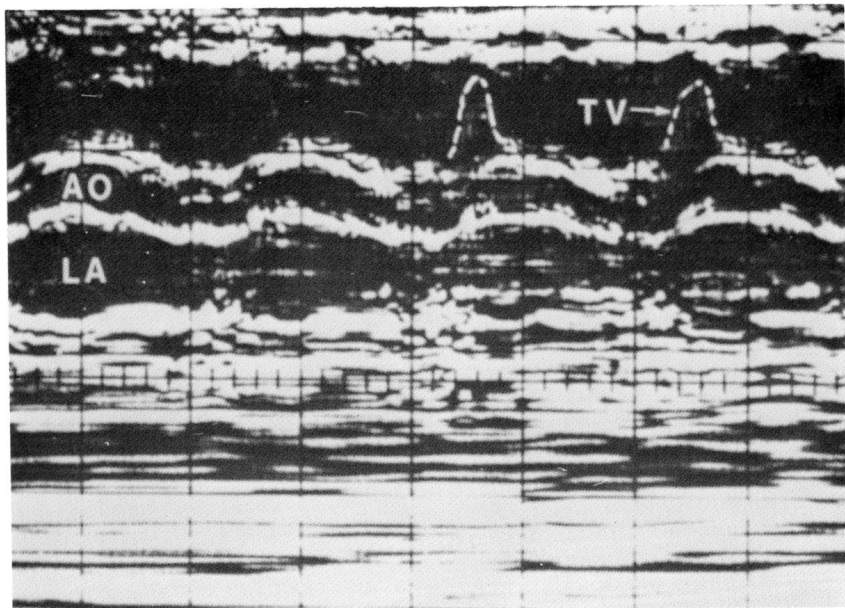

Figure 4. Registration of the tricuspid valve (TV), of
the aortic root (AO) and of the left atrium (LA).

The movement of the interventricular septum (IVS),
visualized below the mitral valve at the level of the
chordae tendineae, has been studied in 55 cases. Of the
25 fetuses, which were recorded during 38 - 41 weeks of
gestational age, 19 cases showed during systole a movement
of the IVS against the posterior wall, with an increase of
its systolic thickness (Fig. 5). A pattern of paradoxical
motion of the IVS against the anterior wall of the right
ventricle during systole, has been noted in the other six
cases. In these fetuses, it was also observed that the
right side of the septum exhibited a larger paradoxical
motion than did the left one (Fig. 6). In the 30 fetuses,
during 34 - 38 weeks of pregnancy, the septal motion was
normal in 19 cases, showed a paradoxical pattern in 10

cases, and a flat pattern in 1 case.

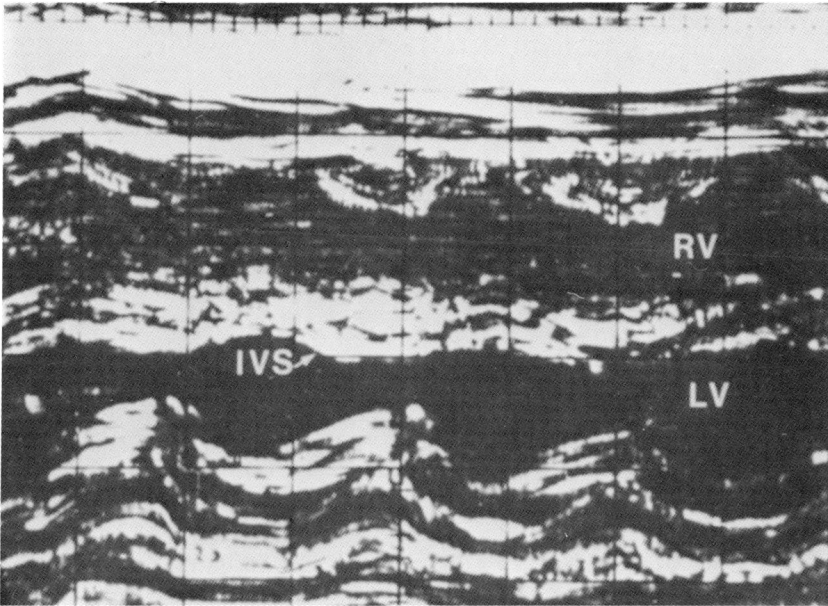

Figure 5. Registration of the right ventricle (RV), of the left ventricle (LV) and of the interventricular septum (IVS) in a fetus at 36 weeks.

At term of pregnancy the end-diastolic thickness of the interventricular septum was 3-4.5 mm.

The combined cardiac output of the right and left ventricles calculated in 10 fetuses at term of normal pregnancy with normal IVS movement averaged 750 ml/minute (range 500-1000 ml/minute). Considerable variations of the values can be encountered associated with fetal breathing movements and with incorrect inclination of the transducer (Fig. 1).

In three fetuses at 39 weeks has been noted that, during fetal breathing movements, the right atrial dimension increased concomitant with the inspiration and the left atrial dimension decreased slightly. However, further investigations are necessary to confirm this finding, because of the very small number of fetuses studied (Fig. 7).

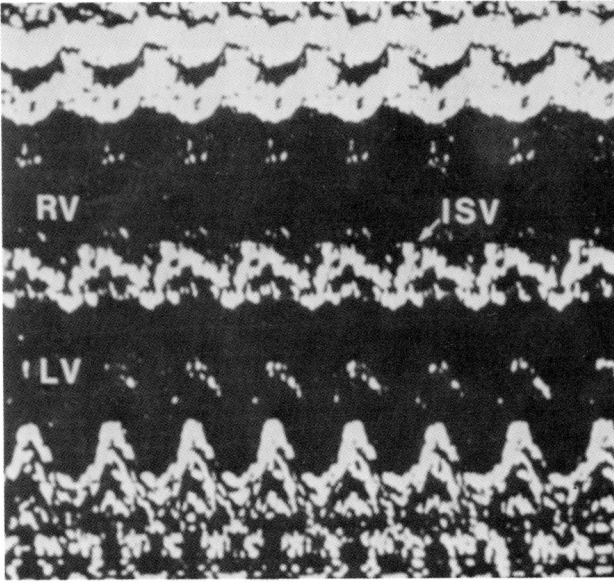

Figure 6. Echocardiographic tracing in TM-mode in a fetus at 39 weeks. A pattern of anterior paradoxical motion of the interventricular septum (IVS) during systole is visible. The right side of the IVS shows a larger paradoxical motion than does the left one.
Right ventricle (RV); left ventricle (LV).

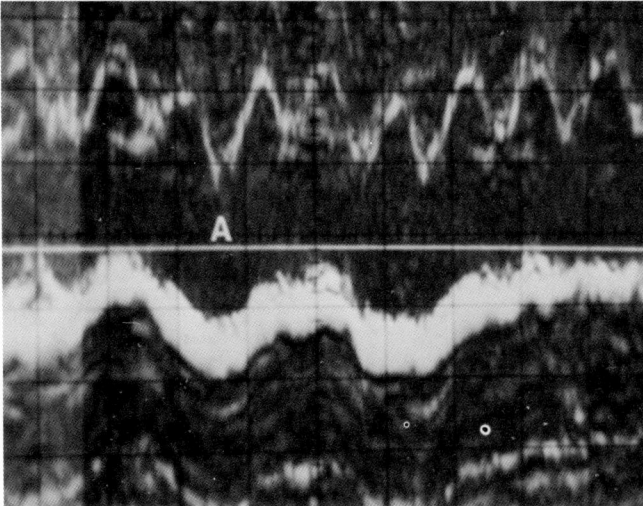

Figure 7. Fetal breathing movements inducing variations of the size of the left atrium (A).

COMMENT

By employing a real-time scanner it has been possible
to identify several fetal heart structures: the mitral
valve, the tricuspid valve, the aortic root, the pulmonary
artery, the ventricular walls, the interventricular
septum, and the interatrial septum with the foramen ovale.

With the aid of this direct observation, some of the
single cardiac structures have been selected for a study
in a TM-mode scanning display and several of their ultrasonic movements have been quantified. As in adults, the
easiest structures to be recognized in the fetus are the
mitral valve and the aortic root.

Most of the morphologic and dynamic features of the
heart of fetuses at term resemble those of newborn infant
(3,10). In particular, the E-F slope velocity of the
mitral valve and of the tricuspid valve is almost equal to
those obtained in newborn infants and reported in the
literature.

At term of normal pregnancy, the two fetal ventricles
have almost equal volumes. The movement of the interventricular septum during systole is normal at term of pregnancy in 76 % of the cases. A paradoxical pattern, presumably due to the right ventricular volume overload during
the fetal period, is present in 24 % of the cases. In the
earlier stages of pregnancy, from 34 to 38 weeks, paradoxical septal motion were observed in 36 % of the cases.
Our findings do not agree with those referred by Hobbins
et al (4), who have noted a normal septal motion only in
2 of 16 fetuses between 25.5 and 40 weeks gestation. The
discrepancy could be explained by the different stages of
pregnancy studied and by a possible different transverse
section of fetal heart recorded.

The cardiac output calculated from heart dimensions
in human fetuses in uncomplicated pregnancies may be compared with the data reported on blood flow in fetal lambs
obtained by invasive techniques using radionuclide-
labelled microspheres (9).

Nevertheless, it should be pointed out that estimations of the combined cardiac output in human fetuses
using ultrasonographic values of heart dimensions must be
confirmed with further investigations and by using other
methods. Thus, the values reported here suffer from the
lack, due to technical difficulties, of a fetal external
electrocardiogram or phonocardiogram registered concomi-
tantly with the echocardiographic tracings. The importance
of the phase relationship of the ultrasonographic tracing
with other parameters, especially with the QRS complex of
an ECG, is well known.

211

REFERENCES

1. Edler, I. and Gustafson, A. (1957): Acta Med. Scand.,
   159, 85.
2. Friedewald, V.E. (1977): In: Textbook of Echocardiography. W.B. Saunders Company, Philadelphia.
3. Hagan, A.D., Deely, W.J., Shan, D. et al. (1973):
   Circulation, 48, 1221.
4. Hobbins, J.C., Kleinman, C. and Creighton, D. (1978):
   Lecture presented at the Poster Session in the 25th
   Annual Meeting of the Society for Gynecologic Investigation, Atlanta, Georgia, USA.
5. Ianniruberto, A., Iaccarino, M., De Luca, I. et al.
   (1977): Atti III Congresso Nazionale S.I.S.U.M.,
   Terlizzi. Suppl. RAYS-International Journal of
   Radiological Sciences, Vol. 1, p. 285. Editors: C.
   Colagrande, A. Ianniruberto and B. Talia.
6. Lee, F.Y.L., Batson, H.W.K., Alleman, N. et al.
   (1977): Am. J. Obstet. Gynecol., 129, 503.
7. Leopold, G.R. (1974): In: Modern Perinatal Medicine,
   p. 179. Editor: L. Gluck. Year Book Medical Publ.,
   Inc., Chicago.
8. Murata, Y., Takemura, H. and Kurachi, K. (1971): Am.
   J. Obstet. Gynecol., 111, 287.
9. Rudolph, A.M. and Heymann, M.A. (1973): In: Foetal and
   Neonatal Physiology, p. 89. Editors: K.S. Comline,
   K.W. Cross, G.S. Dawes et al. Cambridge University
   Press, London.
10. Solinger, R., Elbl, F. and Minhas, K. (1973):
    Circulation, 47, 108.
11. Winsberg, F. (1972): Invest. Radiol., 7, 152.

FETAL HEART ELECTROMECHANICAL INTERVALS - The influence
of labour and relationship to fetal blood gas values.

A.H. Adam, J.R. Doig, J.E.E. Fleming, N.C. Smith,
Anne Houston, Katherine Adam and T. Aitchison.

Department of Midwifery (Queen Mother's Hospital) and
Department of Statistics, University of Glasgow,
Glasgow, Scotland.

SUMMARY

    A study of measured electromechanical intervals
of the fetal heart from one hundred and three unselected
human fetuses in labour is reported. The mean values,
with standard deviations in parenthesis, for the four
intervals studied PEP 76.01 ($\pm$ 9.93) ms; IVC 41.56
($\pm$ 8.51) ms; LVET 156.23 ($\pm$ 16.58) ms and R to R 450.48
($\pm$ 58.76) ms were consistent with previous reports.
The intervals did not consistently alter during the
course of labour and only the R to R interval
significantly increased during uterine contractions.
Correlation of the four intervals and ratio PEP/LVET
with fetal arterial pO_2, pCO_2 and pH failed to identify
consistent relationships although three fetuses showed
shortening of PEP in association with severe acedaemia
and a further fetus with nuchal cord entanglement
exhibited prolongation of PEP interval.

INTRODUCTION

    Over the last two decades, the pioneering work
from Hon, Caldeyro-Barcia, Quilligan, Paul and Kubli
amongst others has made continuous fetal heart
monitoring of the human fetus in labour standard
practice. Despite the many publications describing
the interpretation of cardiotocographic tracings, the
application of specific patterns of fetal heart
deceleration to clinical causation and their
significance as predictors of fetal asphyxia remains
controversial (1, 2, 3). An excellent review article
by Ott (4) discusses tracing interpretation difficulties
and advocates a suitable classification which
incorporates the ideas of several authors.
    There is little doubt that continuous FHR monitoring
has decreased the perinatal and neonatal mortality rate
(5, 6, 7, 8) but increasing concentration on the "at
risk" fetus will, it is hoped, reduce perinatal and
neonatal morbidity still further. Over recent years
adult cardiologists have begun to study and correlate
the electrical and mechanical events in the cardiac

cycle and have asserted that measurement of these electro-mechanical intervals aid clinical management (9, 10, 11). These techniques have been applied to fetal cardiac assessment in animal studies by Organ et al (12) in Toronto, Morgenstern et al (13) in Dusseldorf and Murata et al (14) in Los Angeles and to human fetuses by the groups in Toronto and Los Angeles as well as by our group in Glasgow (15, 16, 17, 18).

The electro-mechanical intervals (EMI's) which have commanded most attention and which were recorded in this study are pre-ejection period (PEP); the phase of isovolumetric contraction (IVC); the left ventricular ejection time (LVET) and the interval between successive QRS complexes (R to R). The PEP is the time interval in milliseconds from the Q wave (septal depolarization) of the fetal electrocardiogram (ECG) to the opening of the aortic valve, that is Q to Ao, and like the IVC is a measure of myocardial contractility (19). The IVC is the time interval between mitral valve closure and aortic valve opening, Mc to Ao, and is the time taken for the myocardium to build up tension isometrically until intraventricular pressure equals intra-aortic pressure. LVET is the time interval recorded between aortic valve opening and its closure, Ao to Ac, and is a function of stroke volume and peripheral resistance. The R to R interval provides a measure of short term baseline beat to beat variability (see Figure 1).

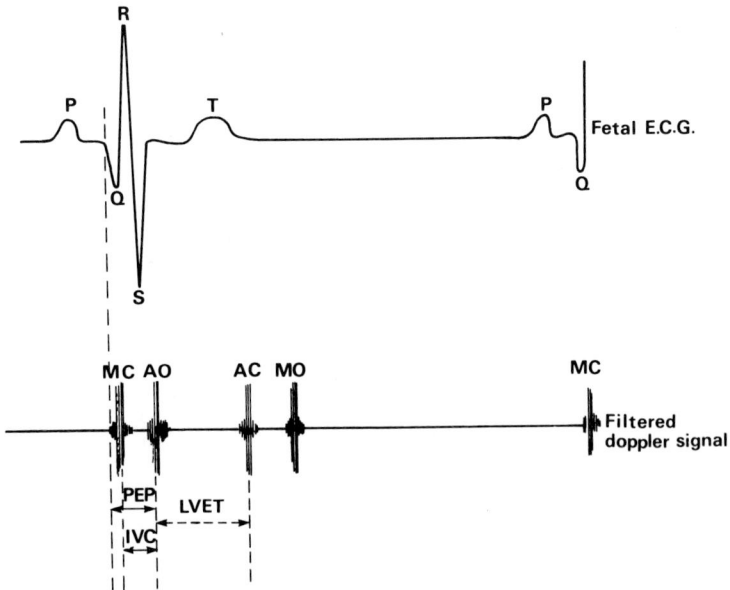

Figure 1. Measurement of fetal electro-mechanical intervals in labour.

It is important when comparing reports of measured EMIs from different sources to note the technique used, since systematic errors are introduced if the Q to R interval is ignored or when the timing of ventricular ejection is assessed by phonocardiographic detection of heart sounds as compared with pulse propagation or if valvular motion is detected by Doppler frequency shift as utilized in this study. Morgenstern et al (13) have summarized the methodology and discussed the limitations of each technique most succinctly.

In this study the authors sought to explore further the relationship between measured fetal electromechanical intervals, the influences of labour and fetal blood gas values in the hope that this technique may provide useful additional information enabling earlier detection of fetal distress.

METHOD

The equipment utilized in this study has been described in detail in an earlier report (18). Essentially it consists of a synchronous display on an oscilloscope of filtered signals from a fetal ECG, obtained via direct scalp electrode, and from the ultrasonic Doppler frequency shift caused by valvular movement detected by a transducer placed on the maternal abdomen. An audio output is also provided which assists identification of the four major high amplitude (high-pitched) valvular signals and an ultraviolet strip chart recorder which is activated after signal verification (Plate 1 and 2).

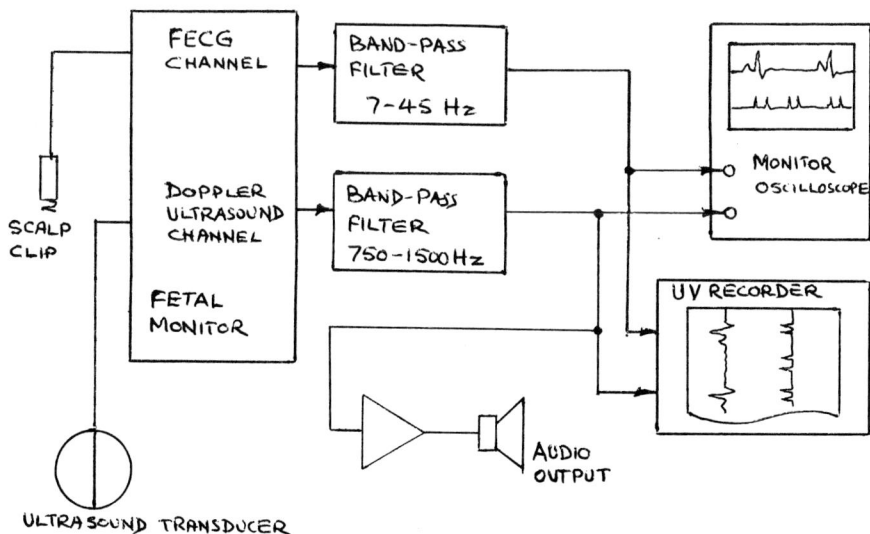

Figure 2. Block diagram of basic EMI recording system.

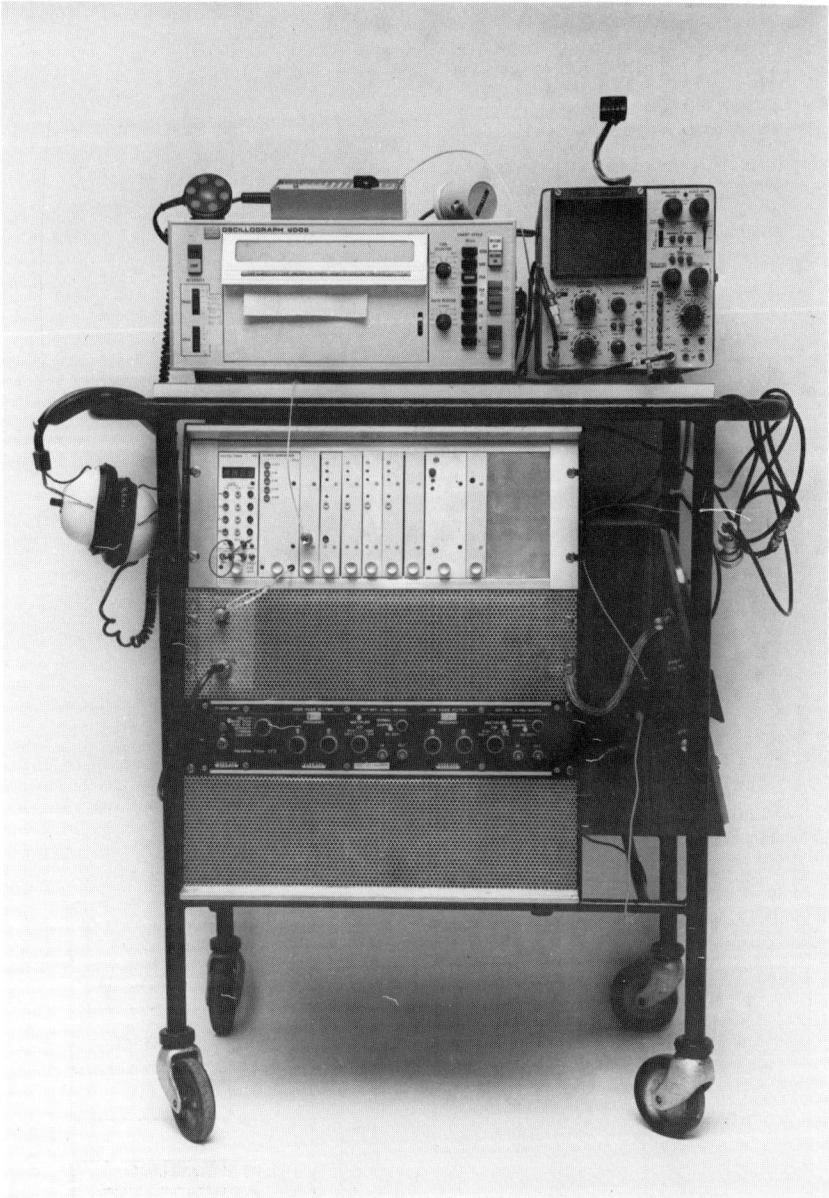

Plate 1.

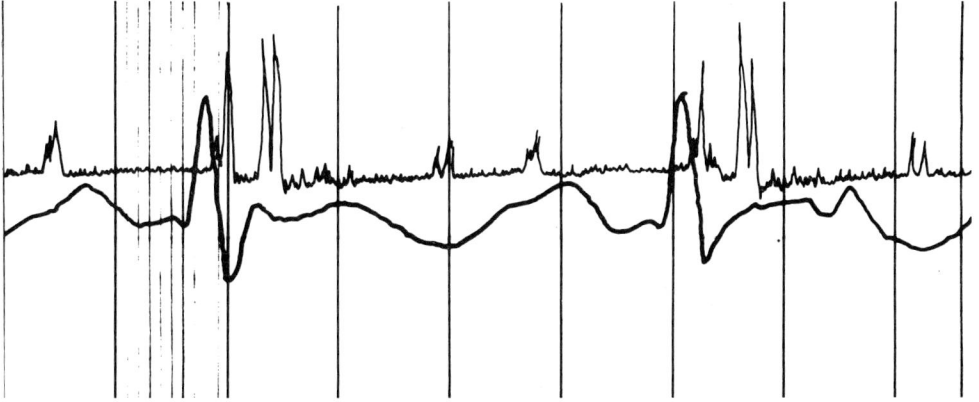

Plate 2.

This paper reports a study of electromechanical interval recordings from one hundred and three unselected human fetuses in labour. The phase of labour and presence of uterine contractions during recording was noted. The latent phase of first stage was defined as less than 6 cm cervical dilation, the active phase as equal to or greater than 6 cm cervical dilatation until full cervical dilatation. In almost all recordings analysed at least 20 consecutive cardiac cycles were measured.

Immediately after EMI recordings in labour, fetal scalp capillary blood samples were obtained from the hyperaemic fetal scalp (20). The recordings made during the second stage of labour were correlated with umbilical cord arterial and venous blood samples. All fetal blood samples were analysed in an AVL 936C blood gas micro-analyser and wherever possible pO_2, pCO_2 and derived values were reported in addition to fetal blood pH.

RESULTS

The measured electromechanical intervals and fetal blood gas values together with basic clinical data were stored in a computer memory and subjected to statistical analysis.

The mean and standard deviation values for the four measured EMIs from the complete population sample were –
PEP 76.01, s.d. 9.93 ms
IVC 41.56, s.d. 8.51 ms
LVET 156.23, s.d. 16.58 ms
R to R 450.48, s.d. 58.76 ms

The influences of stage and phase of labour and of uterine contractions were examined by derivation of appropriate means. Slight increases were observed for the mean intervals of PEP, IVC, R to R and for the ratio PEP/LVET throughout labour and with uterine contractions. Only for the effect of uterine contractions on the R to R interval in latent and active phases of labour was a statistically significant increase observed (Students 't' test p = 0.05) see Table 1. Since the data may not be distributed normally the medians and the overall range of values were examined using 'box plots' (21). This confirmed the impression given by the mean values.

TABLE 1. Electromechanical Intervals (ms), Labour & Uterine Contractions. Standard deviations in parenthesis.

	IVC	PEP	LVET	R to R	PEP/LVET
1st Stage Latent	without 38.92 (6.07)	without 73.27 (8.16)	without 158.38 (17.2)	without 431.8 (45.2)	without 0.467 (0.065)
	with 40.27 (6.18)	with 74.40 (7.46)	with 157.82 (13.7)	with * 451.9 (61.2)	with 0.473 (0.050)
1st Stage Active	without 40.74 (8.94)	without 75.00 (10.4)	without 154.43 (14.0)	without 431.6 (49.1)	without 0.487 (0.071)
	with 42.34 (8.91)	with 76.78 (12.7)	with 155.43 (14.7)	with * 467.1 (88.1)	with 0.497 (0.098)
Second Stage	without 42.61 (10.4)	without 78.43 (11.6)	without 157.89 (18.4)	without 452.5 (82.8)	without 0.503 (0.091)
	with 42.07 (10.50)	with 78.17 (9.86)	with 153.54 (23.0)	with 466.0 (97.7)	with 0.520 (0.099)

* significant at 5% confidence level

Correlation coefficients measured between all the
4 EMIs demonstrated consistently positive r values only
for PEP with IVC and for LVET with R to R interval (see
Table 2).

TABLE 2. Correlation Coefficients for Electromechanical
Intervals.

	PEP	LVET	R R
IVC	0.756 * 0.787 0.700	0.142 0.425 0.329	0.289 0.598 0.085
PEP		0.142 0.295 0.017	0.390 0.549 0.169
LVET			0.606 * 0.774 0.723

* consistent positive correlations

No consistent relationships were confirmed when the
EMI data was correlated with fetal blood, pO_2, pCO_2 or
pH values from either capillary blood samples or from
the umbilical cord (see Table 3).

TABLE 3. Correlation of Electromechanical Intervals and
Fetal Blood Gas Values.

	Stage in Labour	IVC	PEP	LVET	R-R	PEP/LVET
pCO_2 Fetal Scalp Umb.Art.pCO_2	Latent	+0.15	+0.07	+0.09	+0.08	−0.04
	Active	−0.16	−0.21	+0.01	−0.10	−0.25
	Second	−0.13	−0.18	+0.16	−0.06	−0.26
pO_2 Fetal Scalp Umb.Art.	Latent	+0.25	+0.09	+0.06	−0.05	+0.05
	Active	+0.33	+0.33	−0.31	+0.38	+0.49
	Second	+ 0.01	+ 0.04	−0.11	−0.02	+0.08
pH Fetal Scalp Umb.Art.	Latent	+0.13	+0.29	+0.03	+0.02	+0.23
	Active	+0.67	+0.61	+0.60	+0.42	+0.45
	Second	+0.32	+0.27	−0.30	−0.32	+0.40

It is, however, of interest that three severely acidaemic
fetuses recorded mean pre-ejection period values (PEP)
markedly less than the means for the appropriate phase of
labour (see Table 4).

TABLE 4. Pre-Ejection Periods and Fetal Acidosis.

	LATENT	ACTIVE	SECOND STAGE
Patient 9	pH = 7.278 PEP = 70 (without) 65 (with)	-	pH = 7.09 PEP = 60 (without)
Patient 18	PEP = 50.0 (without)	PEP = 45.0 (without) 50.0 (with)	Cord pH = 6.7
Patient 29	-	-	pH = 7.090 PEP = 70 (without) 80 (with)
Mean Pre-Ejection Periods (millisecs)	73.27 without 74.40 with	75.0 without 76.78 with	78.43 without 78.17 with

Their summarized case histories follow.

PATIENT 9. M.C.

This 38 year old Para 1 + 0, previously delivered by
Caesarean section for fetal distress, drained meconium
stained liquor at amniotomy in spontaneous labour. An
EMI recording and fetal blood sample were taken with the
cervix 2 cm dilated. Normal values in parenthesis.

PEP, without contraction   70 ms (73.3, s.d.8.16)
PEP, with contraction   65 ms (74.4, s.d.7.46)
LVET, without contraction 155 ms (158, s.d.17.2)
LVET, with contraction   165 ms (157, s.d.13.7)
R to R   450 ms (451, s.d.61)
pO_2 30.9 mm Hg

220

$$pCO_2 \qquad\qquad 33.9 \text{ mmHg}$$
$$pH \qquad\qquad 7.278$$

After 13 hours in labour she progressed to a spontaneous vertex delivery of a healthy female 3.73 Kg, Apgars 9 at 1 and 5 minutes which required minimal resuscitation. The EMI recording in second stage gave a PEP of 60 ms (78.43, s.d. 11.6) whilst LVET and R to R at 150 and 422 ms respectively remained in the normal range. The umbilical cord arterial blood analysis showed $pO_2 = 10.6$ mmHg, $pCO_2 = 78$ mmHg and pH = 7.09.

PATIENT 18. C.N.E.

This 38 year old Para 2 + 0 had previously required Caesarean section for fetal distress in association with cephalo-pelvic disproportion and had been delivered 10 years before the current pregnancy after a 30 hour labour. Following the development of hypertension at 36 weeks gestation and a period of rest, a consultant decision to deliver by elective Caesarean section was refused by the patient who went into spontaneous labour after a painless antepartum haemorrhage at thirty eight weeks.

Severe fetal distress developed during labour and again the patient refused to accept delivery by Caesarean section. An EMI recording between contractions at 5 cm cervical dilatation showed marked shortening of PEP to 50 ms (73.27, s.d. 8.16) whilst LVET at 160 ms (158.4, s.d. 17.2) and R to R at 420 ms (431.8, s.d. 45.2) were within the usual range. A further EMI recording taken during the active phase gave PEP of 45 ms between and 50 ms with contractions, again markedly depressed when compared to the mean values for that phase. Three and a half hours post amniotomy, whilst preparations were being made for forceps delivery, spontaneous vertex delivery occurred of a fresh stillborn female infant weighing 2.40 Kg. Although aggressive resuscitation efforts were made, there was no response. Analysis of an umbilical cord arterial blood sample immediately obtained at delivery disclosed a pH value of 6.70.

In the immediate postpartum period persistent fresh bleeding in association with a positive finding of blood at abdominal paracentesis necessitated laparotomy which disclosed a posterior uterine corpus vertical rupture 5 cm long which did not communicate with the intact uterine lower segment scar or cervix. Haemostasis was achieved by subtotal hysterectomy.

PATIENT 29. E.C.J.

This 33 year old Para 2 + 1 laboured on syntocinon after spontaneous rupture of the membranes at 38 weeks gestation. In late first stage deep variable decelerations were observed and an EMI recording in second gave

PEP intervals of 70 ms between and 80 ms with contractions. Subsequently, a healthy female baby weighing 3.42 kg, Apgar scores 9 and 10 at one and five minutes was delivered by S.V.D. The umbilical cord arterial pH = 7.09 and a loose true knot was observed.

In addition to these three acidaemic fetuses where reduced PEP intervals were recorded, a further acidaemic fetus was found to have lengthening of the mean PEP interval.

PATIENT 7. E.M.C.

Mrs. C., a 27 year old Para 1 + 0, underwent fore-water amniotomy and oral prostaglandin administration to induce labour for postmaturity. Rapid progress ensued, but fetal heart decelerations of 'variable' type were observed during second stage and an EMI recording was taken. Easy spontaneous vertex delivery was achieved of a healthy male infant weighing 3.63 kg and with Apgar recordings of 9 and 9 at 1 and 5 minutes respectively, but nuchal cord entanglement was noted.

The mean PEP values of 88,between,and 85 ms with contraction were at the upper limits of the usual range for second stage and the umbilical cord arterial pH = 7.083. The LVET of 156.5 and 150 ms and R to R intervals of 455 and 460 ms were again within the normal ranges for second stage of labour.

DISCUSSION

The mean values for the four electromechanical intervals (EMIs) measured in this study were comparable to those reported by our group previously (18), and to those in other reports (15,22) when differences in measurement endpoints are noted (see Table 5).

TABLE 5. Electromechanical Interval Means from Various
         Studies (milliseconds)

	ADAM et al 1979	ROBINSON et al 1978	ORGAN et al 1973a	MURATA et al 1974
Phase of Isovolumetric Contraction IVC	41.56 (8.51)	38.9 (5.8)		41.3 (3.31)
Pre-Ejection Period PEP	76.01 (9.93)	73.6 (4.7)	73.0 (10)	70 (2.4)
Left Ventricular Ejection Time LVET	156.23 (16.58)	155.2 (9.6)		
Time between successive QRS Complexes R-R	450.48 (58.76)			
Conditions of Study	Pooled throughout labour	Not in labour		38-40 weeks gestation

The standard deviations calculated from the data presented
in this paper are wider than those found in our earlier
study. This may reflect the fact that the analysis was
made on collected measurements from 103 unselected
patients, the influence of gestational age on EMIs was
not considered (22) and recognition of the point of onset
of valvular movement when masked by background noise is
a subjective decision which may vary between observers.
     The study of the relationships between the four
measured EMIs (here expressed as correlation coefficients)
produced predictable results. The strong positive
correlation between PEP and IVC reflects the fact that the
former, the time between Q wave onset and aortic valve
opening (Q to Ao), includes the IVC interval (Mc to Ao)
in its measurement. It has been shown (19) that myocardial contractility as measured by the maximum rate of
rise of intraventricular pressure dp/dt max is inversely
proportioned to PEP. This relationship has also been
confirmed (12) on the exteriorized fetal lamb. Similarly
the lack of correlation between the two intervals PEP and
IVC with the R to R interval may support the contention
that these intervals (PEP and IVC) are not significantly

related to fetal heart rate in normal labour (23,14,18).
Conversely the strong positive correlation between LVET
and R to R interval confirms that LVET will increase
linearly with increasing R to R interval and that LVET is
therefore inversely proportional to fetal heart rate.
Animal studies (13) and work in humans (22) and from our
own unit (18) have also demonstrated this inverse
relationship between LVET and FHR. However, when FHR falls
below 115 beats per minute the relationship fails and LVET
remains constant (13,22,24). It is possible that lengthening of LVET with fetal heart deceleration is an attempt
to increase stroke volume and maintain a constant cardiac
output (13,25). Garrard et al (10) in a study of adults
with cardiac disease have studied the PEP/LVET ratio and
found that this correlates closely with ejection fraction
and therefore reflects cardiac output. It seemed
certainly worthy of further study as an additional means
of evaluating fetal cardiac function.

   Although it has been found (17) that antepartum
measurements of PEP were 9.5% shorter than those measured
intrapartum, the present study showed no significant
alteration in mean PEP, IVC, LVET, R to R intervals or the
ratio PEP/LVET when recorded during the latent, active
phases or second stage of labour. Similarly, the study we
reported in 1978 of 22 patients recorded serially during
normal labour also suggested EMI stability (18). Comparison of intervals recorded between and during uterine
contractions showed a significant increase only for the
R to R intervals recorded in the first stage of labour.
The increasing R to R intervals recorded during contractions may result from the inclusion of patients exhibiting
FHR decelerations in the data analysis. It is important
to note that the presence of contractions did not preclude
successful EMI recording which may aid interpretation of
pathological cardiotocographic tracings. Murata and
others (17) described four fetuses in whom PEP lengthened
after contraction stress testing. Although this lengthening is attributed to the effect of uterine contractions,
the recordings were made before and after testing not
during the actual contraction.

   The analysis of EMI recordings and results of fetal
blood sampling in our 103 patients could not show a
consistent association for any interval with fetal
arterial oxygen tension, carbon dioxide tension nor with
arterial pH. The scientific literature contains conflicting reports about EMI relationships (in particular PEP and
LVET) with intrapartum parameters of fetal distress.
Murata and Martin (22) found prolongation of PEP in
patients with FHR abnormalities and in a later study
demonstrated that antepartum PEP prolongation was highly
correlated with a subsequent abnormal perinatal course
(17). In a study of fetal rhesus monkeys, the same
authors (14) reported a strong negative correlation

224

between PEP and arterial blood pH whether acidaemia was of respiratory or metabolic origin. Similarly, our earlier report (18) described four human fetuses where PEP lengthened with acidaemia. In contrast, Organ et al (12) in the exteriorized sheep fetus, demonstrated that hypoxaemia was associated with consistent shortening of PEP intervals irrespective of heart rate changes. The same study also demonstrated that experimental umbilical cord occlusion produced prolongation of the PEP interval. Additionally, the Toronto group found shortening of PEP in association with evidence of uteroplacental insufficiency in three human fetuses in labour and PEP prolongation in seven other patients, three of whom had variable decelerations on FHR tracings normally attributed to umbilical cord occlusion (26). The four case histories summarized in this report tend to corroborate these findings.

Morgenstern et al (13) utilizing acute fetal sheep preparations have performed a comprehensive series of experiments, exploring the relationship between systolic time intervals and various stress events. They have demonstrated that early fetal heart decelerations produced in response to fetal head compression were accompanied by prolongation of PEP in proportion to the applied pressure. This effect was attributed to increasing vagal tone and baroreceptor stimulation (27). Umbilical cord occlusion prolonged PEP confirming the work by Organ et al (12) and was thought to result from the combined effects of increased aortic diastolic pressure (increased afterload) and decreased venous return. Morgenstern's group have also demonstrated that fetal hypoxaemia was consistently associated with shortening of the PEP interval and have attributed the shortening of the interval seen following the release of umbilical cord occlusion to a hypoxic stimulus. Rasmussen et al (28) have demonstrated in dogs, with intact autonomic nervous systems, that hypoxia causes a diminution in PEP/LVET ratio simultaneously with hypertension and bradycardia and claimed that the ratio (PEP/LVET) was a sensitive index of fetal hypoxaemia and that the changes reflect combined sympathetic and vagal activity. The group also demonstrated that hypoxaemia initiates catecholamine release from the adrenal medulla as earlier described (29). The decrease in PEP/LVET ratio in association with fetal hypoxaemia is indicative of increasing myocardial contractility secondary to inotropic effects of the catecholamines released.

Organ et al (26) have diagramatically summarized these influences on pre-ejection period (see Fig 3).

```
┌─────────────────────────────────┐
│      THE PRE-EJECTION PERIOD     │
│         is affected by the       │
│    INOTROPIC STATE and LOADING   │
│          of the heart            │
└─────────────────────────────────┘

┌──────────────────────┐   ┌──────────────────────────┐
│   UTEROPLACENTAL      │   │    UMBILICAL CORD         │
│   INSUFFICIENCY       │   │      OCCLUSION            │
│        ↓             │   │        ↓                  │
│   HYPOXAEMIA          │   │  INCREASED AFTERLOAD      │
│        ↓             │   │  (Increased Aortic/       │
│   RELEASE of          │   │   Diastolic Pressure)     │
│   CATECHOLAMINES from │   │        and                │
│   ADRENAL MEDULLA     │   │  DECREASED PRELOAD        │
│        ↓             │   │  (Decreased Ventricular   │
│   POSITIVE INOTROPIC  │   │   End Diastolic Pressure) │
│   EFFECT              │   │        ↓                  │
│        ↓             │   │                           │
│   PEP SHORTENED       │   │  PEP PROLONGED            │
└──────────────────────┘   └──────────────────────────┘
```

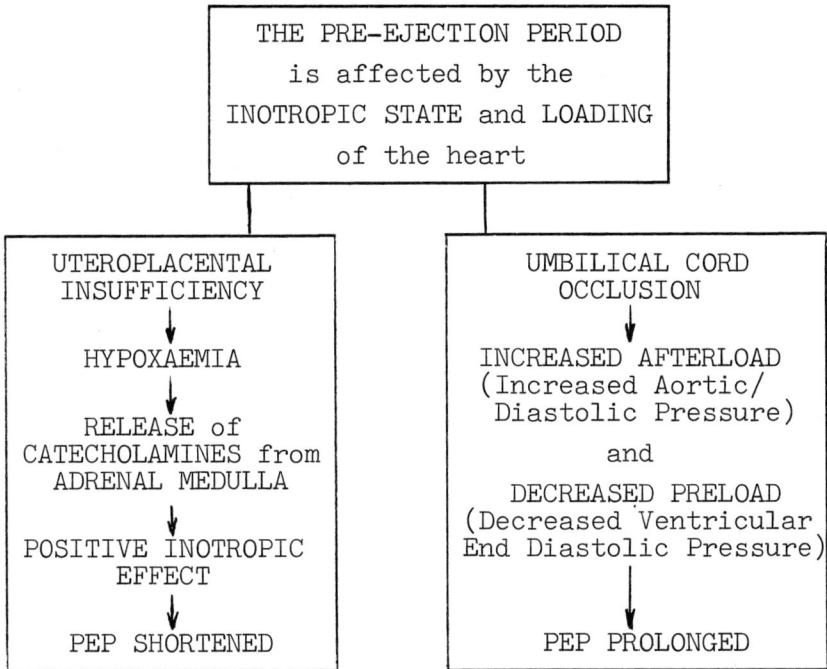

Figure 3. Proposed Mechanism of PEP Change during Fetal Distress (Organ et al 1974)

PEP is primarily influenced by the inotropic state and loading of the heart. Utero-placental insufficiency causes hypoxaemia which stimulated catecholamine release from the adrenal medulla, exciting a positive inotropic effect thus decreasing PEP. Umbilical cord occlusion increases aortic diastolic pressure (increases afterload) and additionally decreases venous return - decreasing ventricular end diastolic volume (decreased preload) thus PEP becomes prolonged.

We believe that the study of electromechanical intervals of the fetal heart continues to offer the possibility of improving the interpretation of FHR patterns and may allow discrimination between the causes of fetal distress. We have therefore embarked upon an investigation of 'high-risk' fetuses in labour and will explore the relationships between EMIs and other intra partum parameters of fetal wellbeing (e.g. FHR, blood lactate, pH and blood gas values) and perinatal outcome. The recent development in our unit of a semi-automated 'on-line' system for recording and measuring EMIs should relieve the tedium of visual measurement, reduce data variability and may in the future lead to continuous EMI recording from the 'high risk' fetus in labour (30).

ACKNOWLEDGEMENTS

The authors wish to thank Professor C.R. Whitfield for
advice and encouragement, the nursing staff of the Labour
Suite for their willing cooperation, Miss Margaret Davidson
and Mrs. Helen Mackenzie for their secretarial assistance,
the Departments of Medical Records and Medical Illustration,
and the Medical Research Council for their support (Grant
G977/284/C).

REFERENCES

1. Thomas, G. (1975): Brit. J. Obstet. Gynaec., 82, 121.
2. Tejani, N., Mann, L.I. and Bhakthavathsalam, A. (1976):
   Obstet. & Gynec., 48, 460.
3. Low, J.A., Pancham, S.R. and Worthington, D.N. (1977):
   Am. J. Obstet. Gynec., 127, 729.
4. Ott, W.J. (1976): Obstet. & Gynec. Survey, 31, 339.
5. James, L. (1974): In: Controversy in Obstetrics &
   Gynecology, II, Reed & Christian, Saunders.
6. Paul, R.H. (1972): Am. J. Obstet. Gynec., 113, 573.
7. Quilligan, E.J. and Paul, R.H. (1975): Obstet. & Gynec.,
   45, 96.
8. Hon, E.H., Zannini, D. and Quilligan, E.J. (1975):
   Am. J. Obstet. Gynec., 122, 508.
9. Weissler, A.M., Peeler, R.G. and Roehll, W.H. (1961):
   Am. Heart J., 62, 367.
10. Garrard, C.L., Weissler, A.M. and Dodge, H.T. (1970):
    Circulation, 42, 455.
11. Perloff, J.K. and Reichek, N. (1972): Circulation, 45,
    929.
12. Organ, L.W., Milligan, J.E., Goodwin, J.W. and Bain,
    M.J.C. (1973b): Am. J. Obstet. Gynec., 115, 377.
13. Morgenstern, J., Czerny, H., Schmidt, H., Schulz, J.
    and Wernicke, K. (1978): J. Perinat. Med., 6, 173.
14. Murata, Y., Martin, C.B., Ikenoue, T. and Petrie,
    R.H. (1978b): Am. J. Obstet, Gynec., 132, 285.
15. Organ, L.W., Bernstein, A., Rowe, I.H. and Smith, K.C.
    (1973a): Am. J. Obstet. Gynec., 115, 369.
16. Bernstein, A., Organ, L.W., Eisner, L.E., Smith, K.C.
    and Rowe, I.H. (1976): Am. J. Obstet. Gynec., 126, 238.
17. Murata, Y., Martin, C.B., Ikenoue, T. and Lu, P.S.
    (1978a): Am. J. Obstet. Gynec., 132, 278.
18. Robinson, H.P., Adam, A.H., Fleming, J.E.E., Houston,
    Anne and Clark, D.M. (1978): Brit. J. Obstet. Gynaec.,
    85, 172.
19. Metzger, G.C., Chough, C.B., Kroetz, F.W. and Leonard,
    J.J. (1970): Am. J. Cardiol., 25, 434.
20. Smith, N.C., Quinn, M.C., Soutter, W.P. and Sharp, F.
    (1975): Early Human Development, 3, 89.
21. Tukey, J.W. (1977): In: Exploratory Data Analysis,
    Addison & Wesley.
22. Murata, Y. and Martin, C.B. (1974): Obstet. & Gynec.,
    44, 224.

23. Goodlin, R.C., Girard, J. and Hollmen, A. (1972):
    Obstet. & Gynec., 39, 295.
24. Kelly, J.V. (1965): Am. J. Obstet. Gynec., 91, 1133.
25. Weissler, A.M., Harris, W.S. and Schoenfeld, C.D.
    (1968): Circulation, 37, 149.
26. Organ, L.W., Bernstein, A., Smith, K.C. and Rowe, I.H.
    (1974): Am. J. Obstet. Gynec., 120, 49.
27. Paul, W.M., Quilligan, E.J. and MacLachlan, T. (1964):
    Am. J. Obstet. Gynec., 90, 824.
28. Rasmussen, J.P., Bech-Jansen, P. and Kann, T. (1974):
    Acta Anaesth. Scand., 18, 5.
29. Comline, R.S., Silver, I.A. and Silver, M. (1965):
    J. Physiol., 178, 211.
30. Fleming, J.E.E. and Doig, J.R. (1979): In preparation.

FLOW VELOCITY IN THE VENOUS RETURN FROM THE PLACENTA

R.W. Gill*, G. Kossoff*, B.J. Trudinger**, P.S. Warren***

  * Ultrasonics Institute, Sydney, Australia
 ** The Westmead Centre, Sydney, Australia
*** The Royal Hospital for Women, Sydney, Australia

This paper will discuss the application in obstetrics of a previously described technique for the non-invasive measurement of blood flow in relatively small and deep-lying vessels (2). The table below lists the characteristics and limitations of the Doppler/B-mode system used.

Ultrasound Frequency	3 MHz
Pulse Repetition Rate	2 kHz
Doppler Signal Processing	$\sqrt{\omega}$ directional mean frequency demodulator
Velocity	$v \cos \theta$ = 1-25 cm/sec
Vessel Diameter	d = 3-10 mm
Flow	Q = 5-600 ml/min
Accuracy:	$v \cos \theta$ ±2%
	θ ±0.5°
	d ±0.5 mm

NORMAL PREGNANCIES

To date the principal application of this technique has been in the fetal umbilical vein. The results obtained in a series of 50 normal pregnancies ranging from 22 weeks gestation to term are shown elsewhere in this volume (3).

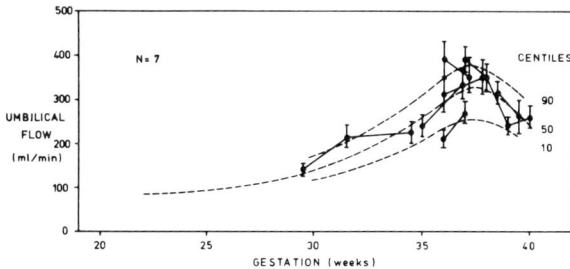

Figure 1. Serial measurements of umbilical vein flow in 7 normal patients. The bars indicate the estimated standard error of the data, while the broken lines indicate the normal range.

Flow increases steadily with increasing fetal size, reaching a maximum at about 38 weeks gestation, after which there is a definite decrease in flow over the last two weeks of pregnancy. This fall-off near term, which appears to coincide with a slowdown of ultrasound growth, is also seen on serial studies of individual patients (Figure 1), demonstrating that it is a real phenomenon, not a statistical artifact.

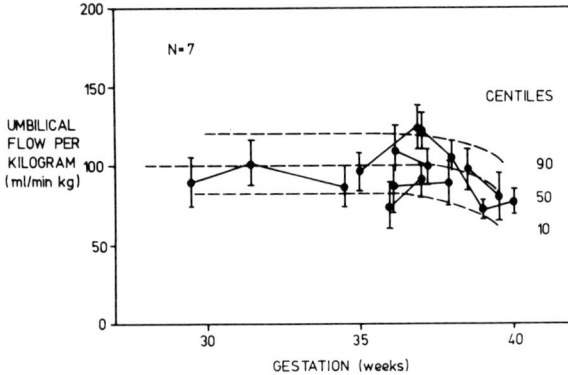

Figure 2. The same data as in Figure 1, but normalised for fetal weight.

These flow results can be normalised by dividing the umbilical flow by estimated fetal weight (Figure 2). The fetal weight is taken as the median value for a normal fetus of the appropriate gestational age, with the age being determined by ultrasound size measurements. These weights are subsequently corrected for actual birth weight wherever necessary. Until about 38 weeks gestation, flow per kilogram remains constant at 100 ml/kg min. (It should be noted that we have previously reported a somewhat higher value for this, due to the use of non-Australian fetal weight charts. This new value was obtained using Australian figures). Previous investigators have reported values of 110 ml/kg min in the second trimester (1,5) and 75 ml/kg min immediately following normal delivery at term (6). These measurements were, however, taken under abnormal physiological conditions and therefore provide a somewhat unsatisfactory comparison. There are no known human fetal flow measurements taken under normal physiological conditions with which the present series can be compared.

ABNORMAL PREGNANCIES

Attention has now been turned to abnormal pregnancies. An obvious group of interest is those pregnancies in which the fetal weight at birth is markedly below the normal value (for the known gestational age). As Figure 3 shows, in 11 patients where the fetal birth weight was below the 5th

230

percentile, flow values were also markedly low, except where some other complication of the pregnancy (such as hypertension) was also present. Looking at these results on a per kilogram basis (Figure 4) again shows (with one exception) that flow values fall within or below the normal range except where other complications exist. More data must be collected before we can address such questions as which of these are low growth-potential babies, and whether the low flow values are the cause or result of growth retardation.

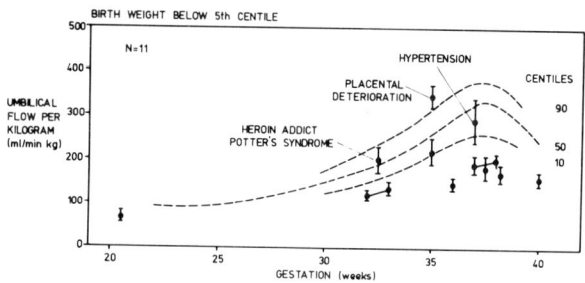

Figure 3. Umbilical vein flow in small-for-dates babies.

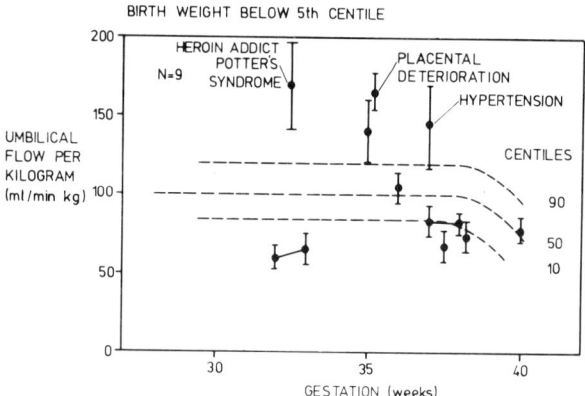

Figure 4. Umbilical vein flow per kilogram in small-for-dates babies.

Another category of interest is maternal diabetes, where abnormally high flow values have generally been observed. In hypertension, however, the situation is far less simple. Even if the PET group is singled out, a clear pattern does not emerge; some flow values are below the normal range, some fall within it and in cases of fetal growth retardation the flow values per kilogram have been above the normal range. Clearly more data are required and a better classification of this group of problem pregnancies is needed.

One final aspect of the umbilical vein flow deserves mention. In cases of fetal breathing, flow is found to be strongly modulated by the breathing (Figure 5). This is presumably caused by the large fluctuations in thoracic and abdominal pressures associated with the breathing movements (4). Umbilical vein flow measurement therefore presents a method of obtaining a hard copy record of fetal breathing movements which can be used for subsequent analysis of the rate, variability and pattern of those movements. This has some obvious advantages over the approach using visual monitoring of a real-time B-scanner with a stop-watch or other manual recorder.

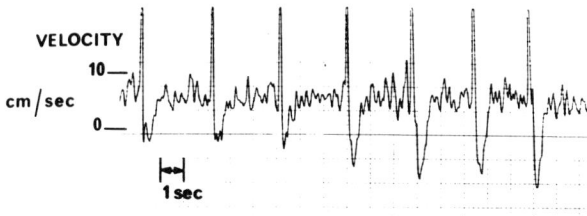

Figure 5. Modulation of umbilical vein flow by fetal breathing

SUMMARY

We have described the application of a fully non-invasive quantitative method for measuring blood flow to the fetal umbilical vein. The range of normal flow values from 22 weeks gestation to term has been determined. Some initial observations on abnormal pregnancies have been made, indicating significant deviations from the normal range of flow values. More results are required before definite conclusions can be reached.

REFERENCES

1. Assali, N.S., Rauramo, L. and Peltonen, T. (1960): Measurement of uterine blood flow and uterine metabolism. Am. J. Obst. & Gynec., 79, 86-98.
2. Gill, R.W. (1978): Quantitative blood flow measurement in deep-lying vessels using pulsed Doppler with the Octoson. In: Ultrasound in Medicine, Vol. 4. Editor D. White, Plenum Press, New York.
3. Kossoff, G. (1979): Look into the future of diagnostic ultrasound. Proc. II Int. Symp. Recent Advances in Ultrasound Diagnosis. Excerpta Medica (in press).
4. Poore, E.R. (1978): The ultrasound measurement of fetal breathing. D. Phil. Thesis, University Press, Oxford.
5. Rudolph, A.M., Heymann, M.A., Teramo, K.A.W., Barrett, C.T. and Raiba, N.C.R. (1971): Studies of the circulation of the previable human fetus. Pediat. Res., 5, 452-465.
6. Stembera, Z.K., Hodr, J. and Janda, J. (1965): Umbilical blood flow in healthy newborn infants during the first minutes after birth. Am. J. Obst. & Gynec., 91, 568-574.

ULTRASONIC MEASUREMENTS OF HUMAN FETAL BLOOD FLOW IN AORTA AND UMBILICAL VEIN: INFLUENCE OF FETAL BREATHING MOVEMENTS.

S.H. Eik-Nes*, K. Maršál*, A.O. Brubakk** and M. Ulstein**

*Department of Obstetrics and Gynecology, University Hospital, Malmö, Sweden
**Department of Clinical Physiology and Department of Obstetrics and Gynecology, University of Trondheim, Trondheim, Norway

So far, no noninvasive method has been available for studying fetal blood flow in utero. Information on human fetal circulation is thus very scarce and is based only on measurements on early abortions (1,2) and on newborns immediately after delivery (3,4).

In 1977, Fitzgerald and Drumm (5) published a method which combined compound B-mode ultrasonography and continuous Doppler to obtain signals of blood velocity in the umbilical cord in utero. Recently, Gill and Kossof (6) demonstrated how flow in the umbilical vein could be quantified by means of pulsed Doppler ultrasound measurement. Their method did not permit, however, measurement of blood velocity in the fetal aorta.

METHOD

For transcutaneous measurement of human fetal blood flow in the aorta and in the intraabdominal part of the umbilical vein we combined real-time B-mode ultrasonography with pulsed Doppler ultrasound technique. The use of real-time ultrasonography makes it possible to visualize the fetal vessels, e.g., the aorta and the intraabdominal part of the umbilical vein. The Doppler ultrasonic technique enables measurement of blood velocity without interfering with the flow. The use of pulsed Doppler instead of continuous Doppler makes it possible to measure flow within a vessel at a selected depth.

For the combined use, the Doppler transducer was attached to the linear array real-time transducer (ADR) at a fixed angle of 52° (Fig. 1). The process of measuring blood velocity was to adjust the real-time transducer parallel to the vessel of interest. The distance from the real-time transducer to the vessel (d) was measured and with a known angle (α) between the two transducers, the distance from the Doppler transducer to the vessel (D) was calculated. The vessel diameter was estimated by taking the mean of 10 measurements made on the B-mode screen. When the vessel was correctly localized, the real-time transducer was turned off and the Doppler transducer turned on. This was done due to interference between the two transducers.

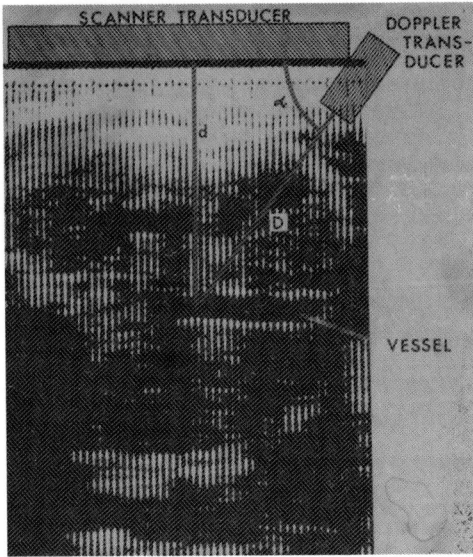

Figure 1. Two-dimensional real-time image of cross-sectional area of fetal abdomen with the umbilical vein. Superimposed is a schematic picture showing the combination of the two ultrasound transducers.

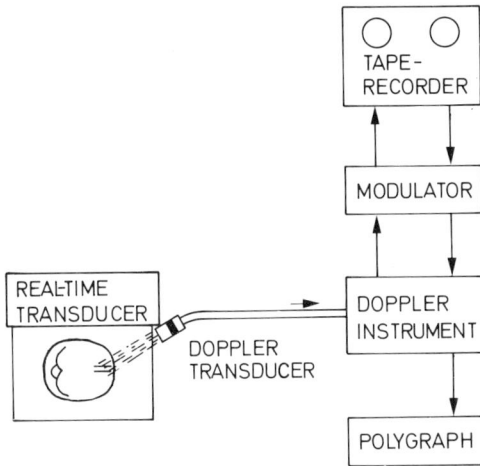

Figure 2. Set-up for the ultrasonic measurements of fetal blood flow.

Fig. 2 shows the set-up for fetal blood velocity measurement. The Doppler instrument (PEDOF) (7) emits ultrasound pulses at a 2 MHz frequency with a duration of 10 μsec and a repetition rate either 6.5 or 9.75 kHz. Thus, blood velocities up to 1.7 m sec^{-1} can be estimated down to a depth of 6.0 cm below the transducer and velocities up to 1.0 m sec^{-1} can be measured between 6 and 10 cm of depth. After the transmission of the pulse, the sample gate closes for 1 μsec at fixed time set by the sample position control. Thus, velocity signals at a pre-set distance from the Doppler transducer can be measured. To eliminate signals from slowly moving tissues in the path of the beam, high-pass filters with selectable cut-off frequencies are inserted. The Doppler shifts can be processed immediately; they can also be stored on tape. They are then led through a single side-band modulator, which permits the storage on a regular stereo tape recorder together with spoken comments. For calculations, the stored signals are demodulated and fed into a maximum and mean velocity estimator within the Doppler instrument. The estimators convert the signals into analogue voltage proportional to the maximum- and the mean velocity in the region of observation. The instrument also provides the derivative of the velocity (i.e., the acceleration), and the integral under the velocity curve. The four output signals of the Doppler instrument, the acceleration, the maximum-, the mean velocity and the integral under the velocity curve, are recorded graphically (Fig. 3).

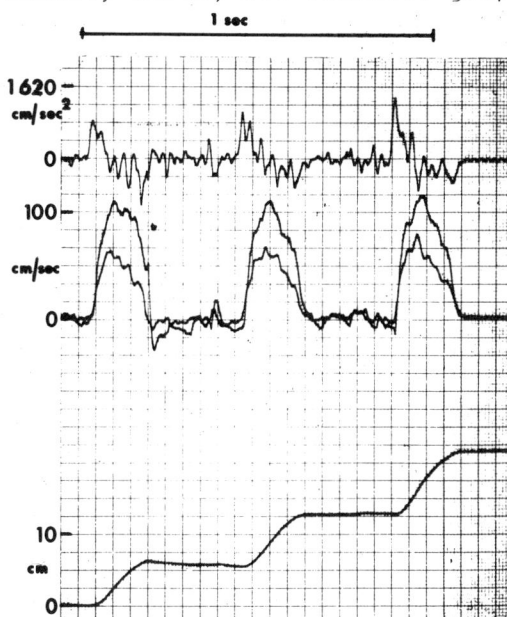

Figure 3. Polygraphic record of the four output signals from the Doppler instrument obtained from the human fetal aorta. The upper tracing: the blood flow acceleration (cm/sec^2). The mid-tracings: the maximum and mean blood flow velocity (cm/sec). The lower tracing: the integral under the maximum velocity curve (cm).

The blood flow in the aorta (Qa) was calculated according to the formula

$$Qa = \frac{I \cdot A \cdot HR}{\cos \alpha}$$

where I is mean integral rise based on 10 heart beats, A vessel area, HR heart rate, α angle between the two transducers.

The blood flow in the umbilical vein (Qv) was calculated according to the formula

$$Qv = \frac{V \cdot A}{\cos \alpha}$$

where V is the mean velocity for a period of at least 15 sec.

235

FETAL BLOOD FLOW IN NORMAL PREGNANCIES

The method was first applied to 26 normal pregnancies in the last trimester. Blood velocities were estimated in the descending part of the fetal aorta and in the intra-abdominal part of the umbilical vein. Fetal weights ranged from 1780 to 4330 g. Where birth took place within 1 week after the measurement, the birth weight was registered. Otherwise, the weight was estimated by means of the ultrasonically measured biparietal diameter and the abdominal transverse diameter. This weight estimation method has a standard deviation of predicted errors of 250 g (8).

TABLE I. Results of the fetal blood flow measurements in normal pregnancies.

	n	Mean velocity $(cm\ sec^{-1})$	Maximum velocity $(cm\ sec^{-1})$	Blood flow $(ml\ min^{-1}kg^{-1})$ based on mean vel.	max. vel.
Descending aorta	26	73	109	132	191
Umbilical vein	20	13	–	110	–

Table I gives the results of the measurements. When calculating blood flow in the <u>umbilical vein</u>, we assumed a parabolic flow profile within the vessel; the calculation was based on the mean velocity. The mean blood flow for the study group was 110 ml $min^{-1}kg^{-1}$.

Several indirect methods have been used for estimating of human umbilical blood flow. Assali et al. (1) analysed umbilical blood flow in early abortions with electromagnetic cuff and obtained a mean value of 110 ml $min^{-1}kg^{-1}$. Štembera et al. (3) used local thermodilution method for measurement of the umbilical blood flow immediately after delivery. The mean blood flow in their study was 75 ml $min^{-1}kg^{-1}$. McCallum (4) used the same method and attained comparable results. Dawes (9) calculated the minimum blood flow needed in the human umbilical vein to be 90 ml $min^{-1}kg^{-1}$. His calculation was based on O_2 consumption. The results obtained in our study exceed the calculated minimum flow and are obviously within the physiological range.

In the <u>descending aorta</u>, we estimated the maximum and mean velocity. The index between them was 1.5. The blood flow in the descending fetal aorta was 191 ml $min^{-1}kg^{-1}$ when calculated from the maximum velocity and 132 ml $min^{-1}kg^{-1}$ when calculated from the mean velocity. When basing flow calculation in the aorta on the maximum blood velocity, one is assuming a flat flow profile and this assumption would probably lead to a slight overestimation of the blood flow. When the flow calculation is based on the mean velocity, the value could be affected by the interference from the near lying veins, which would reduce the resulting value. The mean velocity is also more dependent on a precise aiming, because the vessel has to be completely within the sample volume of the Doppler instrument to make estimation of a true mean value possible. Thus, possible errors when estimating flow in the aorta based on mean velocity will lead to an underestimation of the true blood flow.

No previous reports on blood flow in human fetal aorta are available. Comparison with values obtained on fetal animals is difficult and must be done with care (10).

THE INFLUENCE OF FETAL BREATHING MOVEMENTS ON THE BLOOD FLOW PATTERN IN VENA UMBILICALIS

In 1976, Boyce et al. (11) detected Doppler shifts synchronous with fetal breathing movements (FBM) in human. First, these signals were thought to originate from lung fluid movements. In 1977, the Oxford group analysed the Doppler shift signals during FBM in lamb preparations and also in human pregnancies and concluded that the signals emanated from the blood flow changes in the inferior vena cava (12). Mantell (13) in New Zealand used the same technique but the audible signals were out of phase and had a character different from those obtained by the Oxford group. In a collaborated study, the recordings from Oxford and New Zealand were compared, and the signals obtained by the New Zealand method were identified as originating from the umbilical cord within the amniotic pool (13). Thus, it was demonstrated that during fetal inspiration a momentary increase in the inferior vena cava flow velocity and a decrease in umbilical vein flow velocity occurred.

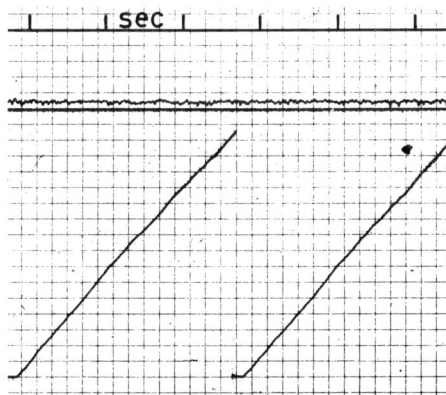

Figure 4. Mean blood velocity curve in the umbilical vein (upper tracing) during fetal apnea. The integrals under the velocity curve (lower tracing) are straight and parallel thus indicating steady blood flow.

Different patterns of FBM with large variations in the frequency and amplitude have been described (14). The type of FBM can change even several times during the recording session. During a period of high amplitude FBM,

the umbilical blood velocity is profoundly changed with
each fetal breath (Fig. 5a). When a period of high amplitude FBM was followed by fetal apnea, continuous undis-
turbed blood flow was recorded (Fig. 5b). The calculated
blood flow was on average 20-30 % increased during periods
of high amplitude FBM compared with the periods of apnea.
Low amplitude FBM also affected the velocity curve (Fig. 6)
but did not quantitatively change the blood flow.

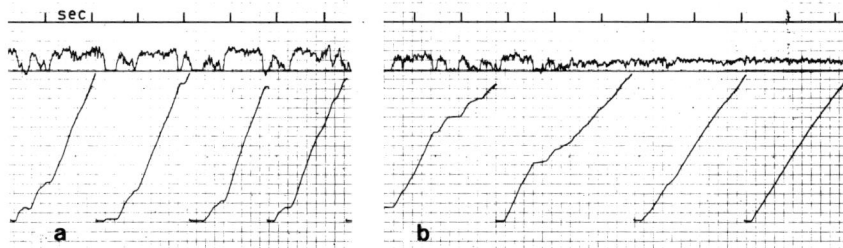

Figure 5. Blood velocity curve in the umbilical vein during high amplitude FBM (a) and 30 sec later during fetal
apnea period (b). The change of the integral slope indicates reduction of blood flow during apnea compared with
the period of high amplitude FBM.

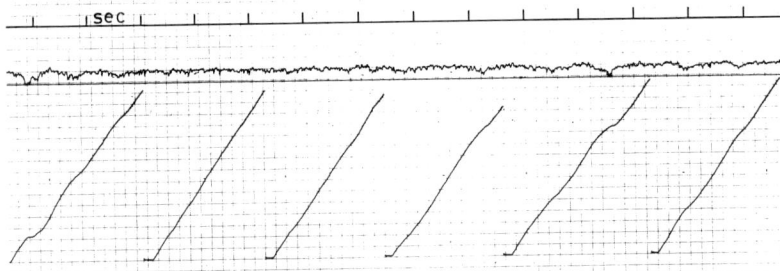

Figure 6. Blood velocity curve in the umbilical vein
(upper tracing) during apnea (left) and low amplitude FBM
(right). The integrals (lower tracing) are parallel indicating unchanged blood flow during the observation period.

To establish the time-relation between the FBM cycle
and the short-term changes in the umbilical blood flow
velocity, an additional real-time transducer was employed
for visualization of the thoracic movements. It could be
concluded that a decrease in blood velocity occurred during the inspiratory phase and was followed by an increase
during expiration.

Recently, Rudolph et al. (15) using electromagnetic
flowmeters measured the blood flow in the thoracic part of
the inferior vena cava in fetal lambs. During FBM, he
found a profound effect on the flow patterns. Our results
suggest that the same is true concerning the flow pattern
in the umbilical vein of the human fetus. In a discussion
of the purpose of FBM, the antenatal training of the respiratory muscles has been accepted as the most plausible

238

explanation. It is, of course, tempting to speculate on a possible role of the FBM in regulating fetal blood flow. More quantitative data on umbilical blood flow during periods of different FBM types are necessary before any conclusions are reached.

SUMMARY

For transcutaneous analysis of fetal blood flow, we combined real-time ultrasonography with pulsed Doppler ultrasound. By this method, blood flow in fetal aorta and umbilical vein can easily be detected and measured. The application of this noninvasive method for studies of fetal hemodynamics during various maternal and fetal conditions appears feasible. The finding of the changes in umbilical blood flow during FBM suggests, that we can expect new facts about fetal physiology to be revealed.

ACKNOWLEDGEMENTS

This study was supported by the Aalesund Central Hospital and the Medical School, University of Trondheim, Norway. The ultrasonic equipment was kindly provided by Kranzbühler u. Sohn, Solingen, Germany, and Nycotron, Drammen, Norway. The valuable advices and friendly help by Kjell Kristoffersen and Olav Bakken are greatly acknowledged.

REFERENCES

1. Assali, N.S., Rauramo, L. and Peltonen, T. (1960): Am. J. Obstet. Gynecol., 79, 86.
2. Morris, J.A., Hustead, R.F., Robinson, R.G., Haswell, G.L., Morgan, C.A. and Gobuty, A. (1974): Am. J. Obstet. Gynecol., 118, 927.
3. Štembera, Z.K., Hodr, J. and Janda, J. (1965): Am. J. Obstet. Gynecol., 91, 568.
4. McCallum, W.D. (1977): Am. J. Obstet. Gynecol., 127, 491.
5. Fitzgerald, D.E. and Drumm, J.E. (1977): Br. Med. J., 2, 1450.
6. Gill, R.W. and Kossof, G. (1979): In: Real-Time Ultrasound in Perinatal Medicine, p. 139. Editor: R. Chef. S. Karger, Basel.
7. Angelsen, B.A.J. and Brubakk, A.O. (1976): Cardiovasc. Res., 10, 368.
8. Eik-Nes, S.H. and Gröttum, P. (1979): In: Proceedings 1st International Berlin Meeting on Perinatal Medicine, Berlin, 1979. Editors: E. Schmidt, J.W. Dudenhausen, E. Saling. (In press.)
9. Dawes, G.S. (1968): In: Dawes, Fetal and Neonatal Physiology, p. 76. Year Book Medical Publishers, Inc., Chicago.

10. Lind, J. (1977): Eur. J. Card., 5, 265.
11. Boyce, E.S., Dawes, G.S., Gough, J.D. and Poore, E.R. (1976): Br. Med. J., 2, 17.
12. Gough, J.D. and Poore, E.R. (1977): J. Physiol., 272, 12P.
13. Goodman, J. and Mantell, C.D. (1978): In: Proceedings 5th Conference on Fetal Breathing, p. 106. Editor: T. K.A.B. Eskes. Nijmegen.
14. Maršál, K. (1978): Obstet. Gynecol., 52, 394.
15. Rudolph, A. (1979): In: Proceedings 6th Conference on Fetal Breathing, Paris, 1979. Editor: C. Tchobroutsky. (In press.)

COMMENTS

G. Gennser

The papers in this section present a wealth of new
data from the human fetus, thereby unequivocally announ-
cing the dawn of a new era in which the fetus will be
accessible to noninvasive and acceptably safe ultrasound
techniques. We shall in the near future be able to found
our clinical evaluations and decisions, not on cardiovascular evidence borrowed from experimental animals but
on relevant measurements on the particular fetus under
investigation. That is the important message carried by
these formidable studies.
The echocardiographic report by Wladimiroff and his
associates demonstrates how rapidly the heart of the newborn adjusts to the altered cardiovascular dynamic situation after birth. Not only the configuration of the heart
but also the contractility of the ventricles reflect the
postnatal closure of the fetal by-passes and the decreased
resistance in the pulmonary circulation. All three papers
on the fetal heart report data.from normal gestations
(although four cases of complicated delivery are included
in the study of the electromechanical intervals). Naturally, further studies on fetuses at risk are awaited
with interest. This pertains to the configurative development of the heart after birth when the respiratory adaptation is disturbed; also to the measurement of the myocardial contractility. In this context it is appropriate
to recall that the fetal myocardium depends on glucose for
its energy metabolism. This is reflected in the demonstration that the contractility of the fetal myocardium in
vitro is lowered by hypoxia and hypoglycemia and that the
reduced contractility is corrected by a tenfold increase
in glucose concentration despite continued hypoxia (Fig.
1). Thus, measurements of the contractility of the fetal
heart might reveal important information on the current
state of energy stores in the fetus.
A major achievment is the quantitation of the blood
flow in large fetal vessels. The two studies using pulsed
Doppler ultrasound give remarkably similar values of the
umbilical blood flow per kg fetal mass; the differences
might be largely due to difficulties in measuring the
calibre of the vessel and in estimating the fetal weight
at the time of the examinations. It is interesting to note

that the values of umbilical blood flow reported here only by 20 % exceeds what has been earlier calculated as the minimum flow necessary for the human term fetus (1). If this estimate of a narrow margin proves to be correct, it suggests that the umbilical flow measurements will in future be of great importance in supervising the growth-retarded fetus.

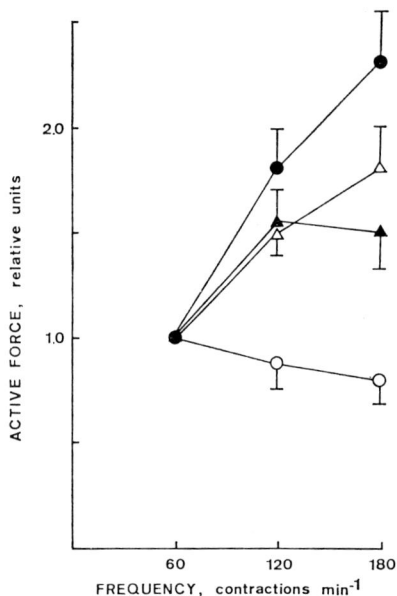

Figure 1. Relation between contraction frequency and maximum active force of adult (solid symbols) and neonatal (open symbols) rabbit papillary muscles during perfusion with 3.3 mmolar glucose with 95 % nitrogen (circles), and 33 mmolar glucose with 95 % nitrogen (triangles) (n = 8 in all muscle groups). Force at 60 contractions $\cdot$ min^{-1} = 1.0. (From Gennser, G.: Influence of hypoxia and glucose on contractility of papillary muscles from adult and neonatal rabbits, Biol. Neonate 21: 90-106, 1972.)

The attempt to estimate the combined cardiac output from the ventricles by measurements of the difference between the diastolic and the systolic values of the transverse diameter suffers from the coarse approximation of one length parameter to the volume of a complexly shaped space. This method must await confirmation by dynamic 3-dimensional studies of the fetal heart chambers before its clinical application.

The very recent character of these reports has to be appreciated: some of the data have come directly from the research laboratories. A few of the presented results are unexpected and should be controlled in larger series. The found decline of the umbilical blood flow per kg fetal weight during the last few weeks before term is contradictory to the recent finding that the velocity of growth is linear up to term and also up to four months post term. This is evidenced when birth weights in a normal population are calculated for gestational ages, which are corrected by fetal ultrasonic morphometry performed early in gestation (P.H. Persson, personal communication). Future work will have to disclose whether the relative fall in umbilical flow during the end of gestation is compensated for by an altered extraction of nutritive compounds.

Both groups of observers found that fetal breathing movements influence the umbilical blood flow. This has been reported earlier from animal studies (2) and seems to be an important feature of fetal physiology. It suggests a possibility for the fetus to alter the blood flow velocity from the placenta and, all other factors remaining constant, thereby to influence the transfer of gases and solubles across the placenta. This discovery has several implications: among others, it might serve to explain the recent, seemingly paradoxical, finding in the fetus of oscillations in the breath-to-breath intervals during periods of continuous fetal breathing movements (3). Similar undulations in the breathing of the newborns have been ascribed to oscillations of a negative feed-back regulated control system due to the time lag between changes in alveolar gas composition and their detection by chemoreceptors. The oscillations in the fetal breathing rate are compatible with the hypothesis that a fetus can, to some extent, influence its own oxygenation, but further studies are needed to clarify this important point.

The methods presented here are still at various stages of experimentation and development; a word of caution might be needed. Because all promise to become useful tools for examining and monitoring the fetus, it is necessary to give these methods time to be thoroughly evaluated and tried clinically in carefully planned studies. The methods are still being researched and are potentially far too valuable to be spoilt by early misuse.

REFERENCES

1. Dawes, G.S. (1968): In: Foetal and Neonatal Physiology. Year Book Publ., Chicago.
2. Rudolph, A. (1979): In: Proceedings of the 6th Conference on Fetal Breathing. Editor: C. Tchobroutsky. Paris (in press).
3. Gennser, G. and Hathorn, M.K.S. (1979): The Lancet, i, 1298.

J.W. Wladimiroff

PRESENT STATUS OF FETAL DYNAMICS

Fetal dynamic behaviour plays an essential role in everyday obstetrics. The observation of fetal movements by the mother and fetal heart activity by the obstetrician is important in the assessment of fetal well-being. It was only after the advent of ultrasound that more detailed studies on various aspects of fetal dynamics could be initiated. It was convential B-scanning which supplied the first data on dynamic parameters such as fetal heart rate in very early pregnancy and fetal bladder function in late pregnancy. Real-time visualization of the fetus has resulted in an explosion of studies on fetal dynamic behaviour. This chapter will provide a true picture of the present status of fetal dynamics as experienced by various experts in this field. The first three papers will deal with fetal motor behaviour in early and late pregnancy. Fetal motor behaviour can now be accurately visualized and therefore, their pattern more reliably studied. Interest in fetal motor activity has particularly been shown in early pregnancy, since it is only during this period that the entire fetus can be made visable. Dr. Reinhold from Vienna will give a detailed account on the observation of fetal motor behaviour and reflex response, and as well provide a qualitative description of body movements under normal and pathological circumstances in early pregnancy. Dr. Henner from St. Gallen, Switzerland in cooperation with Dr. Haller and Dr. Kubli has embarked on early fetal motor activity in a more quantitated manner. They particularly paid attention to the velocity and acceleration of fetal body movements in normal and complicated early pregnancy.

Our insight into fetal motor behaviour would be incomplete if the work of Marsal, Lindström and Ulmsten from Malmö was not included. Ultrasound is of limited value in the assessment of fetal motor activity in late pregnancy, due to the fact that only parts of the fetus can be visualized. Marsal et al. offer an interesting alternative method for objective recording of fetal movements in late pregnancy by means of a fetal movement detector consisting of four piezo-electric crystals placed in various positions on the maternal abdomen depending on the fetal lie. The clinical value of this device needs further evaluation.

247

Fetal breathing movements have aroused the interest of the perinatologists for quite some time. Its dependency on various factors, i.e. circadian rhythm, maternal plasma glucose levels and gaseous exchange, drug administration and cigarette smoking, has made this dynamic parameter a popular subject of investigation. Marsal and Gennser from Malmö will discuss the present state of research and the possible clinical applications of fetal breathing movements.

The last two papers deal with two entirely different exciting fields of dynamic behaviour. Studies on fetal stomach filling and emptying patterns have provided interesting information on fetal stomach activity. Fetal swallowing has been observed. Visualization of the upper intestinal tract has lead to the antenatal diagnosis of oesophageal, as well as duodenal atresia. Vandenberghe from Leuven will present the results of his studies in this particular field. Kurjak will close this chapter with a clear account on fetal bladder function and fetal urinary production in normal and diabetic pregnancy as well as in small-for-dates. The relationship between fetal urinary production and amniotic fluid volume will also be discussed.

FETAL MOTOR BEHAVIOUR

E. Reinold

Department of Obstetrics and Gynaecology, University of
Vienna, Austria

A great, perhaps the greatest advantage of real-time
scanning is the possibility and opportunity of the demonstration and observation of fetal movements and fetal motor behaviour. Intrauterine movements of the fetal body
are signs of fetal life and well-being, given by the fetus
itself. Many other diagnostic tests are only indirect and
are influenced by many other facts and circumstances which
are often not necessarily associated with the fetus.
They are felt by the pregnent woman during the second
half of gestation and have served as indicators of fetal
vitality throughout the ages. That fetal movements also
occur during the first half of gestation was, however,
discovered fairly recently. Less than a 100 years ago fetuses aborted during the first half of pregnancy were reported to make twitching movements with their extremities.
At that time, this was apparently a new and fascinating observation. No more than 50 years ago systematic fetoneuro-
logic investigations were begun, stimulating fetuses aborted alive to shed light on the development of neural
function. Systematic experimental studies of elicitable fetal reflexes under standardized conditions in nutrient media were only initiated some 25 years ago.

SONOGRAPHIC METHODS FOR MONITORING FETAL BODY MOVEMENTS

The development of ultrasonography provided research
with the object of visualizing fetuses in utero and monitoring their movements.

A-scan (amplitude modulation) technique

This technique, which is basically unidimensional and
serves to measure distances, gives a rough idea of movements in the body. Changes of the shape and position of
the so-called heart spike, which is generated by the pul-
sating fetal heart, constitute a typical and characteristic
finding, while configurational and positional changes of
echoes reflected from moving fetal parts are unspecific and
uncharacteristic, since they may be referable to artefacts.

T-M-mode (time-motion) technique

This technique produces a continuous trace of the

movements made by sound-reflecting structures which are shifted with a fixed velocity. The curves generated by the rhythmically moving fetal heart structures are typical and characteristic, while the patterns obtained from moving fetal parts are variable, less typical and uncharacteristic.

Compound scan

This two-dimensional tomographic technique helps to assess movements of the fetal body by comparing tomograms recorded in one and the same plane. The 2 consecutive tomograms will readily show the extent of change in fetal position.

Real-time scan

This tomographic technique records echoes on a real-time scope and produces a continuous scan with changes in fetal position on the screen. Pattern, rate, extent and nature of fetal movements can be monitored continuously (Fig. 1).

While A-scans and T-M-mode patterns document the presence or absence of fetal movements, they fail to produce any more detailed information. As the fetal body moves, the reflecting structure visualized at a given moment is lost by ultrasound beam, while other parts of the reflecting interface are exposed to it and are, as a result, displayed on the screen.

Compound scanning gives some idea of the fetal parts involved in fetal motion and also shows the scope of movements, while their rate and type are missed.

On real-time scanning a useful three-dimensional display of the interior of the maternal body is readily obtained by moving the applicator in different directions, while watching the oscilloscope screen. This particularly shows the size, position, orientation and posture of the fetal body (2). In addition, the optimum scanning plane for monitoring fetal movements is readily identified. As a rule, fetal movements are best visualized along that plane in which the longitudinal axis of the fetal body and/or the fetal extremities are displayed. A useful three-dimensional representation of fetal movements is equally obtained by keeping the ultrasound applicator stationary, while watching shifts of the position of the scanning plane produced by the moving fetal body. From the motor patterns thus generated the fetal movements can be evaluated by different criteria.

Owing to the design of current real-time scanners, the section of the human body reproduced on the sonogram is about 20 cm in size. While this is sufficient for completely visualizing the gestational sac with its contents during the first months of gestation and most or all of the fetal body during the second trimester, only parts of the fetal body can be displayed towards the end of pregnancy.

250

SPATIAL RELATIONS AND DIFFERENTIATION OF FETAL MOVEMENTS

The quality of monitoring fetal movements is closely correlated to fetal age.

(1) In early pregnancy there is sufficient space for extensive fetal movements in the gestational sac. However, the space available for movements becomes progressively smaller with advancing gestation so that, towards the end of pregnancy, fetal movements are limited in scope.

(2) In early pregnancy the fetal body is completely reproduced on the tomograms so that missing fetal movements is unlikely. With increasing fetal size, visualization is confined to some parts of the fetal body; as a result, the likelihood of missing fetal movements is increased.

(3) In early stages of fetal development fetal motion involves the entire fetal body. As the fetus matures, the motor patterns become more differentiated and often involve single muscle groups only.

In describing spontaneous fetal motor behaviour, a distinction between the first and second half of gestation would, therefore, appear to be appropriate.

IDENTIFICATION OF SPONTANEOUS FETAL MOVEMENTS

(a) First half of gestation

Shifts in fetal position can be visualized at about 8 weeks of gestation (from the first day of the last period in normally menstruating females). These first spontaneous fetal movements are of the total pattern type, i.e. they involve the entire fetal body, and are reminiscent of twitches which are not associated with any major displacement of the fetal body in the gestational sac. In further course of neuromuscular development the motor patterns become increasingly differentiated, i.e. they are confined to more or less large muscle groups. Contraction of these muscles produces flexion, extension, lateral flexion and rotation of various parts of the fetal body, which start to become functional at about 10 weeks of gestation (4).

Accordingly, fetal body movements are increasingly diversified so that they can be evaluated by a number of criteria, including:
- the scope of movements (i.e. the body parts involved in the movement);
- the extent of the movement (i.e. the largest distance travelled by the fetal body during a movement);
- the nature of movements (i.e. the speed with which movements are executed);
- the rate of movements (i.e. their number in unit time) (Fig. 2);
- the density of movement (i.e. their distribution and sequence in unit time);
- the duration of movements (i.e. the active and inactive intervals).

As the motor behaviour of the fetus is determined by all of these factors, its description and interpretation is an extremely onerous exercise. Theoretically, any one of these criteria can be taken as a basis for classifying movements. In the last analysis, no such classification will, however, be completely satisfactory, as it disregards various factors whose implications are still poorly understood (5).

For diagnostic purposes in clinical routine a simple and uncomplicated classification proved to be quite useful. The characterization of the motion pattern is based on the onset, the extent and the effect of the movements. Spontaneous movements are graded qualitatively as 'brisk' or 'strong' and 'slow' or sluggish' (4).

For quantitative purpose the number of movements in unit time (e.g. 5/min), can be recorded.

(b) Second half of gestation

During this period only parts of the fetal body are visualized on the sonogram and fetal movements are extremely differentiated. Consequently, an assessment based on the above criteria is useless. Moreover, the chance that spontaneous movements involve muscle groups which, at a given point in time, do not present in the scanning plane is high. During this period different fetal parts may execute different types of flexion, deflexion and rotation. On the sonogram these are often incompletely visualized. To establish fetal vitality during this period of gestation forceful palpation to elicit reflex movements has been very helpful.

In late pregnancy the extremities of the fetus can be successfully monitored: twitches, flexions and extensions may be observed. The fetal head often demonstrates rotations and sometimes flexions.

Dr. Marsal will discuss fetal motor activity in this period of pregnancy in more detail.

OBSERVATION OF STIMULATED REFLEX RESPONSE (MOTOR PROVOCATION TEST)

Spontaneous unelicited fetal movements, which can be assessed both in qualitative and quantitative terms, should be distinguished from reflex movements, which are elicited by tactile stimulation in the gestational sac. Thus, the fetus which floats in the amniotic fluid and is virtually unaffected by the gravity pull, is passively moved when the uterus is forcefully palpated transabdominally so that the fetal body makes contact with the amniotic wall or the umbilical cord. The resultant tactile stimulus may elicit reflex movements. Their assessment is analogous to that of spontaneous movements. This is easily understood considering that the shift in fetal position following spontaneous movements and the resultant tactile stimulus may equally elicit reflex movements consecutive to the spontaneous motor activity (4).

252

In late pregnancy reflex responses are not easily elicitable.

PHYSIOLOGICAL FETAL MOTOR BEHAVIOUR

The total spontaneous fetal movements and motionless periods in between is called 'fetal motor behaviour'. In the first trimester of pregnancy physiologically jerky and strong fetal body movements may be observed. Most of them are of the total pattern type, i.e. the whole fetal body is involved in the motion. The number of movements may vary over a wide range (Fig. 2).

One underlying reason of this wide range is the presence of a more or less long sequence of movements which are often elicited by tactile stimulation during the previous movement.

In the second trimester of pregnancy physiologically strong trunk flexion and extension, sometimes rotation may be observed. Besides, body movements twitches of the extremities may be present.

The number of movements may also vary over a wide range but shows a continuous increase up to about more than 100 movements per 24 hours (1).

In the third trimester of pregnancy physiologically slow but forceful extension and flexion of the extremities may be observed. Flexion and extension of the fetal trunk are more rare. Sometimes there are rotations of the fetal head.

The number of movements show an increase until the 32nd gestational week up to a daily mean of more than 100 movements per 24 hours. With continuing pregnancy to term there is a decrease in the number of movements to less than 100 movements per day. This phenomenon is associated with a decrease in the width of the range.

CLINICAL INTERPRETATION AND SIGNS OF DISTURBANCES IN DE-VELOPMENT OR WELL-BEING

The difficulties in interpretation of fetal motor behaviour are due to the lack of parameters for direct correlations. Clinical abnormal findings referable to the maternal organism need not necessarily mean a disturbance in fetal development or condition or well-being. And, vice-versa, a disturbance of fetal development or condition or well-being need not be correlated with abnormal clinical findings referable to the gravida. Hormonal tests, like estriol or HPL, are only indirect parameters regarding the fetus. The outcome of pregnancy and the condition of the newborn can be used for correlations; but there are a lot of other facts which may falsify the results.

In the first trimester of pregnancy absence of spontaneous fetal movements or the presence of only slow, sluggish and rare movements were considered as signs of fetal disturbances. The application of the 'motor provocation test' exhibit no reflex response or only a slow movement as a result of a tactile stimulus.

In the second trimester of pregnancy the interpretation of spontaneous fetal motor behaviour is very similar. A low number of spontaneous fetal movements are often associated with high-risk pregnancies with clinical signs of risks (7,8). But without clinical signs a decrease of spontaneous movements may be a very early indication of impending fetal death (Fig. 3).

In the third trimester disturbances were often associated with intrauterine growth retardation. Decreased fetal movements indicated chronic fetal asphyxia and were associated with a poor fetal outcome (3). Acting on the reduction of fetal movements, pregnancy could be terminated by means of induction of labour or caesarean section (1,9).

The actual observation of fetal movements by ultrasonic techniques during this period of pregnancy is rather unsatisfactory. The underlying reasons are the limited space in the gestational sac for fetal movements and the demonstration of only small parts of the fetal body by the scan. In addition fetal movements are highly differentiated and involve only small groups of muscles.

REFERENCES

1. Ehrström, Ch. (1979): Acta Obstet. Gynec. Scand., Suppl. 80.
2. Henner, H., Haller, U., Wolf-Zimper, O., Lorenz, W.J., Bader, R., Müller, B. and Kubli, F. (1975): Excerpta Medica International Congress Series No. 363.
3. Mathews, D.D. (1975): Obstet. Gynec., 45, 488.
4. Reinold, E. (1976): In: Ultrasonics in Early Pregnancy. S. Karger, Basel.
5. Reinold, E. (1979): Contr. Gynec. Obstet., 6, 29.
6. Reinold, E. (1979): Contr. Gynec. Obstet., 6, 123.
7. Sadovsky, E. and Yaffe, H. (1973): Obstet. Gynec., 41, 845.
8. Sadovsky, E. and Polishuk, W.Z. (1977): Obstet. Gynec., 50, 49.
9. Sadovsky, E., Laufer, N. and Allen, J.W. (1979): Brit. J. Obstet. Gynaec., 86, 10.

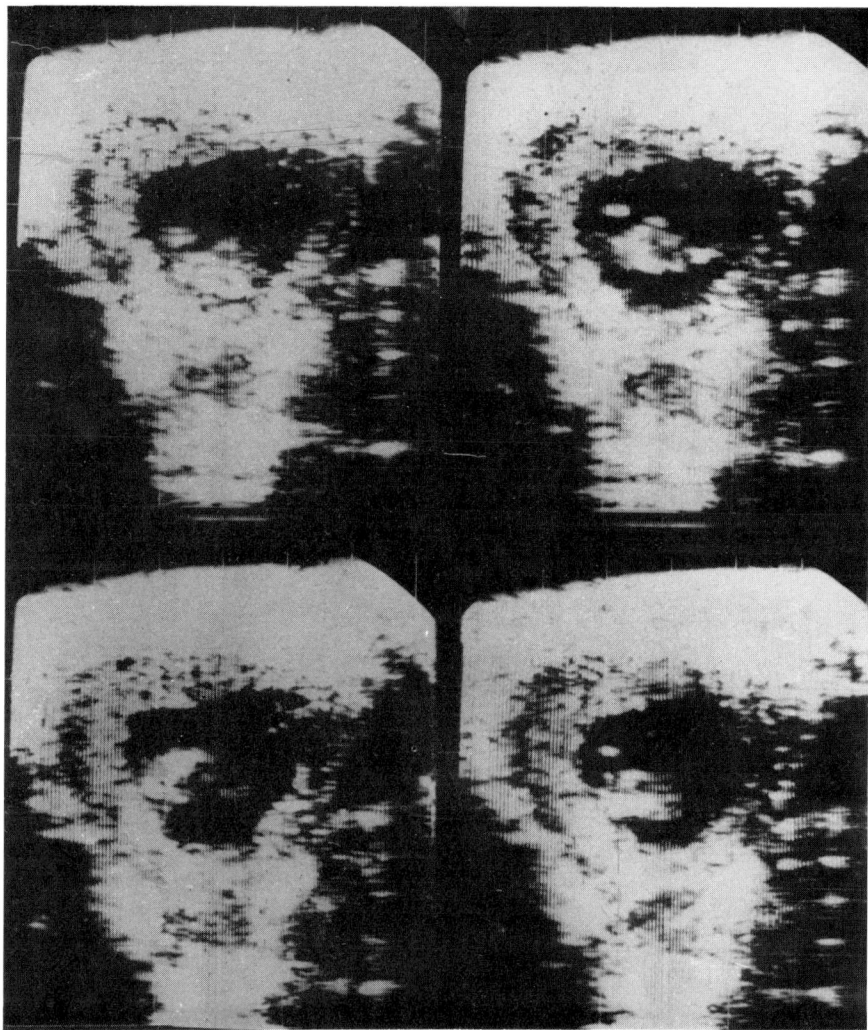

Fig. 1. Fetal body movement in the gestational sac shown on 4 consecutive frames.

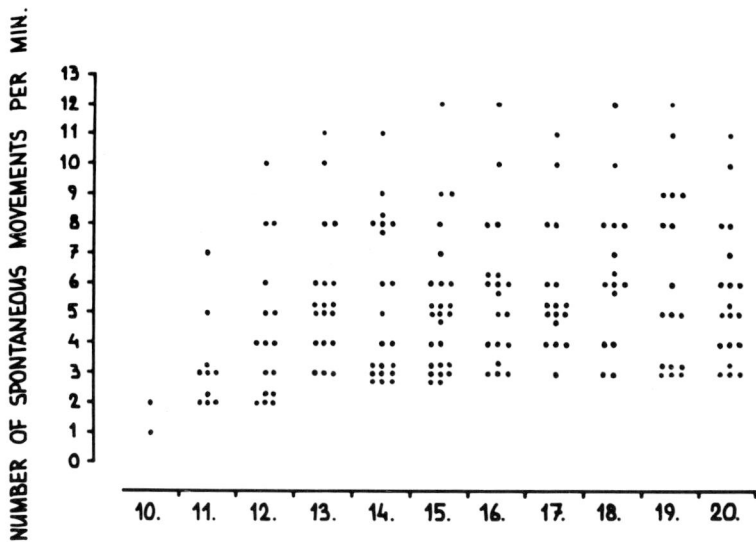

Fig. 2. Number of spontaneous fetal movements per minute
in uncomplicated pregnancies between 10 and 20 weeks of
gestation (n = 180).

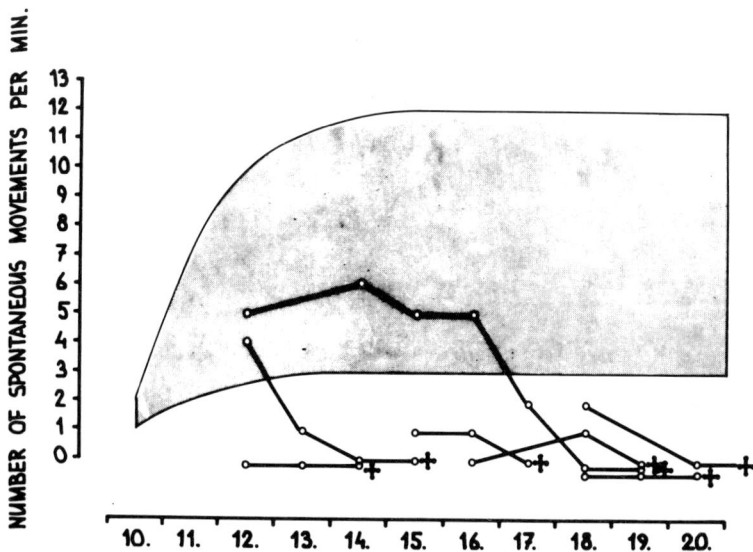

Fig. 3. Normal range of spontaneous fetal movements and the
number of fetal movements before the fetus dies (n = 7).

ACTIVE FETAL BODY MOVEMENTS IN EARLY PREGNANCY

H. Henner

Department of Obstetrics and Gynecology, Kantonsspital,
St. Gallen, Switzerland

During the last few years, various investigators were able to find a rather strong relationship between fetal movements and pregnancy outcome in the early period of gestation. The results of Reinhold (7,8,9), Hollaender(5) and Kratochwil (6) were obtained from purely qualitative studies. In our group Schmid (Fig.1) found that in cases of pathologic body movements, the abortion rate is 10 times higher than in pregnancies where normal fetal body movements were observed. However, like with all biophysical parameters, qualitative evaluation is subject to the observer's experience and therefore limited in reproducibility. We attempted to quantify fetal body movements in two pilot studies performed some time ago in Heidelberg. This report will give a review of our results obtained between 1973 and 1978. The first study (1,2) was performed in 24 normal patients (55 examinations) and 18 cases of threatened abortion (28 examinations) between the 9th and 21st week of pregnancy, with a total examination time of 415 min and evaluation of 1.116 active fetal movements. Examinations were done with the Siemens real-time scanner Vidoson, data was stored on magnetic videotape and analyzed off-line under slow motion.

The following parameters were determined: a) movement frequency, i.e. number of movements per 5 min of examination b) relative duration, i.e. total time of movements per 5 min examination expressed as percentage of recording time. The following results were obtained:

1. The frequency of movements in the normal control population increases significantly with increasing gestational age (correlation coefficient of 0.42 between the movement frequency and gestational age). The same holds true for relative duration of the movements.
2. With threatened abortion this correlation is lacking.
3. It can be shown, however, that the frequency distribution of the movement is significantly different between the normal and the abnormal group, with a peak of 7.5 per 5 min in the control group against 2.5 movements in the pathologic population.
4. In Figure 2 individual values of the abnormal group are plotted against mean+SD of the control population. Of special interest are 3 cases ending in fetal death between 15 and 20 weeks of pregnancy. In all 3 cases low

and/or decreasing frequencies of body movements were observed, pathological frequencies being observed up to 2 weeks before fetal death.

In this study, the type and pattern of fetal movements were evaluated semiquantitatively. The frequency of different types of movements was assessed quantitatively; the classification of the types of movements, however, was done purely qualitatively and subjectively. Two typical examples are shown in Figures 3 and 4.

PREGNANCY - OUTCOME				
		N (tot.)	Term. Deliv.	Abortion	Ab. Freq.
		3515	3356	159	4,5 %
normal		3424	3297	127	3,7 %
patholog.		91	59	32	35,2 %
path. Freq.		2,6 %	1,75 %	20,1 %	

FETAL - MOVEMENTS (FM)

Fig. 1. Correlation between type of fetal movements and pregnancy outcome (Schmid, 1978).

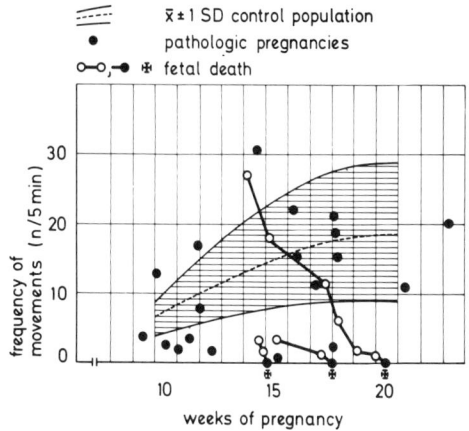

Fig. 2. Three individual cases ending in fetal death plotted against the control population (Haller et al. 1973).

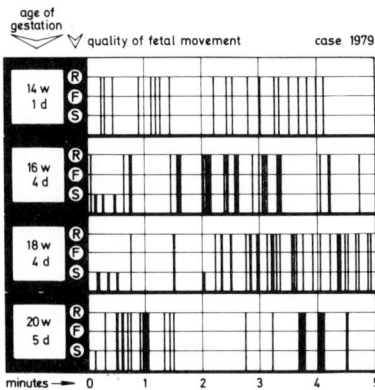

Fig. 3. Serial study of fetal movements in case of uncomplicated pregnancy: 4 examinations (w=weeks of gestation d=days of gestation). Height of bars represents type of movements. R=rapid, F=fluctuating, S=slow. Width of bars represents duration of movement (Haller et al. 1977).

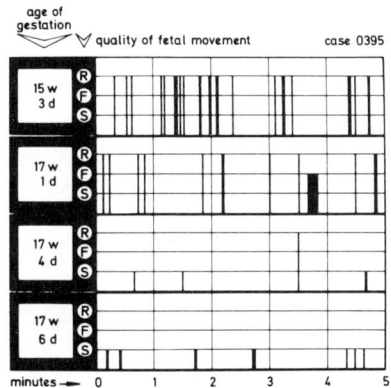

Fig. 4. Serial study of fetal movements in case ending in fetal death: 4 examinations (w= weeks of gestation, d=days of gestation). Height of bars represents type of movements. R=rapid, F=fluctuating, S= slow. Width of the bars represents duration of movement. Fetal death occurred within 3 days after last exam. (Haller et al. 1973).

258

Figure 3 demonstrates four examinations between 14 and 20 weeks in a normal patient. Each fetal movement is represented by a bar; normal rapid movements by a large bar, pathologic slow movements by a small bar. In this case, the movement pattern is characterized by a high frequency of rapid movements at each examination. Slow movements rarely occur.

Figure 4 demonstrates in the same manner a pregnancy ending in fetal death at 17 weeks. Two weeks before fetal death a lower incidence of movements and predominance of pathologic slow movements can be shown.

In order to classify the type of movements on a more objective basis, a second study (3,4) was done in a limited series of 47 periods of 5 min duration including 310 fetal movements of normal and abnormal pregnancies with threatened abortion. In this study the two-dimensional representation on the TV screen of the in vivo three-dimensional movement was analyzed in more detail.

Figure 5 is a diagram of the equipment used to quantify fetal movements. The following parameters were described and evaluated (Fig. 6). The first one called 'loop excursion' is defined as the course of fetal movement in utero, i.e. the path followed during fetal movement. The second parameter termed 'loop area' is defined as the area covered by the fetal movement during a loop excursion. In an open loop the area is demarcated by the shortest line between start and end of the registered fetal movement. The third parameter termed 'movement amplitude' is defined as the sum of the largest right angle distances of fetal excursion from a zero line connecting the start and end point.

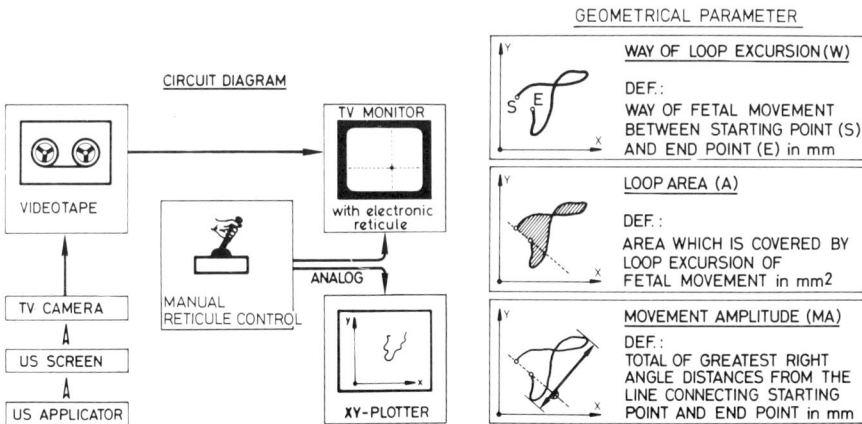

Fig. 5. Diagram of the equipment used to quantify fetal movements (Henner et al. 1975).

Fig. 6. Three geometrical parameters to quantify fetal movements; i.e. way of loop excursion, loop, area, and movement amplitude (Henner et al.1975).

259

In the total normal population we could show that all three parameters increase as gestational age preceeds, which does not hold true for the pathologic population where all cases ended in spontaneous abortion before the 19th week of gestation. For the parameter 'loop area' the differences are statistically significant. (Figure 7).

From our experience we felt that the characteristics of fetal body movements should be revealed in an even more dynamic way than as described above. Therefore we finally introduced the two parameters, 'velocity' and 'acceleration'.

From the videotape the fetal movements were played back in time motion followed with the electronic reticule and drawn out again on the XY plotter. As shown on Figure 8, for every time interval of 0.2 sec the position of fetal movement was marked and the distance by the fetal movement calculated for each interval.

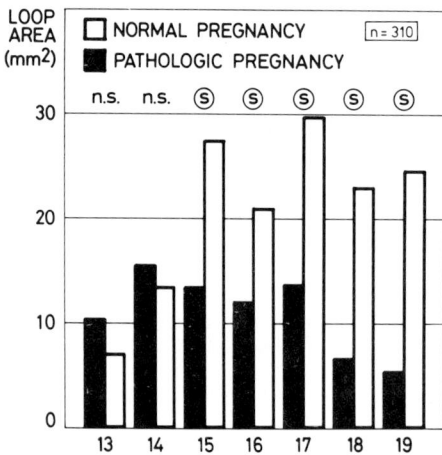

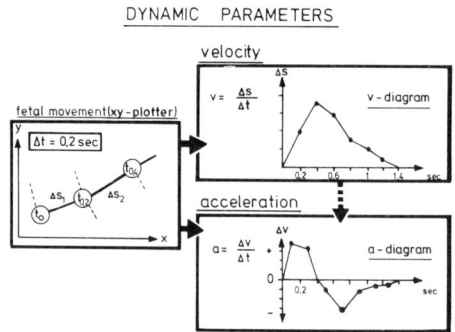

Fig. 7. Behaviour of loop area for normal and pathologic pregnancies(Henner et al. 1975).

Fig.8. The dynamic parameters velocity and acceleration (Henner et al. 1976).

From these noted distances velocity and acceleration were computed and registered in a velocity and acceleration diagram. In Figure 9 typical examples of two individual cases are demonstrated. On the left side of the Figure the velocity and acceleration diagram of a single fetal movement from the 17th week of gestation in normal pregnancy is demonstrated. As a comparison, the velocity and acceleration diagram from a pathologic case is seen on the right side of Figure 9.

The following differences are observed:
1. The velocity of fetal movement is slower in pathologic than in normal pregnancies. In practical terms this means a slow and short movement in pathologic situations.
2. Pathologic movements show more changes from acceleration to deceleration. This is probably a quantitative description of the jerky nature of the pathologic movement.

260

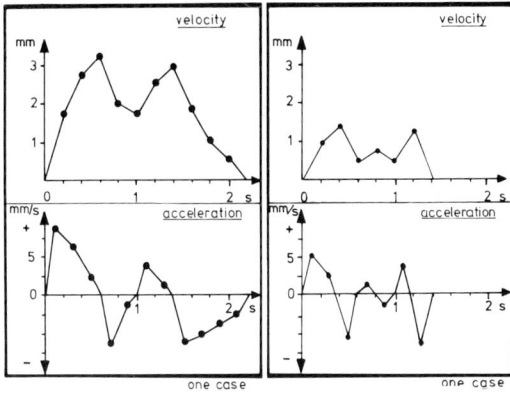

Fig. 9. Movement velocity and acceleration in a normal
(left) and pathological case (right) at 17 weeks of ges-
tation(Henner et al. 1976).

In conclusion, we can say that the results of the two
pilot studies described above, provide more detailed information on the various aspects of fetal body movements than
the findings based on purely qualitative evaluation. However, the methodology applied is far too time-consuming for
futher research studies in a larger population. Computerized
recording and evaluation directly from the TV screen is not
yet possible. It is therefore that these parameters are not
yet application in clinical obstetrics.

REFERENCES
1. Haller, U., Rütgers, H., Wille, F., Heinrich, D., Müller, P. and Kubli, F. (1973):Gynäk. Rdsch. 13, 118.
2. Haller, U., Rütgers, H., Wille, F., Müller, P., Heinrich, D. and Kubli, F. (1973): In: Dudenhausen und
   Saling, Perinatale Medizin, v. 30. Thieme Verlag.
3. Henner, U., Haller, U., Wolf-Zimper, O., Bader, R.,Mül-
   ler, B. and Kubli, F. (1975): In: Proceedings 2nd Eur.
   Congr. Ultrasound in Medicine, Munich.
4. Henner, H., Haller, U., Rütgers, H. and Kubli, F.(1976):
   Proc. VIIth Wld. Congr. Gynec. Obstet., Mexico City.
5. Hollander, H.J.(1974): In: Ultraschalldiagnostik in
   er Schwangerschaft, Urban & Schwarzenberg.
6. Kratochwil, A.(1968): In: Ultraschall-Diagnostik in Geburtshilfe und Gynäkologie, Thieme, Stuttgart.
7. Reinold, E. (1971): Z. Geburtsh. Gynäk. 174, 220.
8. Reinold, E. (1971): Pädiat. Pädol. 6, 274.
9. Reinold, E. (1972): Perinatal Medizin, vol. IV, p. 25
   Thieme, Stuttgart.

FETAL BREATHING MOVEMENTS EXAMINATIONS: RESEARCH TOOL AND/OR CLINICAL TEST?

K. Maršál and G. Gennser

Department of Obstetrics and Gynecology, University Hospital, Malmö, Sweden

In 1977 at the International Symposium on Recent Advances in Ultrasound Diagnosis in Dubrovnik, fetal breathing movements (FBM) were the subject of a round-table discussion (1). The then state of the knowledge of FBM physiology, as observed both in animal and human fetuses, the methodology of FBM recording by ultrasound, and the possible role of FBM examinations in clinical practice was thoroughly reported. Interest is still focused on this antenatal activity, a subject of numerous studies. Some of the experience gained in these works has forced us to reconsider earlier concepts. The present report gives a short account of some recent developments in research on FBM and presents the scope and limitations of clinical application of FBM examinations.

RECORDING TECHNIQUE

For examining FBM, the real-time B-mode technique became a method of choice (2). It offers a detailed two-dimensional image of the fetal chest and abdomen, in which FBM can be easily recognized. The most widely used method for quantification of FBM visualized by this technique is a simple observing of the screen of the scanner and marking each FBM cycle manually by an event marker (3). This can be done either on-line or off-line from image sequences stored on video-tape. The method is relatively rough, but still shows good reproducibility and sufficient accuracy in clinical studies evaluating FBM incidence (3). When applied for more detailed analysis, it appears subjective and the need for an objective recording from the real-time image is obvious.

At present, the only systems in practical clinical use for objective FBM recording are those extracting FBM signals from the echo information of one of the selected lines in the real-time image. These systems use either a TM-mode display of the echo signals (4) or perform an automatic measurement of the momentary changes in fetal chest or abdomen diameter along the selected line, so called time-distance recording (TD-recording) (5). Of these two methods, the TD-recorder offers the advantage of being semi-automatic and yielding an analogue signal ready for further processing (Fig. 1). The principle of TD-recording has been subject to further improvement by adding a phase-lock echo tracker in the combined A- and B-mode scanning, thus increasing the ability to resolve small movements of the target (6). Another possibility is offered by the multiple TD-recording along several image lines (7).

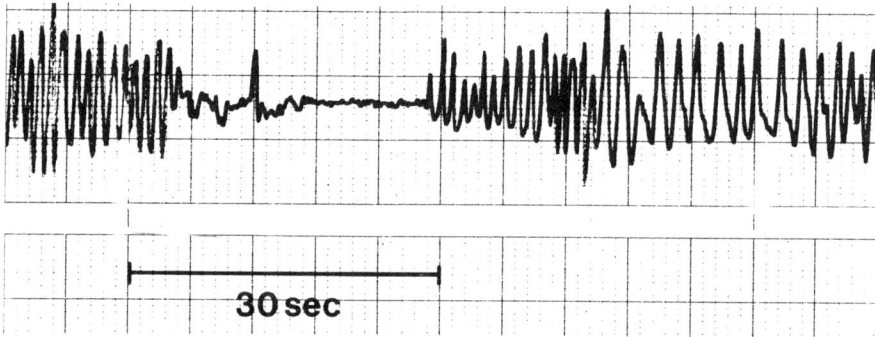

Figure 1. Fetal breathing movements recorded by the TD-recorder. Changes in the thorax diameter of the fetus are automatically measured in the real-time image and dis-played as an analogue signal.

The use of the Doppler principle is another approach to the problem of recording FBM (8). When using Doppler ultrasound in pulsed mode, different fetal structures have been chosen as targets indicative for breathing movements, e.g., the fetal chest wall (9) or undefined tissues with-in the fetal chest (10). Recently, measurements of blood flow velocities in the umbilical vein have revealed typi-cal breath-dependent changes (11).

MORPHOLOGICAL CHANGES DURING FETAL BREATHING MOVEMENTS

The present opinion among physiologists is that the central event of fetal breathing movements in experimental animals is the contraction of the diaphragm, as evidenced by EMG (12). Observations of the human fetus by real-time ultrasound suggest that the same is true in man (13). It was early observed that the breathing movements of human fetal chest and abdominal wall predominantly display the inverse or paradoxical pattern (13) also apparent in the premature newborn infants. This can be illustrated by using two TD-recorders, recording simultaneously the dia-meters of the fetal chest and fetal abdomen. The obtained signals displayed on an XY oscilloscope, create a Lissa-jous figure (Fig. 2). A typical inverse movement with the expansion of the fetal abdomen and simultaneous retraction of the fetal chest during inspiration can thus be demonstrated. During expiration, the fetal structures move in the reverse direction. In some fetuses, it could be observed that sometimes a simultaneous expansion of both the fetal abdomen and fetal thorax occurs during the inspiratory phase (14). This finding suggests a possibility that the chest wall might be transitorily stabilized by activated intercostal muscles during such atypical breath cycles and that the amniotic fluid would enter into the fetal lung as a consequence of a decreased intrathoracic pressure. This is opposed to the early opinion which stated that, during FBM, there is no active exchange between the amniotic pool and the lung fluid (15).

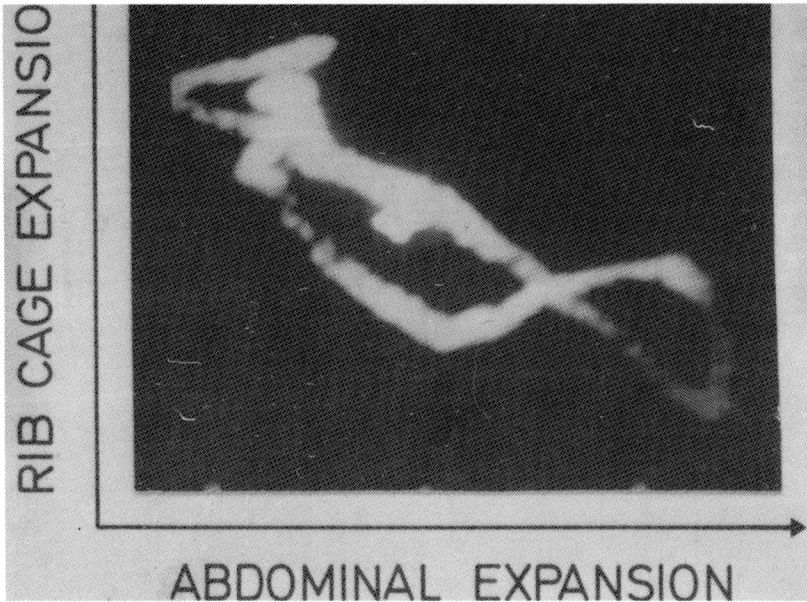

Figure 2. Lissajous figure demonstrating the reverse movement of the fetal abdominal and thoracic wall during one FBM cycle. The displayed signals correspond to the chest and abdominal diameter of the fetus measured simultaneously in the real-time image by two TD-recorders.

Recently, Miyake et al. reported on a successful recording by a pulsed Doppler technique of rhythmic movements of the fluid in the fetal trachea (16). Application of this technique might in the near future answer the question of the existence of a tidal flow in the upper airways of the fetus.

METHODS FOR EVALUATING THE FBM RECORDS

In early animal studies, the fetal breathing was quantified as the amount of time spent breathing (17). A similar method was, from the beginning, applied to the

human investigations by the ultrasound A-mode method and
has been continued because the scanning quality was insufficient for more detailed analysis and because the
information gained by this method was regarded as satisfactory for the clinical purpose. This was based on the
presumption of fetal breathing being a physiological
activity and the time of non-breathing (fetal apnea)
being directly related to the degree of fetal compromise.
This concept, however, was shattered by two groups of new
experience: first: the variable, intermittent character
of FBM with a diurnal pattern of incidence (3,18), second:
the pathological significance of a very high incidence of
regular FBM (19).

A pattern analysis of the FBM was early attempted to
gain more qualitative information from the FBM records
(20). The analysis was based on an evaluation of breathing
in the neonatal period (21). Breathing movements during
20-sec. epochs were classified in regular, irregular,
periodic, or apneic types (Fig. 3).

Types of FBM

Regular	nearly equal breath-to-breath intervals
Irregular	unequal intervals
Periodic	2 apneic periods of ≥3 sec within 20 sec
Apnea	apnea of ≥6 sec within 20 sec

|← 20 sec →|

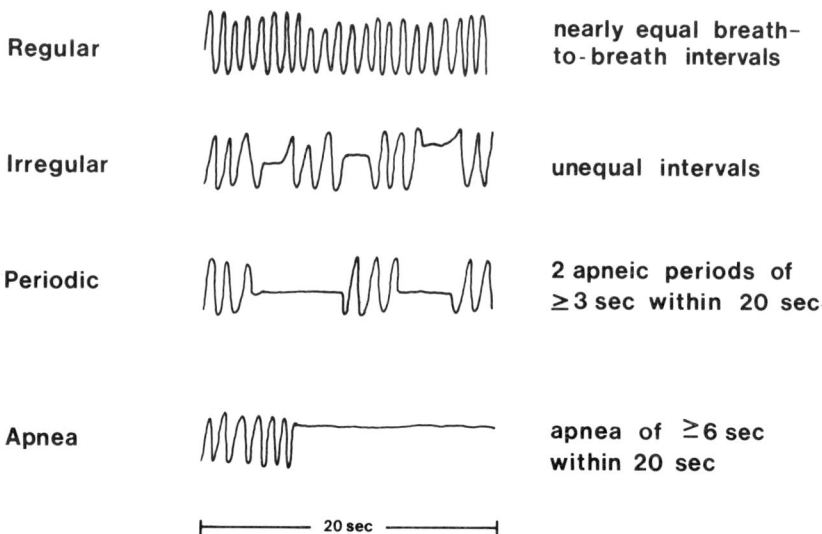

Figure 3. Definitions and examples of the FBM types used
in pattern analysis of FBM records.

265

Other methods of the FBM evaluation include the calculation of the incidence of FBM and fetal trunk movements (fetal total activity) (22) and evaluation of the time course of the FBM (Table I). Of these, the analysis of the breath-to-breath interval variability has been used for comparison between the regulation of fetal and neonatal breathing (23).

TABLE I. Current methods for evaluating fetal breathing recordings

	Reference
Incidence - per cent of time spent breathing	
- 30 min	(13,25,27)
- 60 min	(33)
Presence or absence of FBM ($\geq$ 30 sec. during 30 min)	(28)
Total fetal activity - incidence of FBM + incidence of FM	(22)
Pattern analysis in 20 sec. epochs - regular	(20)
- irregular	
- periodic	
- apneic	
Breath-to-breath interval - 4 min period	(34)
Breath-to-breath variation	(23,29)
Breathing rate	(34)
Ratio active movement/cycle duration	(31)

The fetal total activity has been shown to be less influenced by the intra-day variations than FBM alone and therefore it might be of more significance in clinical work (22). It can be expected that, in future, some qualitative analyses will succeed the present utilization of the percentage incidence as a dominant FBM parameter.

APPROPRIATE RECORDING TIME

Most published clinical studies evaluated the percentage incidence of FBM during 30 min recording time (19, 24,25). The 30-min duration of the recordings was chosen mainly for practical reasons, as longer recording often causes discomfort to the patients and is very demanding on the concentration of the operator. As mentioned above, Patrick et al. (3) and Roberts et al. (18) described the

existence of repetitive patterns in the incidence of FBM
when recording for 24 hours. This makes it difficult to
correctly evaluate clinical FBM records. The existing
variability in the incidence both inter- and intra-indi-
vidually complicates the evaluation still further. In an
attempt to analyse the applicability of the 30-min recordings and the stability of the incidence levels on consecutive days, the following two studies were performed.

30-min recordings

Six pregnant women hospitalized for prophylactic
reasons were examined four times each day on 5 consecutive
days. None of the women smoked and none took any drug
known to influence FBM. Mean gestational age of the group
was 35 weeks (range 33-36 weeks). The examination took
place at 0800, 1100, 1300, and 1500 hours; each recording
lasted for 30 minutes. The patients had their usual meals
at 0730 and at 1200 hours. FBM were recorded by the TD-
recorder connected to the linear array real-time scanner
(ADR). Thus an outsignal of the changes of the fetal chest
(or abdominal) diameter was recorded graphically and could
be evaluated quantitatively later. Fetal body movements (FM)
were marked on the chart record manually by the operator
observing the screen of the scanner. All records were
analysed for the incidence of FBM and FM for each minute
of the recording. Thus, according to the design of the
study, 120 30-min recordings, i.e. 3.600 one-min epochs,
should be recorded, but owing to 3 drop-outs, only 3.510
epochs were obtained.

In individual recordings, large variations in the FBM
and FM incidence were observed. No constant pattern in the
incidence could be revealed. The only significant relation
to be found was the negative correlation between the FBM
and FM incidence. This means that usually the two types of
movements substituted for each other and only rarely were
they present at the same time. This agrees with our observation
in other material that FBM and FM occurred simultaneously
only in 2.4 % of the recording time (unpublished). Fig. 4
presents the mean incidence of FBM for the whole group and
each hour. A considerable variability and no constant
pattern between the different times and days could be observed. On 3 days, the incidence of FBM was highest at
1300 hours. The mean incidence of FBM for each hour was
36 % at 0800 hours, 34 % at 1100 hours, 36 % at 1300
hours, and 30 % at 1500 hours.

Table II summarizes the variance analysis of the FBM
results. It gives the percentual proportion of the variance, as related to the different variables. The table
might be interpreted as follows: In a clinical situation,
we are looking for possible differences between the populations of the patients. We can control the time of day
by examining all patients at the same time, e.g., at 1300
hours. The day of the week did not influence the results.

However, the residual was very large (51 %) and might
include factors we are unaware of and which cannot be
controlled. Therefore, the clinical usefulness of such
quantitative FBM examination based on 30-min recordings of
FBM incidence will be limited.

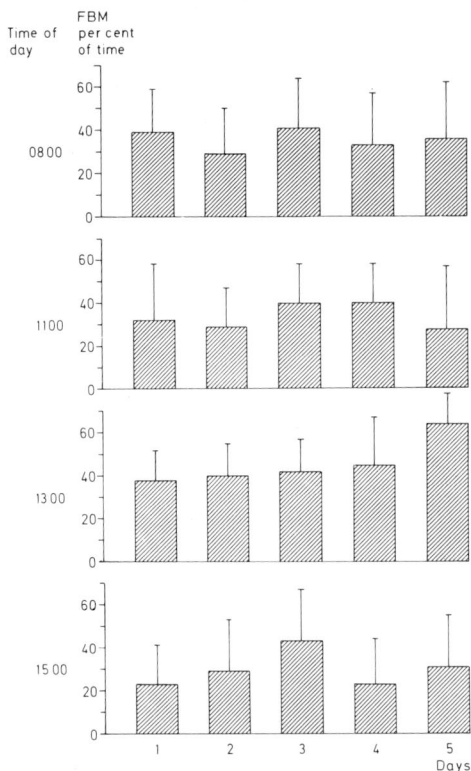

Figure 4. Incidence of
FBM at different re-
cording sessions. Each
column represents the
mean ($\pm$ SD) of 6 30-
min recordings.

TABLE II. Variance analysis of the FBM incidence in 117
30-min recordings registered in 6 fetuses.
(See text for details.)

Source of variation	Variance (per cent)	Significance
Patient	5	$p < 0.05$
Day	4	N.S.
Time of day	40	$p < 0.001$
Residual	51	
Total	100	

60-min recordings

To further analyse the problem of a proper recording time, we examined 10 randomly chosen pregnant women, who were fully active and had uncomplicated pregnancies. All were in the 32nd week of gestation. None smoked or took drugs. FBM recordings were performed for 60 min starting at 1300 hours, i.e. one hour after the women had lunched. All the FBM records were analysed on the basis of one minute epochs.

The incidence of FBM for the whole group was 27 $\pm$ 20.5 % (mean $\pm$ SD). No pattern in the FBM incidence could be recognized on this basis. Therefore a method of moving average evaluation was applied, which might accentuate a possibly hidden cyclicity. When a moving average of the 10-min periods was plotted for each patient, distinct cycles could be seen. In Fig. 5, the plotted curves of all patients were centred around the top point of each curve, disregarding the time position. In this compiled diagram, an active period similar for most of the patients could be distinguished. No such cycle pattern was observed in the FM records analysed in the same way (Fig. 6). The length of the FBM active period was 25-30 10-min periods, which represents the 34-40 min time. This suggests that, compensating for the short-term cycles, the recording time should be at least twice as long as hitherto, i.e. 70-80 min, even if the recording is made at the time of day found in the previous study as the most convenient (at 1300 hours).

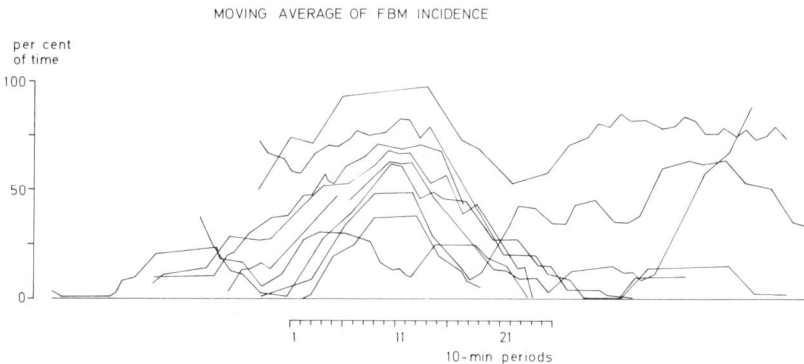

Figure 5. Moving 10-min average of fetal breathing movements incidence based on 60-min recordings in 10 normal pregnancies of 32 weeks gestational age.

To summarize: the results of both the 30-min and the 60-min studies showed that:

1) 30-min recordings of FBM are of limited value when only the FBM percentage incidence is considered.

2) The variance analysis revealed that the residual, which we are unable to control, is too large and therefore makes difficult the possible discrimination between different groups of patient populations.
3) On average, the highest incidence of FBM was found when the recording was performed at 1300 hours, i.e. one hour after the maternal lunch. This is consistent with the reports showing increased FBM incidence after maternal meals (3) or glucose ingestion (26).
4) 70-80 min duration of FBM recordings seems to be necessary to cover one cycle of the FBM incidence and to allow a pattern recognition.

MOVING AVERAGE OF FM

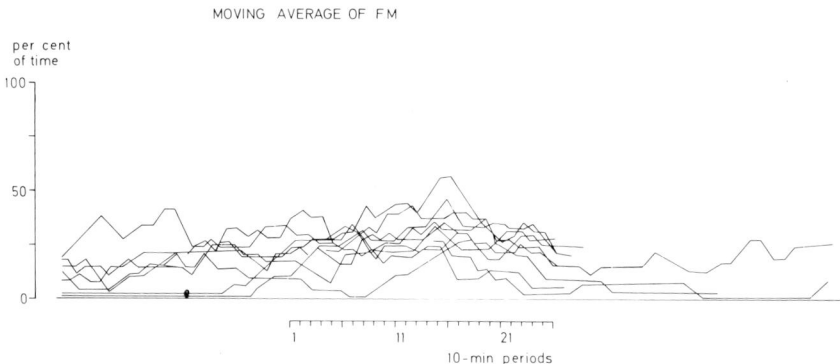

Figure 6. Moving 10-min average of fetal movements incidence based on 60-min recordings in 10 normal pregnancies of 32 weeks gestational age.

CLINICAL STUDIES

In 1978, Maršál published a study analysing the possible relation between FBM incidence and clinical course of pregnancy (13). 100 consecutive pregnancies were examined in the last trimester. Real-time ultrasound method was used for 30-min recordings of the percentage incidence of FBM. 76 pregnancies were normal and 24 women had various disorders of pregnancy. In 92 % of the observations with FBM incidence more than 17 % of the recording time, this finding indicated an uncomplicated pregnancy. In 64 % of the recordings with low incidence or apnea, this was indicative of a pregnancy complication. The results suggest that the presence of FBM might be a sign of fetal well-being. On the other hand, the finding of fetal apnea seems to have less clinical significance. In that study, no correlation was found between the FBM incidence and the subsequent course and outcome of pregnancy. This was probably due to the long interval between FBM monitoring and parturition.

Platt et al. (27) examined 124 high risk pregnancies within 2 weeks of delivery. They found a significant relation between the FBM — classified as present or absent — and the outcome of pregnancy judged by Apgar score and birth weight. The same group of authors (28) analysed the FBM in a number of pregnant women subjected to contraction stress test and suggested that the interpretation of the abnormal or equivocal contraction stress test could be modified by the results of the FBM examination. Recently, Trudinger et al. (29) performed a comparative analysis of the prognostic value of the FBM incidence (and FBM variability) and of the routine methods for fetal monitoring (CTG, biochemical tests, ultrasound measurements of the fetal growth). They found that FBM analysis had a sensibility surpassing that of the biochemical methods.

A group of studies have explored the relation between FBM incidence and fetal growth retardation. Trudinger et al. (19) found that most fetuses with subsequent birth weight below the 5th percentile had a lower incidence of FBM than the normal fetuses. Some of the growth retarded fetuses, however, had a highly increased breathing activity and breath-to-breath intervals with lower variability than normal. This observation is of profound importance as it seems equivalent to the finding of "picket-fence breathing" in dying sheep fetuses (30) and thereby points to a quality of FBM — apart from the incidence — suitable for monitoring. Bots et al. (31) on the other hand, found no difference in breathing incidence between normal fetuses and those born with low birth weight; this result might be ascribed to the selection of the study group (below the 25th percentile). In the study of Roberts et al. (32) asymmetrically growth retarded fetuses showed a significant reduction in FBM incidence; fetuses with symmetric growth retardation had a breathing activity within the normal range. This agrees with the results presented by Persson and Maršál (24) demonstrating that FBM recordings could not distinguish between fetuses later born small-for-gestational age (all except one fetus being symmetrically retarded) and fetuses born appropriate-for-gestational age. In this study, the pregnant women with growth retardation and urinary estriol excretion below -2 SD of normals had on average a lower FBM incidence than was found in the group with normal estriol. However, there was no predictive capacity of the FBM incidence in the individual cases.

CONCLUSIONS

The technical problems of ultrasonic monitoring of FBM in human are largely solved. Relatively inexpensive and efficient real-time scanners are now more generally available, and breathing movements can be easily visualized. However, the interpretation of the FBM results is difficult because our understanding of many features of the FBM in normal fetuses is far from complete. The episodic irregular character and the nyctohemeral pattern of FBM force the examiner to take special precautions when evaluating the FBM records. As demonstrated, the percentage incidence of FBM depends on the duration of the recording and on the time of day, which makes the reproducibility of the results questionable. Furthermore, it has been shown that a high incidence of FBM might be a finding of abnormality, thus destroying the concept of a linear relation between increasing FBM incidence and fetal well-being.

The future methods of improving the diagnostic and prognostic value of the FBM recordings might include combined recording of FBM and other fetal parameters (e.g. fetal movements, CTG, amount of amniotic fluid), and also measuring qualities of FBM other than the incidence. Moreover, various load tests might increase the discriminatory power of the FBM monitoring.

It is pertinent to warn against uncritical use of the FBM monitoring for supervising the fetus. The clinical interpretation of the FBM records must consider the limitations and pitfalls mentioned in this paper, lest the method will soon be discredited. The place of FBM monitoring in clinical obstetrics is, due to the time and personell consuming character of the method, at present restricted to a small number of departments.

As a research tool, the FBM study is promising. In recent years, investigations have confirmed the interrelation between FBM and maternal blood glucose level and various physiological rhythms have been revealed. The oscillations of breath-to-breath intervals and the influence of FBM on the umbilical blood flow are other new achievements of this research field. It is striking, however, that many aspects of the physiology and the regulation of FBM in the human still need clarifying. Our belief is that, for some time to come, FBM examinations should be regarded mainly as a research tool in the field of fetal physiology.

REFERENCES

1. Fetal breathing movements (Round table discussion) (1978): In: Recent Advances in Ultrasound Diagnosis, p. 187. Editor: A. Kurjak. Excerpta Medica, Amsterdam.
2. Maršál, K. (1979): In: Ultrasound in Perinatal Physiology. Editor: D.N. White. Research Studies Press, Forest Grove, Oregon. (In press.)
3. Patrick, J., Natale, R. and Richardson, B. (1978): Am. J. Obstet. Gynecol., 132, 507.
4. Wladimiroff, J.W., Ligtvoet, C.M. and Spermon, J.A. (1976): Brit. Med. J., 2, 975.
5. Maršál, K., Gennser, G. and Lindström, K. (1976): Lancet, 1, 718.
6. Korba, L.W., Cousine, A.J., Cobbold, R.S.C. and Gare, D. (1978): In: San Diego Biomedical Symposium Proceedings. Academic Press, New York.

7. Bots, R.S.G.M., Hopman, J.C.W., Rijken, C.J. and Jongsma, H.W. (1978): Proceedings 5th Conference on Fetal Breathing, Nijmegen, June 26-27, p. 111. Editor: T.K.A.B. Eskes. Nijmegen.
8. Boyce, E.S., Dawes, G.S., Gough, J.D. and Poore, E.R. (1976): Brit. Med. J., 2, 17.
9. Tremewan, R.N., Aickin, D.R. and Tait, J.J. (1976): Brit. Med. J., 1, 1434.
10. McHugh, R., McDicken, W.N., Bow, C.R., Anderson, T. and Boddy, K. (1978): Ultrasound Med. Biol., 3, 381.
11. Eik-Nes, S.H., Maršál, K., Brubakk, A.O. and Ulstein, M. (1979): In: Proceedings of the International Symposium on Recent Advances in Ultrasound Diagnosis, Dubrovnik, October 1-7. Editor: A. Kurjak. Excerpta Medica, Amsterdam. (In press.)
12. Harding, R., Johnson, P., McClelland, M.E., McLeod, C.N. and Whyte, P.L. (1977): J. Physiol., 272, 14P.
13. Maršál, K. (1978): Obstet. Gynecol., 52, 394.
14. Gennser, G. (1979): In: Central Nervous Control Mechanism in Breathing, p. 375. Editor: C.v.Euler. Pergamon Press, Oxford.
15. Boddy, K. and Dawes, G.S. (1975): Br. Med. Bull., 31, 3.
16. Miyake, K., Chiba, Y., Imai, S. and Kurachi, K. (1979): Proceedings 2nd Meeting of WFUMB, 4th World Congress on Ultrasonics in Medicine, July 22-27, Miyazaki, Japan, p. 314. Scimed Publications Inc., Tokyo.
17. Dawes, G.S., Fox, H.E., Leduc, B.M., Liggins, G.C. and Richards, R.T. (1972): J. Physiol., 220, 119.
18. Roberts, A.B., Little, D. and Campbell, S. (1978): In: Recent Advances in Ultrasound Diagnosis, p. 189. Editor: A. Kurjak. Excerpta Medica, Amsterdam.
19. Trudinger, B.J., Lewis, P.J. and Pettit, B. (1979): Br. J. Obstet. Gynaecol., 86, 432.
20. Maršál, K., Gennser, G. and Ohrlander, S. (1975): Life Sci., 17, 449.
21. Parmelee, A.H., Stern, E. and Harris, M.A. (1972): Neuropädiatrie, 3, 294.
22. Roberts, A.B., Little, D., Cooper, D. and Campbell, S. (1979): Br. J. Obstet. Gynaecol., 86, 4.
23. Gennser, G. and Hathorn, M. (1979): Lancet, 1, 1298.
24. Persson, P.H. and Maršál, K. (1978): Acta Obstet. Gynecol. Scand., Suppl. 78, 49.
25. Fox, H.E., Hohler, C.W., Jaeger, H., Steinbrecher, M. and Peco, N. (1977): Proceedings 3rd Conference on Fetal Breathing, June 8, p. 56. Editors: G. Gennser, K. Maršál, T. Wheeler. Malmö.
26. Lewis, P.J., Trudinger, B.J. and Mangez, J. (1978): Br. J. Obstet. Gynaecol., 85, 86.
27. Platt, L.D., Manning, F.A., Lemay, M. and Sipos, L. (1978): Am. J. Obstet. Gynecol., 132, 514.
28. Manning, F.A. and Platt, L.D. (1979): Am. J. Obstet. Gynecol., 133, 590.

29. Trudinger, B.J., Gordon, Y.B., Grundzinskas, J.G., Hull, M.G.R., Lewis, P.J. and Lozana Arrans, M.E. (1979): Brit. Med. J., 2, 577.
30. Patrick, J.E., Dalton, K.J. and Dawes, G.S. (1976): Am. J. Obstet. Gynecol., 125, 73.
31. Bots, R.S.G.M., Broeders, G.H.B., Farman, D.J., Haverkorn, M.J. and Stolte, L.A.M. (1978): Eur. J. Obstet. Gynecol. Repr. Biol., 8, 21.
32. Roberts, A.B., Little, D. and Campbell, S. (1978): In: Recent Advances in Ultrasound Diagnosis, p. 192. Editor: A. Kurjak. Excerpta Medica, Amsterdam.
33. Wittmann, B.K., Davison, B.M., Lyons, E., Frohlich, J. and Towell, M.E. (1979): Br. J. Obstet. Gynaecol., 86, 271.
34. Wladimiroff, J.W. (1977): In: Poor Intrauterine Fetal Growth, p. 261. Editor: B. Salvadori. Centro Minerva Medica, Parma.

ULTRASONIC ASSESSMENT OF FETAL STOMACH FUNCTION. PHYSIOLOGY AND CLINIC.

K. Vandenberghe and F. De Wolf.

Department of Obstetrics and Gynecology, Academic Hospital
Sint-Rafaël, University of Leuven, Leuven, Belgium.

Swallowing of amniotic fluid by the fetus constitutes
an important aspect of its functional development, and represents one of the mechanisms regulating amniotic fluid
volume and turnover. The stomach being the first station
for the swallowed amniotic fluid, assessment of fetal stomach volume and volume changes seems appropriate. The echographic visualisation of the fetal stomach has improved
progressively with the increasing capabilities of ultrasonic techniques (4,2,5).

METHODS

The apparatus used are a real time system, Toshiba
Sonolayergraph SAL-10A, and a compound scanner, Diasonograph NE 4102-Emisonic with PEP 500 scan converter. The
sound velocity calibration is 1530 and 1540 m/sec. respectively; the frequency 3.5 MHz. Linear measurements are
performed with electronic calipers on the screen, and on
photographs.

The fetal stomach is mostly visualized during fetal
trunk measurement techniques (2) (Fig. 1 and 2); important
landmarks are : vertebral column, umbilical vein, gallbladder, occasionally the descending and transverse colon
(Fig. 3 and 4), the diaphragm and the heart. By scanning
in different planes the largest diameters of the stomach
are determined in three dimensions perpendicular to each
other. The longitudinal axis of the fetal stomach is oriented from the upper fundal part, cranial, left and dorsal,
to the lower pyloric part, caudal, medial and ventral (Fig.
1 and 2). To calculate the approcimate stomach volume, the
ellipsoid formula ($V = 0,52$ abc; a, b and c standing for
the three diameters) was first applied (5). The ultrasonographic appearance and a few observations in autopsy specimens were however supportive of the cyclinder model
($V = 0.785$ abc); the overestimation because of the rounded
poles of the stomach is likely to be compensated by the
fact that the pyloric part is not completely included.

The fetal stomach can be visualized from 12-14 weeks
on in most instances. In about 5 % of subjects, where it
was not possible to visualize the stomach at routine examination, it was not always easy to differentiate between
intrinsic reasons (real empty stomach) and extrinsic reasons (e.g. shadowing of vertebral column, or, insufficient
penetration in obesity). Repeated examinations are essential to assess absence of fetal stomach filling.

DYNAMIC ASPECTS

In a trial phase several continuous observations were made with periods of one to four hours in order to define timing, duration, rhythm and degree of filling and emptying of the fetal stomach. By scanning through the fetal face, in a sagittal plane from forehead to chin, the process of drinking at the level of the fetal mouth was also studied.

In most of the 20 observation periods in 8 subjects (pregnancies between 26 and 32 weeks) no large volume changes were observed; only in some a quick filling was noted, suggesting a large-volume swallowing episode; emptying was sometimes observed, but slower and never complete. Together with the interference of extrinsic factors such as compression, body movements and respiratory movements, no clear patterns were demonstrated. During fetal breathing movements pronounced changes were seen in the form of the stomach mostly caused by contractions of the diaphragm; however differentiation between passive changes in form and intrinsic contraction waves can be questioned.

At the level of the fetal mouth two or three types of drinking or swallowing movements can be observed. One type shows very small movements of lips and chin, and sometimes of the tongue, with suggestion of fluid transition to the pharynx; these fish-like biting movements often occur in repeated serial episodes of 1 to 14 bites with between episodes intervals of 15 seconds to half a minute. More expansive and continuing biting or chewing mandibular movements, accompanied with tongue movemens and occasional protrus ion of the tongue, present another type; this type

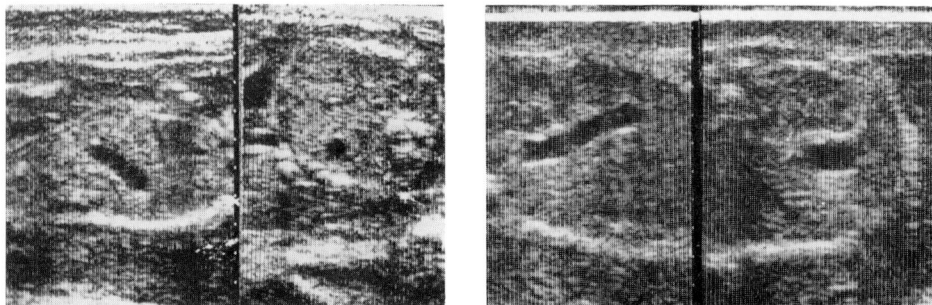

Figure 1. Fetal stomach on longitudinal and transverse tomogram in pregnancy of 24 weeks duration.

Figure 2. Fetal stomach on longitudinal and transverse tomogram in pregnancy of 37 weeks duration.

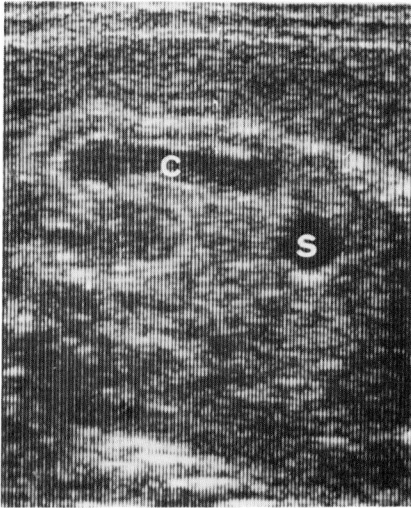
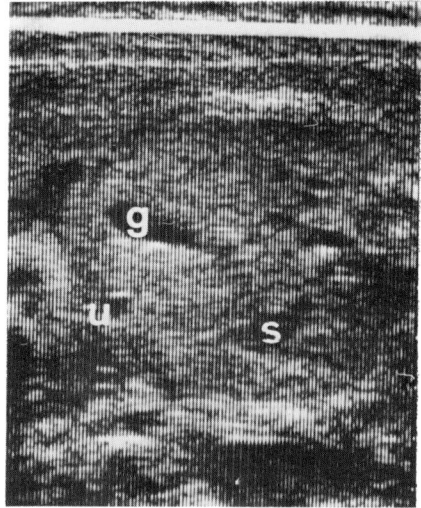

Figure 3. Fetal colon descendens (c), close to fetal stomach (s) in pregnancy of 33 weeks duration.

Figure 4. Fetal gallbladder (g) at the right side of the
mobilical vein (u) with fetal stomach (s) left and dorsal
pregnancy of 32 weeks.

occurs more frequently in later pregnancy. Some very wide
mouth opening movements were occasionally observed with
some repetitions at 1 to 3 minutes, often with extension
and retroflexion of the head; the observer spontaneaously
associates this type of movement with yawning movements.
Incidentally thumb sucking is noted.

LARGE SCALE CROSS-SECTIONAL DATA

      In a next approach a large scale cross-sectional
study was planned with single shot and short term observations; although stomach function is dynamic, this more
static approach can give useful information on the possible range of stomach volumes in the course of normal pregnancy and in some pathological conditions, and it can also
orientate further research.
      In a study of 299 single normal pregnancies between
12 and 38 weeks, the total range and the mean values of
stomach volume measurements are plotted against gestational
age (Fig. 5 and 6).

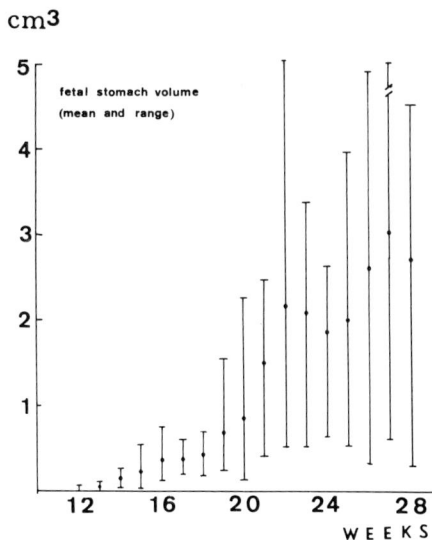

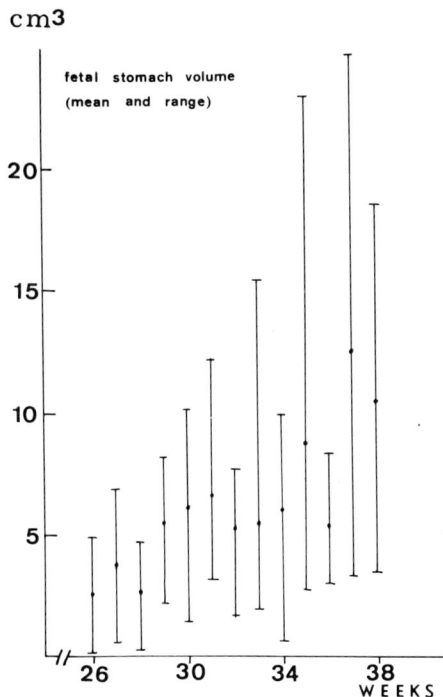

Figure 5. Fetal stomach volumes in the second trimester of pregnancy : mean and total range of 180 measurements, from 12 to 28 gestational weeks.

Figure 6. Fetal stomach volumes in the third trimester of pregnancy : Mean and total range of 165 measurements, from 26 to 38 gestational weeks.

CLINICAL ASPECTS

On some occasions the location of the stomach can be of utmost importance; on one occasion the diagnosis of congenital absence of the diaphragm with herniation of the stomach in the thoracic cavity was missed; it should however be possible with present day techniques. A case of situs inversus was correctly diagnosed prenatally.

The stomach volume estimations obtained in a series of clinical situations have been plotted against the normal range ($\pm$ 2 SD), in order to detect certain trends.

The distribution of stomach volumes measured in 5 cases of anencepahly (Fig. 7 and 8) seems normal.

Five cases of definitely proven premature rupture of membranes were observed : all stomach volumes were to be found in the very low range (Fig. 8). In five consecutive cases of definite or extreme oligoamnion, not in relation with premature rupture of membranes the fetal stomach vol-

278

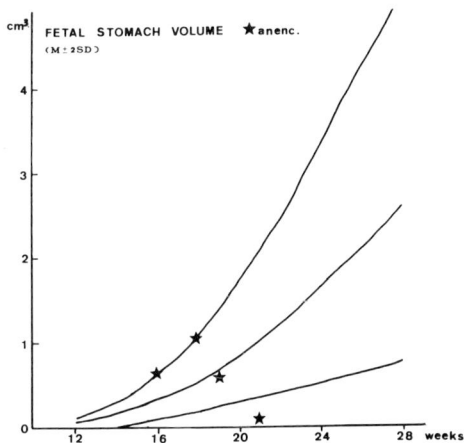

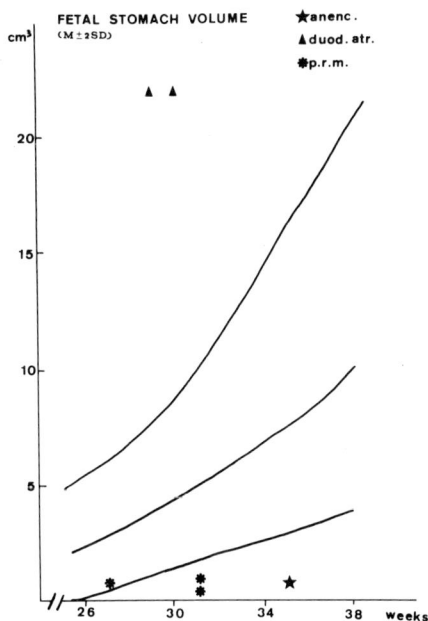

Figure 7. Fetal stomach volumes in the second trimester of pregnancy (mean and ± 2 SD). Stomach volume assessments in four cases of anencephaly are plotted.

Figure 8. Fetal stomach volumes in the third trimester of pregnancy (mean and ± 2 SD). Estimations of fetal stomach volume in premature rupture of membranes (p.r.m.), duodenal atresia and anencephaly are indicated.

umes are distributed in the lower range (Fig. 12).

In 25 consecutive cases of definite or extreme polyhydramnion, ultimately not caused by mechanical obstruction of the fetal G.I. tractus, the distribution of the fetal stomach volumes was normal (Fig. 11). In 2 cases of polyhydramnion with a very large fetal stomach volume (22 cm^3), examined at 29 and 30 weeks, fetal duodenal atresia was diagnosed correctly (Fig. 8, 9 and 10). Four cases of polyhydramnion, where no fetal stomach filling could be demonstrated, at repeated examinations and with sufficient visualisation of the stomach region, turned out to give : an esophagal atresia, a mixed thyroid-thymus tumor, a floppy infant syndrome, and a lethal cardiopathy.

DISCUSSION

Already from the twelfth gestational week on the fetal stomach appears to be fluid filled, and can be demonstrated by echography in most instances. The function of

279

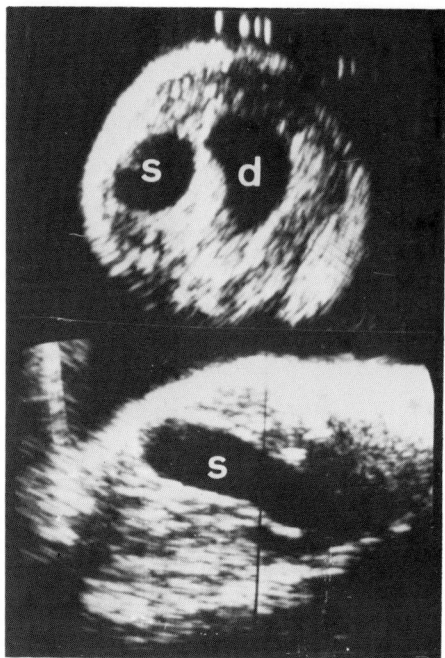

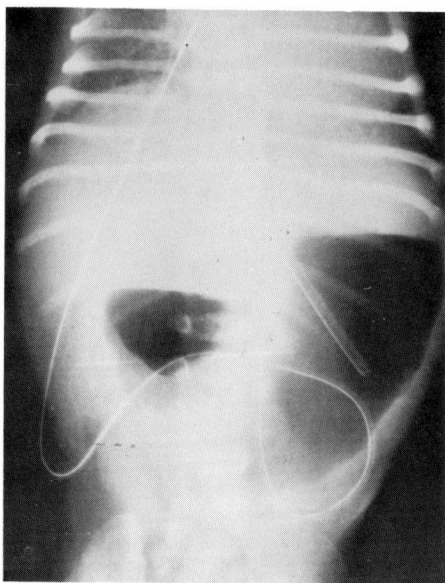

Figure 9. Duodenal atresia. Ultrasonic diagnosis at 24 weeks of pregnancy : polyhydramnion, enlarged fetal stomach volume (s) and first duodenal loop (d).

Figure 10. Duodenal atresia. Radiography in premature newborn (same as fetus in Fig. 9), confirms ultrasonic diagnosis.

swallowing is already established in the early second trimester (3), but gastric secretion might also play a role. More quantitative data are needed on individual long period observations, at different ages of gestation, to evaluate dynamics and patterns of fetal stomach filling and emptying. The observations on fetal mouth movements are also to be extended and quantified. Our preliminary observations, mainly bearing on the 26-32 weeks pregnancy period, suggest that the fetus is swallowing fluid with small quantities over longer periods, with only occasionally a large volume swallowing episode. A different pattern migt be expected in later pregnancy, with a better defined stomach filling and emptying rhythm, and with contraction waves (6).

From our limited data on anencephalics it is so far not possible to draw any firm conclusion, but our data

280

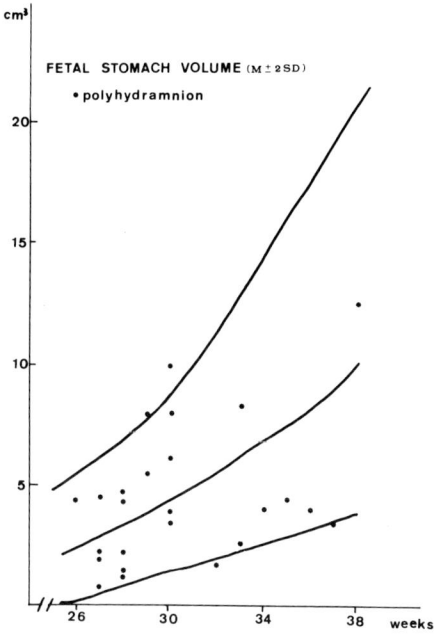

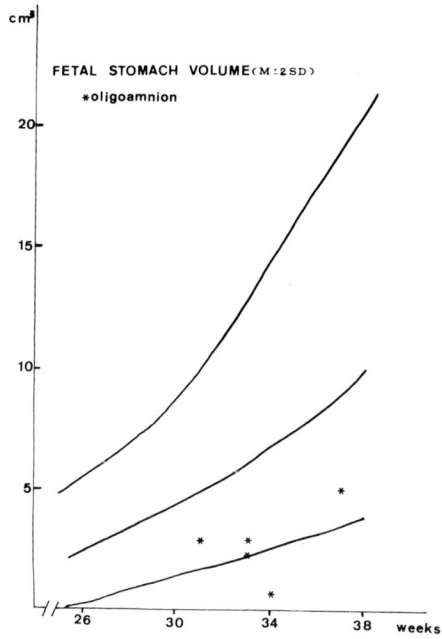

Figure 11. Fetal stomach volume in polyhydramnion; estimations of fetal stomach volume in 25 cases of polyhydramnion, not caused by gastro-intestinal obstructive pathology in the fetus, are plotted against normal values.

Figure 12. Fetal stomach volume in oligoamnion. Estimations of fetal stomach volume in 5 cases of oligoamnion, not caused by premature rupture of membranes, are plotted against normal values.

are not in disagreement with earlier experimental findings (1). The observations in premature rupture of membranes and in oligoamnion of other origin show that fetal stomach volumes seem to be small when there is not very much amniotic fluid available. In polyhydramnion ultimately not caused by obstruction of the fetal G.I.tractus, no special trend was observed in fetal stomach volumes. Extremely large stomach volumes very strongly suggest intestinal obstruction. With permanent absence of stomach filling, and polyhydramnion, a mechanical obstruction above the level of the stomach or a severe functional disturbance can be expected.

    The reported data and observations can offer a frame work for further research in fetal stomach function.

ACKNOWLEDGEMENT

The authors are indebted to Prof. Dr. E. Eggermont, neonatol., Prof. Dr. A. Van Assche, obst., Dr. J.P. Frijns, hum. genet., and Dr. P. Goddeeris, path., for their constructive suggestions and assistance in different parts of the study.

REFERENCES

1. Abramovich, D.R. (1978) : In : Amniotic Fluid. Research and Clinical Application. p. 31. Editors : D. Fairweather & T. Eskes. Excerpta Medica, Amsterdam, 2nd edition.
2. Campbell, S. and Wilkin, D. (1975) : Brit. J. Obst. Gyn., 82, 689.
3. Humphrey, T. (1978) : In : Perinatal Physiology, p. 667. Editor : U. Stave, Plenum, New-York.
4. Kossoff, G. and Garrett, W.J. (1972) : Obst. Gyn., 40, 299.
5. Vandenberghe, K. and De Wolf, F. (1978) : In : Abstracts 3rd European Congress on Ultrasonics in Medicine. p. 417. Bologna, Ed. Centro Minerva Medica.
6. Wladimiroff, J.W. (1979) : In : Proceedings 2nd Meeting of the WFUMB, Japan. In press.

ULTRASONIC ASSESSMENT OF FETAL RENAL FUNCTION IN NORMAL AND COMPLICATED PREGNANCY

Asim Kurjak

Department of Obstetrics and Gynecology, University of Zagreb, Zagreb, Yugoslavia

Thanks to ultrasound we are now sure that human fetuses void and this fact is now generally accepted as a part of normal intrauterine activity. However, this idea is by no means new since Hipocrates believed this to be so in his time. Scientific evidence supporting this physiological fact has accumulated very slowly and before ultrasound was introduced, this fetal activity was confirmed only by animal experiments and indirect analyses of urine passed by aborted or preterm delivered babies.

In 1973 Campbell, Wladimiroff and Dewhurst (1) described an ultrasonic technique for estimating the hourly fetal urine production rate (HFUPR) in the human fetus. This technique has made it possible to study fetal renal function in normal and complicated pregnancies. Antenatal measurement of fetal urine production was introduced in our Ultrasonic Center in 1974 by Wladimiroff. A number of papers have already been published in this field. In this report we present final results from our 4-year study period in Zagreb (6,7,8).

HFUPR IN NORMAL AND COMPLICATED PREGNANCY

We essentially followed Campbell's measuring technique in our investigations(1,4).

In the initial part of our study, we examined a total of 106 antenatal patients between 32 and 41 weeks of pregnancy. Each patient was certain of the date of her last menstrual period. All pregnancies were uncomplicated; birth weights of the babies were above the tenth percentile for gestation according to the tables of Thompson et al(3). Correction was made for maternal parity and fetal sex.

As our research progressed, we were able to identify the fetal bladder as early as 22 weeks of normal pregnancy. Fetal urinary production was then studied in 255 normal pregnancies from 22 to 41 weeks of gestational age. The 255 HFUPR estimations between 22 and 41 weeks were plotted against the menstrual age of the fetus and the regression line was drawn. There was a highly significant positive correlation between urinary production and gestational age (r=0.94)(2).

The ultrasonic measurement of fetal urinary production

has made it possible to study fetal renal function not only under physiologic but also under pathologic conditions.

Hundred and thirty eight patients were studied during complicated pregnancy; 62% of these cases had hypertensive disorders. Whereas our normal curve showed that in normal pregnancies HFUPR varies from a mean value of 2.2 ml at 22 weeks to 26.3 ml at 40 weeks, it became clear that in 24% of the complicated pregnancies the hourly fetal production rate was below the 5th percentile of the normal curve. Almost all of the 25 small-for-dates had significantly reduced production rates below the normal range.

In an additional study, hourly changes of bladder volume were measured in 56 small-for-date babies, i.e. a fetal birth weight below the 10th percentile for gestational age. Sixty-eight percent of the mothers who delivered small-for-date babies had EPH gestosis. HFUPR was reduced in 81.8%.

It is known that in diabetic pregnancy the incidence of polyhydramnios is very high; some authors report 20 to 50%. The etiology of this complication in diabetic pregnancy is still unknown. Since well-controlled diabetes is usually associated with normal amniotic fluid volume, some authors suggested that increased production of amniotic fluid was the result of maternal hyperglycemia and fetal polyuria.

The hourly fetal urinary production rate was measured in 42 diabetic patients. In the group of insulin-treated patients, 11 had normal HFUPR values, 10 had values above the 95th centile, while 6 fetuses had values below the 5th centile when compared to our normal standard. Five fetuses from this last group were delivered as small-for-dates, whereas only one normal weighing baby had low fetal bladder volume values.

When the fetal bladder volume was compared with the birth weight of the newborn, it was obvious that the babies with high birth weights regularly had high urinary values.

In the group of patients on diet, only one baby had low fetal bladder volume values and its birth weight was between the 5th and 10th centile. Nine fetuses from this group had normal values while 4 fetuses had values above the 95th centile. If all the investigated fetuses are analyzed together, 19 fetuses had normal values, 16 had values above the 95th centile and 7 had values below the 5th centile.

In our previous study a good correlation was found between HFUPR in complicated pregnancies and birth weight of the newborns. Larger babies produced higher values of fetal urine and vice versa. We came to the same conclusion in the investigation of the diabetic pregnant patient. In spite of the severity of the disease, fetal renal function is not significantly affected by maternal diabetes. Sixteen out of the 42 investigated fetuses produced urine with values above the 95th centile. These findings, however, should not be attributed to the increased glomerular filtration or decreased tubular reabsorption rate of the fetuses (5). We

284

have already stressed that the results obtained had a direct correlation with the size of the baby, i.e. its birth weight.

From these results, it is justifiable to conclude that polyhydramnios in diabetic pregnancy should not be attributed to polyuria. The pathophysiologic mechanisms which cause polyhydramnios are still unknown.

Eleven cases of anencephaly were diagnosed by means of ultrasound and HFUPR was measured. Our results obtained on fetal urinary production in anencephaly were either normal or even below the normal range. So it seems highly unlikely that polyhydramnios in anencephalics is caused by fetal polyuria.

Fifteen cases with polyhydramnios were also investigated. We found nearly normal HFUPR values in almost all of them. Polyhydramnios was defined as an amniotic fluid volume of more than 1500 ml judging by the clinical examination.

URINARY SYSTEM ABNORMALITIES

Fetal kidneys can usually be visualized during the last trimester of pregnancy. Even as early as 20 weeks, the fetal bladder can be shown and bladder volume measured. Enlargement of the fetal kidney by polycystic disease or hydronephrosis can be differentiated. Failure to demonstrate kidneys or to see bladder filling over a period of several hours is strong evidence of renal agenesis. We have diagnosed two cases of Potter's syndrome where bladder filling could not be detected for four to six hours.

Evaluation of the fetal urinary system is of more than theoretical importance. The sporadic occurrence of renal agenesis in a general population is one in 2000 pregnancies. If this condition occurs, however, on a genetic basis, there is a 25% recurrence rate after one pregnancy has been affected.

Routine ultrasonic examination is recommended between the 34th and 36th week of gestation for all pregnant women who have had a previous family history of a urinary tract anomaly. Diagnosis in the fetal stage allows prompt surgical treatment at birth before further structural damage has occurred. Parents who have had a baby with renal agenesis can be greatly reassured by the information that the current pregnancy shows normal-looking kidneys and normal fetal bladder filling.

In conclusion, the possibility of directly measuring fetal urinary production has lead to a better understanding of fetal renal function in normal and complicated pregnancies. Before Campbell and Wladimiroff introduced their method of measuring HFUPR, the assessment of fetal urine production was possible only indirectly or by comparison with the results obtained from animal studies. The findings obtained by Campbell, Wladimiroff and ourselves may also help in increasing our understanding as to what extent amniotic fluid volume is dependent on fetal urinary output.

REFERENCES

1. Campbell, S., Wladimiroff, J.W. and Dewhurst, C.J.
    (1973): J. Obstet. Gynaecol. Brit. Cwlth., <u>80</u>, 680.
2. Kurjak, A.(1977): Combined ultrasonic-biochemical as-
    sessment of fetal renal function in normal and compli-
    cated pregnancies. Doctor's thesis. Uni. of Beograd.
3. Thompson, A.M., Billewicz, W.Z., and Hytten, F.E.(1968):
    J. Obstet. Gynaecol. Brit. Cwlth., <u>75</u>, 903.
4. Wladimiroff, J.W. and Campbell, S.(1974): Lancet, <u>1</u>,
    151.
5. Wladimiroff, J.W. (1978): In: Handbook of Clinical
    Ultrasound, p. 203, Editor, M. de Vlieger, Wiley, New
    York.
6. Kurjak, A., Latin, V.(1975): IRCS Medical Science,
    <u>3</u>, 9.
7. Kurjak, A., Latin, V.(1978): Medicina Fetale, Simposio
    Internazionale, pp. 105-109, Monduzi Edizioni, Bologna.
8. Kurjak, A., Latin, V., Breyer, B. (1977): In: Ultra-
    sound in Medicine. ed. D. White and R. Brown, pp. 691.
    Plenum Publishers, New York.

9. RECENT ADVANCES IN ECHOCARDIOGRAPHY

I. Cikes, Chairman

STUDY OF LEFT VENTRICULAR RELAXATION AND FILLING BY ECHOCARDIOGRAPHY

D.G. Gibson

Brompton Hospital, London, England

INTRODUCTION

Filling is as important to the function of the left ventricle as ejection. When heart rate is high there is progressive abbreviation in the time that the mitral valve is open, so that the mean velocity of blood into the ventricle during diastole comes to exceed that into the aorta during ejection. Filling is thus likely to be a highly organized process, and interference by disease to cause impairment of overall cardiac function to an extent comparable with that of the much more widely recognized disturbances of systole. It is the purpose of this presentation to demonstrate how echocardiography is of value in analyzing such abnormalities(1).

We take relaxation to mean a change in the properties of the myocardium manifesting itself as a reduction in tension at constant length. We are not concerned with its biochemical or ultrastructural manifestations but rather to show how it can be studied from direct measurement of pressure, wall thickness or cavity dimension or valve movement. A number of approaches are possible. Of these the oldest is that formalized by Wiggers (2), who defined three phases of diastole: protodiastole, as the time of aortic pressure drop, ending with closure of the aortic valve, isovolumic relaxation, the period between aortic valve closure and mitral valve opening, and finally filling, following opening of the mitral valve. The present account will be concerned with left sided events, although analogous definitions can be formulated to apply to the right side of the heart.

There is now little disagreement that the time of aortic valve closure can be satisfactorily assessed from the timing of the onset of the first high frequency vibration of the aortic component of the second sound (3). The exact timing of mitral valve opening is more difficult to assess. A number of definitions have been proposed, which have been reviewed in detail elsewhere (1). The most satisfactory appears to be the timing of separation of anterior and posterior mitral valve cusps as measured by M-mode echocardiography. It seems likely, however, that mitral valve opening does not occur instantaneously in all regions of the valve, with consequent difficulties in arriving at a satisfactory definition of its exact timing.

A second approach to the study of diastole is to use observations of the ventricular wall and their relation to the pressure pulse. Here, relaxation is regarded as part of the pressure-dimension loop, which itself gives fundamental information about regional pump function. Although either method may be used in isolation, their interrelations provide considerable insight into mechanisms operating during this important phase of the cardiac cycle.

ISOVOLUMIC RELAXATION

Although measurement of the duration of isovolumic relaxation would seem to be useful in studying relaxation in man, it has been little studied. A number of workers have assumed that the onset of mitral valve opening corresponds with the "O" point of the apexcardiogram. Such estimates, however, are open to serious error, since the "O" point may follow mitral valve opening by up to 120 msec (4), and so they will not be considered further. Mean valves in normal subjects are in the range of 50-70 msec (5,6), and are weakly correlated with heart rate. Isovolumic relaxation time is increased in left ventricular hypertrophy, whether primary, as occurs in hypertrophic cardiomyopathy or secondary as in aortic stenosis or hypertension. In coronary artery disease also, isovolumic relaxation time may be prolonged, but less consistently than in left ventricular hypertrophy. Isovolumic relaxation time is short in mitral stenosis, and may be zero or even negative in patients with severe left ventricular disease in whom left atrial pressure is high. A similar abnormality occurs in patients with transposition of the great arteries after Mustard's operation, provided that the left ventricle is ejecting into a normal pulmonary vascular bed. The results of animal experiments suggest that it may be shortened by drugs with a positive inotropic effect or by elevation of left atrial pressure, and lengthened by an elevation of systemic arterial pressure.

Abnormal left ventricular wall movement may occur during isovolumic relaxation, and M-mode echocardiography is a particularly suitable means of studying this in view of its repetition rate of 1000/sec. Normally, there is an increase of left ventricular dimension of 1-2 mm during isovolumic relaxation, due to thickening of the posterior wall. The onset of mitral valve opening corresponding within 20 msec to minimumcavity dimension (Figure l). In patients with either left ventricular hypertrophy or coronary artery disease, mitral valve opening may be delayed with respect to movement of the posterior wall (Figure 2). In patients with left ventricular hypertrophy, this delay is merely a reflection of prolongation of isovolumic relaxation time. In patients with coronary artery disease, however, its mechanism is more complex. In a minority, it again reflects prolonged isovolumic relaxation. However, this is relatively uncommon. In the majority, aortic valve closure is also

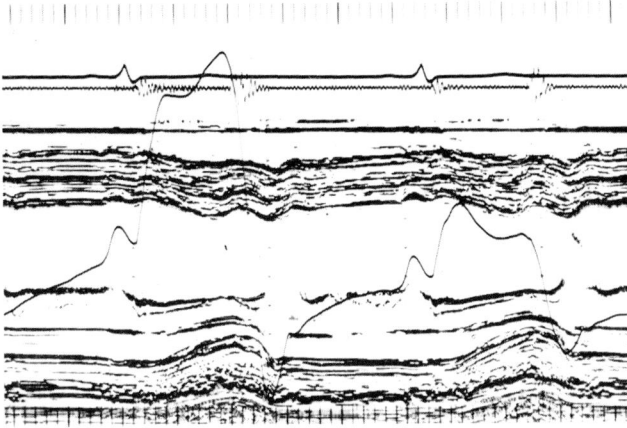

Fig. 1. Normal left ventricular echocardiogram with simultaneous phono- and apexcardiogram recorded. Isovolumic relaxation time can be measured from A2 to the onset of mitral valve opening (Reproduced by permission of the Editor, British Heart Journal).

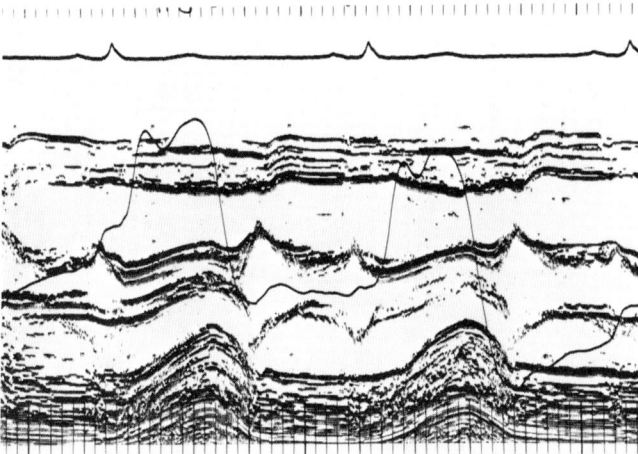

Fig. 2. Left ventricular echocardiogram from a patient with coronary artery disease. The onset of mitral valve opening is delayed with respect to peak inward movement of the posterior left ventricular wall, and minimum transverse dimension.(Reproduced by permission of the Editor, British Heart Journal).

delayed, and now comes to coincide with minimum cavity dimension, isovolumic relaxation time itself being normal. In some patients, both disturbances are present (6). Investigation of the mechanism of this relative delay in aortic valve closure has demonstrated that it is closely correlated with the presence of abnormal wall movement during the period of isovolumic contraction. It seems likely that such abnormalities are due to the presence of segments of myocardium in whom the onset of contraction is delayed but otherwise normal, so that tension still persists in them when the remainder of the ventricle is relaxing. This results in a delay in the fall of the ventricular pressure and thus in A2 with respect to normal regional of the cavity. Such abnormalities are aggravated by propranolol suggesting that the drug increases the disturbance in regional function (7).

Abnormalities of wall movement during isovolumic relaxation can also be detected by their relation to the pressure pulse. This is best demonstrated by constructing pressure-dimension loops. The normal pressure-dimension loop is rectangular (Figure 3), with little change in dimension during the upstroke or the downstroke. This shape represents the most efficient condition for transferring energy from the myocardium to the circulation. In patients with coronary artery disease, significant dimension changes occur during the downstroke, leading to distortion of the loop and thus to inefficient energy transfer (Figure 4). Similar, but qualitative information can be obtained if the apexcardiogram is substituted for the pressure trace, since the timing of the two is virtually identical during the upstroke and the downstroke of the pressure (8). This method of detecting incoordinate relaxation has been shown to have approximately 80% sensitivity and specificty in comparison with left ventricular angiography, using a computer-based method for demonstrating regional wall movement.

Abnormal endocardial movement during isovolumic relaxation can be understood more completely if the corresponding changes in wall thickness are studied, using the technique of digitization of the original echocardiograms (8). Normally, inward movement of endocardium during systole is due primarily to wall thickening rather than to epicardial movement. In normal subjects, peak wall thickness is attained at the time of onset of mitral valve opening. During rapid filling of the ventricle, the posterior wall shows a corresponding period of rapid thinning, at a peak velocity approximately twice that of its peak rate of thickening during systole (Figure 5). In patients with coronary artery disease, however, the abnormal dimension increase during isovolumic relaxation is due to premature wall thinning. Since rapid wall thinning can occur before mitral valve opening, it clearly cannot be regarded as a manifestation of filling, and is therefore likely to be a property of the posterior wall itself. This conclusion is strengthed by the observation that the extent to which it occurs varies with position in the ventricle, and that it does not occur on the septum or in the free wall of the right ventricle. Further, even in the posterior wall of the left ventricle, the extent to which it occurs varies with position. These results indicate that rapid thinning is not a property of all myocardium, but that it probably resides in the complex fibre structure of the normal left ventricle (9).

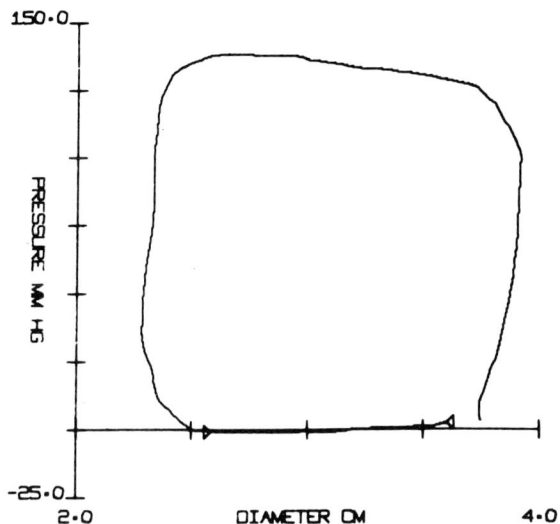

Fig. 3. Normal, rectangular pressure-dimension loop. (Reproduced by permission of the Editor, British Heart Journal).

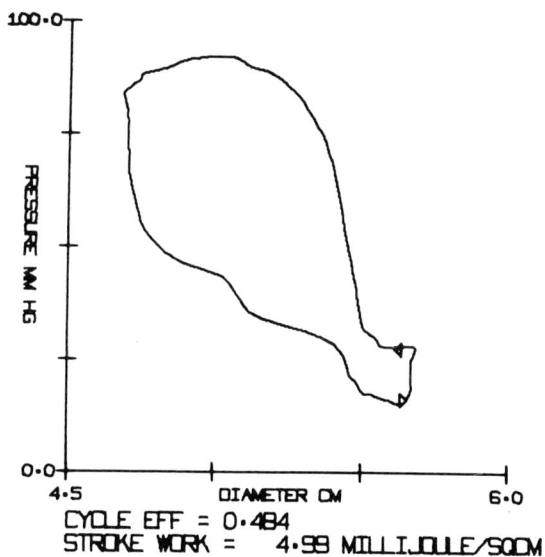

CYCLE EFF = 0·484
STROKE WORK = 4·99 MILLIJOULE/SQCM

Fig. 4. Distorted pressure-dimension loop, from a patient with coronary artery disease (Reproduced by permission of the Editor, British Heart Journal).

Filling of the left ventricle is assumed to start at the time of onset of separation of the two cusps of the mitral valve. Dimension changes during this period are very characteristic. In normal subjects, there is an early diastolic period of rapid filling, when the rate of dimension increase rapidly reaches a peak value of 12-20 cm/sec, returning to 20% of its peak valuve within 120-200 msec (8). This normal pattern is also seen when the change in a transverse dimension of the cavity is studied by angiography, and both peak values and also the timing of the onset and the termination of the rapid filling period can be shown to correspond closely to events on the curve of area against time. In patients with left ventricular inflow tract obstruction, the pattern of dimension change is very abnormal. Peak values are reduced, and the early diastolic period of rapid inflow is either prolonged, or in more severe cases, is lost altogether. These observations can be made the basis of a definition of mitral stenosis, allowing the condition to be defined independently of any anatomical abnormality of the valve itself (8). It can also be used to define malfunction of mitral prostheses.

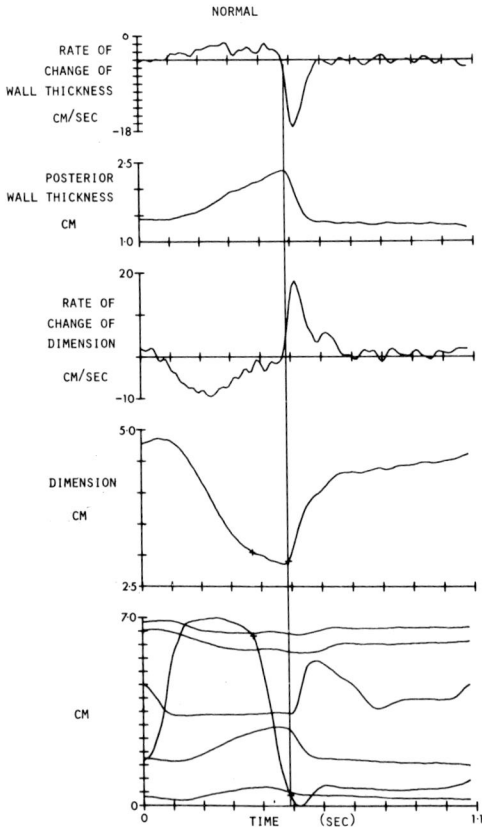

Fig. 5. Digitized echocardiogram showing changes in left ventricular cavity dimension and wall thickness, along with their respective rates of change. The vertical line represents the timing of mitral valve opening, which corresponds to the minimum cavity dimension. The cross on the dimension trace is the timing of A2, taken from the phonocardiogram. (Reproduced by permission of the Editor, British Heart Journal).

Abnormal dimension changes also occur during left ventricular filling in patients with left ventricular hypertrophy. Although systolic function is usually normal, there is a consistent reduction in the peak rate of dimension increase, exactly similar to that seen in mitral stenosis (Figure 6). The two conditions differ, however in the duration of the period of isovolmic relaxation. In mitral stenosis it is short, due probably to a high left atrial pressure. In left ventricular hypertrophy, from whatever cause, it is prolonged, suggesting that the reduced rate of dimension increase reflects a primary abnormality of relaxation rather than mechanical obstruction to inflow due for example to extreme septal hypertrophy.

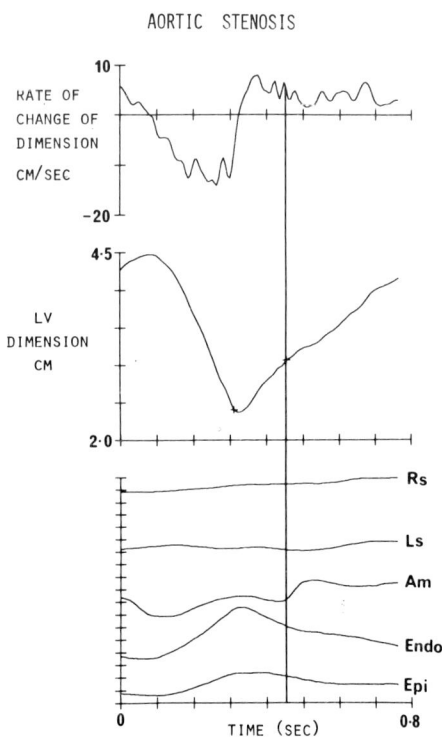

AORTIC STENOSIS

Fig. 6. Changes in left ventricular dimension in a patient with aortic stenosis. Isovolumic relaxation is prolonged, mitral valve opening delayed and peak rate of dimension increased,with prolongation of the early diastolic period of rapid dimension increase.(Reproduced by permission of the Editor, British Heart Journal)

PASSIVE DIASTOLIC PROPERTIES

Echocardiography can be also used to assess the passive elastic properties of the left ventricle during diastole. This can be performed by simultaneous measurement of left ventricular pressure, wall thickness and cavity dimension, so that stress strain curves can be constructed. These are characteristic. They show an early period of increasing cavity size when stress drops, reflecting the well known ability of left ventricular filling to start while relaxation is still taking place. During mid-diastole, there is a per-

295

iod when wall stress remains constant although cavity size
increases. The mechanism underlying this rather unexpected
behaviour is discussed elsewhere: we believe that it is a
manifestation of rapid ventricular thinning, rather than a
manifestation of visco-elastic properties of the wall (1).
Finally, during late diastole, there is a period of elastic
behaviour, when both wall stress and strain increase together. During this period, an elastic modulus can be calculated, and this has been shown to be increased in patients
with cardiographic evidence of left ventricular hypertrophy.
It must be pointed out, however, that this period is only
demonstrable when heart rate is slow and the diastolic filling period prolonged, so that an abnormally stiff ventricle
is unlikely to be a cause of limitation of exercise tolerance unless, for some reason, heart rate is low and fixed.

CONCLUSIONS

It is clear from this brief account that diastole in
the human heart cannot be regarded as a simple or a passive
process. It is highly organized, as might be deduced from
simple considerations of transmitral flow when heart rate
is high. It appears that echocardiography is a very satisfactory means of studying it in the normal subject, and in
defining abnormalities that may occur in disease. These
latter may well prove to be at least as significant as those
occurring during systole in causing impairment of overall
cardiac function, although the attention that they have received has been very much less.

REFERENCES

1. Traill, T.A., and Gibson, D.G.(1979): In: Progress in
   Cardiology, Ed. Yu P and Goodwin, J.F., Vol. 7 (in press)
2. Wiggers, C.J.(1921): American Journal of Physiology.
   56:415-438.
3. Mills, P and Craige, E. (1978): Progress in Cardiovascular Diseases. 20:337-358.
4. Prewitt, T.A., Gibson, D., Brown, D. and Sutton, G.
   (1975): British Heart Journal. 37:1256-1262.
5. Sahn, D.J. (1977): In: Echocardiology. Ed. N. Bom.
   Martinus Nijhoff. The Hague pp 83-93.
6. Chen, W. and Gibson, D.G. (1979): British Heart Journal
   42:51-56.
7. von Bibra, H., Gibson, D.G. and Nityanandan, K. (1979):
   British Heart Journal. 42: (in press).
8. Upton, M.T. and Gibson, D.G. (1978): Progress in Cardiovascular Diseases. 20:359-384.
9. Gibson, D.G., Greenbaum, R., Marier, D.L. and Brown, D.J
   (1979): European Journal of Cardiology. In press.

CHANGE OF CONCEPT IN HYPERTROPHIC CARDIOMYOPATHY

J. Gehrke

Department of Medicine, Division of Cardiovascular Disease, Clinical Cardiology, Royal Postgraduate Medical School, Hammersmith Hospital, London, United Kingdom

M-scan echocardiography made a major impact on the non-invasive diagnosis of hypertrophic cardiomyopathy (HCM), and it is the purpose of this communication to show that it is again echocardiography, however, the more refined technique of real-time B-scanning, which seems to revise earlier concepts of this disease.

The earliest description of asymmetrical septal hypertrophy goes back to the year 1907 when the pathologist Schmincke (1) from the University of Würzburg, Germany, described two post-mortem cases with the typical anatomical abnormality of left ventricular hypertrophy, predominantly involving the superior interventricular septum asymmetrically in contrast to the otherwise concentric hypertrophy of the rest of the left ventricle. He called this entity 'primary muscular conus'.

These findings were later confirmed by Teare (2) who in addition described a distortion of the mitral valve, which, however, appears clearly to be due to acquired mitral valve disease. Brock (3,4) in 1957 described a condition of functional obstruction of the left ventricle due to hypertrophic changes in the left ventricular outflow tract. He observed left ventricular outflow tract gradients without being able to palpate any anatomical obstruction on digital exploration of the left ventricular outflow tract during operation. Angiographic findings of a systolic lucent line in the outflow tract led to the theory of systolic anterior motion of the mitral valve producing the gradient or obstruction and also the concomitant mitral regurgitation (5,6,7). Thus it was unavoidable that the first systolic anterior moving echo structures in patients with HCM (8,9) were interpreted as re-opening of the mitral valve in systole for a long time, so that no further thoughts about the mechanisms of gradient production and mitral regurgitation could develop. It was also understandable that an attempt was made to non-invasively assess the magnitude of left ventricular outflow tract gradients by form analysis of the 'SAM' structures in the mitral echogram (10,11).

Early M-scan findings (12) in 1973 seemed to contradict the prevailing explanations of left ventricular outflow tract obstruction. It was possible to obtain one recording where we could observe the mitral valve echo pat-

tern together with structures moving through this complex
during diastole and being in continuity with the 'SAM' complex in systole. Triggered B-scan recordings at that time
also showed anteriorly bulging subvalvular structures while
the anterior mitral valve leaflet was in an already more
closed position in early systole (12). These early one- and
two-dimensional findings convinced us that the M-scan
echographic 'SAM' was produced by chordae tendineae rather
than by the mitral valve leaflets themselves. This idea was
supported by observing 'SAM' in many other conditions than
HCM (13) and recording complete 'SAM' structures touching
the interventricular septum in systole in patients who did
not show any mitral regurgitation during LV angiocardiog-
raphy.

After realising that 'SAM' was no longer reliable for
Real-time B-scanning, with which we started in 1974
(14), enabled us to observe the mitral valve leaflets during the entire cardiac cycle. In none of our patients with
HCM have we ever seen re-opening of the mitral valve. However, we observed structures between the MVL and the prominent papillary muscles to move in opposite direction to
that of the anterior mitral valve leaflet. These echoes
were interpreted as systolic anterior motion of chordae
and/or papillary muscles traversing the single ultrasonic
beam in systole and producing the M-scan echographic 'SAM'
in patients with HCM. The mechanism of 'SAM' is believed
to be the hyperkinetic apical left ventricular posterior
wall motion. These observations were initially presented
in 1975 (15) but unfortunately could be fully published only much later (16), since they did not comply with the
present schools of thought.

After realising that 'SAM' was no longer reliable for
diagnosing HCM (17) we paid particular attention to another
echographic hallmark of HCM, the asymmetric septal hypertrophy of Schmincke (1), which can be visualised and related to left ventricular posterior wall thickness (10,11).
Experience has shown that this sign is not reliable either,
since many interpretations are possible with the single
beam echo technique. These findings were subsequently reported (13) and not well received.

Another sign, the 'immobile interventricular septum'
(18,19), which was reported to be a characteristic finding
in HCM, was initially investigated next and found to be an
M-scan echographic illusion (20,21). Real-time B-scanning
revealed that the upper septal bulge moves forcibly towards
the cardiac apex, while the lower part of the septum moves
normally towards the left ventricular posterior wall. The
motion of the upper septum is more or less perpendicular
to the usual direction of the single ultrasonic beam in M-
scanning and can therefore not be appreciated according to
its true amplitude of motion. The change in upper septal
bulge motion may have an underlying pathophysiological
mechanism (22) in order to prevent further left ventricular
outflow tract obstruction during systole, and may, because
of this motion, contribute considerably to hyperkinetic

298

left ventricular ejection and thus to the development of
a left ventricular outflow tract gradient. The malalign-
ment of myocardial fibres within the upper septal bulge,
which appears as a relative damping of the myocardium adjacent to the bright septal endocardium, may be the histological manifestation of this mechanism (16,22).

The implication of this so-called 'immobile septum'
for the M-scan echographic evaluation of left ventricular
function, using left ventricular internal diameters, has
recently been discussed (23). With only slight changes in
transducer angulation different values for dimensions and
calculated functional indices between 13 and 93% may be obtained.

Another very early observation was obtained by M-scan
echocardiography. In the same patient, in whom the first
chordal structures were observed to move through the diastolic mitral valve echo pattern, different amplitudes of
'SAM' could be recorded with different transducer angula-
tions, ranging from no 'SAM' to a complete 'SAM'. When
angling the transducer more to the base of the heart, still
in the same patient, the 'SAM' disappeared completely and
we were able to record a mitral valve prolapse. This made
us believe that mitral valve prolapse may be the mechanism
of mitral regurgitation in hypertrophic cardiomyopathy (24).
We have since observed many cases of hypertrophic cardiomyopathy with one- and two-dimensional signs of 'localised
mitral valve prolapse' (25), which may be one of the primary pathophysiological mechanisms of HCM.

The first publication from America confirming our findings appeared recently in Circulation (26). It is interesting to note that the schools of thought, which had impeded
the publication of our earlier work in a major American
journal several months prior to the submission of that paper, are beginning to change in the United States. Although
this paper confirms nearly all our findings, the authors
have chosen a rather complicated way of describing the same
changes with different interpretations. Though the only
significant contradiction seems to be the contention that
the unusual echo pattern of the septal bulge produces a
denser (and not a relatively lighter) echo pattern than the
rest of the myocardium, many points of their interpretations
are worth discussing in the light of their findings and displayed evidence.

DIFFERENT VELOCITIES OF 'SAM' AND POSTERIOR WALL MOTION

The authors observed the most hyperkinetic wall motion
basally to the anteriorly bulging chordae and conclude this
to be evidence that chordae are not pushed anteriorly by
the myocardium. Besides blood, only two structures, the anterior mitral valve leaflet and anterior papillary muscle
may influence the kinetics of the anterior chordae tendineae. Their Figures 5, 6a,b,c and 9, display both the anterior mitral leaflet and part of the papillary muscles in

a posterior position. All scans in this paper fail to show
the entire ventricle, and the chordal anterior motion and
posterior wall excursion are therefore compared in an incomplete or restricted view, since the amplitude of motion
clearly increases towards the apex in M- and real-time B-
scanning. In our experience, where the entire left ventricle
is visualised the apex appears the most hyperkinetic portion
of the left ventricle, and often exhibits a squeezing pattern of contraction, which correlates very well with the
earlier observed apical cavity obliteration (27), which was
later believed to produce artificial left ventricular outflow tract gradients (28). Is it not that the apical antero-
lateral left ventricular wall, which displaces the anterior
papillary muscle and anterior chordae tendineae (16), lies
in a plane different from the usual long axis cross-section
shown, and that therefore an unrelated velocity of motion
between the posterior wall and anterior chordae at 'SAM'
level is compared by the authors? Furthermore it is easily
understandable that distal parts of a whip-strap move faster
than proximal ones, but there are, of course, some correlations between these two relative velocities. Indeed, M-
scanning very clearly shows a good correlation between the
velocity of posterior chordal motion near the posterior
papillary muscle and that of the apical posterior wall (see
Fig. 1).

SLACKENING OF CHORDAE AND VENTURI EFFECT

     The momentum of the anterior chordae following the an-
terior papillary muscle during diastole and the motion of
the anterior mitral leaflet during systole may well be responsible for their anteriorly billowing configuration,
which may also be facilitated by the momentary relative
slackening which occurs with the apex to base contraction
of the left ventricle in early systole, as well as by the
suction of the hyperkinetic flow in the left ventricular
outflow tract. The traction produced by the rapidity build-
ing up high left ventricular pressure brings the chordae
immediately into a straight line again, and whatever slack
remains, due to apex to base contraction or to fibrotic
changes and lengthening of chordae, will contribute to mitral valve prolapse. This may be the main mechanism of mitral regurgitation in hypertrophic cardiomyopathy (16,24),
and has been observed both in our laboratory in an increasing number of patients, and in others (29). The prolapse is
often very localised, and a careful search may be necessary
to visualise this effect. With regard to the Venturi effect,
suggested as an explanation by the authors, can the high
velocity of chordal systolic anterior and posterior motion,
often seen in M-scanning (Fig. 1)[*] ever be produced by a
passive motion of chordae floating in a hyperdynamic left

_____
[*]All figures by courtesy of GHRF London.

ventricle? Such velocities can probably be generated by forces of the anterior mitral leaflet and papillary muscle motion. How would the authors explain that the chordal 'SAM' touches the interventricular septum? The hyperdynamic flow and pressure in the left ventricle would impede the anteriorly floating chordae from trespassing this hyper- kinetic current in the left ventricular outflow tract. It seems unlikely that the suction created by the rapid flow in the left ventricular outflow tract may overcome these originating forces.

UNUSUAL BRIGHTNESS OF SEPTAL MYOCARDIUM

Fig. 3 and panels C and D of Fig. 6 in the authors' publication seem to show what is found by others, viz. a strong endocardial border on both ventricular sides of the septum, and myocardium in between relatively lighter (30, 31). In secondary septal hypertrophy in particular, we of- ten find another bright line in the middle of the septum, which looks like a fibrous separation of myocardium, as in our Fig. 2*, but the myocardium is less bright. In all scans of the authors, except for Fig. 1, the near gain seems too bright to separate the 'artefacts', which may, in fact, be properly visualised as anterior heart wall, as in their Fig. 1 and in our Fig. 3*. Their statement about relative brightness must be validated by comparison against anterior structures with comparatively less brightness. It therefore seems possible that the conclusions about relative brightness may be due to the particular scanning mode used, since the scans of Henry et al. (32), referred to in the authors' paper, and M-scanning anyway, indicate similar results to our obser- vations. Unfortunately no proof was given for the statement that the same enhanced brightness was observed when the septal bulge was translocated posteriorly in the ultrasonic image, as can well be demonstrated in an apical view. In our experience with both sector and linear scanners, the same textures remain in the apical view, and the relative clarity of this presentation makes for a better differentia- tion between the denser fibrous lines and plaques and the lighter myocardial areas (see our Fig. 4*). These findings, however, may also be seen in any secondary form of hyper- trophy, and differ only in the extent of their distribution.

AKINETIC SEPTUM AND COMPENSATORY FREE WALL HYPERKINESIS

The septal bulge in HCM moves jerkily towards the car- diac apex, which is at right angles to the direction of the single ultrasonic beam when scanning through the long axis of the heart, as explained earlier, and also to the trans- verse cross-section of real-time B-scanning. This is more difficult to see when working with a sector, as compared to a linear real-time B-scanner. It is surely the case that

---

*All figures by courtesy of GHRF London.

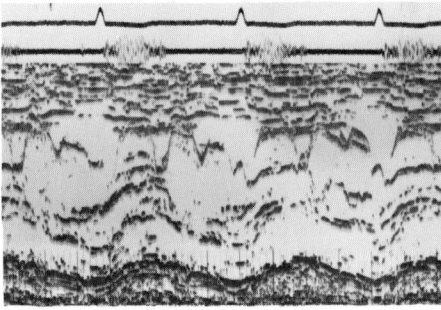

1

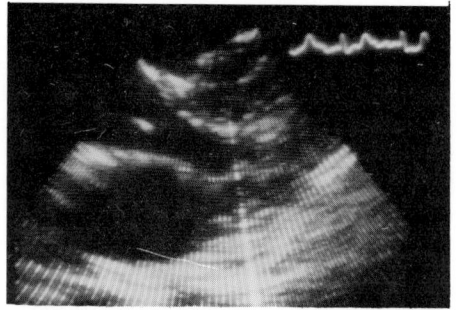

2

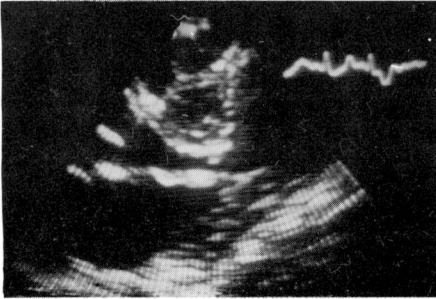

3

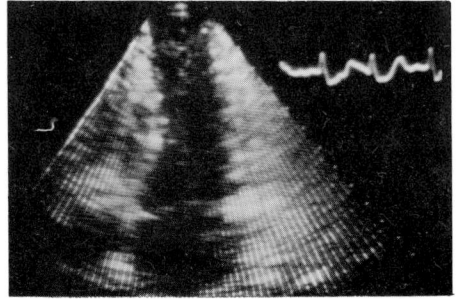

4

the hyperkinetic left ventricular contraction is not a
compensation for the 'akinetic' septum, but is in fact the
underlying pathology of this disease.

Furthermore the authors, despite experience of over
3000 patients cling to the expression of 'SAM', and the impression left with the reader, after studying the authors'
work, is that 'SAM' should still be regarded as a specific
feature of HCM. In fact, 'SAM' is what it denotes: a systolic anterior motion of any structure - and there are
many - e.g. the posterior wall, aortic root, chordae, and
papillary muscles. 'SAM' of the subvalvular mitral apparatus may be seen in any hyperkinetic situation associated
with hyperdynamic apical contraction of the left ventricle
(13,16,34). If one restricts the nomenclature 'SAM' and
also 'ASH' (asymmetrical septal hypertrophy) to the description of pathognomonic features, many conditions will
continue to be misdiagnosed by echocardiography, and particularly by M-scanning.

Another point: real-time B-scanning seems to have been
able to clarify the selective apical hypertrophy of the
septum, which has recently been believed to be another subset of hypertrophic cardiomyopathy. We believe that this
one- and two-dimensional echographic feature should be included into the criteria of right ventricular volume overload (35). An additional real-time B-scan criterium is the
'see-saw motion' of the interventricular septum with or
without increase in left ventricular internal diameter. It
is postulated that selective increase in apical septal hypertrophy may be the result of long-standing stroke work
of the lower septum to compensate for the haemodynamic loss
of the reversed upper septal motion ('RUSM'), thus serving
as a differential diagnostic sign in right ventricular volume overload of recent onset (35).

The final point regards the mechanism of left ventricular outflow tract obstruction in HCM. In recent work (36),
one- and two-dimensional echographic measurements of left
ventricular posterior wall thickness, septal thickness,
'SAM' amplitude, left ventricular and right ventricular
outflow tract size have been correlated with the severity
of left ventricular outflow tract gradients. None of the
measurements, including left ventricular outflow tract size,
were found to correlate significantly with the haemodynamic
findings. These results strongly suggest that the force of
left ventricular wall contraction in combination with the
recently described forceful movement of the septal bulge
towards the apex are the primary factors of outflow tract
gradients in HCM.

The implications of our recent one- and two-dimensional echocardiographic research for diagnosis, therapy, and
terminology have recently been discussed (12). The term
'obstruction' has confused the issue of terminology for
some time. Our work has shown that it would seem to simplify the issue if one no longer applied this term 'obstructive' to two different situations, to haemodynamic and ana-

tomical left ventricular outflow tract obstruction,and use it, as was suggested earlier from our department (37), as hypertrophic obstructive cardiomyopathy (HOCM) only in its original meaning (lat. obstruere), to merely describe the anatomical abnormality. The initial terminology of HOCM, but with the subdivision into HOCM with fixed, labile, or no left ventricular outflow tract gradients would leave space for such future cases which we see in increasing numbers and in whom a gradient but no obstruction is found.

This brief review on hypertrophic cardiomyopathy shows the complexity of this disease and a great deal of research seems necessary to solve the many questions which are still open in this fascinating disease.

REFERENCES

1. Schmincke, A. (1907): Dtsch. Med. Wschr., 33, 2082.
2. Teare, D. (1958): Brit. Heart. J., 20, 1.
3. Brock, R.C. (1957): Guy's Hosp. Rep., 106, 221.
4. Brock, R.C. (1959): Guy's Hosp. Rep., 108, 126.
5. Fix, P. and Moberg, A. (1964): Acta Radiol., 2, 177.
6. Dinsmore et al. (1966): New Engl. J. Med., 275, 1225.
7. Simon, A.L. (1967): Circulation, 36, 852.
8. Pridie, R.B. and Turnbull, T.A. (1968): Proceedings of the Vth European Congress of Cardiology, Athens, September 1968.
9. Shah, P.M. et al. (1968): Circulation, 37 and 38, Suppl. VI.
10. Henry, W.L. et al. (1973): New Engl. J. Med., 288, 989.
11. Epstein, S.E. et al. (1974): Ann. Int. Med., 81, 650.
12. Gehrke, J. (1979): Proceedings of the 2nd Meeting of the WFUMB, Miyazaki, Japan, 1979. Excerpta Medica, in press.
13. Gehrke, J. (1977): Amer. J. Cardiol., 39, 270.
14. Gehrke, J. and Leeman, S. (1975): Brit. J. Radiol., 48, 510.
15. Gehrke, J. (1976): Brit. Heart J., 38, 314.
16. Gehrke, J. and Goodwin, J.F. (1978): Clin. Cardiol., 1, 152.
17. Gehrke, J.: Ultraschall-Diagnostic 76, Heidelberg.
18. Feizi, O. and Emanuel, R. (1975): Brit. Heart J., 37, 1286.
19. Rossen, R.M. et al. (1974): New Engl. J. Med., 291, 1317.
20. Gehrke, J. (1977): Z. Kardiol., 66, 556.
21. Gehrke, J. (1978): Brit. Heart J., 40, 475.
22. Gehrke, J. (1979): Basic Research in Cardiol., 74, 95.
23. Gehrke, J. (1978): Ultraschall-Diagnostik 77. Thieme Verlag, Stuttgart, p. 308.
24. Gehrke, J. (1976): Book of Abstracts of the 7th European Congress of Cardiology, Amsterdam.
25. Gehrke, J. (1979): Submitted to Brit. Med. Ultrasonic Soc. Edinburgh, Sept.
26. Martin, R.P. et al. (1979): Circulation, 59, 1206.

27. Criley, J.M. et al. (1965): Circulation, 32, 881.
28. Wigle, E.D. et al. (1967): Circulation, 35, 1100.
29. Isshiki, T. et al. (1979): Book of Abstracts of the 2nd Meeting of WFUMB, Miyazaki, Japan, 1979.
30. Gehrke, J. et al. (1976): Proceedings of the International Congress of the European Society for Clinical Respiratory Physiology and European Society of Cardiology. Cor Pulmonale Chronicum, Munich.
31. Gehrke, J. (1977): Ann. Radiol., 20, 409.
32. Gehrke, J. (1975): Amer. J. Cardiol., 35, 337.
33. Gehrke, J. (1978): Verh. Dtsch. Ges. Kreisl., 44, 242.
34. Gehrke, J. (1979): Ann. Radiol., 22, 4, 315.
35. Gehrke, J. (1978): Brit. J. Radiol., 51, 645.
36. Gehrke, J. and Goodwin, J.F. (1978): Book of Abstracts of the 8th World Congress of Cardiology, Tokyo, 1978.
37. Cohen, J. et al. (1964): Brit. Heart J., 26, 16.

TWO-DIMENSIONAL ECHOCARDIOGRAPHY IN THE DIAGNOSIS OF PERICARDIAL EFFUSION AND ADHESIVE PERICARDITIS

Ivo Cikes

Institute of Cardiovascular Diseases, School of Medicine, University of Zagreb, Zagreb, Yugoslavia

The value of M-mode echocardiography in the diagnosis of pericardial effusion is widely recognised (1,2,3,4). It is the most reliable, safest and simplest method currently available in the diagnosis of pericardial effusion. However, its role in the diagnosis of fibrinous pericarditis is still limited. The variety of described echocardiographic signs are not specific (5,6,7). There are only a few articles in literature on the role of two-dimensional echocardiography in the diagnosis of pericardial disease (8,9). To the best of our knowledge pericardial and pleuropericardial adhesions have not previously been described by echocardiography. These structures could not be directly visualized in vivo by other methods except during cardiac surgery, or later at autopsy.

The purpose of this study was to evaluate the role of two-dimensional echocardiography in the detection and localization of pericardial effusion in comparison with M-mode echocardiography. Following our first observation of pericardial adhesions and villous epicardial deposits in a patient with systemic lupus erythematosus in October 1978 (10), in the current study we paid special attention to the possibility of echocardiographic detection of pericardial and pleuropericardial adhesions as well as epicardial deposits in our patients with pericardial and pleural effusions.

MATERIALS AND METHODS

The study group comprised 34 patients with pericardial effusions of various etiology, ranging in age from 1 to 66 years. In 10 (29.4%) out of 34 patients a coexistent left pleural effusion was present. Diagnosis of pleural effusion was made by a standard chest X-ray examination.

M-mode echocardiograms were performed using a Smith-Kline Ekoline 20A or Irex System II ultrasonoscope and 2.25 MHz transducer focused on 7.5 cm. An approximate quanitification of pericardial effusion was done by the cubed volume method of Horowitz (4). Two-dimensional echocardiograms were obtained using a Varian V-3000 ultrasonoscope with a 2.25 MHz fixed focus transducer. Multiple long and short axis views were performed from left parasternal, apical and subxyphoid approach (11). The illustrations used in this article are Polaroid pictures of desired single frame image from video tape monitor. These images are of significantly lower quality than the display in real-time, since they consist of a single field of a two-field video frame. Thus only half of the information from the video tape is displayed by this procedure.

RESULTS

In our study group of the 34 patients with pericardial effusion by gross semiquantification we found 12 patients (35.3%) with minimal effusion, 14 (41.2%) with moderate and 8 patients (23.5%) with large pericardial effusion.

In all 34 patients pericardial effusion was identified using both one- and two-dimensional technique. Wide angle cross-sections in long and short axis from different approaches enables better visualization of pericardial space and distribution of pericardial fluid than the conventional M-mode technique. Pericardial thickness can be imaged very well in cases with coexistent pericardial and pleural effusion (Fig. 1).

In 12 patients with small pericardial effusion pericardial fluid could be easily identified behind the posterobasal left ventricular wall near the atrioventricular groove (Fig. 2).

In 14 patients with moderate pericardial effusion pericardial fluid could be seen not only posteriorly, but also around the left and right ventricles, cardiac apex as well as the anterior to the right ventricle (Fig. 3). In contrast to Martin's observation (8) of echo-free space cranial to the posterior A-V groove in all his 11 patients with moderately sized effusions, we were able to notice such a finding in only 3 of our patients with moderate effusions.

In 8 patients with large effusion more fluid was present around the right and left ventricle permitting the heart to move freely within the pericardial sac (swinging heart); the heart floated in the pericardial fluid. In 5 patients the phenomenon of invagination of anterior right ventricular wall was present. In 1 patient this phenomenon was very striking at the right atrial wall (Fig. 4). In 3 patients with cardiac tamponade reciprocal changes in ventricular diameters were seen: during inspiration the left ventricle diminishes, while the right ventricle increases in size.

We were unable to observe pericardial and pleuropericardial adhesions by one-dimensional echocardiography in any patient from our study group. Using the two-dimensional technique pericardial or pleuropericardial adhesions were found in 4 (11.8%) out of 34 patients with pericardial effusion. The first 2 patients had pericardial adhesions, while the other 2 had pleuropericardial adhesions.

Case 1

A 15-year-old girl with systemic lupus erythematosus

was admitted to the hospital, because of cardiomegaly and pericardial rub with signs of inflow obstruction. M-mode echocardiography revealed large pericardial effusion. Nothing striking was observed on either the epicardium or pericardium or in the pleural fluid. By two-dimensional technique, in a four-chamber view, we first noticed a small strand on the epicardial surface of the left ventricular posterior wall floating in pericardial fluid (Fig. 5). On the short axis section at the level near the cardiac apex we could clearly see the adhesive strand in the large pericardial effusion extending from the epicardium to the pericardium, which moved chaotically during the cardiac cycle (Fig. 6). In diastole the strand was shaky, while in the systole it was tight. In Figure 7 obtained in a section along the short axis of the heart at the level of the papillary muscles, a change in the appearance of the left ventricular epicardium during the systole and diastole can be seen. During the systole epicardial deposits made the epicardial surface more villous (which we called 'hairly epicardium'), while during the diastole epicardium was less irregular. In the real-time image these shaggy epicardial deposits vibrated impressively in the pericardial fluid. In the same sections we were able to image very thick lumpy deposit also moving chaotically in the pericardial fluid (Fig. 8).

By pericardiocenthesis 600 ccm of fluid was obtained and the pericardial rub immediately disappeared. With the appropriate treatment of corticosteroids and azathioprine, the pericardial effusion did not reappear and signs of pericardial constriction did not develop in the follow-up year.

Case 2

A 9-year-old boy was sent for echocardiographic examination on suspicion of pericardial effusion in the course of autoimmune thyroid disease. M-mode echocardiography revealed the common feature of a large pericardial effusion. In the long axis view on two-dimensional echocardiography around the cardiac apex numeroud tiny strands fluttering in the pericardial fluid were observed (Fig. 9).

Case 3

A 53-year-old man was implanted with an artificial valve in the mitral position. Two weeks later he developed pericardial rub with pleural effusion on X-ray examination. Two-dimensional echocardiography revealed a small pericardial effusion and a large pleural effusion. The pericardium was clearly seen between them separating these two effusions (Fig. 10). In this patient we were able to visualize two pleuropericardial adhesions. Because of the tightening of the pericardium by adhesive strands in systole the small pericardial effusion became a little enlarged. Four weeks later both the pericardial and pleural effusion had disappeared as well as the pericardial rub.

Case 4

A 14-year-old boy with Marfanoid habitus was treated for streptococcal pleuropneumonia with a large pleural effusion. X-ray showed a left pleural effusion spreading up to the clavicula with the mediastinum shifted to the right side. By two-dimensional echocardiography with transducer placed in the second left intercostal space in midclavicular line the pleuropericardial adhesion was imaged extending from the cardiac surface up to the pleura (Fig. 11). After the removal of 1700 ccm of pleural fluid by pleural puncture and 3 weeks of appropriate antibiotic therapy the patient recovered.

In the present study we found the subxyphoid approach very useful with regard to deciding on therapeutic or diagnostic pericardiocenthesis, because the width of echo-free space between the diaphragm and the right ventricle is crucial for safe pericardiocenthesis.

DISCUSSION

Echocardiography is the best available method for detection of pericardial effusion, but it is still of limited value in the diagnosis of fibrinous pericarditis. The majority of articles published on echocardiographic diagnosis of pericarditis are based on the results of M-mode echocardiography, while only a few consider the role of two-dimensional echocardiography in pericardial disease.

Recently, Martin and associates reported on the role of two-dimensional echocardiography in the localization of pericardial effusion (8). Matsuo and co-workers described the rotational excursion of the heart in massive pericardial effusion (9).

With regard to the localization of pericardial effusion with two-dimensional echocardiography, our observation was similar to that of Martin and co-workers (8). Wide-angle cross-sections in long and short axis from different approached provide better visualization of pericardial space and distribution of pericardial fluid than the conventional M-mode technique. By two-dimensional echocardiography we could readily detect pericardial effusion in all our 34 patients even in cases with very small effusions diagnosed previously by M-mode technique. In cases with co-existent pericardial and pleural effusions pericardial thickness could be easily measured. In small pericardial effusions pericardial fluid was localized behind the posterobasal left ventricular wall. In moderate effusions more even distribution of fluid was found. In large effusions the heart floated in profuse pericardial fluid, moving freely in the pericardial sac. This type of motion abnormality was initially described using M-mode technique (3) and is known as swinging heart syndrome. The phenomenon of invagination of the anterior right ventricular wall could be seen in large pericardial effusion as well. In one case

with large effusion marked invagination was noticed on the
right atrial wall (Fig. 4).

Subxyphoid approach gives unique anatomic data for
safe pericardiocenthesis: the width of the echo-free space
between the diaphragm and right ventricle can be imaged,
which is essential in deciding on therapeutic or diagnostic
pericardiocenthesis.

Besides better visualization and localization of pericardial fluid two-dimensional echocardiography provides
direct observation of pericardial and pleuropericardial adhesions as well as epicardial shaggy or lumpy fibrinous deposits, which is not possible by any other method in vivo.
Using one-dimensional echocardiography these structures
could not be seen. To our knowledge pericardial and pleuropericardial adhesions have not previously been described by
echocardiography.

In the first patient with systemic lupus erythematosus
we heard the pericardial rub which is rather unusual in
large pericardial effusions. As soon as pericardiocenthesis
was carried out, the rub disappeared. Listening to the rub
during the real-time display, we observed that the pericardial rub occurred simultaneously with systolic stretching
and tightening of the pericardial adhesions and their cha-
otic movement. We could assume, therefore, that these movements are the cause of the pericardial rub in large effusion and not the friction between the epicardium and pericardium or some extrapericardial origin as previously supposed (12).

It is obvious that echocardiographic findings of fibrinous epicardial deposits and pericardial adhesions suggests that the natural course of pericarditis could progress
toward a constriction. Therefore early echocardiographic
finding of these structures is of clinical importance, since
it should indicate more active therapy to avoid the development of a constriction. With further experience in echocardiographic detection of pericardial adhesions and epicardial deposits, the specificity and sensitivity of these
findings remains to be confirmed.

REFERENCES

1. Edler, I. (1955): Acta Med. Scand., 152 (Suppl. 308),
   32.
2. Feigenbaum, H., Waldhausen, J.A. and Hyde, L.P. (1965):
   J. Amer. Med. Ass., 191, 711.
3. Feigenbaum, H., Zaky, A. and Grabhorn, L.L. (1966): Circulation, 34, 611.
4. Horowitz, M.S., Schultz, C.S., Stinson, E.B., Harrison,
   D.C. and Popp, R.L. (1974): Circulation, 50, 239.
5. Feigenbaum, H. (1976): Echocardiography, 2nd Ed., Lea
   and Febiger, Philadelphia, PA.
6. Chandraratna, P.A.N. and Imaizumi, T. (1978): Cardiovasc.
   Med., 3, 1279.
7. Horowitz, M.S., Rossen, R. and Harrison, D.C. (1979):
   Amer. Heart J., 97, 420.

8. Martin, R.P., Rakowski, H., French, J. and Popp, R.L. (1978): Amer. J. Cardiol., 42, 904.
9. Matsuo, H., Matsumoto, M., Hamanaka, Y., Ohara, T., Shohichi, S., Michitoshi, I. and Abe, H. (1979): Brit. Heart J., 41, 513.
10. Cikes, I., Cikes, N. and Pustisek, S. (1979): Zbornik radova sastanka kardioloskih sekcija SLD i ZLH, in press.
11. Tajik, A.J., Seward, J.B., Hagler, D.J., Mair, D.D. and Lie, J.T. (1978): Mayo Clin. Proc., 53, 271.
12. Spodick, D.H. (1971): Amer. Heart J., 81, 114.

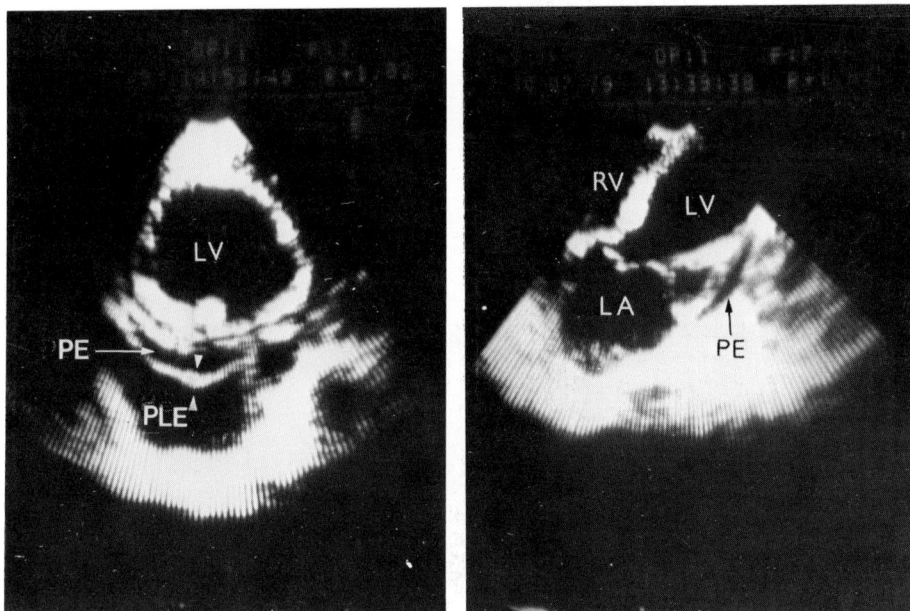

Fig. 1. Two-dimensional echocardiogram in the short-axis view from a patient with coexistent pericardial (PE) and pleural (PLE) effusions. The thickened pericardium (between two arrows) lying between the pericardial and pleural effusion is well seen. LV = left ventricle.

Fig. 2. Two-dimensional echocardiogram in apical view showing the small pericardial effusion (PE) behind the postero-basal left ventricular wall. LV = left ventricle; RV = right ventricle; LA = left atrium.

311

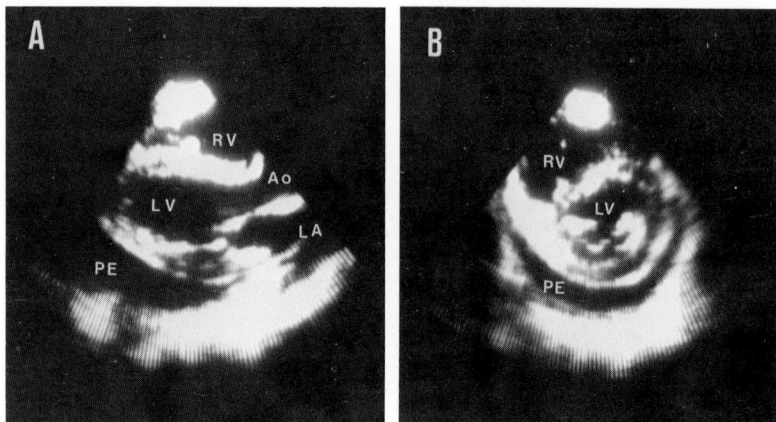

Fig. 3. Two-dimensional echocardiogram in long- (panel A) and short-axis (panel B) views from a patient with moderate pericardial effusion. Besides posteriorly, the effusion is seen toward the cardiac apex (panel A) and around the left and right ventricles (panel B). LV = left ventricle; RV = right ventricle; Ao = aorta; LA = left atrium; PE = pericardial effusion.

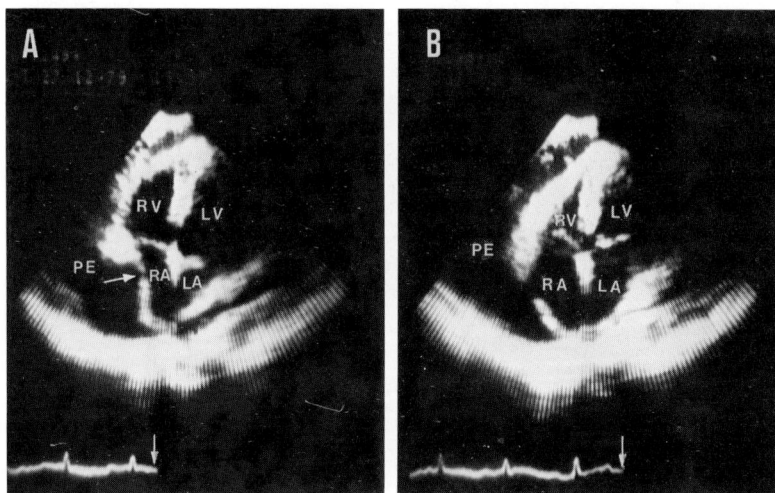

Fig. 4. Two-dimensional echocardiogram from a patient with the large pericardial effusion (PE) showing the phenomenon of invagination of the right atrial wall (arrow) in systole (panel A). The right atrial cavity (RA) is compressed with invaginating right atrial wall in systole, while in diastole (panel B) it shows normal configuration. LV = left ventricle; RV = right ventricle; LA = left atrium; RA = right atrium; PE = pericardial effusion.

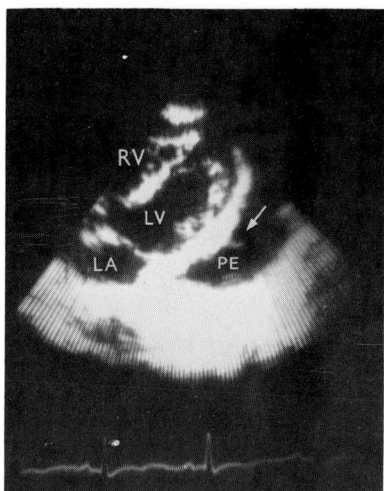

Fig. 5. Four-chamber view from patient 1 showing small strand (arrow) on epicardial surface of the left ventricular posterior wall. During the real-time imaging the strand vibrated in pericardial fluid. LV = left ventricle; RV = right ventricle; LA = left atrium; PE = pericardial effusion.

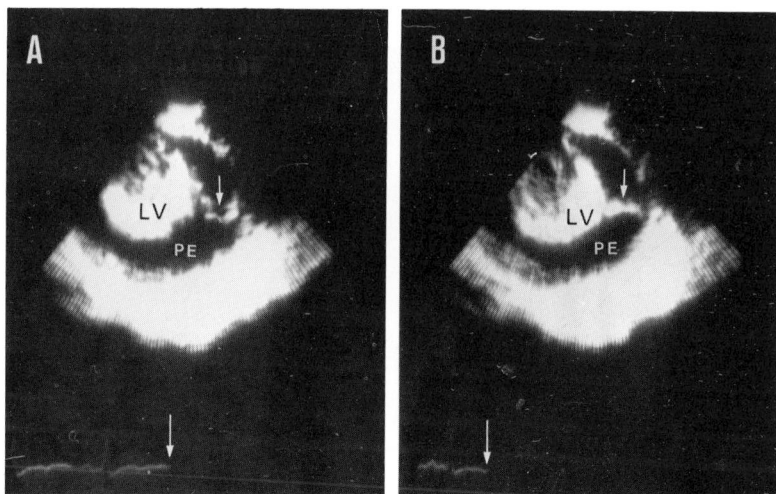

Fig. 6. Short-axis section at the level near the cardiac apex from patient 1. In the profuse pericardial effusion (PE), the large adhesive strand (arrow) extending from epicardium to pericardium can be clearly seen. During the diastole (panel A) the strand is shaky, while in systole (panel B) it is tight. LV = left ventricle.

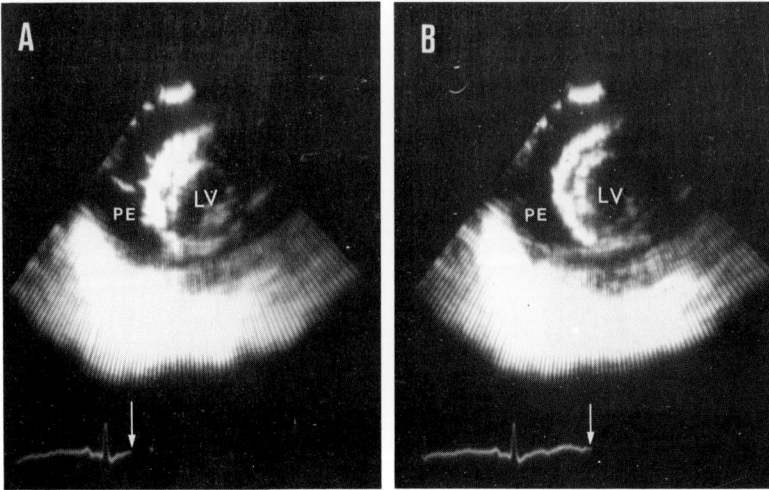

Fig. 7. Short-axis section at the level of the papillary muscles from patient 1 showing a change in the appearance of epicardial deposits during the systole (panel A) and diastole (panel B). During the systole epicardial deposits made the epicardial surface more villous, shaggy; in diastolic frame the epicardium is less irregular. During the real-time imaging shaggy epicardial deposits vibrate in pericardial fluid. LV = left ventricle; PE = pericardial effusion.

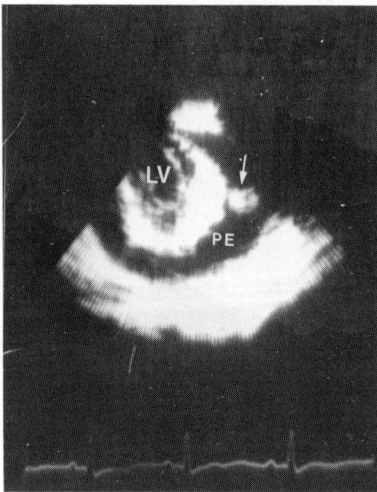

Fig. 8. Short-axis section at the level of the papillary muscles from patient 1 showing thick, lumpy epicardial deposits (arrow). LV = left ventricle; PE = pericardial effusion.

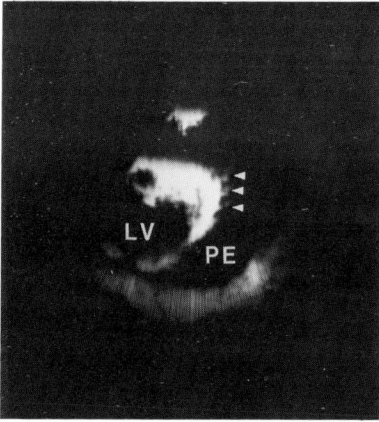

Fig. 9. Two-dimensional echocardiogram in the long-axis view from patient 2 showing tiny strands (arrows) around the cardiac apex fluttering in the pericardial fluid. LV = left ventricle; PE = pericardial effusion.

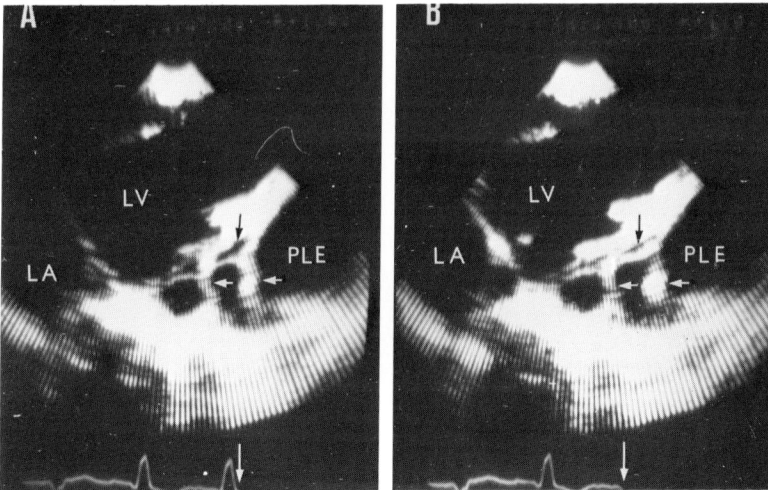

Fig. 10. Two-dimensional echocardiogram from patient 3 with small pericardial effusion (black arrow) and large pleural effusion (PLE). Two white arrows point at two pleuropericardial adhesions. During the systole (panel A) the small pericardial effusion becomes little enlarged due to the tightening of the pericardium by adhesive strans. LV = left ventricle; LA = left atrium.

315

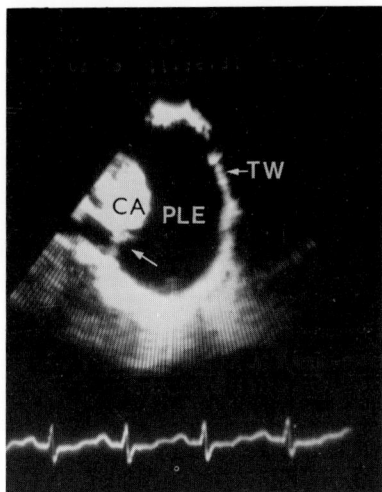

Fig. 11. Two-dimensional echocardiogram from patient 4 with large pleural effusion (PLE) performed with transducer placed in the second left intercostal space in midclavicular line. The pleuropericardial adhesion (arrow) extends from the cardiac surface up to the pleura. TW = thoracic wall; CA = cardiac apex.

CROSS-SECTIONAL ECHOCARDIOGRAPHY AND PROGRESSIVE
CONSTRICTIVE PERICARDITIS

Sonia Chang and John K. Chang

Echocardiography Laboratory, Medical College of Ohio, Toledo
and Echocardiography Laboratory, Riverside Hospital, Toledo
Ohio, USA

In the presence of clinical constrictive pericarditis,
M-mode echocardiography is primarily used for detection of
pericardial effusion and pericardial thickening. The value
of abnormal wall motion or quality of systolic function is
often minimized by associated disease. We arc presenting
a patient with constrictive pericarditis in whom pericardial
thickening and quantity of effusion on the M-mode echocardiogram stabilized early in the disease process. Cross-
sectional echocardiography was more definitive of an active
adhesive pericarditis which finally required surgical intervention.

A 58 year old, white male was known to have chronic
renal failure, amyloidosis, systemic hyerptension and severe
anemia for the past three years. He was on chronic hemodia-
lysis with a Scribner shunt in the left wrist since November
of 1978. Regular blood transfusions were required.

In late February of 1979, an A-V fistula was established
between the radial artery and cephalic vein at the level of
the left wrist. A week later, the patient complained of bilateral chest pain, fever and chills during dialysis. The
symptoms receded during several days of observation. An
echocardiogram revealed a large pericardial effusion for the
first time (Figure 1). Epicardial thickening was suspected
based upon the unusual echo-reflective qualities of this
structure even at low levels of signal amplification. Cross--
section echocardiography showed a large quantity of pericar--
dial effusion with adhesive strands connecting the lateral
left ventricular epicardium to the partial pericardium
(Figure 2).

In late March, the patient was admitted to the hospital
for persistent fever and hypotension during dialysis. A paradoxical pulse of 16 mm Hg was present. Constrictive pericarditis was confirmed by cardiac catheterization. All
right heart diastolic pressures were elevated and equalized
at 20 mm Hg. A paradoxical pulse of 35 mm Hg was present.
Two hundred and fifty milliliters of sanguinous, nonclotting
fluid was obtained by pericardiocentesis with relief of symptoms.

Over the next two weeks, the patient again became hypotensive each time he was dialyzed, requiring dopamine and
blood transfusions to maintain pressure. The quantity of

pericardial effusion and pericardial thickening had stabilized and was unchanging on serial M-mode echocardiograms (Figure 3). However, serial cross-sectional echocardiograms demonstrated increasing numbers of adhesive strands emanating from the lateral left ventricular epicardium. The surface of the epicardium became progressively more lumpy and irregular (Figures 4,5).

At surgery, the partial pericardium was thickened and adherent to underlying structures, enclosing a large quantity of sanguinous fluid. The surface of the heart was cleaned of grumous material disclosing a very thick, tough epicardium which was also removed. The patient subsequently recovered and no longer has hypotensive episodes during dialysis.

CONCLUSIONS

Cross-sectional echocardiography allowed visual quantification and localization of increasing adhesion and lumpy deposits on the epicardial surface indicating an active disease process undetected by M-mode echocardiography. While identification of adhesive strands and pericardial effusion does not necessarily indicate constriction, their presence may indicate the potential for effusive-constrictive physiology.

ACKNOWLEDGEMENTS

We wish to thank Mrs. Julie Arthur, echocardiographer; Richard Leighton, M.D., cardiologist; and Terrance Davis, M.D., surgeon, for their definitive diagnosis and treatment of this patient.

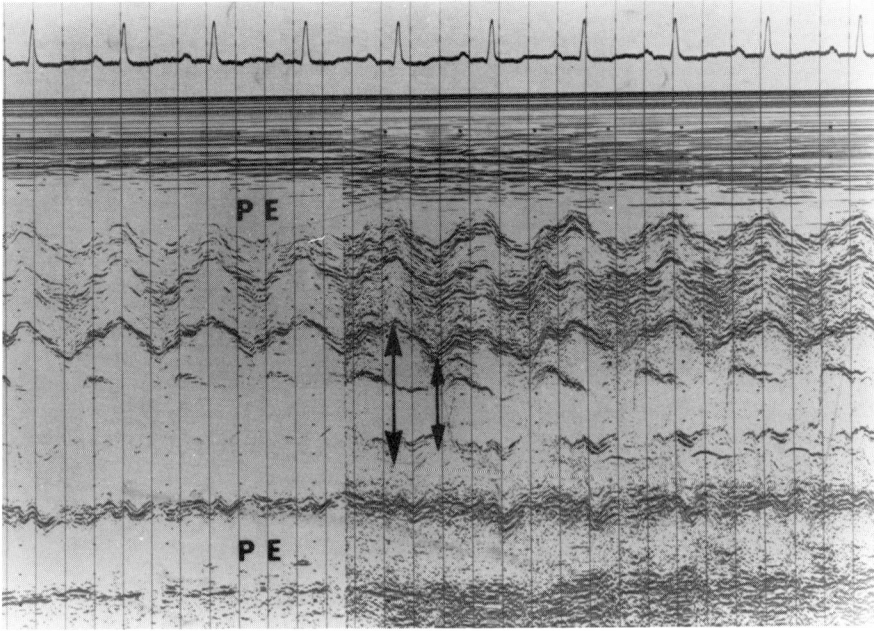

Fig. 1. M-mode echocardiogram from 58 year old male with chronic renal failure, amyloidosis, hypertension and severe anemia. Tracing exhibits large pericardial effusion (PE) anterior and posterior to heart. An unusual quantity of echoes are reflected from epicardial surface suggesting thickening of this structure. Arrows, Diastolic and systolic left ventricular dimensions.

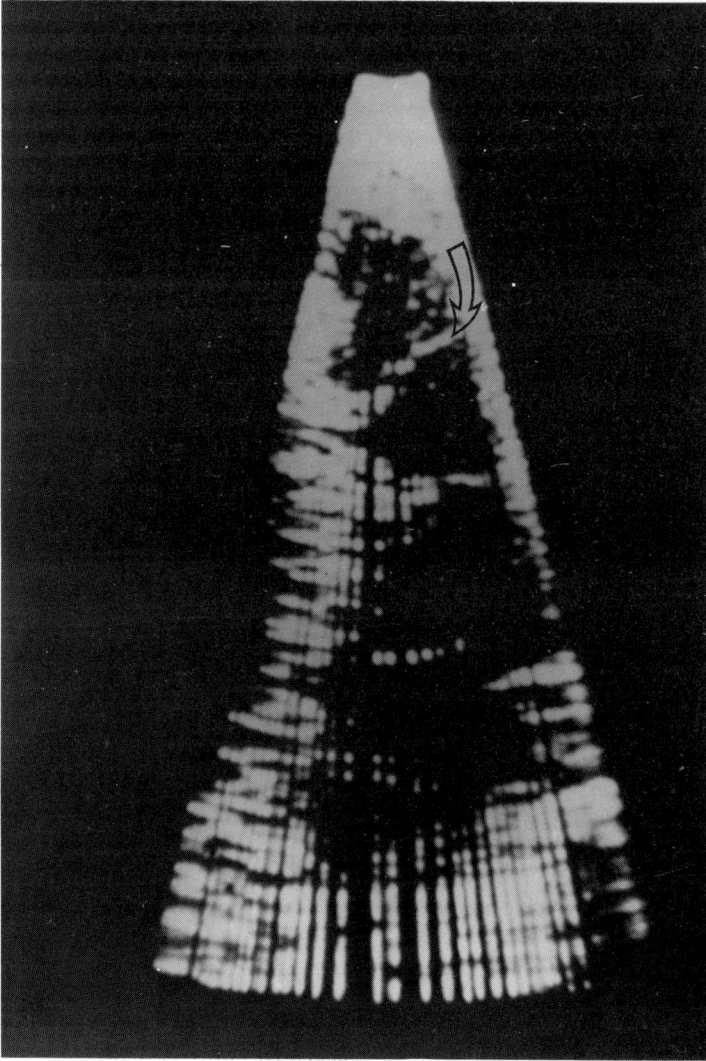

Fig. 2. 30° cross-sectional echocardiogram, apical view. Tracing presentation shows apex located anteriorly, left ventricular base located posteriorly. Adhesive strands (arrow) connect epicardial surface of left ventricular lateral wall to pericardial surface through a large quantity of pericardial effusion.

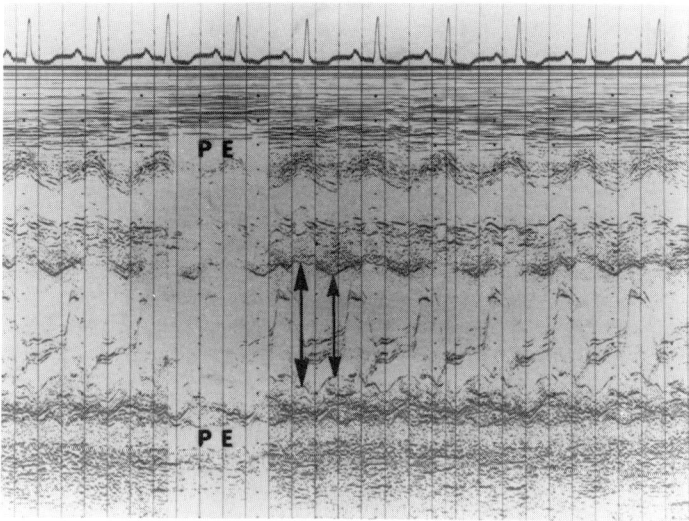

Fig. 3. Representative M-mode echocardiogram of quantity of pericardial effusion (PE) and pericardial "thickening" which was evident throughout latter phase of this patient's disease prior to surgical removal of epicardium and partial pericardium. Arrows, Diastolic and systolic dimensions of left ventricle.

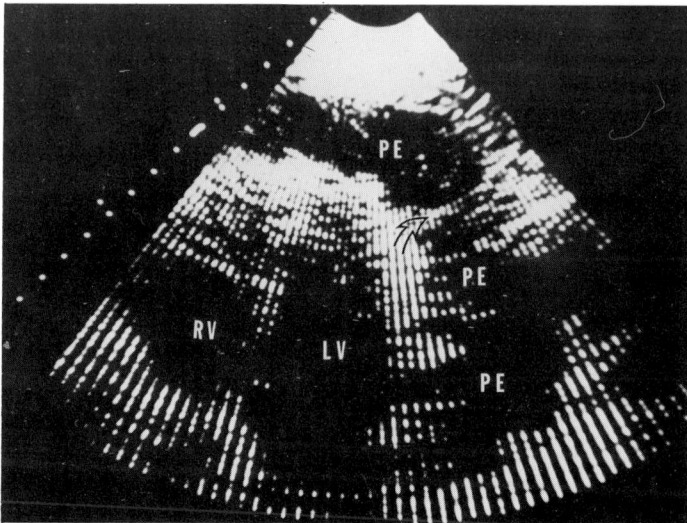

Fig. 4. 80° cross-sectional echocardiogram, apical view, shwoing large quantities of pericardial effusion (PE) with adhesive strands through effusion. Tracing presentation shows apex located anteriorly with adhesive strands emanating from lateral wall of left ventricle (arrow). RV, right ventricle; LV, left ventricle.

321

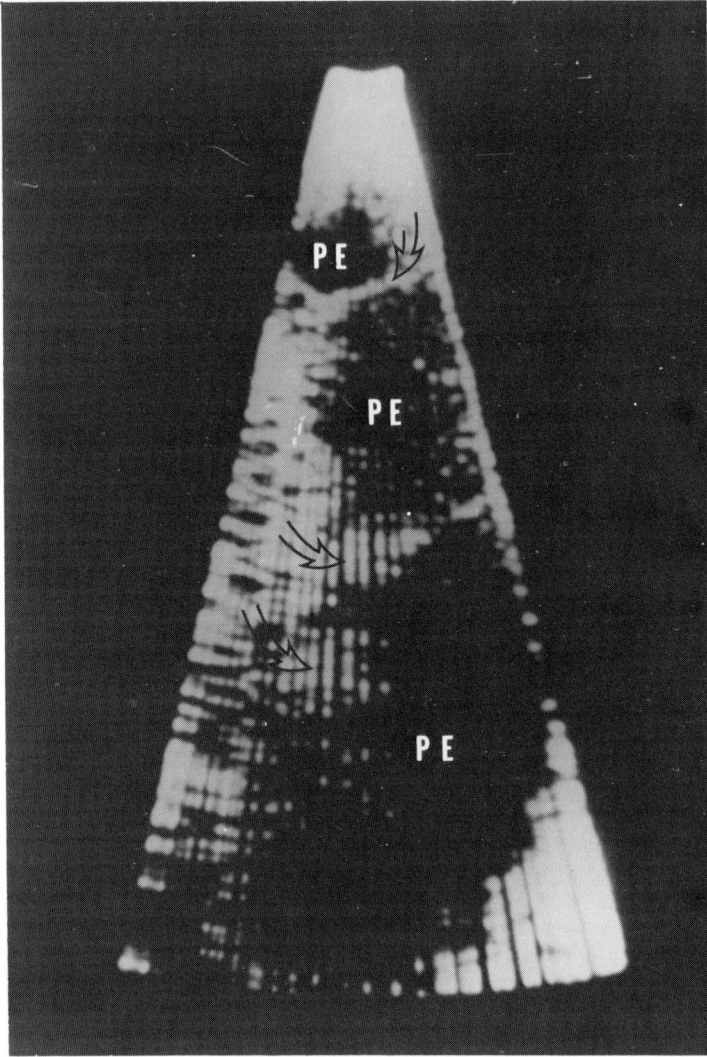

Fig. 5. 30° cross-sectional echocardiogram of lateral left ventricular wall. Improved signal resolution shows strong adhesions (arrows) between epicardium and partial pericardium. Lateral left ventricular wall's surface is irregular and lumpy, unlike smooth contour seen in earlier stages of disease (Figure 2). PE, Pericardial effusion.

EVALUATION OF TRICUSPID REGURGITATION BY CONTRAST ECHOCARDIOGRAPHY. COMPARATIVE ONE- AND TWO-DIMENSIONAL STUDY

M. Klicpera, J. Mlczoch, J. Kaliman, M. Weissel, F. Kaindl

Department of Cardiology, University of Vienna, Vienna Austria

Tricuspid regurgitation as an isolated primary valve disorder is rather a rare condition but usually does not create diagnostic difficulties. In the majority of cases, however, tricuspid regurgitation is due to changes in the right ventricular architecture and tricuspid valve complex secondary to volume or pressure overload of the right ventricle. It so represents a frequent finding in various forms of heart disease such as shunt lesions, congestive cardiomyopathy or severe mitral valve disease.

The presence of hemodynamically significant tricuspid regurgitation is usually recognized on the basis of clinical findings. But moreoften the detection utilizes time-honored assessment and even then the clinical findings might be inconclusive.

Lieppe et al. have first shown the possibilities of contrastechocardiography in detecting tricuspid incompetence (1). Using a two-dimensional device they discussed the method as being specific and sensitive by direct visualization of valve incompetence with back and forward movement of microcavitations across the tricuspid valve and by systolic appearance of bubbles in the interior vena cava. Further reports demonstrated the usefulness of the M-mode technique in observing the inferior vena cava (2-4). The purpose of our study was threefold:
a) to prove the specificity and sensitivity of contrastechocardiography in evaluating tricuspid regurgitation by correlating the echoresults with those of other invasive and noninvasive techniques; b) to compare the diagnostic power of contrast echocardiography in evaluating the tricuspid valve and the inferior vena cava;and c) to assess the sensitivity of conventional M-mode studies in the inferior vena cava approach compared to the two-dimensional technique.

METHODS

A total number of 41 persons were included into the study, assigned to three groups (table 1) in reference to Lieppe et al.(1). Group I and II consisted of 31 consecutive patients with either clinical signs diagnostic for tricuspid regurgitation (group I with 13 pts.) or findings suggestive of tricuspid regurgitation (group II with 18 pts). Group III included control patients, 4 normal persons and 6 patients with atypical chest pain and no evidence of heart disease.

The echocardiographic findings were correlated with rheographic tracings and right atrial pressure curves in all group Group I and II patients. The control patients have been referred to an echocardiographic and rheographic study only. All examinations were performed within five days of each other.

The echocardiographic studies were performed with a commercially available M-mode ultrasonoscope and a dynamically focussed phased array sector-scanner. Two dimensional recordings from the tricuspid valve were obtained from various cross-sectional planes including the long axis view of the right ventricle, a short axis view in the plane of the great vessels and an apical four chamber view (Fig.1). The inferior vena cava was examined from subxyphoid in cross-section and with the M-mode technique (Fig.2/A+B,3/A).

Echocardiographic contrast was produced by rapid injection of normal saline into a peripheral vein (5,6). With repeated injections images from the right heart with the tricuspid valve and the plane of the inferior vena cava were obtained and reviewed with regard to the systolic appearance of microcavitations in the inferior vena cava(Fig.

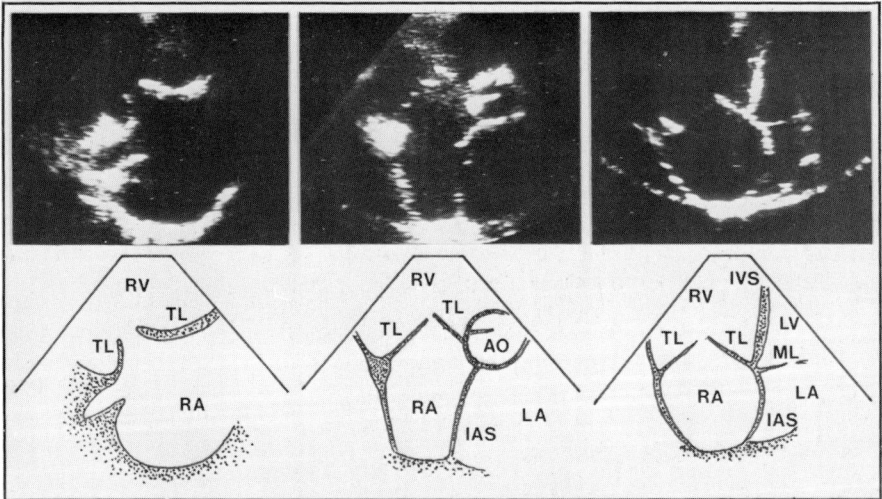

Fig. 1. Cross-sectional planes for examination of the tricuspid valve. For details, see text. RA=right atrium; RV= right ventricle; LA=left atrium; LV=left ventricle; IVS= interventricular septum; IAS=interatrial septum; AO=aorta with the aortic valve; TL=tricuspid leaflet; ML= mitral leaflet.

2/C+D, 3/B+C) and back and forth movement across the tricuspid valve. The study was done in a certain sequence with
the 2-D tricuspid valve approach at the beginning, followed
by the M-mode recording of the inferior vena cava before the
2-D echocardiogram was performed in this cross-section.

The rheographic examination was performed as impedance
plethysmography with leads on both arms and interpreted with
reference to the observation of a regurgitant wave, which
has been considered diagnostic for tricuspid regurgitation
(fig. 4)(7).

The pressure in the right atrium was measured with a
flow directed catheter. In recording care was taken for a
rapid withdrawal into the right atrium after registration
of the pulmonary artery and right ventricular pressure. The
atrial pressure curve has been considered positive, if a
prominent and early starting v-wave was found, which tended
to obliterate the x-descent and terminated in a steep de-
scent (fig.5) (8,9).

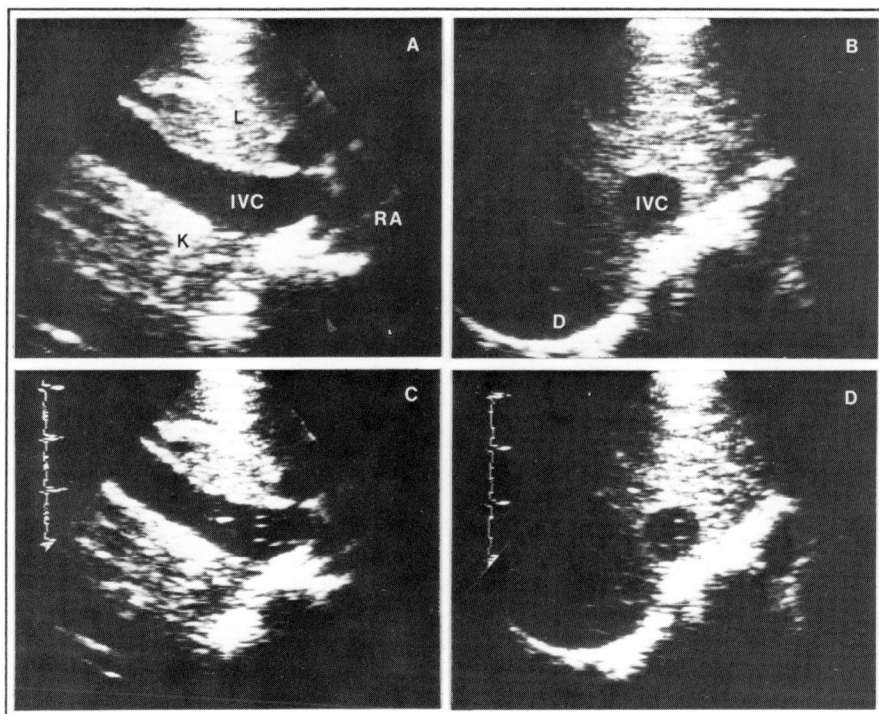

Fig. 2. Cross-sectional images of the inferior vena cava in
long axis (panel A and C) and short axis (panel B and D).
Systolic appearance of microcavitations in the inferior vena
cava in patients with tricuspid regurgitation(panel C and
D). IVS=inferior vena cava; K=kidney; L=liver; D=diaphragm.

RESULTS

Comparing the three techniques used in evaluating the group I and II patients, the echocardiographic contrast-study has shown the most positive results compared to the rheographic study and right atrial pressure tracing (table 2). In all group I patients the echo-study was positive, while negative in all control patients. All group I patients had further also a positive right atrial pressure tracing and only one had a negative impedance plethysmography. In group II 14/18 pts. showed positive echo-studies, but there were significantly less positives with rheography or right atrial pressure tracing.

PATIENTS

GROUP	N	DISEASE	HOLOSYSTOLIC MURMUR	TR-MURMUR	HEPATOMEGALY	PULSATILE LIVER	POS.JVP
I	13	8 MV 5 CCM	13/13	10/13	11/13	11/13	13/13
II	18	9 MV 6 CCM 2 PH 1 EBSTEIN	12/18	0/18	10/18	0/18	0/18
III	10	4 NP 6 ATYP.PAIN	0/10	0/10	0/10	0/10	0/10

TABLE 1. Patients
Abbreviations:TR-MURMUR=murmur typical of tricuspid regurgitation, JVP=jugular venous pulse,MV=mitral valve disease, CCM=congestive cardiomyopathy, PH=pulmonary hypertension, NP=normal person

POSITIVE RESULTS (IN %)

	GROUP I	GROUP II	GROUP I+II
ECHO	13/13 (100)	14/18 (78)	27/31 (87)
RHEO	12/13 (92)	11/18 (61)	23/31 (74)
RA	13/13 (100)	8/18 (44)	21/31 (68)

TABLE 2. Positive results
Abbreviations: ECHO=contrast echocardiography, RHEO=rheography, RA=right atrial pressure contour

326

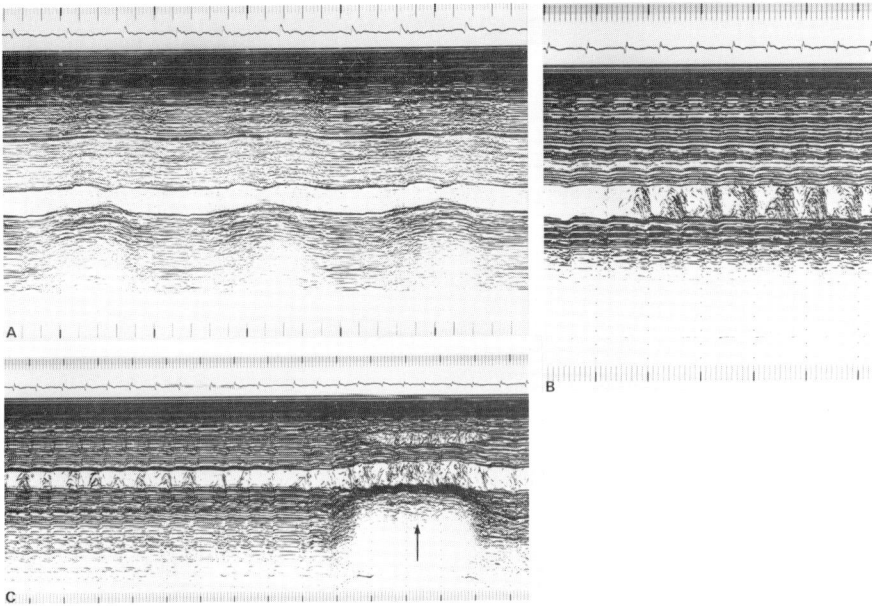

Fig. 3. M-mode recording of the inferior vena cava. Note the partial collapse during inspiration (A) and the systolic appearance of microcavitations indicating tricuspid insufficiency (B) with increase in density during deep inspiration (C) (17).

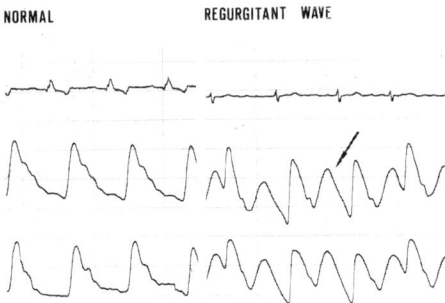

Fig. 4. Impedance plethysmography in a normal person and in a patient with tricuspid regurgitation. The arror indicates the regurgitant wave following the arterial pulse wave.

Comparing the results of all three techniques with each other the echocardiographic study has shown good conformity with each of both other methods, which was much better than the conformity between rheography and right atrial pressure contour (fig.6). This can also be appreciated in the graphic illustration in the bottom of the figure with a special marked sector for the non-corresponding patients and best correlation between echo- and rheography.

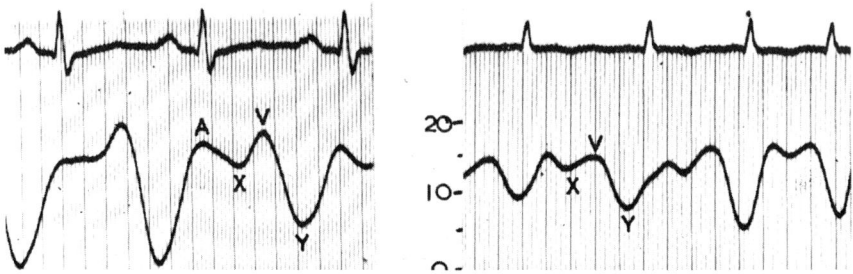

Fig. 5 An example of the right atrial pressure contour considered diagnostic for tricuspid regurgitation in a patient with sinus rhythm (A) and atrial fibrillation (B). For details, see text.

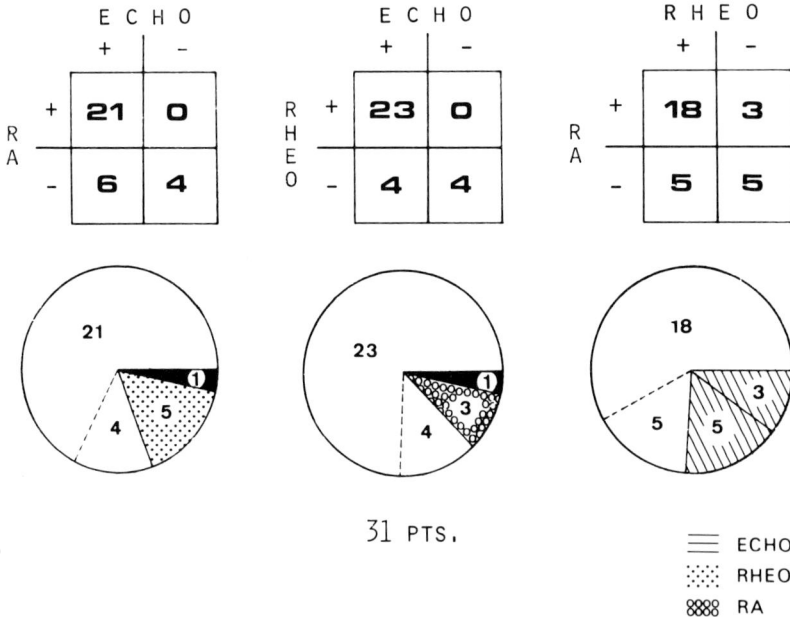

31 PTS.

Fig. 6. Comparison of the three different methods used: (A) 2-2 contingency tables, (B) graphic illustration of corresponding and non-corresponding results. For detail, see text.

5/6 patients with positive echocardiogram but negative right
atrial pressure contour had positive rheographic findings,
only one showed a negative result here too. 3/4 patients
with negative rheography but positive contrast echocardiogram had positive right atrial pressure tracing (only one
patient was negative) and finally of the 8 patients, in
whom we could not achieve a conformity between rheography
and right atrial pressure tracing (but who had one positive
examination), all had a positive echo study.

Figure 7 illustrates the correlation of all three techniques simultaneously. Two facts should be pointed out:
a) no patient with negative echocardiogram had a positive
study with one of the other techniques and b) there was only one patient with a positive echocardiogram without a second positive result.

Comparing the diagnostic power of the tricuspid valve
approach with the examination of the inferior vena cava
(table 3), we found a distinct predominance of positive results observing the inferior vena cava (IVC). Registrating
the tricuspid valve(TV) we could not achieve positive results in more than 56% of the positive IVC-studies (15/27).
There was a predominance of positives in the group I patients
with 11/13 compared to 4/14 in group II.

Table 4 illustrates the sensitivity of the M-mode recording of the inferior vena cava compared to the two-dimensional exploration. As noted before the echo-study was performed with the M-mode recording and interpretation before
the inferior vena cava was studied two-dimensionally. The
sensitivity of contrast M-mode echocardiography thereby was
92% for group I (12/13 positives with just one patient missed)
and 79% for group II (11/14 pts) with an overall sensitivity
of 85%.

ECHO

		RA +	RA −	RA +	RA −
RHEO +		18	5	0	0
RHEO −		3	1	0	4

Fig. 7. 2-4 contingency table. For detail,see text.

DISCUSSION

Clinical evaluation of tricuspid regurgitation has long been attempted on the basis of physical findings, right a- trial or jugular venous pressure levels and contours. The presence of physical signs however usually reflects gross regurgitation, while with trivial or moderate tricuspid re- gurgitation sensitive methods of detection and confirmation are necessary (11). Contrast echocardiography has been po- stulated as a new promising technique. In the initial re- port, Lieppe et al. showed a high specificity and sensitivity by correlating their echocardiographic results with physical findings and right ventricular angiography(1). Two positive contrast studies in patients with negative right ventricular angiography were a surprising finding in this report, since angiography has been considered to be a sensitive means of proving the absence of significant tricuspid incompetence (9). This stresses the problem of lacking a reliable stand- ard of reference to prove the sensitivity of a new technique (10). With this fact in mind we correlated our findings with rheographic studies and right atrial pressure curves, thereby postulating that the appearance of a regurgitant wave (in absence of constriction pattern) and the criteria we required for a positive pressure contour were diagnostic for tricuspid regurgitation.

There was only one patient in our series who showed no regurgitant wave and had a negative pressure pattern despite a positive contrast echocardiogram. All other patients with positive echo studies had at least a second positive test with one of the other techniques. This and the fact, that all group I patients had positive and all controls negative echo studies supports the results of Lieppe et al., that contrast echocardiography is indeed a specific and sensitive

POSITIVE RESULTS (TV/IVC)

	GROUP I	GROUP II	GROUP I+II
TV	11 (85%)	4 (29%)	15 (56%)
IVC	13	14	27

TABLE 3. Postive echo results obtained with the tricuspid valve approach (TV) and inferior vena cava approach (IVC).

method in evaluation of tricuspid regurgitation.

Muller and shillingford studied the direction of right atrial and caval blood flow using calibrated differential pressure records (12). In normal subjects the forward blood flow reached its maximum in midventricular systole, stopped at endsystole, restarted to a lesser degree in early systole when there was a small backward flow. This normal flow pattern was greatly modified in patients with tricuspid regurgitation, since forward blood flow decreased during ventricular systole and was replaced by a reversed flow.

Identical results have been gained with catheter velocitimeters (13), catheter mounted (14) and external directional Doppler system (15).

M-mode recording of the inferior vena cava allows exact timing of the appearance of microcavitations in relation to the cardiac cycle by easy correlation to the electrocardiogram (4). This certainly makes it superior to the two-dimensional approach as far as timing is concerned. The importance of this ability can be demonstrated in patients with constrictive pericarditis or huge pericardial effusion with appearance of microcavitations in the inferior vena cava during atrial systole (fig.8). This way M-mode helps to avoid false positives, which could occur with hasty interpretation of a two-dimensional study with slow speed recording of the electrocardiogram.

Two-dimensional approach on the other hand does have an advantage as far as spatial orientation is concerned. The simultaneous visualization of the right atrium and vena cava with its entrance into the atrial cavity allows demonstration of even mild regurgitation with slight reflux of microcavitations into the caval vein. Furthermore patients with right heart failure and high venous pressure with tense vena cava show attenuation or absence of inspiratory collapse of the inferior vena cava (16) such lacking a help in differentiating the vena cava from the abdominal aorta in the M-mode recording. The lack on spatial orientation might be compensated in part by continuous sweeping the transducer toward the right atrium with demonstration of direct contin-

POSITIVE RESULTS (M-MODE/2-D)

	GROUP I	GROUP II	GROUP I+II
M-MODE	12 (92%)	11 (79%)	23 (85%)
2-D	13	14	27

TABLE 4. Positive echo results obtained by observing the inferior vena cava.

uity between the right atrial wall and right atrial cavity
and the caval tube (fig.9 and 10). Despite all limiting
factors M-mode echocardiography provided an acceptable high
sensitivity of 85% for all our patients compared to our two-
dimensional studies.

Detection of tricuspid regurgitation by observing the
systolic backward motion of microcavitations across the
atrioventricular valve is a time-consuming procedure and
seems to be less sensitive than the vena cava approach.
While in patients with significant regurgitation the systolic backward flow can be recognized with certainty in the

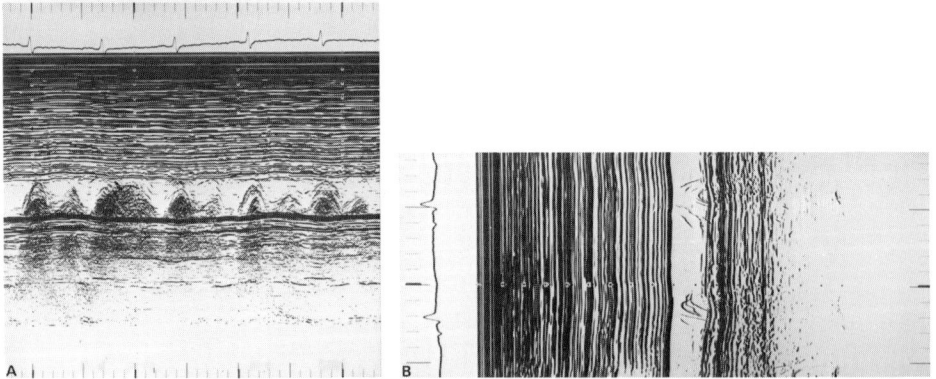

Fig. 8. Presystolic appearance of microcavitations in the
inferior vena cava in a patient with constrictive pericardi-
tis(A) and a patient with huge pericardial effusion (B).

majority of cases, reliable judgment in mild regurgitation
with conformity of more observers seems to be often impossible. Swirling of microcavitations within the right atrium
makes it quite frequently impossible to differentiate between true systolic backward flow from the right ventricle
and swirling due to atrial filling from the venous pool.

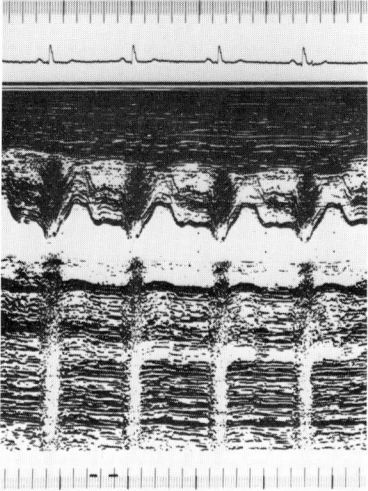

Fig. 9. M-mode recording of the right atrium. Note the typical pattern of atrial wall motion directed away from the
transducer during atrial contraction and toward the transducer during ventricular systole due to atrial filling(from
the venous pool in a normal person or due to systolic backward flow in patients with atrioventricular valve incompetence respectively).

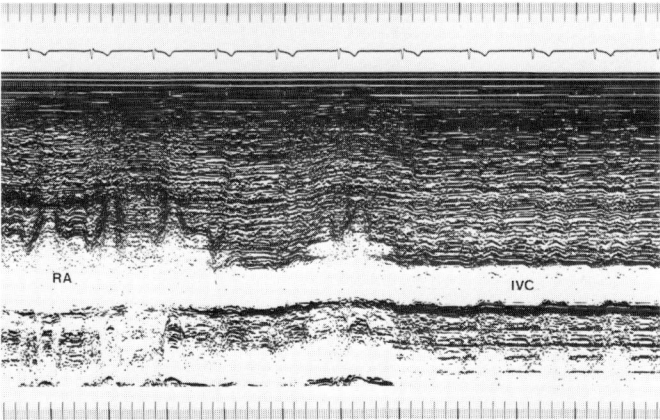

Fig. 10. Continuous sweep form the right atrium toward the
inferior vena cava. RA=right atrium; IVC=inferior vena cava.

CONCLUSIONS

Summarizing the results of the present study we suggest that in evaluation of tricuspid regurgitation (a) contrast echocardiography is a highly specific and sensitive techqniue, (b) contrast echocardiography is more sensitive than right atrial pressure contour and rheography (c), the diagnostic power of assessing the inferior vena cava is superior to the tricuspid valve approach and (d) contrast M-mode echocardiography provides and acceptable high sensitivity in analyzing the inferior vena cava compared with the two-dimensional approach.

ACKNOWLEDGMENT

The authors wish to acknowledge the technical assistance of Ms. Ingrid Teufelhart.

REFERENCES

1. Lieppe,W., Behar, V.S., Scallion, R., Kisslo, J.A. (1978): Circulation, 57:128.
2. Myers, A., Kisslo, J.A., Fraker, T.D. (1978): Proceedings of the American Institute of Ultrasound in Medicine. 1:16.
3. Klicpera, M., Mlczoch, J., Kaliman, J., Kaindl, F. (1979): Zeitschrift für Kardiologie. 68:276.
4. Kisslo, J.A. (1979): In: Echocardiology, edited by Lancée ChT., Martinus Nijhoff Publishers, bv, The Hague/Boston/London.
5. Bove, A.A., Ziskin M.C., Mulchin, W.L. (1969): Invest Radiol. 4:236.
6. Seward, J.B., Tajik, A.J., Hagler, D.J., Ritter, D.G. (1977): Am.J.Cariol. 39:202.
7. Kaindl, F., Polzer, K., Schuhfried, F. (1959): In: Rheographie, Dr.D.Steinkopff Verlag, Darmstadt.
8. Tavel, M.E. (1972): Clinical phonocardiography and external pulse recording. Ed. 2. Chicago, Year Book Medical Publishers.
9. Müller, O., and Shillingford, J. (1954): Br. Heart J 16:195.
10. Cairns, K.B., Kloster, F.E., Bristow, J.D., Lees, M.H. Griswold, H.E. (1968): Am. Heart J. 75:173.
11. Wooley, ChF. (1975): In: Physiologic principles of heart sounds and murmurs. edited by Leon D.F. and Shaver, J.A.,Am. Heart Assoc. Monograph Nr. 46, New York.
12. Müller, O., Shillingford, J.. (1955): Br. Heart J 17:163.
13. Nolan, S.P., Bottero, L.M., Inocencio,E.C., Rawitscher R.E., Lee, R.J. (1971): Circ. 43 (Suppl I). 57.
14. Benchimol, A., Barreto,E.C., Tio, S. (1970): Am. Heart J. 79:603.
15. Kalmanson, D. et al.,(1974): Bri.Heart J., 36:428.
16. Weill, F., and Maurat, P.(1974): J.Clin.U. 2:27.
17. Wexler, L. et al. (1968): Circ. Res. 23:349.

TWO-DIMENSIONAL ECHO-DOPPLER VELOCIMETRY IN MITRAL AND TRICUSPID VALVE DISEASE

Daniel Kalmanson, Colette Veryrat and Guy Abitbol

Department of Cardiology, Fondation A. de Rothschild, Paris, France

The advent of one dimensional Echo-Doppler, i.e. stand-ard echocardiography combined with pulsed Doppler has open-ed an entirely new field of noninvasive investigation of blood flow within the heart and large vessels, leading to noninjurious methods for diagnosing and evaluating cardiac disease. In particular, the combination of an analog read-out to such a technique has made feasible the recording of blood flow velocity patterns and has turned out to be an ex-tremely useful tool for diagnosing and assessing the sever-ity of valvular lesions (1,5,7,9,11,12).
  Practical though it may be, such a technique is however limited by the lack of accuracy in localizing spatially the recorded blood sample with respect to the cardiac or vessel wall structures. A first step toward overcoming this short-coming has been more recently achieved by the combination of real-time two-dimensional echocardiography with pulsed Dop-pler involving the use of two separate transducers and a display of the velocity frequency spectrum, either for the vessels (Baker(10)) or the heart (Nimura (10)). An alter-native approach consists in the use of one single transdu-cer both for the echo and the Doppler techniques and has led the Advanced Technology Laboratories (Bellevue, Wash.,USA) to devise a new device, the Cardiac Duplex Scanner, a proto-type of which we have been currently investigating (8).
  We present herewith a preliminary report on the clini-cal applications of this prototype, using an analog readout which allows the recording of blood flow velocity traces, for investigating mitral and tricuspid valve diseases.

PATIENTS STUDIED

36 patients, 7 male and 29 female, ranging in age from 20 to 72 years (mean 41 years) as well as a control group of 10 subjects, either whose heart was normal or in whom an atrio-ventricular valve anomaly had been ruled out using the classical procedures. The lesions included 26 pure mitral stenosis (MS), 5 pure mitral regurgitation (MR), 6 combined mitral stenosis and regurgitation (MS+MR), and 5 pure tri-cuspid regurgitation (TR). All MS, MS + MR lesions were of rheumatismal origin. One MR was due to ischaemic heart di-sease, 3 TR were due to congestive heart failure, one TR was due to bacterial endocarditis, and one was of congenital ori-

gin and associated with a ventricular septal defect. In all cases, but 8, the diagnosis was established by cardiac catheterization, dye dilution technique and/or surgical findings whenever appropriate. The severity of the disease was assessed in all cases but 8 using the Gorlin formula and/or surgical findings for mitral and tricuspid stenosis, atrial pressure curves, dye dilution technique, angiography and/or surgical findings for mitral and tricuspid regurgitation and was established on a 3 grade scale for each type of lesion, namely, mild, moderate and severe.

The remaining cases involved patients who had undergone closed heart commissurotomy prior to the ultrasonic investigation. They were not submitted to invasive procedures but the nature and degree of severity of the lesion was assessed and evaluated on the clinical picture, ECG, Chest X-rays and phonomechanocardiography.

TECHNIQUES AND APPARATUSES

We used an ATL Cardiac Duplex Scanner Doppler prototype which included: a) a 501 A Pulsed Doppler equipment, operating at 3.0 MHz, the description, specifications and clinical use of which has been previously described (1,5,6); b) an ATL 851 90° angle mechanical sector scanner; c) both were connected to a single probe (Fig. 1), which included the scanhead together with the Doppler probe. Also built-in was the adjustment system of the Doppler range gate including a lever, with one degree liberty, that could be tilted to and fro from an axial position, and allowed the Doppler beam to be moved in the plane of the sector scan. At its free extremity was a knob, which enabled to adjust in depth the position of the Doppler gate (i.e. of the recorded blood sample which measured 2 x 4 mm) along the Doppler beam at any given point from 3 to 17 cm from the chest wall. In addition, we used 2 video monitors, one for the real-time scanning, and the other for the Doppler display. The real-time imaging together with the schematic visualiation

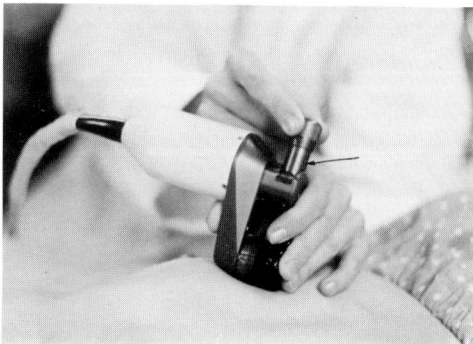

Fig.1. The Duplex(Scanner-Doppler)Probe. The single, cylindric (2.5 cm in height,2.5 cm in dia.) ultrasonic transducer is laid in contact with the skin by its rounded surface. The Doppler beam can be swept across the scan by tilting to and fro the lever (arrow), to the top of which is connected a knob(between thumb and index), that allows the Doppler gate to be moved in depth along the Doppler beam.

of the Doppler beam axis and of the Doppler gate were recorded on a magnetic tape using the NTSC/PAL/SECAM compatible SONY video tape recorder. Hard copies of real-time
images were obtained on a Tektronix recorder or by simple
photography. Doppler analog flow velocity curves, T-motion
echocardiographic tracings, Doppler spectral displays as
well as simultaneous ECG Lead 2 and frequency selecting pho-
nocardiograms were recorded on an IREX(Inc.,Mahwah,N.J.,USA)
fiberoptics recording system.

RECORDING METHOD

The Duplex recording always requires a sequentially
two-fold procedure, including successively the real-time
scanning and the Doppler recording. They were made on the
patient reclining on his back or on his left side, the head
slightly elevated, and in apnea or very light respiration.

A.MITRAL VALVE RECORDINGS

The mitral valve was first visualized in real-time according to the standard procedure and therefore several approaches were successively used: short axis, long axis, apex
(or 4 chamber) view, apex view centered on the left ventricle, and subxiphoid approach, to mention the most common
ones. For each of these approaches, when a satisfactory i-
mage was obtained with a proper gain setting, the latter was
freezed, while the apparatus automatically switched to the
Doppler system. The axis of the Doppler beam, visualized
as a straight and continuous white line, was then swept
across the scan plane, using the above mentioned lever,until
it transsected the mitral valve under the desired angle.
Thereafter, the Doppler gate was adjusted in depth along that
line using the afore described knob of the probe until it was
properly located at the desired site of the mitral valve:
centre, posterio-medial and antero-lateral commissure. A
prerequisite for making correct Doppler recording was to obtain a typical "Doppler sound" corresponding to blood flow
detection. The latter is quite recognizable from the different, harsh and strident noise originated by cardiac structures and particulary heart valve leaflets. When the "Doppler sound" was present, the recording could be readily
made, however great care was taken not to move the transducer during the Doppler procedure, and it was our policy
to cross   check several times that the correct position
had not been lost by a slight hand move or by the patient's
respiration. If the Doppler sound could not be obtained,
then the Doppler gate had to be slightly displaced, or a
slightly different scan plane had to be tried, implying a
new start of the whole procedure from the beginning. In certain cases, various respiratory states had to be tried before
a recording could be made.
Short Axis. This approach is particularly suitable for exploring the different sites of the mitral valve: centre, antero-lateral and posterio-medial commissures. It thus allows
the differentiation of the various flow disturbances with re-

spect to their localization (Figs.2 to 4, 8 to 10, 13 to 15).
Long axis. This approach is useful for investigating flow
patterns at the site of above and below the mitral annulus
(Figs.5,12,16 and 18). Tilting the probe externally allows
also the exploration of the postero-medial commissure, whereas tilting interiorly enables the exploration of the antero-
lateral commissure.
Apex (or Four Chamber) view. This approach is particularly
well suited since the Doppler beam can then be "threaded"
through the mitral valve almost parallel to the direction
of blood flow(Fig. 6 and 17). Centre, septal and lateral
points may also be explored.
Subxiphoid approach. This approach is best suited when the
apex view is difficult to obtain.

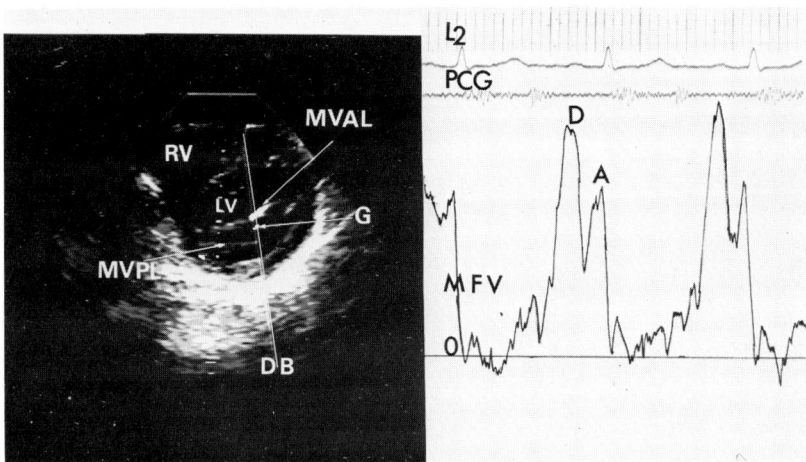

Fig. 2. Short axis Doppler-Scanner recording of the flow
velocity at the centre of the mitral valve(normal).
Left: Duplex recording. Right: Mitral valve flow velocity
pattern. The Doppler beam (DB) is visualized by a continuous white line, the Doppler gate (recorded blood sample site)
by a round dot. LV: left ventricle, RV: right ventricle,
MVAL: mitral valve anterior leaflet, MVPL: mitral valve posterior leaflet. L2: ECG lead 2. PCG: phonocardiogram, Interval between two successive bars equals to 0.04 sec. D: initial filling wave of the left ventricle. A: end-diastolic
filling wave of the left ventricle due to atrial systole.
IC: negative deflection due to isometric contraction. MVF:
mitral flow velocity pattern. Note the smooth aspect of
both limbs of the D and A waves.

B. TRICUSPID VALVE RECORDINGS

The approaches of choice are the apex view and the subxiphoid approach (Fig. 7 and 20), but a parasternal approach
may sometimes be used.

Results. In all patients, although not all the above mentioned approaches were always possible, a sufficient set of
curves was, as a rule, possible to be recorded, in order to

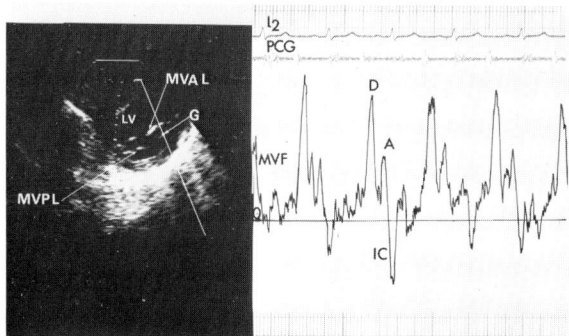

Fig. 3. Short axis Scanner-Doppler recording of the flow
velocity at the antero-lateral commissure of the mitral
valve. Same legend as in Fig. 2. Note the position of the
gate (G) at the antero-lateral commissure.

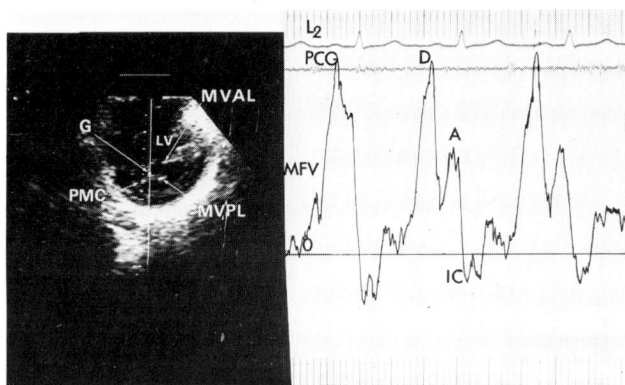

Fig. 4. Short axis Scanner-Doppler recording of the flow velocity at the postero-medial commissure of the mitral valve
(normal). Same legend as in Fig.2. PMC: postero-medial commissure of the mitral valve.

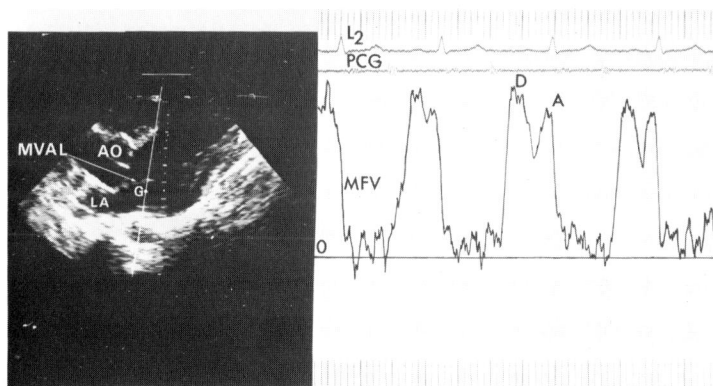

Fig. 5. Long axis Scanner-Doppler recording of mitral valve
flow velocity. Same legend as in Fig. 2. AO:aorta. Normal valve.

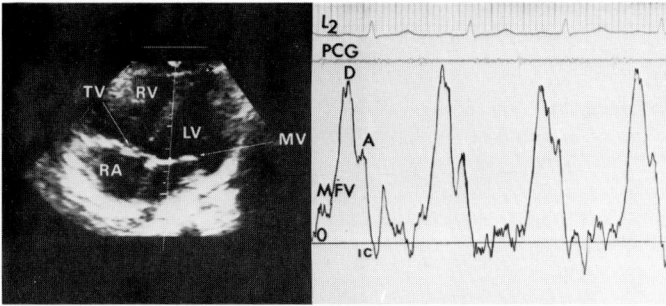

Fig. 6. Apex Scanner-Doppler recording of mitral flow velocity. MV: Mitral valve. LA: Left atrium. Normal valve

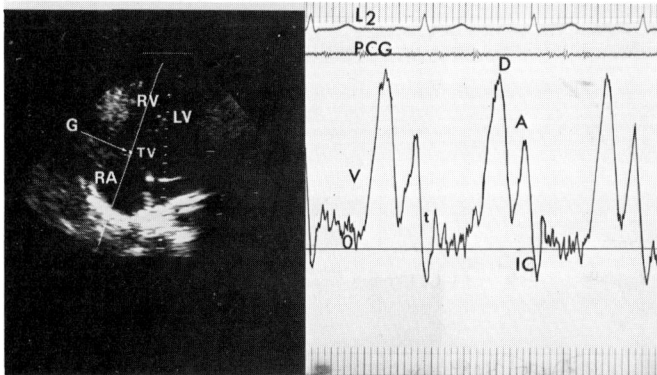

Fig. 7. Apex Scanner-Doppler recording of tricuspid flow velocity (normal). The Doppler beam transsects the tricuspid valve along the direction of blood flow. RA: right atrium, TV: tricuspid valve, TVF: tricuspid flow velocity.

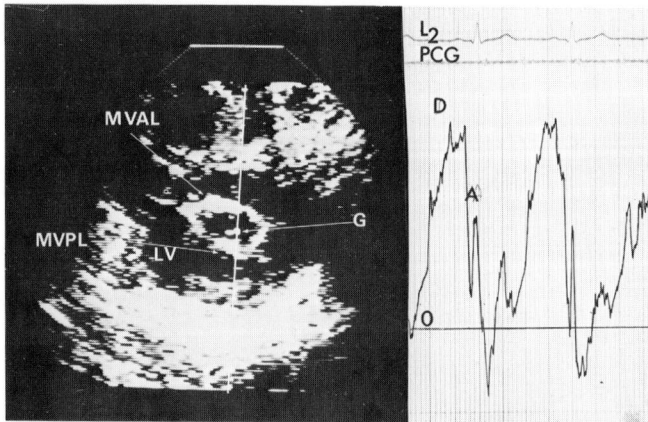

Fig. 8. Short axis duplex recording of central mitral flow in moderately severe mitral stenosis (pre-op. recording). Same legend as in Fig. 2. Left: both commissures are fused. Mitral valve area: 1.3 cm^2. Right: The ascending limb of the D wave presents typical indentations.

340

provide the desired information.

In all cases, as could be expected, the recorded analog flow velocity tracings, as well as the spectral displays,
were found similar to those found using the 1-D echo-Doppler
technique, both for the mitral and the tricuspid valves, in
normal and diseased states, and which were previously published (1,4-7,11,12).

Normal subjects. (Figs. 2-7). Both mitral and tricuspid flow
velocity tracings showed a more or less conspicuous, but
sometimes absent, early systolic negative deflection during
isometric contraction, followed by a systolic segment oscil-
lating slightly along the baseline (zero line). Thereafter,
the diastolic part of the curve showed an initial, triangular shaped, positive wave (initial filling wave) labelled
D, followed in patients with sinus rhythm, by an end diastolic positive, usually smaller, triangular shaped wave, due
to atrial contraction and labelled A wave, whose time relationship with the P wave of the ECG was constant. Both
limbs of the D and of the A wave were smooth, and their summit sharp and well defined. In cases of atrial fibrillation,
even when the valve was normal, the possibility occurred of
small negative oscillations after the initial filling wave.
Depending on the heart rate, the D and A summits were more
or less distant, but could become more or less fused in
cases of tachycardia. The distance between the two summits
varied also during respiration, whenever the heart rate was
affected (Figs. 2-7).

PATIENTS WITH MITRAL VALVE DISEASE

1. Mitral stenosis. The major feature of the recordings was
the occurrence of characteristic indentations on the ascending limbs, at the summit or on the descending limb of the D
wave. In mild stenosis, these indentations were slight, and
occurred only close to the anatomic lesion, i.e. at the commissures whereas the curve recorded at the centre remained
unaffected and normal or almost normal. In severe stenosis,
whatever the site of recording may be, the trace disclosed
important and coarse indentations on the ascending limb and
on the summit which whenever it remained well defined, was
delayed. In most cases, actually, this summit was replaced
by an irregular plateau, and more or less fused with the A
wave. In some instances, in patients with sinus rhythm, the
A wave was found of greater amplitude than the D wave (Figs.
8 to 12). After commissurotomy, (Figs. 13 to 17), the D
wave came back to an almost normal pattern, although small
indentations may remain on the summit of the D wave. It was
possible, in the post-operative controls, to differentiate
the improvements of blood flow of the commissures (Figs. 13
to 15, as compared to Figs. 8 to 10).

2. Pure mitral and tricuspid regurgitation. The major feature was the existence of a reversal, i.e. negative flow
wave during part or all of systole (Figs. 18 to 20). Using
the amplitude, the duration and above all, the anatomic extension of this negative wave, a first approximation of the

severity of the lesion could be obtained.
3. Combined mitral stenosis and regurgitation. The recorded curves either on the same recording or on separate ones
disclosed both types of lesion.

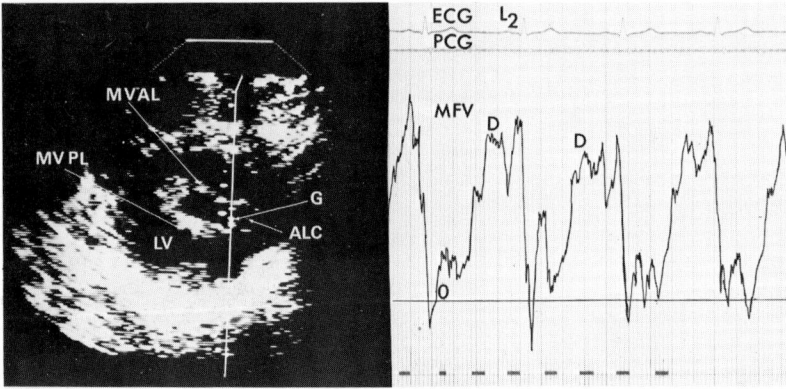

Fig. 9. Short axis duplex recording of mitral flow velocity
at the antero-lateral commissure. (Mitral stenosis). ALC:
antero-lateral commissure of the mitral valve. Right:the summit of the D wave is erased and replaced by a coarse, irreg-
ularly indented plateau.

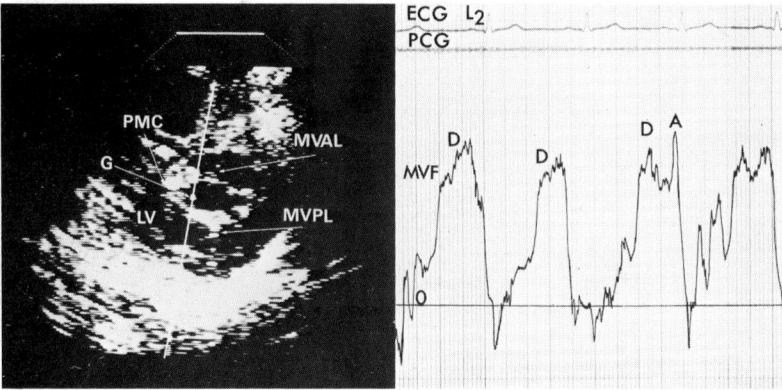

Fig. 10. Short axis duplex recording of mitral flow velocity
at the postero-medial commissure (Mitral stenosis). Same
legend as in Fig. 2. Right: typical aspect of the D wave due
to turbulence originated by the stenosis. The summit of the
D wave is replaced by a shaggy, irregular plateau.

COMMENTS

Although a non quantitative technique, one-dimensional
Echo-Doppler velocimetry has been clearly demonstrated to be
a highly reliable method for non invasively establishing the
diagnosis and assessing the severity of valvular heart disease, based on pattern recognition: detection of turbulence
for stenosis, demonstration of a negative systolic wave for
regurgitation (6,7,9). The combination of the analog read-

342

out technique with the spectral display method (detection of broadening of the spectrum) still enhances further reliability of the method.

Advantages of the Duplex technique. The basic advantage of the 2-D Echo-Doppler over the 1-D version of the technique relies not so much on its diagnostic capabilities expressed as "yes or no" and on a "mild versus severe" basis, since both are quite similar, rather than on its ability to refine the spatial localization of the flow information with respect to cardiac structures, while simultaneously displaying the latter. Indeed, in view of the considerable achievements already available by the present day non injurious techniques, what is now required--and may ultimately justify the use of sophisticated and expensive devices-- is basically a refinement of the relevant information with respect, not only to the indications for surgery per se, but to the choice of the most appropriate procedure for open or closed heart commissurotomy, valve repair or valve replacement. And this requires a more detailed description of the lesions both in terms of anatomy and of pathophysiology, i.e. flow information. In that sense, 2-D Echo Doppler appears very promising for determing simultaneously localized anatomical and functional impairments of the atrio-ventricular valves. Furthermore, as shown above, it offers a practical, non traumatic tool for checking the functional and anatomical quality of a surgical intervention, and for the patients' follow-up.

Diversity of the Duplex approaches. A) The possibility of obtaining satisfactory flow velocity tracings using the apex view came as no surprise since this is the best orientation of the Doppler beam. It only reproduces the results already obtained using the one dimensional technique. B). One of the most intriguing findings of our study, on the other hand, is the possibility of obtaining valid velocity curves using approaches, which one would expect to be inadequate, if not incompatible. This is particularly the case for short and long axis approaches, in which the Doppler beam appears to be oriented at 90° with the supposed direction of the blood flow, a situation which should entail a Doppler shift equal to zero. The fact that this is just not the case certainly calls for some explanation. Truely, our knowledge about the physics of ultrasound still remains too scarce to readily provide an explanation. However, in the first place, since the recorded velocity is a function of the cosinus of the angle between the Doppler beam and the direction of flow, a certain angle allowance is already compatible with the obtention of an acceptable output signal, even if reduced in amplitude. Furthermore, recent investigations about the scattering of ultrasound (Bom (3)) substantiate that secondary lobes tend to develop and diverge from the axial beam in the commonly used, non focussed ultrasonic emitters,and this might contribute to originating an unexpectedly high output signal.

In addition to these physical considerations, spatial

haemodynamical particularities might also be taken into account. Transvalvular flow is a complex, three dimensional phenomenon, and it is not unlikely that part of the streamlines of blood flow also diverge, up to a certain extent away from the central axis of the mitral annulus, thus contributing to minimize the incidence of the angle of the Doppler equation. Furthermore, and ultimately, it should also be recalled that the described diagnostic method relies only on pattern recognition and not on the accurate value of recorded velocities.

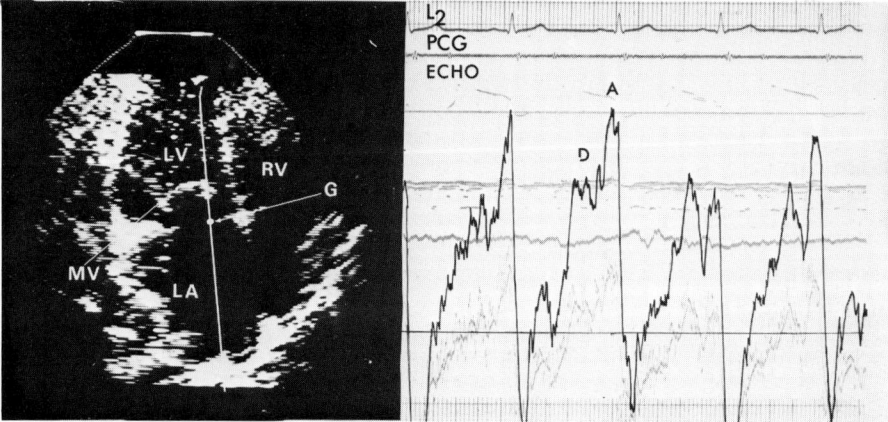

Fig. 11. Apex Duplex recording of mitral flow velocity (mitral stenosis). The Doppler beam is oriented right in the direction of blood flowing into the left ventricle.

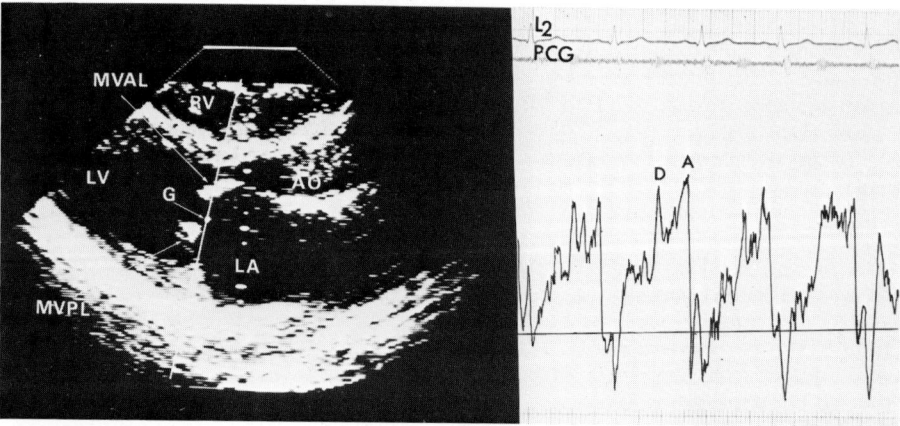

Fig. 12. Long axis Duplex recording of mitral flow velocity (mitral stenosis) (same patient as in Fig. 8 to 11). Left: note the typical bulging of the anterior leaflet of the mitral valve and the dilated left atrium. The direction of the Doppler beam seems perpendicular to the supposed direction of blood flow. Nevertheless, a perfectly adequate flow velocity pattern can be recorded(right), similar to that obtained using other approaches.

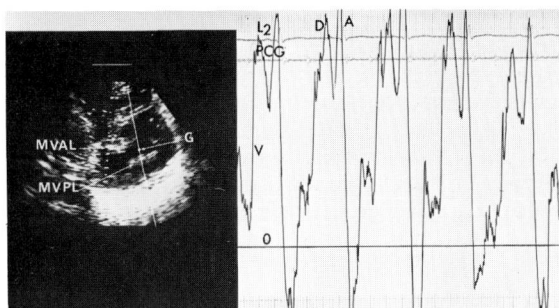

Fig. 13. <u>Short axis Duplex recording of mitral flow velocity</u>
<u>at the centre of the valve.</u> (Post-commissurotomy control).
Same patient as in Fig. 8. Compare with Fig. 8 right and note
the dramatic improvement of the flow velocity pattern which
returns almost to normal, with a much larger D wave, and the
almost total disappearance of the indentations.

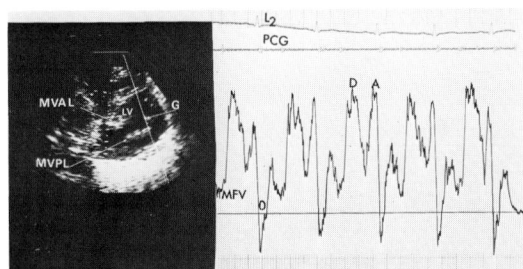

Fig. 14. <u>Short axis Duplex recording of mitral flow velocity</u>
<u>at the antero-lateral commissure</u> (post-operative control re-
cording:cf with Fig. 9.Note in particular the clear cut improvement in pattern: decrease of the indentations of the D
wave, which is much better defined, as well as the A wave.
(Compare with fig.9). In this particular patient, the surgeon
could open satisfactorily the antero-lateral commissure,where-
as nothing could be done to the postero-medial one. See following illustration.

<u>Sensitivity and limitations of the technique.</u> By and
large, and inasmuch as our limited number of studied patients
allows us to draw a valid statement,the sensitivity and reliability of the present ATL Duplex prototype seems of the
same order of magnitude than those of the one dimensional
device. However, further investigation is certainly needed.
Indeed, it should be stressed, that in some cases already,
the ability of the Duplex probe to provide access to specific (and in particular tricuspid) valvular sites appears to
be restricted by the present volume and the cumbersomeness
of the mechanical sector scanhead. The latter entail un-
questionably lesser flexibility and handiness of the probe
with regard to the small available intercostal spaces to be
explored, than those experienced previously by the much

345

smaller 500 A ATL one dimensional transducer. In our view, this calls for future improvements and miniaturization, and perhaps phased array systems might prove to provide some kind of answer to these problems. Much in the same way, additional improvements, including the replacement of the zero crossing technique by a fast Fourier transform, a better signal to noise ratio, as well as a more flexible coupling between the echo and the Doppler transducers would certainly be of benefit.

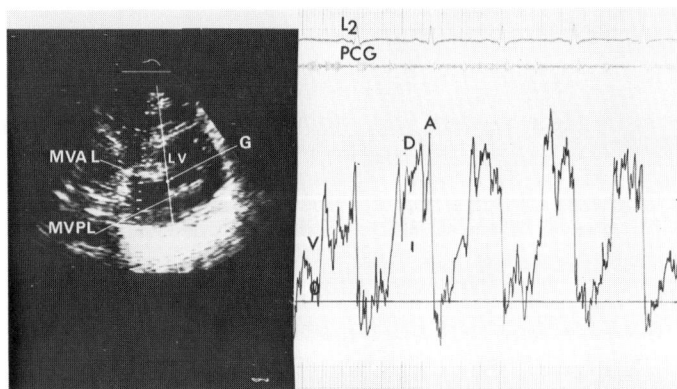

Fig. 15. <u>Short axis Duplex recording of mitral flow velocity at the postero-medial commissure</u>(post-operative control). Compare with Fig. 10, and note the persistence of crude indentations, and of the same pattern as before operation.

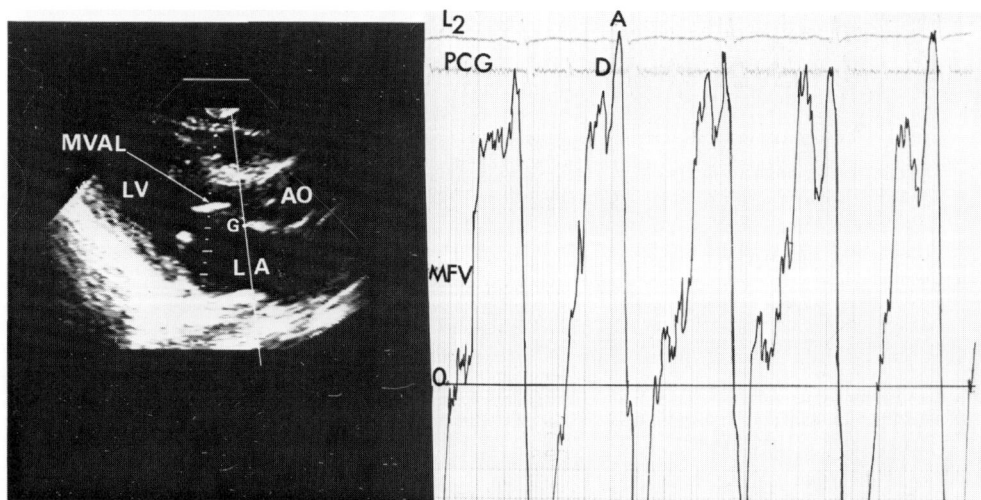

Fig. 16. <u>Long axis Duplex recording of mitral flow velocity at the centre of the valve</u> (post-operative control). Compare with Fig. 12. Note the remarkable improvement in amplitude and flow pattern, similar to that found in Fig. 13. The Doppler gate is placed immediately above the mitral annulus, near the anterior leaflet of the mitral valve.

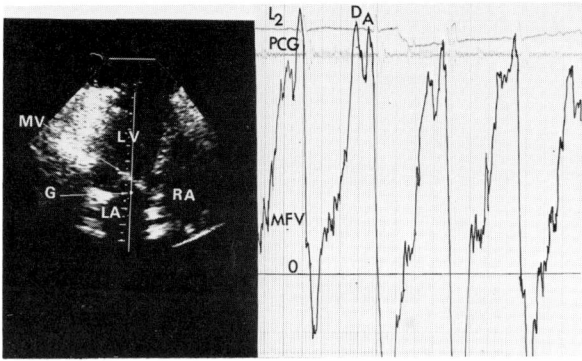

Fig. 17. Apex Duplex recording of the flow velocity at the
mitral valve. Left: The Doppler beam is oriented very close
to the direction of blood flow, and the gate place just at
the mitral annulus. Right: the blood flow pattern is clearly back to almost normal, as in Fig. 16.

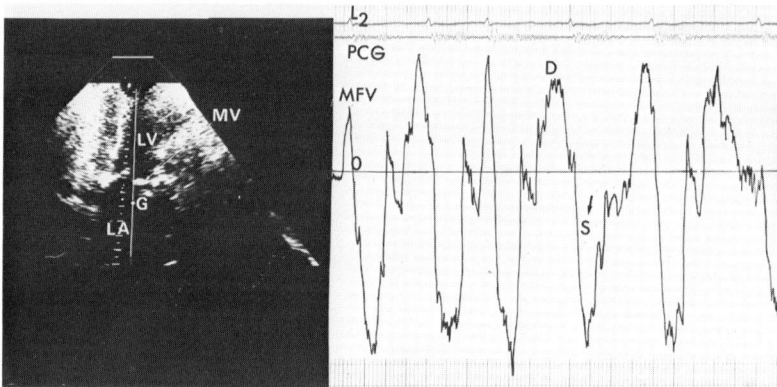

Fig. 18. Apex Duplex recording of mitral flow velocity in
case of massive mitral regurgitation. Left: the Doppler beam
is directed along the direction of blood flow. Right:note
the large negative systolic wave (S:arrow) as well as the
very irregular indentations of the diastolic flow wave.

CONCLUSION

Nevertheless, the above mentioned restrictions should
not overshadow the fact that even in its present state the
Duplex system does represent on its own a remarkable technological breakthrough and already provides improved and refined simultaneous information on the localization both of
anatomic lesions and of flow disturbances, thus far not a-
vailable, in atrioventricular valve diseases. Its practical
value cannot be overemphasized and it already appears to be
very promising for non invasive exploration of the normal
and diseased heart.

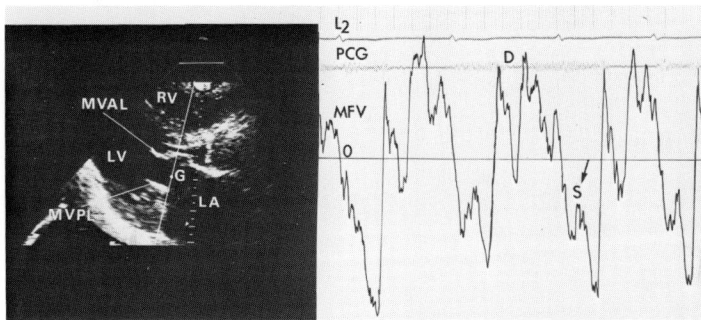

Fig. 19. Long axis Duplex recording of mitral flow velocity
in case of massive mitral regurgitation. (Same patient as
in Fig. 18). Note the large negative systolic wave(S), similar
to that recorded in Fig. 18.

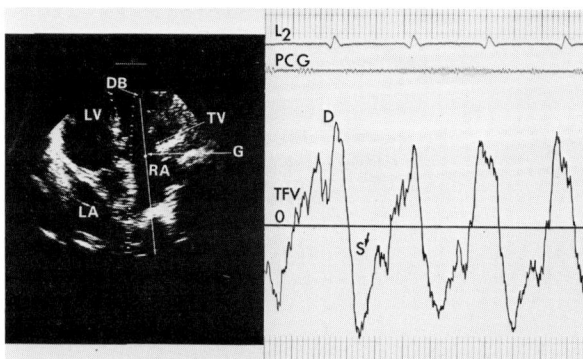

Fig. 20. Subxiphoid Duplex recording of tricuspid flow velocity in case of massive tricuspid regurgitation. Left:subxi-
phoid view of heart. The Doppler gate is positioned at site
of the tricuspid valve(TV). Right:Note a clear cut negative-
systolic wave(S). TFV: tricuspid flow velocity.

REFERENCES

1. Baker D Lorch G, & Rubenstein S.(1977):In: Echocardiology
   N.Bom(ed). Martinus Nijhoff, The Hague, Netherlands,207-221
2. Barber F, Baker D, Strandness D, Mahler G. (1974):Ultrason-
   ic Sym. Proceedings IEEE, cat R74, CHO-896-1 SU.
3. Bom N, Lancee C, Ligtvoet C(1977): Acta Med Scand. 627,41.
4. Johnson J, Baker D,Lute R, Dodge H (1973):Circul.48,810-822
5. Kalmanson D et al.(1976): C.R.Acad.Sci(D),282,937-940.
6. Kalmanson D et al.(1977): Bri Heart J, 39, 517-528.
7. Kalmanson D et al.(1979): In: Quantitative Cardiovascular
   Studies. Ed. N Hwang et al, Uni.Park Press, Ch.17,689-714.
8. Kalmanson D et al.(1979): Proceed. of WFUMB,Japan, July.
9. Pearlman A et al.(1979):In:Echocardiology, Nijhoff,255-260.
10.Matsuo H et al.(1977): Jap Cir J, 41, 515-528.
11.Veyrat C et al.(1979):In: Echocardiology,Nijhoff,261-266.
12.Veyrat C and Kalmanson D(1979):In: Advanced Technobiology,
   ed. B. Rybak, The Netherlands, 317-339.

PULSED DOPPLER ULTRASOUND VESSEL IMAGING USING THE GEC MAVIS

Hylton B. Meire and C.P.L. Wood

Clinical Research Centre, Harrow, England

INTRODUCTION

For the past year we have been performing a clinical evaluation of a new Pulsed Doppler Mobile Artery and Vein Imaging System (MAVIS, GEC Medical Ltd) and have used this to perform non invasive ultrasound angiograms of the carotid, vertebral, femoral and brachial arteries and the leg veins.

This new system consists of a 5 MHz ultrasound probe which can be driven in either a continuous or pulsed mode. The transducer is mounted on the end of a position resolving arm and once a vessel has been located using the continuous wave mode, manual scanning of the transducer over the vessel of interest permits the generation of a vessel image on a bistable storage oscilloscope. The positional information from the transducer can be used to generate either antero posterior, lateral or cross sectional images. With an additional monitor both AP and lateral views can be assembled simultaneously. Since the technique uses ultrasound, it is both painless and harmless and, since it employs the doppler principal it images only those areas in which there is moving blood. The images therefore represent the shape of the blood column within a vessel and atheromatous plaques or stenoses may appear as defects within the image.

Once an image has been generated the probe can be located accurately over any chosen point of a known vessel and velocity information can be obtained to augment the anatomical information. By this technique the haemodynamic effect of stenoses can be assessed and certain image artifacts can be reliably identified or excluded.

The equipment is direction sensitive enabling flow either towards or away from the probe to be selected separately and has the facility to demonstrate vessels with advancing flow on one half of the screen and receding flow on the other half of the same storage oscilloscope. This facility is particularly useful when arteries and veins lie closely adjacent, such as in the groin.

The clinical evaluation has comprised three separate phases: firstly, the development of suitable scanning techniques and approaches; secondly, the evaluation of these on normal subjects and, thirdly, an evaluation of the reliabilty of the technique in the detection of arterial and venous disease.

GENERAL TECHNIQUE

In common with other ultrasound scanners it is necessary to hold the transducer in contact with the area of interest and to apply a suitable contact medium to the skin. Unlike other imaging systems the pulsed doppler vessel images obtained with MAVIS may require several minutes to compile and patient movement during this period will, of course, introduce anatomical distortion and errors. It is therefore frequently necessary to immoblise the area of interest and, whilst this is seldom a serious problem with the arm or leg, it is not infrequently a problem when scanning the extra cranial cerebral vessels. This is particularly so in patients with cerebral vascular disease and we have found the Internuclear vacuum head immobiliser extremely valuable for the comfortable immobilisation of restless patients. It is by no means unusual for patients to fall asleep during the examination!

In common with other compound scanning techniques pulsed doppler vessel imaging is highly dependant on the skill and expertise of the operator who must have a full working knowledge of the vascular anatomy and pathology that he is likely to encounter. The operator must also be able to obtain velocity recordings where necessary to help in the interpretation of the images and we listen invariably to the audio converted doppler shift frequencies throughout the scanning procedure since this may help to detect areas of turbulent blood flow in vessels of relatively normal calibre.

It can be seen therefore that the technique is rather more difficult than imaging vessels with the small modern automatic linear array scanners but these of course will not yield haemodynamic information and cannot be used to compile complex anterior projections.

We will now review briefly our experience with the major vessels and indicate our opinion considering the advantages potential and limitations of MAVIS scanning in several different clinical situations.

THE CAROTID ARTERIES

It is invariably possible to identify and image the carotid arteries when they are patent (Figure 1). Difficulties may arise in both obtaining and interpreting images in those patients where the vessels are extremely tortuous, particularly if flow in one direction is being excluded from the image. This may result in apparent complete gaps in the image, but analysis of the flow characteristics in the segments imaged will confirm functional continuity of the vessel segments. We have imaged the carotid arteries in 102 patients and in many patients have obtained repeat scans after both short and long intervals and have found the images reproducible. In those patients where angiographic confirmation of vascular anatomy has been available this has correlated closely with the MAVIS findings.

350

The clinical value of MAVIS imaging of the carotids is probably greatest in those patients with transient cerebral ischaemic attacks or in patients with incidentally observed bruits within the neck. In the former group of patients it is possible that a surgically correctable lesion may be present in the extra cranial carotid circulation and MAVIS seems capable of reliably detecting or excluding such lesions (Figure 2) and could therefore be used as a screening procedure to select patients for arteriography prior to surgery. It is also valuable to exclude haemodynamically significant stenoses in patients with carotid bruits and in our experience there have been several such patients in whom MAVIS scans have shown normal carotid vessels and a probable cause of the bruit proximal to the carotid origin. The technique is suitable also for the post operative follow-up of patients submitted to vascular surgery. In the small number of patients examined in this group, continued patency of the endartectomy site has been monitored and one post-operative stenosis detected.

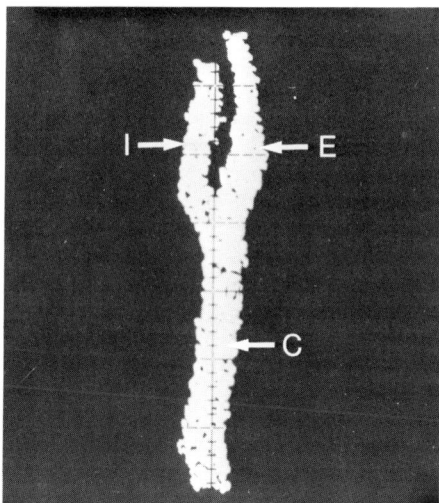

Fig. 1. Anterior view of a normal carotid artery, Common Carotid(C), Internal Carotid (I), External Carotid (E)

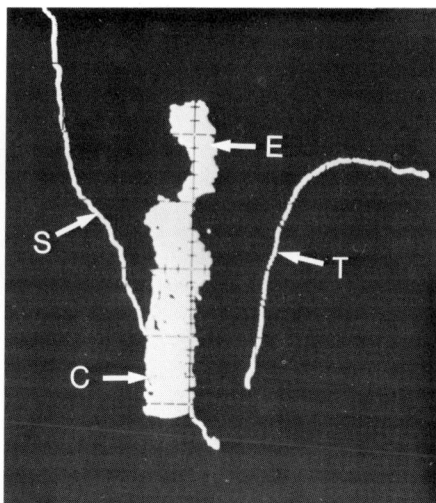

Fig. 2. Anterior scan of a patient with totally occluded internal carotid artery. Thyroid Cartilage(T), Sterno Mastoid Muscle(S), Common Carotid (C), External Carotid (E).

VERTEBRAL ARTERIES

Very few publications have appeared describing ultrasound imaging of the vertebral arteries. The most detailed
paper is that of White (1978) in which he demonstrated the
ability to image short segments of the vessel between the
lateral masses of the cervical vertebrae. In practice most
lesions in the vertebral arteries occur very close to the
origin and we have thus developed a technique for imaging
this part of the vessel. The technique depends upon identification of the subclavian artery and the common carotid
artery in the root of the neck. The vertebral artery is
searched for at the apex of the curve of the subclavian artery and can often be imaged for several centimetres of its
extra osseous course (Figure 3). To date we have attempted
imaging of the vertebral artery in 60 cases and have been
successful in 93 per cent. It is possible that our failures
may be due either to ectopic orgin of this vessel or to total occlusion. We do not yet have angiographic confirmation
in most of these cases. It has been unusual in our experience to identify significant stenoses of the vertebral artery on our images but observation of the flow velocities
within the vessel has permitted identification of haemodynamically significant stenoses and also permitted us to make
an assessment of the distal vascular bed. This form of vessel imaging is particularly useful in patients with transient
ischaemic attacks and vertigo or other symptoms which may be
attributable to vertebro basilar insufficiency. We have so
far identified 2 cases of subclavian steal syndrome and have
excluded the diagnosis in 6 cases. We have also made the
first recorded diagnosis of bilateral intermittent subclavian
steal in a child (Wood, 1980, in press).

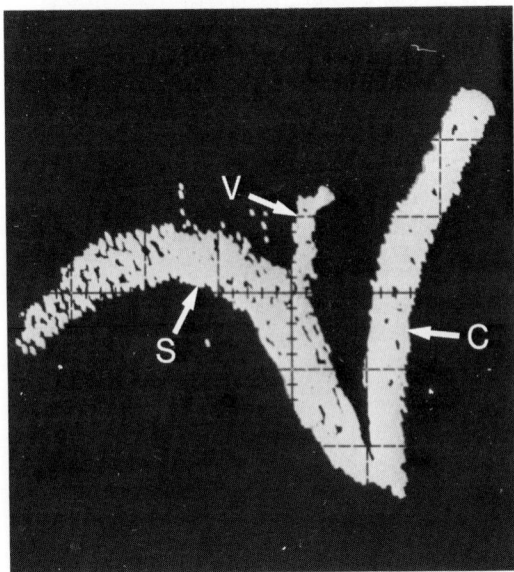

Fig. 3. Anterior Scan
of the vertebral artery
origin (V) from the
subclavian artery (S),
Common carotid artery
(C).

BRACIAL ARTERIES

Atheroma of the brachial arteries is extremely unusual but in our institution there is a large group of patients undergoing periods of 24 to 72 hour ambulatory blood pressure monitoring via indwelling brachial artery catheters. We have performed a study on these patients after removal of the catheters in order to diagnose or exclude evidence of vascular damage subsequent to catheterisation. Satisfactory images have been obtained in all 25 patients and in no case has any vascular abnormality been detected either on the images, the velocity tracings or the doppler ultrasound transit time measurements to a point distal to the catheterised segment. We have been able therefore to confirm that the blood pressure monitoring technique employed does not appear to cause any permanent arterial morbidity.

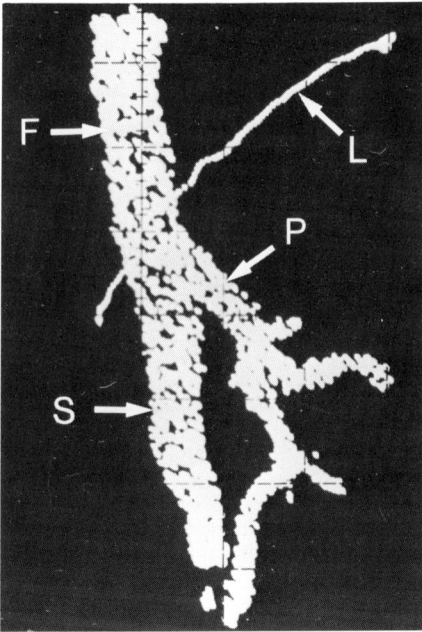

Fig. 4. Anterior Scan of the normal femoral artery at the groin. Common Femoral (F), Superficial Femoral (S), Profunda Femoris (P), Inguinal ligament (L).

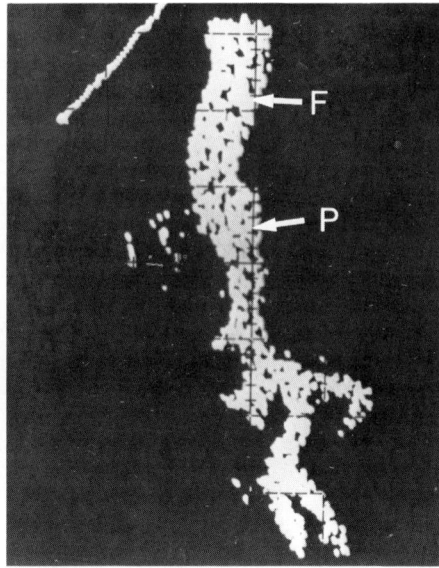

Fig. 5 Anterior Scan of patient with obstructed superficial femoral artery. The profunda femoris and its branches are moderately dilated. Common femoral (F), Profunda Femoris (P).

FEMORAL ARTERIES

Atheromatous disease of the femoral arteries is extremely common and is a frequent cause of morbidity and discomfort.

We have been successful in imaging the common femoral artery in every patient in whom blood flow has been present within this vessel and as our technique has improved the superficial femoral and profunda femoris vessels have been imaged more successfully (Figure 4). Angiographers will be aware that the origin of the profunda femoris artery is notoriously difficult to image reliably by conventional angiographic techniques and yet is of particular interest to the vascular surgeon. Reference to figures 4 and 5 will show that the origin of this vessel is frequently well seen and that the functional dilation of the profunda femoris artery in some patients with obstruction to the superficial femoral can also be demonstrated (Figure 5). The superficial femoral artery can be identified lower in the leg in a high proportion of patients but in highly muscular and obese patients and in those with operation scars over the vessel we have experiences some difficulty in imaging the deeper segments of this vessel. Despite this limitation, we have found MAVIS a useful means of identifying and assessing the short occlusions and tight stenoses which can now be treated by the non operative dilatation techniques such as the Dotter procedure. MAVIS is useful not only for the diagnoses and selection of suitable patients but also, of course, for the follow up of these patients after treatment.

PARA-ARTERIAL MASSES

We have investigated the role of MAVIS in the investigation of patients with masses thought to be of arterial origin, particularly at the site of previous arterial surgery. We have compared the information obtained from a conventional grey scale B scanner with that obtained from the pulsed doppler vessel imaging system in these patients. In a small series we have correctly diagnosed one true aneurysm, one false aneurysm, one thyroid cyst and have excluded an arterial origin for a mass which was subsequently proven to be an abscess. In a further patient we have refuted the clinical diagnosis of a carotid body tumour.

In those patients with thrombus formation within an aneurysm the size of the aneurysm is under estimated by MAVIS, as with conventional arteriorgraphy, and in these patients conventional B scanning has proven to be complementary, as has been the case with B scanning of abdominal aortic aneurysms.

VENOUS IMAGING

The clinical diagnosis of deep vein thrombosis within the leg is often difficult to confirm and yet it is important to establish or refute the diagnosis to allow the accurate selection of patients for anticoagulation. Whilst radioactive fibrinogen studies may be helpful in many patients conventional radiographic contrast venography is usually performed as the confirmatory diagnostic procedure and we are performing a study to compare the diagnostic accuracy of MAVIS with conventional venography. In the first 22 cases ultrasound and venography were in agreement for the diagnosis of DVT in 7 patients and for the exclusion in 10. MA VIS gave false negative results in 3 patients in whom there was minor thrombus formation in the small calf veins. In a further 10 patients not undergoing venography no evidence of DVT was found on MAVIS scanning and the subsequent clinical findings and progress of the patients indicated that venous thrombosis was unlikely to have been present. Since performing this pilot study we have constructed a cyclical calf compressor which has greatly augmented venous return from the lower limb and substantially improved our ability to image the femoral and popliteal veins. Whilst further work clearly needs to be done on this important use of this new non-invasive tool our initial results are extremely encouraging and compare favourably with those obtained by Day et al in 1976.

FUTURE DEVELOPMENT

The first prototype of a microprocessor based blood flow calculation module has just been produced. This additional facility permits the operator to measure accurately volume blood flow within any chosen vessel segment with absolute confidence about the site from which his measurements are being obtained. At the same time information can be obtained concerning flow profile and many other functional parameters which should prove immensely valuable in the diagnosis and management of patients with vascular disease.

SUMMARY

Our first year's work with this apparatus has shown that the results are highly dependent upon the skill of the operator, but when these skills have been learned and are combined with a thorough knowledge of the vascular anatomy and pathology this vessel imaging system is a powerful diagnostic tool. Not only does it permit the better selection of patients for conventional vascular studies but it should also obviate the need for these studies in many patients and also permit us to obtain, without any hazard or discomfort to the patient, a great deal of anatomical and functional information which previously was not available to us.

The ability to obtain blood velocity information from precise sites within the vessel lumen confers a significant advantage upon this apparatus compared with conventional continuous wave doppler systems and, combined with this facility, the subsequent ability to compute volume flow will open up a new and fascinating field of medical investigation.

REFERENCES

1. Day, T.K.,Fish, P.J. and Kakkar, V.V.(1976): British Medical Journal, 1:618-620.
2. White, D.N., Curry, G.R. and Stevenson, R.J. (1978): In: Ultrasound in Medicine 4, Eds. White & Lyon, Plenum Press
3. Wood, C.P. & Meire, H.B. (1980): Br. J. Rad. (in press).

10. NEW CLINICAL APPLICATIONS

G. Kossoff, Chairman

NEW CLINICAL TECHNIQUE WITH THE UI OCTOSON - VISUALISATION OF PAEDIATRIC HEART ANOMALIES

M.J. Dadd, M. McCredie and G. Kossoff

INTRODUCTION

The problem facing the echocardiographer in studying paediatric cardiac anomalies differs significantly from those encountered in adult cardiography. In the adult, there usually exists essentially normal anatomy modified in some way by disease. Commonly functional aspects of the heart are of most relevance and these can be conveniently studies with M mode supplemented by real-time cross sectional scanning. With a suspected paediatric congenital cardiac anomaly, the prime requirement is to establish which of a wide variety of possible anatomical relationships, in both the heart structure and of the viscera, is present. In this complex situation therefore, the overall view of both the thorax and abdomen obtainable with a general purpose compound B scanner, the UI Octoson, has potentially much to offer.

TECHNIQUE

The UI Octoson has been described in detail elsewhere (1,2). Particularly relevant to cardiac examinations is the good coupling to the thorax obtainable with the plastic membrane. This, together with the array of large aperture transducers in the water bath, allows maximum utilisation of the limited acoustic window. The flexibility of the coupling method and the mobility of the scanning arm allow a wide variety of scanning planes to be achieved. Routinely with the patient prone, a series of sections 5 mm apart are taken parallel to the path of the thoracic aorta. This provides a good overall view of the heart, the major vessels and associated viscera, while a series of transverse sections provides a more complete view of the heart chambers and their connections with the great vessels. Oblique sections are taken when appropriate to the particular diagnostic problem. The transducer scan time varies from 2 seconds for a full compound scan, resulting in a diastolic image with some superimposed motion, to less than 1/3 second with simple scanning, resulting in a "freeze frame" effect.

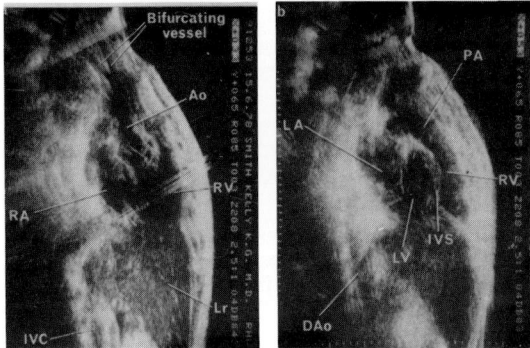

Figure 1. Parasagittal sections of normal heart

NORMAL PATIENTS

In normal parasagittal sections the liver, IVC, right
ventricle, right atrium, aortic valve and the ascending
aorta are shown (figure 1a). Figure 1b is a section taken
2 cm to the left and shows the right ventricle and the right
ventricular outflow tract, pulmonary artery, the interventricular septum, the left ventricle, left atrium and
the path of the aorta. The position of the cardiac valves
can normally be seen but there is little indication of
their condition unless heavily calcified. Transverse sections
in the abdomen provide a convenient record of the relative
positions of the major vasculature, and the position and
shape of the viscera. In the heart, transverse sections
provide a view of the interventricular and atrial septa, the
atrio-ventricular valves and the relative positions of the
great vessels.

DEVELOPMENTAL ANOMALIES

In a series of 75 patients examined by this technique
abnormalities of the atrial septum, atrio-ventricular canal,
interventricular septum, truncus and conus, semilunar valves
and abnormalities in the position of the heart have all been
visualised. The atrial and interventricular septa are best
visualised in transverse sections as shown in Figure 2.
A normal interventricular septum can be seen in the same
section as the atrial septal defect. This view is similar
to the four chamber view commonly used in real time
echocardiography, although in this case the plane is angled
more caudally.

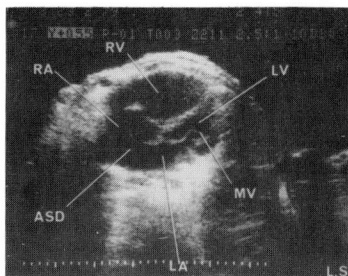

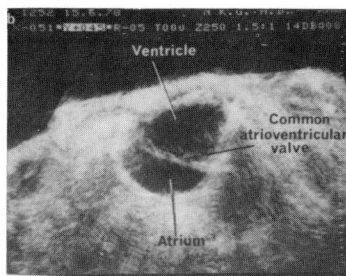

Figure 2. Transverse section of ASD

Figure 3. Transverse section of single ventricle with AV canal defect.

It is essential to be confident of reliably portraying both the atrial and interventricular septa where they exist. For example, in a 12 month old child with a single ventricle and AV canal defect, there existed only a rudimentary interventricular septum. The common AV valve is seen and the two chambers are shown in Figure 3. The low scanning speed used here results in an M-mode like appearance of the valve leaflets. Less extreme forms of persistent atrioventricular canal and ostium primum defects are visualised best in transverse sections.

Abnormalities of the truncus and conus are particularly well displayed as shown in Figure 4 where the relative paths of the aorta and pulmonary artery in a 13 year old boy are demonstrated. The thoracic aorta can be seen passing above a large vessel before joining the heart anteriorly. This vessel arising in the position normally occupied by the ascending aorta and passing out of the scan plane immediately below the aortic arch was shown to be the pulmonary artery in a case of corrected transposition.

In the sagittal echogram in Figure 5 all the major anatomical features of persistent truncus arteriosis are displayed. In this section portions of the left and right ventricles are seen separated by a septum, a VSD immediately below a single valve at the entrance to a large common vessel which bifurcates 2 cm above the valve. The transverse section taken through the truncus demonstrates the right atrium, right ventricle, beginning of the aorta and pulmonary artery with the truncus.

The UI Octoson is particulary suited to detailed visualisation of the abdomen. Therefore it has a special place in determining problems of situs, abnormal position or absence of the viscera and in visualising venous draining. In situs inversus for example, normal transverse echograms are obtained but in mirror image. The ability to study both abdominal and cardiac structures in one examination is of value in defining such conditions. A four year old with a complex histroy including blockage of the superior vena cava and associated veins, was referred to deter-

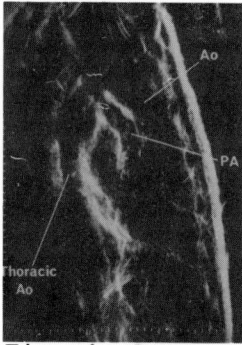

Fig. 4. Corrected
Transposition

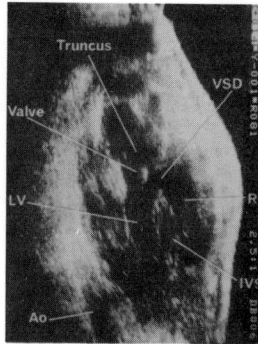

Fig. 5. Truncus

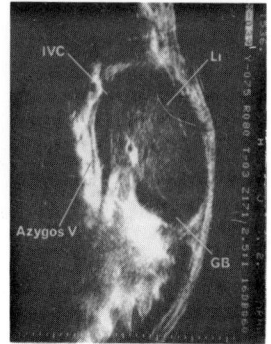

Fig. 6. Abnormal
venous drainage

mine the patency of his venous drainage as repeated cathe-
terisations had failed. It is clear from the sagittal section in Figure 6 that the vena cava was patent down to the
level of the right kidney at which point bowel gas prevented
clear visualisation. Immediately behind the IVC a tubular
structure thought to be a dilated azygos vein was shown.
Other sections revealed a vessel running transversely from
the IVC towards the left of the patient, together with a
cluster of varices behind the aorta. This examination provided information which had not been available from any
other source and in conjunction with radiological examinations, allowed a comprehensive picture of this patient's
venous drainage to be established.

The UI Octoson has been shown capable of providing
high quality images of the cardiac chambers, the great vessels and associated organs. A wide variety of pathological
conditions have been visualised and correlated with angiography and surgical findings. It is particularly suitable
for examination of paediatric patients as the examination
is atruamatic and comfortable. Further experience will
establish its final role in this field but the results to
this point suggest that the UI Octoson can play an important role in the study of paediatric heart anomalies.

REFERENCES

1. Carpenter, D.,Kossoff, G., Garrett, W.J., Daniel, K.
   & Boele, P. (1977): The UI Octoson - A New Class of Ultrasonic Echoscope. Aust. Radiology, Vol. XXI, 1, 85-89.
2. Kossoff, G. (1977): Automated Ultrasonic Scanning Techniques. In: Proc. Int. Symp. on Recent Advances in Ultrasound Diagnosis, Dubrovnik, Ed. A. Kurjak, Excerpta
   Medica.

EXPERIMENTS WITH A HAND-HELD REAL-TIME IMAGING SYSTEM

Klaas Bom, Elma J. Gussenhoven, Jos R.T. Roelandt
and Jura W. Wladimiroff.

Thoraxcenter, Erasmus University, P.O. Box 1738, Rotterdam.
Dept. of Obstetrics/Gynaecology, University Hospital
Dijkzigt Rotterdam and Interuniversity Cardiology
Institute, Rotterdam, The Netherlands.

INTRODUCTION

Real-time imaging is well accepted for diagnostic
use today. The most significant properties of real-time
imaging devices are:

1. the capability to study moving structures.
2. instantaneous echogram display when the transducer is moved over area of interest for any
   moving or non-moving structure study.

A number of apparatus properties may be distinguished
which are important and may become significant for even
wider acceptance of real-time echography in clinical
routine. The properties include the following:

a. Image quality and resolution.
b. Single frame and video documentation capability.
c. Complexity of the system. Simplicity in use.
d. Size and portability.
e. Cost/effectiveness.

Most of the present real-time systems fall in the
class of large, complex and rather expensive machines,
which are permanently installed in the diagnostic ultrasound room and cannot be used for quick decision making
elsewhere. We have therefore developed a new diagnostic
instrument. The main characteristics are its small size,
full portability and battery operation combined with
a real-time imaging technique based on the linear array
principle. The instrument is shown in figure 1.
During the last year studies have been carried
out to test the application of the new instrument. Image
quality was for instance investigated for six cardiac
structures in a group of 58 children. In adult cardiology
comparisons with M-mode recordings were made. The instrument has also been intensively used in the obstetric
ward. Following a description of the most important
technical parameters, experiences obtained in various
clinical areas will be briefly described.

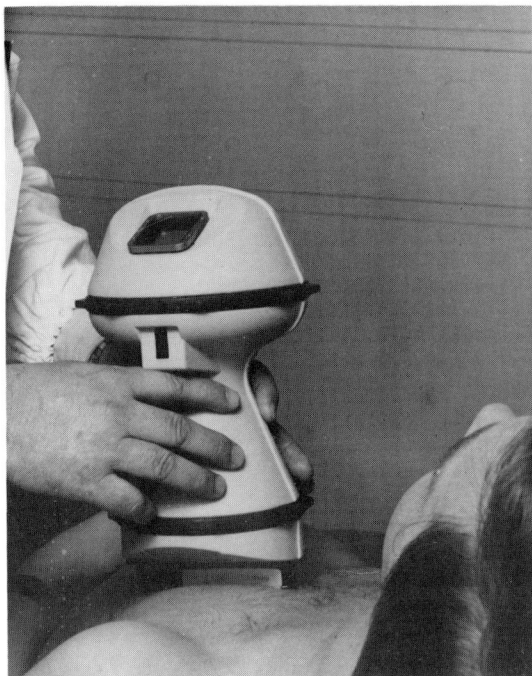

Fig. 1 Photograph of the battery powered hand-held
real-time imaging device*.

TECHNICAL DESCRIPTION

The goal was to develop an instrument with the display tube, the recta-linear scan transducer, the necessary electronics and battery power supply in a single housing. A detailed technical description has been reported
earlier by Ligtvoet et al. (1).

From figure 1 the final toad-stool shape may be
observed. This shape resulted from an excentrically positioned small display tube in combination with the requirement of easy one-hand manouvrability of the instrument.
The center of gravity is in the grip area. The transducer
is incorporated in the center of the bottom area.

Total weight is less than 1.5 kg. The rechargable
batteries permit 1½ hrs of operation without need for
the electrical mains power supply. Single knob operation
has been incorporated by combination of the on/off switch
and gain setting into one knob. This was obtained with

*The Minivisor, Organon Teknika, Oss, The Netherlands.

364

a semi-automatic amplification circuit. The result is utmost simplicity in instrument handling.

On the small display tube a cross-sectional image of 10 x 20 cm is projected with a display format of 2 x 4 cm and a line density of 20 lines per cm.

With this miniaturized real-time ultrasonic two-dimensional imaging system it became possible to obtain, in a very simple way, good quality ultrasonic images for immediate diagnostic examination in the emergency ward, at the bedside, or at any desired location where rapid ultrasonic diagnosis is needed.

PEDIATRIC CARDIOLOGY

The primary goal of this study was to evaluate cardiac structure recognition as obtained in children on the screen of the Minivisor. The standard long axis view over the left ventricular outflow tract and a second transducer position over the right ventricular outflow tract and pulmonary trunk were selected. Investigation was carried out in 58 children under the age of 18. Cardiac structure visibility was specifically studied for six structures (aortic root, left atrium, right ventricle, inter ventricular septum, left ventricle and mitral valve). Visibility was judged as either:

> good = structures well-outlined; seen during
> the complete cardiac cycle.
> fair = structures observed during part of the
> cardiac cycle.
> poor = when no definite conclusion could be made
> about size or motion pattern.

In addition an attempt was made to ascertain specific diagnoses. An echographic example of a cardiac long axis cross-sectional view of a patient with increased aortic root dimensions is shown in figure 2.
This patient was known to have coarctation of the aorta. The left atrium/aorta ratio, which normally approximates unity, is clearly diminished in this case. The evaluation of structure visibility in children under 1 year of age showed that it was sometimes difficult to obtain good separate images of the right ventricle, the interventricular septum and left ventricle. Aorta, mitral valve and left atrium were seen with a high success rate. In the age group between 1 and 18 years visibility has improved for all structures. The quality of the obtained images in this group allowed confirmation of specific diagnoses in many children with a congenital malformation. More information on this study is reported by W.J. Gussenhoven et al (2).

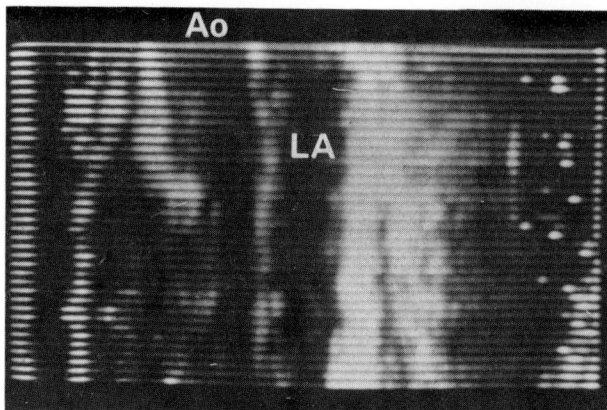

Fig. 2   Long axis cardiac echogram in a patient where the aortic root (Ao) diameter is larger than that of the left atrium (LA).

ADULT CARDIOLOGY

First clinical tests with the minature device were performed on 20 adult cardiac patients. Image quality proved to be good and diagnostic information could be obtained. Thereafter a comparison was made between the Minivisor results in the outpatient department and those obtained in the diagnostic echo laboratory. Image quality was found to be compatable with that of non-focussed conventional linear scanners. As a next step 100 patients were studied independently by two investigators. M-mode measurements were compared with information obtained with the hand-held system. (Roelandt et al.(3)).

Structure visualization was evaluated in this group of adult patients following the previously described procedure. Results are illustrated in figure 3. Apparently the aorta and left atrium are best recognized and problems in visualization of these structures arise in only approximately 5% of the cases. With exception for the aortic cusps, visualization of all structures is qualified in at least 90% of the cases as "fair" or "good".

For further evaluation the calibration dots on the small screen were used for a semi-quantitative assessment (normal, abnormal, enlarged, severely enlarged, etc.) when compared with the M-mode data. Comparison on aortic root dimension, left atrial size and left ventricular size showed that in the majority of cases agreement between the methods existed. When disagreement existed the data derived from the Minivisor tended to slightly overestimate the structure size.

The instrument is now routinely used, particularly in the emergency department and coronary care unit where conventional apparatus is cumbersome. Applications include differentiation between tamponade and dilated left ventricle, monitoring of pericardiocentesis. At the outpatient department it is a substitute of cardiac fluoroscopy.

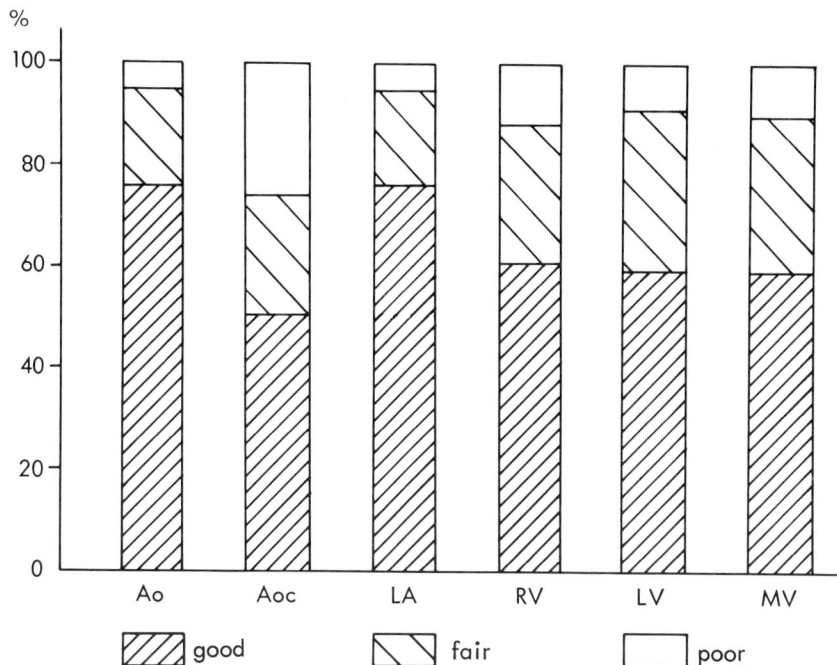

Fig. 3 Cardiac structure recognition as obtained in 100 adult patients. (Ao = aorta, Aoc = aortic cusps, LA = left atrium, RV = right ventricle, LV = left ventricle, MV = mitral valve).

OBSTETRICS

The introduction of a simple, hand-held scanner is a major step forward towards realisation of a screening procedure. This, in combination with the possibility of on-the-spot examination capabilities in cases of acute complications, is one of the major advantages experienced at various stages of gestation. In the first trimester of pregnancy, for instance, on-the-spot visualization

of a viable fetus in case of vaginal haemorrhage rules
out the presence of incomplete or missed abortion or
molar pregnancy. In the beginning of the second trimester
of pregnancy more detailed information on fetal anatomy
becomes available. An echogram obtained with the miniature
device showing early pregnancy is given in figure 4.

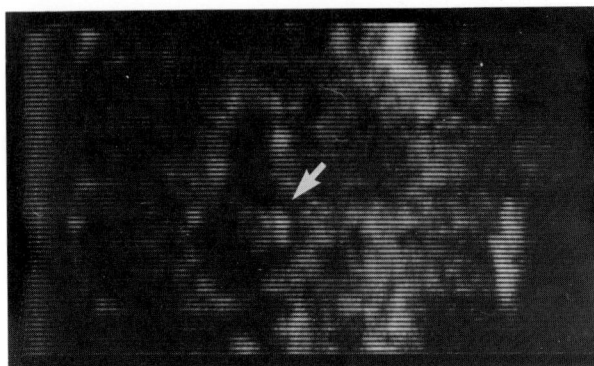

Fig. 4   Echogram demonstrating gestational sac and fetus
at 9 weeks of gestation (The arrow indicates the fetus).

The hand-held device can also provide important information during the procedure of amniocentesis since the
location of the placenta and the position of the needle
relative to fetal structures can be easily followed.
A quick decision on single or multiple pregnancy becomes
possible, anywhere on the obstetrical ward.
        During the latter half of the second trimester
and during the third trimester of pregnancy valuable
information can be obtained on fetal dynamics and fetal
growth. It is well-known that before 28 weeks of gestation
the fetal biparietal diameter provides reliable information on fetal age. Serial cephalometry will reflect
fetal growth. Measurements of the biparietal diameter
as obtained with the hand-held device were tested against
measurements carried out with a standard compound scanning
system. The minature device had been extended with a
hardcopy/ video convertor device for documentation purposes during this study. The incorporated interpolation
circuit doubles the numbers of lines on the display.
Figure 5 shows the resulting image during measurement
of the biparietal diameter.
The calipers were part of the video convertor. The study
showed that no difference existed between measurements
with the conventional compound scanner and the biparietal
diameter as obtained with the miniature device in all
149 patients studied. It is experianced that a small,
battery powered, real-time system when used in obstetrics

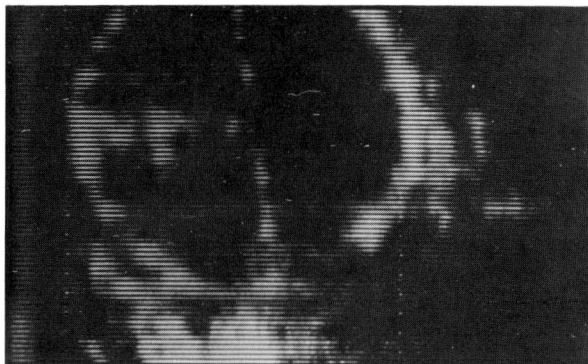

Fig. 5 Echogram showing measurement of biparietal diameter.

has great diagnostic value in on-the-spot diagnosis in case of antepartum haemorrhage. It is a valuable adjunct in the procedure of amniocentesis. Furthermore routine screening of an obstetric population with all the important questions such as single/multiple pregnancy, fetal life, location of the placenta, fetal position and fetal growth and size becomes possible in a simple and very convenient way.

ACKNOWLEDGMENT

     We are grateful to Cees Ligtvoet who was the project leader of the first prototype instrument and who provided some of the photographs for this paper.

REFERENCES

1. Ligtvoet, C.T., Rijsterborgh, H., Kappen, L. and Bom, N. (1978): Ultrasound Med. Biol. Vol. 4, pp. 91-92, Pergamon Press.
2. Gussenhoven, W.J., Kappen, K., Ligtvoet, C.M. and Eggink, J.H. (1979): In press, Ultrasound in Med. & Biol.
3. Roelandt, J.R.T., Bom, N. and Hugenholtz, P.G. (1979) Submitted for publication in Journal of Clinical Ultrasound
4. Roelandt, J.R.T., Wladimiroff, J.W. and Baars, A.M. (1978): Ultrasound Med. Biol. Vol. 4, pp 93-97, Pergamon Press.

ULTRASOUND FETAL MORPHOMETRY

By Hylton B. Meire and Pat. Farrant.

INTRODUCTION

Ultrasound has been used to measure the fetal biparietal
diameter for over two decades now and it can therefore be claimed
that ultrasound fetal morphometry is a well established proven
technique. More recently the occipito-frontal diameter and crown
rump length of the fetus have also been measured and the latter
measurement has proven invaluable in the accurate dating of early
pregnancies. Many other fetal measurements have also been
attempted with the object of assessing the fetal volume or weight
though, it must be confessed, none has yet proven to be clinically
very useful or sufficiently rapid to be widely applied to large
populations on a screening basis.
This report is a preliminary communication concerning a study
initiated to investigate the value of ultrasound in performing
meaningful measurements of other fetal structures which may be of
clinical relevance. We have firstly reviewed the major fetal
malformations to identify which structures are most commonly
abnormal in size or shape. We have concluded that the diameter and
separation of the orbits, the size and shape of the pelvic bones and
the length of the limb bones are all measurements which are
theoretically possible with ultrasound and which may be clinically
useful. Orbital measurements should permit the detection of
microphthalmia and hyper - and hypoteliorism. The morphometry of
the fetal pelvis is abnormal in   several of the chromosomal
disorders and also in a variety of skeletal dysplasias.
The length of the individual limb bones may be affected by the
various forms of primary dwarfism and may also be abnormal in other
syndromes, such as the Ellis Van Creveld syndrome, and may
therefore be used as indicators of this syndrome even though the
cardiac and cerebal malformations cannot be detected at the
present time.
Our experience with orbital and pelvic measurements is still
limited but we have obtained satisfactory preliminary results for
our ultrasound measurements of fetal limb length and these have
already proved useful in several clinical situations. We present
below a brief outline of our technique and results for limb
measurements and a brief analysis of their clinical value.

370

MATERIALS AND METHOD

The patients included in this study were drawn from two sources.
Firstly, patients already being examined as part of a screening
project for fetal abnormalities were used as controls, and secondly
the patients referred in from departments of Clinical Genetics and
Genetic Counselling were used as the high risk group. A particular
effort was made to obtain patients in whom there was an increased
risk of a fetal abnormality in which limb length reduction might
be present.

Initially all scans were performed on a conventional grey scale
B scanner and the majority of our results to date have been
obtained with this equipment. We have found the proximal limb bones
(humerus and femur) the easiest to measure since they most
frequently lie in the same axis as the fetal spine and can
therefore be imaged shortly after the scans taken to confirm the
integrity of the spinal canal. It is important to use a "single
sweep" scanning technique, to ensure that the apparent thickness
of the limb bone is uniform throughout the image, and that
reproducible measurements are obtained on at least three separate
scans of each bone. Having obtained a satisfactory image a
calibration mark is then included on the image and photographic
prints are obtained via a "Vidicam" unit. Measurements can then
be taken at leisure from the permanent images.

We have recently been experimenting with a linear array real
time system with which it is much easier to rapidly and correctly
identify the individual limb bones. With a 'frame freeze' facility
satisfactory images can be obtained and stored very much more
quickly than with a conventional B scanner.

We are performing a comparative investigation of fetal limbs
scanned in a water bath and subsequently x-rayed with a no
magnification technique and have shown that the component of the
fetal limb seen in the ultrasound images is the diaphysis, the
epiphysis not being seen in the ultrasound images. The measurements
obtained with our B scanner correlate very closely with the
measurements from the x-ray images with an error of generally less
than three per cent. It seems unlikely that the real time images
will be so accurate since the lateral resolution of current linear
array systems is less satisfactory than that of a B scanner with
a highly focused transducer. We cannot say yet whether the error
introduced by the real-time systems will be clinically significant.

RESULTS

There are no published data for ultrasound measurement of fetal
limbs in utero with which we can compare our measurements. However,
post mortem examination of aborted fetuses has been performed by
several authors and the normal ranges quoted by these authors show
a fairly wide spectrum and most have not demonstrated any
significant difference in the lengths of the individual limb bones
in the mid trimester of pregnancy (1,2). This may well be because
the exact gestational ages of the fetuses included in these studies
is often uncertain. There is also no universal agreement concerning
the end points between which the measurements should be taken.

371

Our measurements indicate diaphyseal lengths similar to most
of the published data but with a smaller standard deviation and we
have also shown that the lengths of the individual limb bones,
although similar at 15 weeks, becomes significantly different as the
femur becomes disproportionally longer after about 25 weeks. By 28
weeks the femur is 7.5% longer than the humerus and the normal
ranges no longer overlap. These results concur with those
obtained by Mehta and Singh (1972) on aborted fetuses (3). It seems
likely therefore that the ultrasound technique is more accurate than
the previously reported post mortem examinations, though we must
emphasize that this apparent increased accuracy may be due to our
improved confidence in the gestational ages.

Further work is necessary to confirm the normal ranges for the
dimensions of the individual limb bones at different stages in
pregnancy and to improve and consolidate our technique, particularly
with respect to use of the real-time scanner. Despite this
limitation there have been four patients in whom the technique has
proved to be of clinical value in their management. These patients
were referred with a past history of each of the following
conditions: Ellis Van Creveld Syndrome, Thanatophoric Dwarfism,
Achondropla sia and Spondylo Epiphyseal Dysplasia Congenita. In
each case the patients were examined from 12 weeks of pregnancy
onwards and on the initial examination the crown rump length and
fetal biparietal diameter were measured to confirm the gestational
age and attempts were made to measure the limb bone lengths.
Subsequent measurements were taken on several occasions up to the
twentieth week of pregnancy and in all four cases measurements
within the normal range were obtained. All four patients continued
normally to term and delivered normal fetuses with no evidence of the
condition to which they were at risk.

DISCUSSION

Although the newer techniques which we are proposing for
measurement of fetal structures in early pregnancy are still in their
infancy it seems likely that at least some of them will prove to be
of some clinical value. It is, of course, important to emphasize
the need to establish a normal range for the parameters to be
measured and to attempt to examine the fetuses before about twenty
weeks of pregnancy so that therapeutic termination can be considered
if a significant abnormality is discovered.

Although we have included in this study patients with non
lethal conditions such as Achondroplasia and Spondylo Epiphyseal
Dysplasia Congenita we would not normally recommend that patients
at risk from these conditions, and similar non lethal disorders,
should be examined since there is no therapeutic implication in terms
of possible termination of pregnancy. However, these patients do act
as useful examples to permit us to develop and improve our technique
and their help and co-operation in this work is greatfully
acknowledged.

It seems unlikely that the measurements we are proposing can,
or indeed should, be applied to whole populations on a screening
basis. However, with the rapidly expanding use of genetic
counselling services an increasing number of patients at risk for

lethal conditions with detectable fetal morphological abnormalities
are being identified and special ultrasound techniques may well be of
value in these patients.

REFERENCES

1. Nagamori, H., Ebe, M., Sasaki, M., and Kuroda, S. (1965)
   Japanese Journal of Legal Medicine, 19, 422 - 430.
2. Fazekas, I. and Kosa, F. (1966) Ann. Med. Leg., 46, 262 - 272.
3. Mehta, L. and Singh, H. M. (1972) American Journal of Physical
   Anthropology, 36, 165 - 168.

THE USE OF ULTRASOUND IN INTRINSIC GASTRIC DISEASE - A Preliminary
Report

Richard H. Picker, Department of Radiology, Royal North Shore
                   Hospital, Sydney
George Kossoff,   Ultrasonics Institute, Sydney
Peter Warren,   Department of Diagnostic Ultrasound, Royal
                   Hospital for Women, Sydney

During our routine use of the fluid filled stomach as an ultrasonic
window on the Octoson, we have come to recognise the ability of the
technique to demonstrate some pathology which has arisen from the
stomach. This paper presents preliminary findings by the demonstration of several gastric diseases recognised using B-mode
ultrasonography. The presentation consists of examples of both
inflammatory and neoplastic diseases. The published paper demonstrates two cases of malignant disease of the stomach suggesting a
complementary role of ultrasound to conventional radiology by
showing the extent of the disease not shown by radiology.

In Figure 1 we present a transverse echogram through the liver and
fluid filled stomach demonstrating the normal anatomy of the area.
The arrow points to an area on the anterior gastric wall where the
mucosal and muscular layers of the normal stomach wall can be seen.
The mucus layer returns a line of increased reflectivity whilst the
muscular layer is represented by a line of decreased reflectivity.

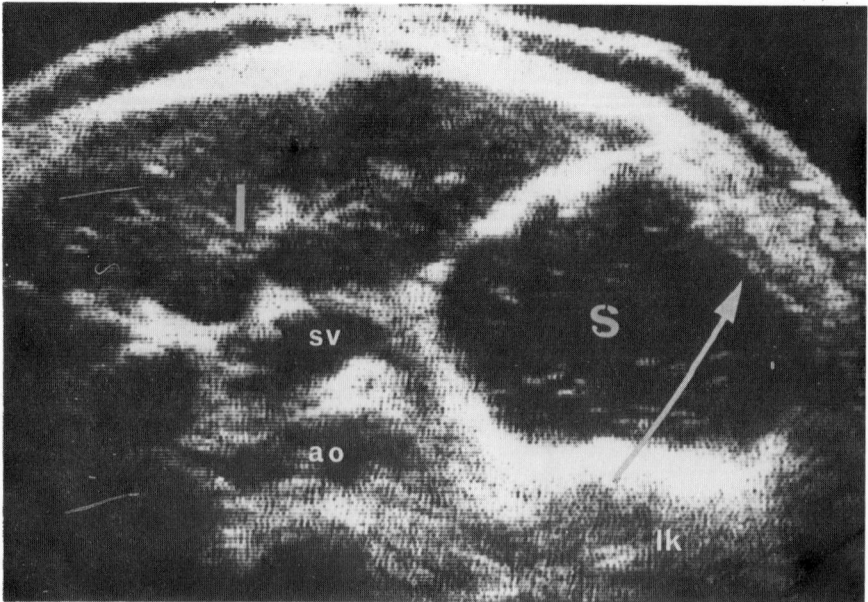

Fig. 1 - Transverse echogram through the normal fluid filled stomach.

In Figure 2, a transverse echogram through the liver and fluid filled stomach, a leiomyosarcoma (m) is seen arising from the posterior gastric wall (arrowed). The stomach is filled with orange juice and lies between the liver (1) and the tumour mass (m). The echogram is able to demonstrate the shape and extent of the tumour which was shown on a barium meal as a filling defect on the posterior wall of the stomach.

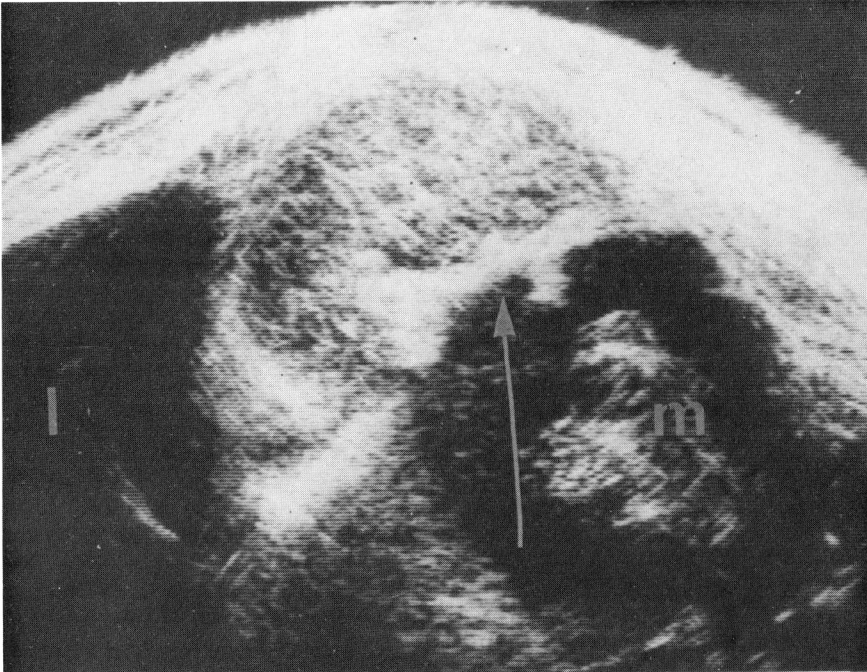

Fig. 2 - Transverse echogram through liver (1) and fluid filled stomach demonstrating a tumour mass (m) arising from the posterior gastric wall.

Figure 3, a longitudinal echogram to the left of the midline through a normal fluid filled stomach demonstrates the stomach (s) containing 1% methyl cellulose allowing visualisation of the left kidney (k) and the tail of the pancreas (p) with the splenic vessels superior to it producing a characteristic indentation in the posterior gastric wall. The contour of the gastric wall, however, is smooth and the mucus layer unbroken to the point where it meets the gas/liquid interface just superior to the pancreas.

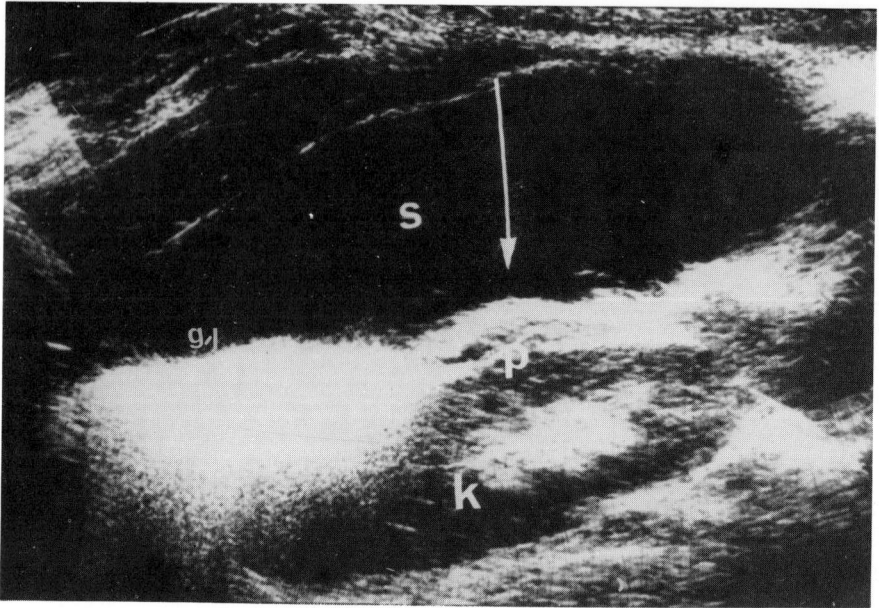

Fig. 3 - Longitudinal echogram through the fluid filled stomach (s) showing the tail of pancreas (p) and left kidney (k).

Figure 4 demonstrates a longitudinal echogram through the fluid filled stomach to the left of the midline in a similar plane as shown in Figure 3. On this occasion there is an adenocarcinoma of the posterior gastric wall high up near the cardia and on the echogram a tumour mass (m) can be seen infiltrating the posterior gastric wall above and behind the tail of the pancreas. There is an irregular break in the mucus line (arrowed) just above the pancreatic indentation. This indicates an area of ulceration in the stomach by the tumour. The findings were confirmed at endoscopy.

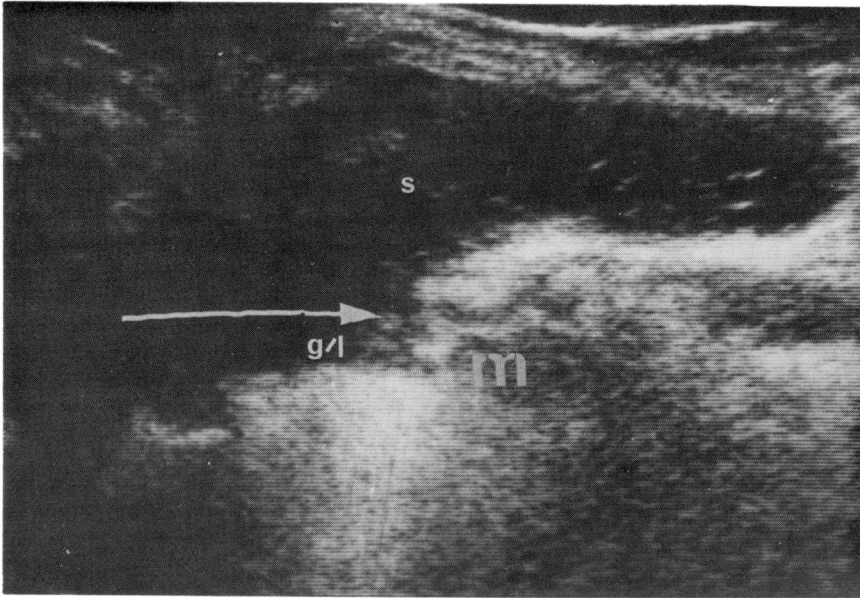

Fig. 4 - Longitudinal echogram through the fluid filled stomach showing a break in the mucosal lining of the stomach (arrowed) by a tumour mass (m). The echogram allows visualisation of the extent of the tumour mass causing the ulceration.

SUMMARY

Preliminary experience with the use of the fluid filled stomach and the Octoson suggests that ultrasound may play a complementary role to conventional radiological techniques by its ability to demonstrate transmural and extragastric involvement in gastric disease. This ability is confirmed by the two illustrative cases presented in this short paper.

IN VIVO DIFFRACTION ANALYSIS

D. Nicholas

Physics Department, Royal Marsden Hospital, Sutton,
Surrey, U.K.

It has previously been demonstrated (Nicholas and
Hill, 1975) that human soft tissues can be characterised
by utilising a diffraction phenomenon analogous to the
Bragg diffraction of X-rays by crystalline structures.
These results showed that, in a pulse echo system, if a
sample of tissue is rotated relative to the beam axis,
the amplitude of the frequency-filtered backscattered
signal, from a small tissue volume located on the axis
of rotation, varied with angle. Moreover, the diffraction
patterns (relationships of echo amplitude to orientation
angle) thus formed were found to characterise differing
tissue types and pathologies (Nicholas, 1976). It has
been postulated by Nicholas and Hill (1975) that the
tissues examined comprise a semi-regular array of
scatterers over the small volume being interrogated,
and that the diffraction patterns result from constructive
and destructive interference of the backscattered signal
from each scatterer. Since many diseases only result in
a subtle change in the structural composition of a tissue
it seems likely that any technique which is capable of
monitoring such changes could have immense diagnostic
implications.

METHODS

The equipment and methods used for laboratory implem-
entation of this technique have been described in earlier
papers and a prototype equipment designed for clinical
application, with the examination performed in a manner
similar to that used for conventional B-scanning, has
been described by Huggins and Phelps (1977). The results
reported here have been obtained using the latter equipment modified to be capable of providing a conventional
B-scan image in addition to the diffraction information.
The present version of the diffraction scanner has completed clinical trials and the stage has been reached
where both it and the in vivo technique can be evaluated
in terms of their limitations, potential and present
diagnostic capabilities.

CLINICAL RESULTS

In this paper the results of a clinical trial involving 70 patients with various hepatic diseases are presented. Investigations have been performed on the two categories of disease best described as diffuse disorders and focal neoplasms. In the former case, organs which exhibit a uniform parenchymal echo pattern (though abnormal) on the conventional B-scan images are examined over as wide a region as possible with diffraction patterns being collected from randomly selected regions of the tissue. For the second case, regions of interest (suspected lesions) are first located using standard scanning techniques, and then diffraction patterns obtained from within the suspected lesions are compared with those from adjacent, supposedly normal, regions of tissue. As this latter case involves a differential analysis it permits an immediate appraisal of tissue normality.

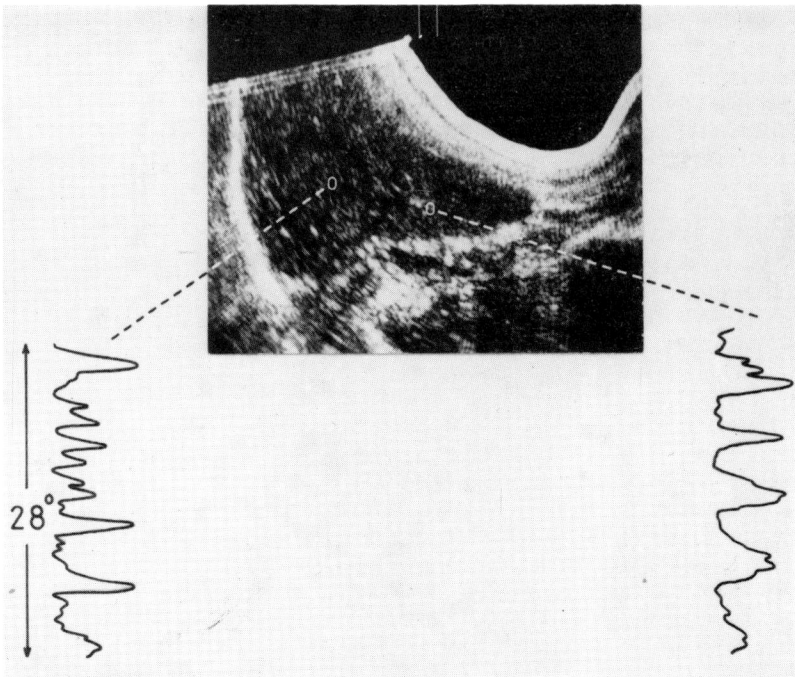

Figure 1. Longitudinal B-scan of the right lobe of the liver depicting an anechoic ring of approximately 3 cm diameter. Accompanying diffraction patterns confirm this as a solid lesion.

Figure 1 illustrates the procedure and results for one particular patient. The longitudinal B-scan of the patient showed an interesting area of about 4 cm diameter in the posterior region of the right lobe of the liver. The enlarged picture of this region indicated that it consisted of a ring of diminished echoes within which the echo pattern was visually indistinguishable from that of the, supposedly normal, adjacent parenchymal echoes. The clinical diagnosis based on this conventional scan and others was inconclusive as to whether this region was metastatic or normal. The ring of diminished echoes was suggestive of a 'target' lesion but these usually display an abnormal pattern of internal echoes. When investigated with the diffraction scanner at a frequency of 2.5 MHz and with a 10μs gate length the region of interest produced a diffraction pattern which differed significantly from the scans associated with the supposedly normal regions. This difference, an increase in the number of diffraction peaks per unit angle of scanning movement, is typical of both the in vitro findings of Nicholas (1976) and previous in vivo results where similar patterns have been associated with neoplastic involvement. Confirmation of these findings was obtained on the following day when a liver scintigram clearly indicated the presence of a large single lesion in the posterior border of the right lobe of the liver.

The main advantage of this method of tissue characterisation is the ease with which the diffraction patterns can be quantified, thus eliminating the need for subjective evaluation. At present the diffraction scanner is connected on-line to a PDP/8e computer, enabling the patterns to be digitised and stored on magnetic tape. Although various analytical approaches are available for quantitation of these scans, the results of this survey were based upon the application of Fourier techniques.

CONCLUSION

The results of our preliminary trial (Nicholas, 1979) can be summarised according to the method of scanning and disease state. Where a differential method can be applied, as in focal disorders of the liver, the technique involves making a diffraction record within the focal abnormality and comparing this with the corresponding record for, supposedly, normal liver tissue. In this situation a 95% success rate was achieved in determining the malignant state of the abnormality. Only 2 cases were incorrectly classified as normal and in each case only a single deposit of diameter between 1.2 and 2.5 cm was involved. The error in diagnosis in these cases may well have been associated with incorrect positioning of the scanning arm, and consequent failure to locate the suspected region.

380

The technique also seems particularly useful in differentiating between fluid filled lesions (containing debris) and degenerating tumours, both of which can produce similar appearances on conventional sector B-scans. The diffraction patterns associated with the former are non-repeatable due to the motion of the debris within the lesion, whilst the latter present some degree of rigidity in structure and thus give patterns which exhibit some repeatable features.

The use of diffraction scanning to characterise specific diffuse disorders has met with varied degrees of success. Diffuse neoplastic liver involvement is easily characterised, with diffraction patterns similar to those associated with focal neoplasms. So far a 100% success rate in detecting malignant infiltration of the liver has been achieved in our investigation of 11 cases (including 5 cases of widespread 'patchy' metastatic involvement) involving 61 diffraction patterns. Of the other types of diffuse disorder only cirrhotic tissue has yet produced a specific disease signature, where a single cycle modulation of the diffraction pattern occurs. Although many patterns have been collected, the variations in disease types have resulted in too few examinations of specific tissue pathologies to do other than group them into broad categories. It is to be hoped that when a larger set of data has been accumulated a more specific differentiation of tissue abnormalities may prove possible.

Many problems specific to in vivo studies must be investigated before the true potential of this technique can be realised. Parameteric studies of quantities such as transmit pulse length, frequency and volume size are at present being performed, whilst an evaluation of the effects of intervening tissue layers of muscle, fat and skin has yet to be performed.

The clinical value of our present apparatus can only be postulated at this stage, but the results indicate that it is capable of providing useful quantitative data to complement the high quality grey-scale scans that are at present attainable.

REFERENCES

Nicholas, D. and Hill, C. R. (1975): Nature, 257, 305.
Nicholas, D. (1976): In: Proc. 1976 I.E.E.E. Ultrasonic Symposium, pp. 64-69, 76CH1120-55u.
Huggins, R. W. and Phelps, J. V. (1977): Ultrasound Med. Biol. 2, 271.
Nicholas, D. (1979): Brit. J. Radiol. (in press).

THE USE OF B MODE SCANNING IN THE OPERATING THEATRE

RODNEY J. LANE M.B., B.S., F.R.A.C.S., F.R.C.S.,F.R.C.S.E

Vascular Fellow, St. Mary's Hospital, London U.K.

Surgeons rely very much on what they can feel to assess what they cannot see - particularly intraoperatively. Intraoperative real time B mode scanning allows insight into the lumena of hollow tubes and solid organs without invading their substance. The main advantage, over intraoperative radiology is the easily repeatable multiplanar images and although the technique is in its infancy it has great practical appeal to the general surgeon. The applications are described in the pancreatico - biliary and arterial trees.

METHODOLOGY

A real time ocular transducer of 10 megahertz (Xenotec U.S.A.) is sterilised with ethylene oxide. The ultrasound machine is isolated with a transformer to allow the use of diathermy and the patient is anaesthetised with a non-inflamable agent. To achieve acoustic coupling the area is flooded with saline after the organ to be examined is exposed.

ULTRASONIC ARTERIOGRAPHY

Stenoses of arteries are never absolutely round so no finite number of longitudinal radiographs can give an accurate estimation of cross sectional area. On table scanning readily provides multiplanar information which therefore refines the preoperative angiogram by defining posterior plaques and has the potential of replacing radiology as the "gold standard" for non-invasive physiological tests particularly in the carotid area (Carotid Phonoangiography, Supra orbital doppler and oculoplethysmography). The profunda orifice is another area consistently underestimated by contrast radiology. Fig. 1 is a profunda orifice (true sagittal section) on ultrasound showing a 50% stenosis which was reported normal on the standard arteriogram.
Detection of technical error post reconstruction by radiology is a time consuming, difficult to organise, procedure that exposes the surgeon to repeated irradiation. It therefore has not received wide acceptance but errors are relatively common - in some series up to 27%. The

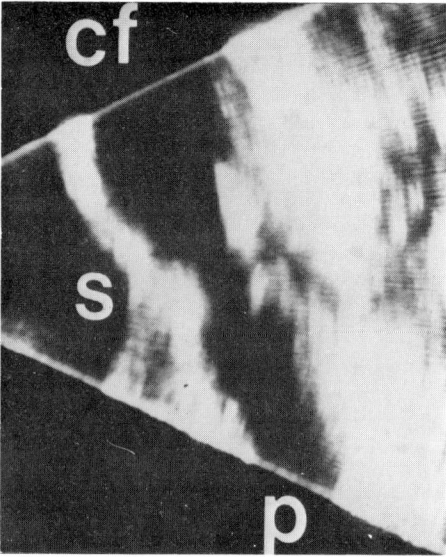

Figure 1: Stenosed profunda orifice. c.f. is common femoral, p is profunda, s is the stenosis.

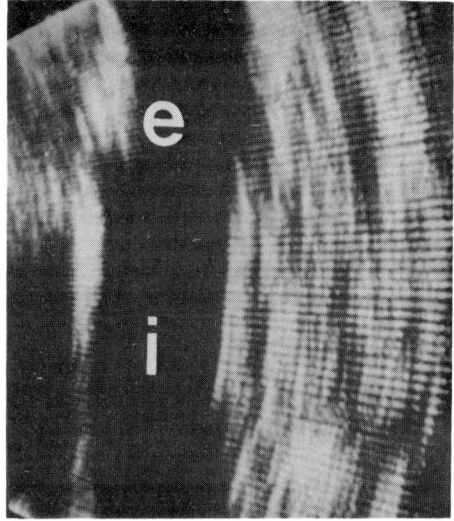

Figure 2: End of endartectomy. i is internal carotid, e is a large step.

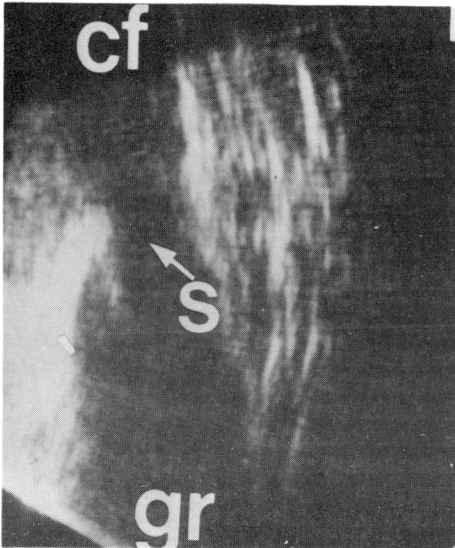

Figure 3: 40% stenosis of anastomosis. gr is the graft, s is the stenosis.

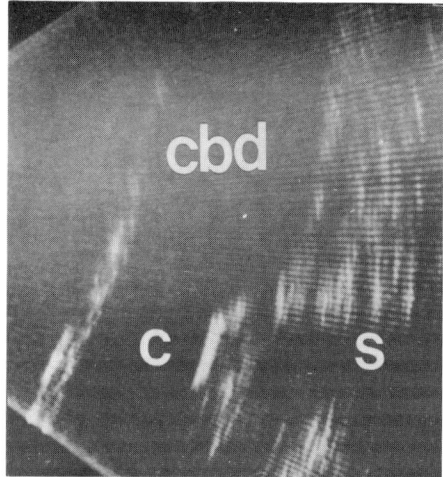

Figure 4: cbd is the common bile duct. c is the calculus. s is the shadow.

commonest errors are those associated with endarter-
ectomies where residual plaques or flaps may provide a lo-
cus for mural thrombosis and embolisation, complete thrombosis or in the long term predisposing to recurrence of
the atheromatous process. Fig. 2 is an abnormal step following a carotid endarterectomy. The critical projections
to detect anastomotic error are the true lateral, to determine inflow-outflow obstructions (in end to side grafts)
and a cross section midway through the anastomosis. Neither of these can be reliably obtained by on-table radiology. Fig. 3 is a stenosis of an aorto-bifemoral graft at
the distal end.

THE BILIARY TREE

Most surgeons perform operative cholangiography with
cholecystectomy to detect unsuspected stones in the common
bile duct. The procedure is unsatisfactory in one third
of cases as there may be difficulties in cannulation, air
bubbles, position and extravasation of dye. Ultrasound
has the potential of providing the same information in less
time. Fig. 4 shows a stone in the dilated common bile duct
casting a posterior shadow whilst fig. 5 shows an impacted
stone at the lower end of the duct which should be compared with the lower end of the normal duct (fig 6). Presently some skill in manipulation and interpretation is required to detect all stones and simplification of the technique involves placing a sonically uniform base (plastic)
behind the mobolised head of pancreas. The stones are indicated by a discontinuity in the linear echo of the plastic (caused by shadowing). This considerably facilitates
interpretation by the general surgeon.

THE PANCREAS

Ultrasonic scanning of the pancreas provides information about the duct, the parenchyma and immediate anatomical relations. Apart from locating small tumours (insuli-
nomas, gastrinomas) determination of portal vein infiltration in neoplastic disease saves the surgeon a time-wast-
ing trial dissection. Fig. 7 shows a carcinoma of the pancreas completely obstructing the portal vein. The ductal
structures are defined in fig. 8 in a patient with chronic
pancreatitis showing the "chain of lakes" phenomenon.

DISCUSSION

The present difficulties are related mostly to probe
design, notably the large size, limited sector angle and
the penetration is restricted to 4 cms. by the 10 meq transducer. Specific types of probes are required for different areas: In the arteries/pancreas a linear array would
allow a longer segment for comparison whilst a 3 meg (liver) and 5 meg (kidney) would allow suitable penetration.

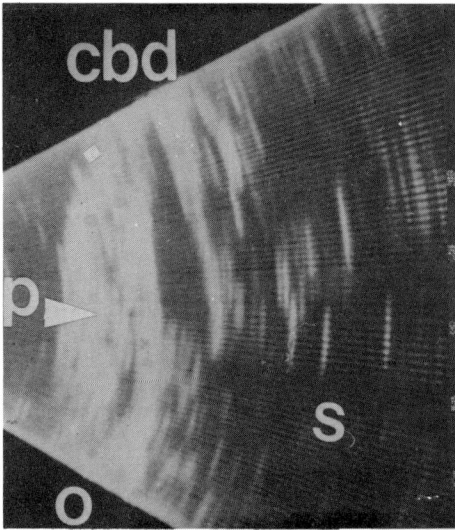

Figure 5: Stone in the end
of the common bile duct cbd
with shadow s. o is the sph-
incter, p is pancreas.

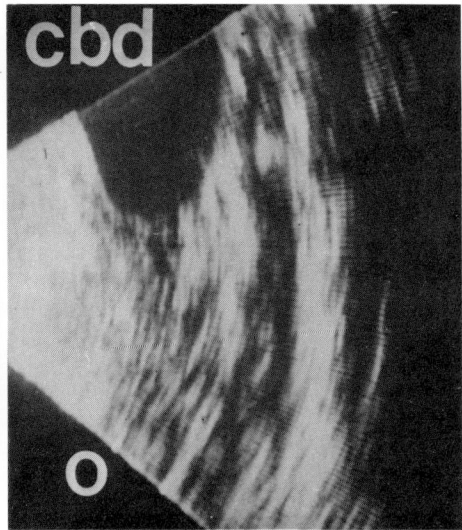

Figure 6: Normal lower end
of the common bile duct.

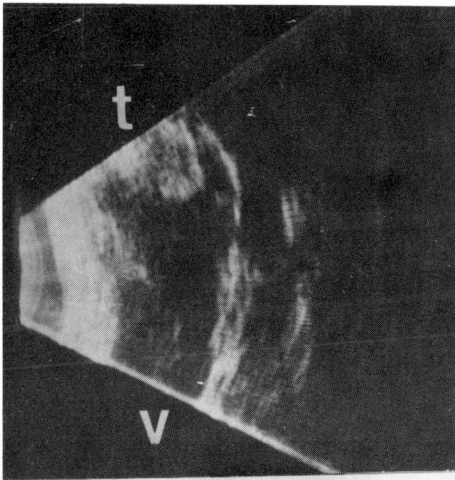

Figure 7: Tumour of the
pancreas, t completely obstructing portal vein v.

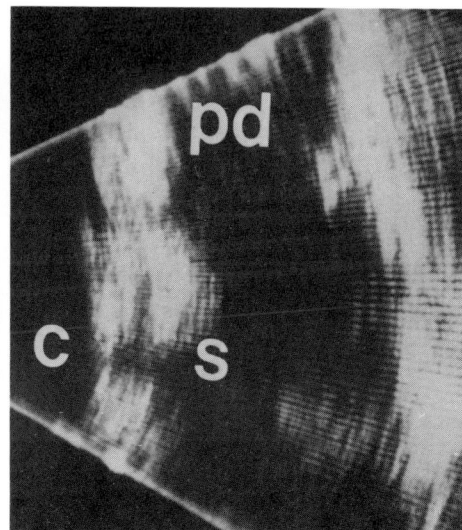

Figure 8: dilated pancreatic duct pd. c is calcifi-
cation with a shadow s.

11. ULTRASOUND MONITORING OF OVARIAN STIMULATION

B. J. Hackelöer, Chairman

Ultrasound Monitoring of Ovarian Stimulation,
by B.J. Hackelöer, Universitäts-Frauenklinik, Marburg,
W-Germany

Members: A. Christie (Scotland), B. Funduk-Kurjak
(Yugoslavia), S.Nitschke-Dabelstein (W-Germany), H.
Persson)Sweden), R. Picker (Australia), R.Terinde
(W-Germany).

Introduction
B.J. Hackelöer

In 1975 we started to monitor follicular growth in
gonadotrophin stimulated patients, based on first reports by Kratochwil concerning ovarian imaging by ultrasound in 1972. First results were published in 1976
and 1977 and were reported on the last Dubrovnik conference in 1977. At this time we started monitoring
normal, physiological cycles, in addition, to see
wether there was a significant discrepancy between the
preovulatory follicular diameter of stimulated cases
compared to those of unstimulated physiological cycles.
This was not the case. At same time other groups started to get their own experience in ovarian and follicular imaging by ultrasound. Different follicular diameter seen preovulatory by other group, when, mostly
originated in different technique of measuring the follicle.
It is nice to have most of the groups, active in this
field and scattered all over the world, represented
here on this round table, in order to hear about their
findings and their difficulties in imaging cyclic
ovarian changes. This will give us a chance to discuss
the reproducibility and possibility of clinical application of this method in the investigation and treatment of the infertile woman.

Ultrasound Monitoring Of Follicular Growth In Hormone
Stimulated Ovaries.

A.D. Christie, Dept. of Obstetrics & Gynaecology, University of Dundee, Scotland.

Introduction: Following the recently reported succes of
follicle visualisation by ultrasound (1), we decided to
investigate the value of ultrasound scanning in patients
undergoing hormone treatment for primary infertility.
As there is always some doubt as to whether or not ovulation has actually taken place, it was felt that visual proof of follicular development through to the cor-

pus luteum stage would be valuable in assessing the
effectiveness of a particular course of treatment. In
our investigations, two groups of patients have been
monitored - those on Clomiphene therapy, and those on
Perganol/HCG stimulation.

METHOD:
The full bladder technique was used and the equipment
a Nuclear Enterprises Diasonograph, 4102 series using
a frequency of 5MHz. All patients were routinely examined at two-day intervals commencing at DAY 8 of the
menstrual cycle until DAY 18. In some cases where hyperstimulation occurred, large follicular cysts were
monitored up to DAY 28 or later - Fig. I and Fig. 2.

RESULTS:
Two groups were studied as follows.
1. 10 Patients undergoing Clomiphene Therapy.
   Having confirmed on a series of 6 normally ovulating
   patients the data reported by Hackelöer (1) concerning the mean follicular diameter for successful
   ovulation, we used these figures as a basis for our
   investigations.
   In our 10 patients we found the following: -
   a) 5 patients ovulated on standard dosage and a
      corpus luteum developed.
   b) 3 patients ovulated on a doubled dosage failed
      to ovulate on 2 standard dose cycles.
   c) 2 patients failed to ovulated on a standard,
      double, and trebled dosage. These are now being
      considered for alternative treatment.
   Of the 8 patients who have now ovulated, 2 have
   recently become pregnant.

2. Perganol/HCG - 4 Patients.
   In this series, hormonal evidence was related to
   ovarian response to stimulation. In one case, erroneous hormone levels were reported (but later corrected !), resulting in hyperstimulation of both
   ovaries.
   a) In 3 patients, 2 cycles have been studied, the
      first of which, in each case, resulted in under-
      stimulation. Increased dosage in the 2nd cycle
      resulted in hyperstimulation of both ovaries with
      development of several follicular cysts in each.
      No HCG stimulation was given in these cases.
   b) In the fourth patient, 3 cycles have been studied.
      In the first both ovaries became hyperstimulated
      after HCG was administered following an incorrect
      hormone assay result. In the 2nd cycle, the per-
      ganol dose was reduced and no ovulation took
      place. In the 3rd cycle, an intermediate dose was
      given and ovulation occurred. Two corpus lutea

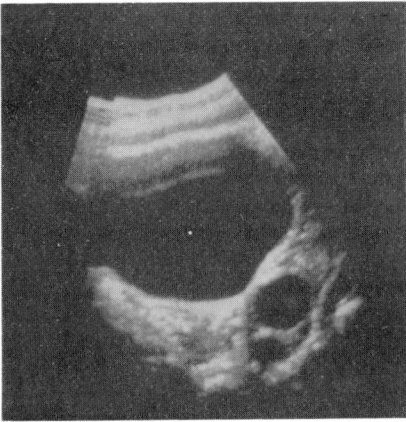

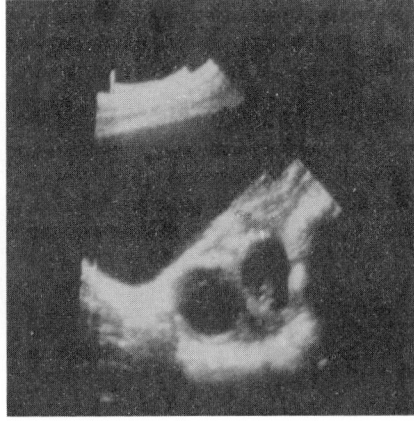

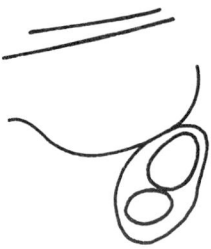

DAY 14   DAY 16

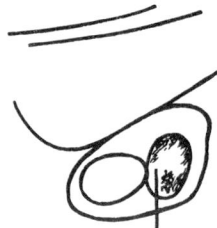

Corpus Luteum

(R) OVARY

Figure 1:

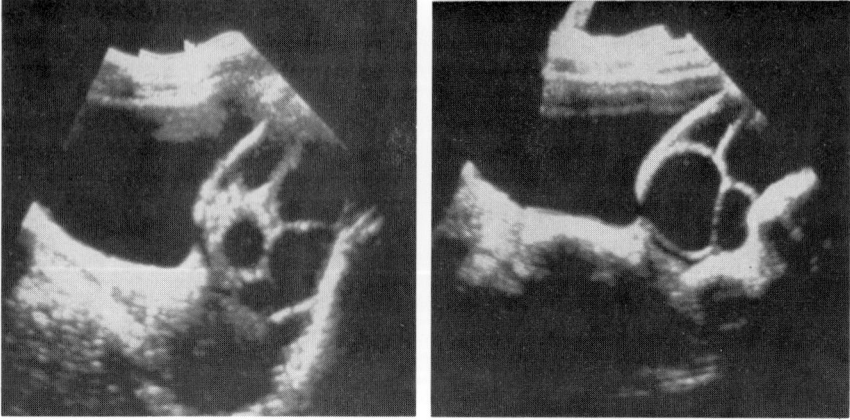

Max d = 38 mm

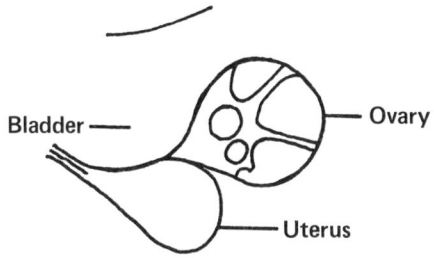

HYPERSTIMULATED OVARY — DAY 26

Figure 2:

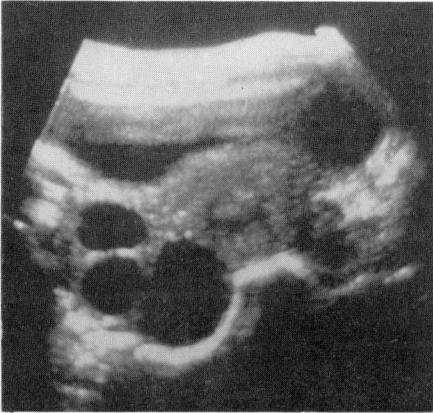

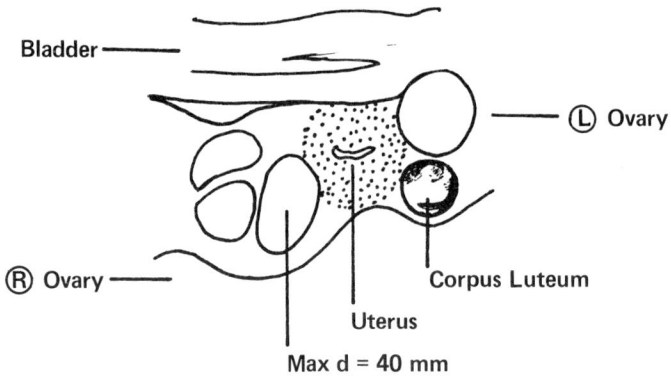

Bladder

(L) Ovary

(R) Ovary

Corpus Luteum

Uterus

Max d = 40 mm

EARLY PREGNANCY – 28 DAYS POST

OVULATION (HCG STIMULATED)

Figure 3:

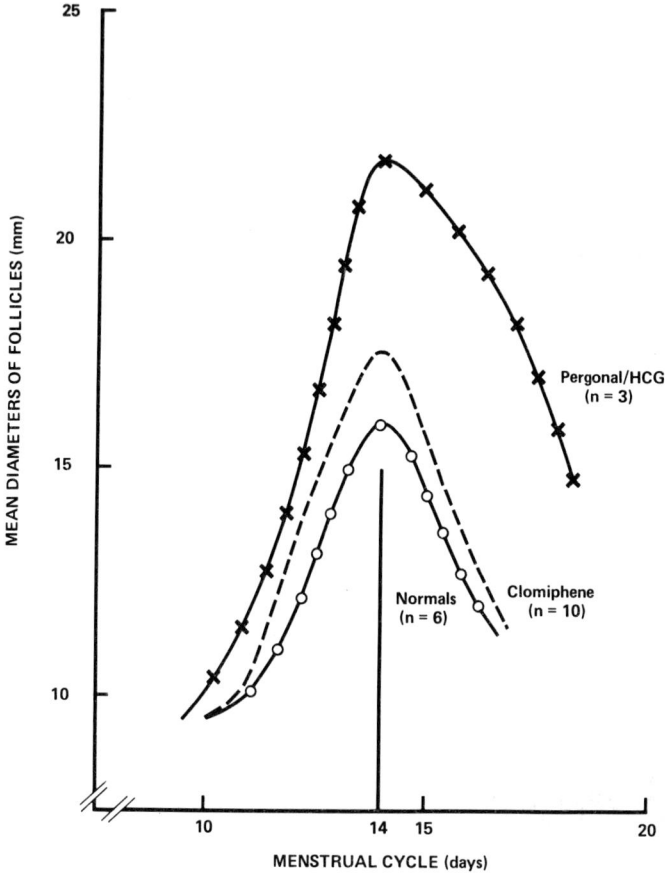

Figure 4:

were identified and this patient now has a twin pregnancy. Fig. 3.

Conclusion:

The results and experience gained from this limited series indicate to us that ultrasound screening of infertile patients undergoing hormone therapy has much to offer in indicating the effectiveness of a particular dose, and in being able to indicate visually those ovaries which produce multiple follicles under stimulation. It is thus a most useful complimentary technique to standard hormone investigatory procedures.

TWO - YEAR EXPERIENCE IN ULTRASONIC MONITORING OF FOLLICULAR GROWTH.

Biserka Funduk-Kurjak.

Stimulated by the impressive results obtained by Hackelöer and his group, we started in October 1977, to ultrasonically monitor the growth and development of ovarian follicles. Between 15 October 1977 and 15 September 1979, we examined 20 patients with a normal menstrual cycle and 85 patients who underwent ovarian stimulation. Sixty of these patients were treated with Clomiphen, 1 with Parlodel and 24 with Gonadotropins. Three hundred and seventy measurements were taken in 134 cycles in the group of stimulated patients, while 102 measurements were made in the group of 20 normal cycling women.
The British machine, Diasonograph 4200 and the full-bladder technique were used for all examinations.
Hackelöer's technique was closely followed for all the other detailed procedures. Ultrasonic visualization of the normal sized uterus and both ovaries is shown in Figure 5.
Figure 6 illustrates the technique of measurement. We used two bright calipers and a direct measurement from the inside to the inside of the follicular cystic structure.
The first results obtained with ultrasonic monitoring of normal cycling women have been published elsewhere (Funduk-Kurjak, Kurjak, 1978 a and b). It was found that approximately 3-4 days prior to ovulation, follicles could be visualized and then measured in almost all cases. The mature follicle just prior to ovulation had a diameter of 18-24 mm.
A linear increase of the mean maximum follicular diameter was seen ranging from 11.5 to 22.6 mm in the second group. There was no significant difference between Clomiphen and Gonadotropins patients. Further details about this were presented at the 3rd World Congress on Ultrasound (Funduk-Kurjak and Kurjak, 1979a). Ultrasonic

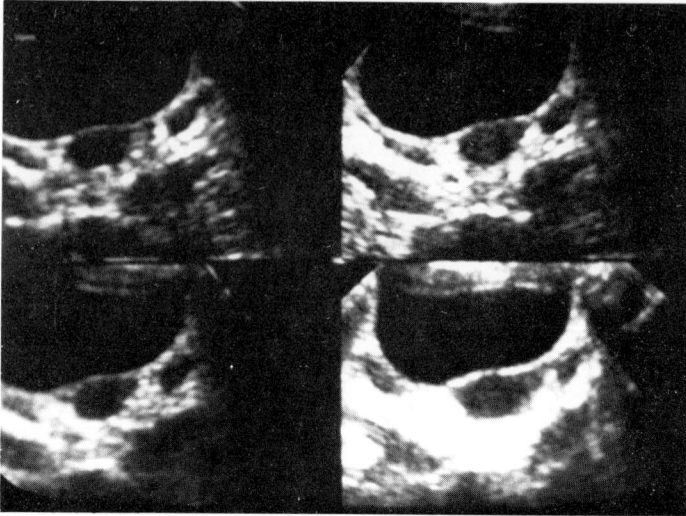

Figure 5:

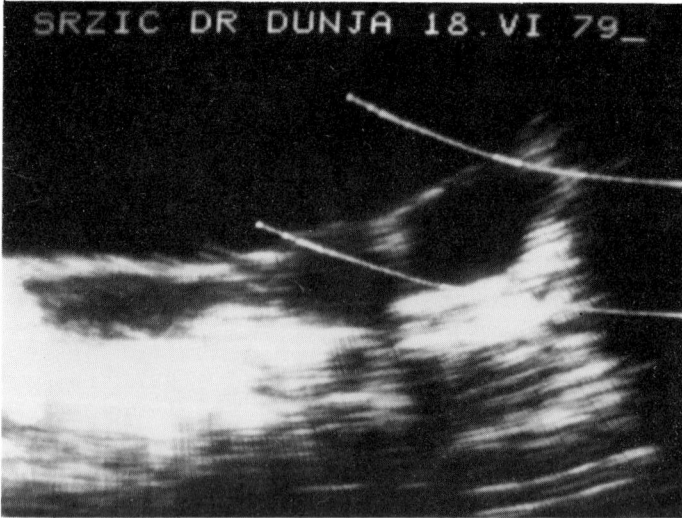

Figure 6:

assessment of early pregnancy after stimulation of
ovulation have also been described recently (Funduk-
Kurjak and Kurjak, 1979b). Seventeen patients became
pregnant and among them there were 10 normal single
pregnancies, 1 triplets, 4 twins and 2 blighted ova.
A successful ultrasonic diagnosis was made in all patients. In multiple pregnancies, more than one follicle
was observed and multiple pregnancies were suspected in
all of them. We had an interesting case of triplets in
which three equally growing follicles were found by
early identification of three embryos. Three healthy
babies were delivered safely at 36 weeks of pregnancy.

After almost two years of practical experience, it is
now our belief that this method is a simple, safe,
clinically reliable means for determining follicular
development and the time of ovulation. It should be
widely used as a routine clinical tool in the monitoring of ovarian stimulation.
However, the technique requires an experienced examiner,
especially in the recognition of the corpus luteum
formation.

Comparison of Ultrasonic and Hormonal Monitoring of
Follicular Growth in Patients Receiving Ovarian Stimulating Therapy.

Nitschke-Dabelstein, S.
University of Marburg, Department of Obstetrics and
Gynecology, West Germany.

Regular ultrasonic monitoring of ovulatory cycles in
the past years has shown that ultrasonography is a well
reproducible method for the observation of follicular
growth. To assess the usefulness of this method in routine clinical practice, the following questions had to
be answered:
1. Whether the follicular size measured by ultrasonics
   is a dependable parameter for prediction of ovulation;
2. whether ovarian stimulating therapy in ovulatory disorders influences the follicular size prior to ovulation,
3. whether multifollicular development alters the size
   of the Graafian follicle;
4. whether ultrasonic monitoring is a safe methode for
   preventing hyperstimulation in multifollicular ovarian reaction in patients treated with gonadotrphins;
5. which procedure in monitoring gonadotrophin treated
   patients will be the best when additional ultrasonic
   monitoring is possible.

In 1977 we started a prospective study of patients receiving various stimulating therapy for ovulatory disorders. For purposes of comparison, at the time of daily ultrasonic examination, which started at the 8th to 10th day of the cycle, corresponding to the 4th to 5th days of stimulation, blood samples were taken for later collective radioimmunological assessment of FSH, LH, 17ß-estradiol and progesterone. Ultrasonic measurements of the follicle were performed in 3 or at least 2 planes: longitudinal, sagittal and transversal (Fig. 7+ 8); the mean diameter was taken as follicular size.

Included in the study were the following cycles, which were considered ovulatory because of a preovulatory LH-peak, following or coinciding with a 17ß-estradiol maximum, and a progesterone elevation starting 1 to two days prior to the typical postovulatory changes of the ruptured follicle demonstrable in ultrasonics (4) (Fig. 9)

<blockquote>
10 epimestrol treated cases (3)
20 clomiphene treated cases (3)
24 gonadotrophin treated cases (5)
 2 bromocryptine treated cases
</blockquote>

<u>Follicular maturation</u> took an average of 3.9 to 4.1 days from the first ultrasonic observation of a follicle exceeding 13 mm in size to a Graafian follicle on the day of the LH-peak or the day of HCG application, resp. 3.9 to 4.1 days on the average.

The <u>mean follicular sizes</u> on the day before typical postovulatory structural changes in ultrasonics revealed ovulation ranged from 20.2 mm (SEM $\pm$ 0.8) in the epimestrol to 22.6 mm (SEM $\pm$ 0.7) in the clomiphene treated cycles with unifollicular development. There was no significant difference in the size of the Graafian follicle either among differently treated patients or when unifollicular and multifollicular cases were compared (Tab.1)

<u>Mean plasma 17ß-estradiol</u> on the day before ovulatory changes were observed ranged from 199 pg/ml (SEM $\pm$ 20.9) in epimestrol treated patients to 320.4 pg/ml (SEM $\pm$ 32.6) in gonadotrophin treated patients with unifollicular cycles. These values were in the range described for spontaneous ovulatory cycles in the literature (1).
In cases with multifollicular development, seen in clomiphene and gonadotrophin treated cases, the mean 17ß-estradiol levels prior to ovulation were significantly above normal (Tab.1).

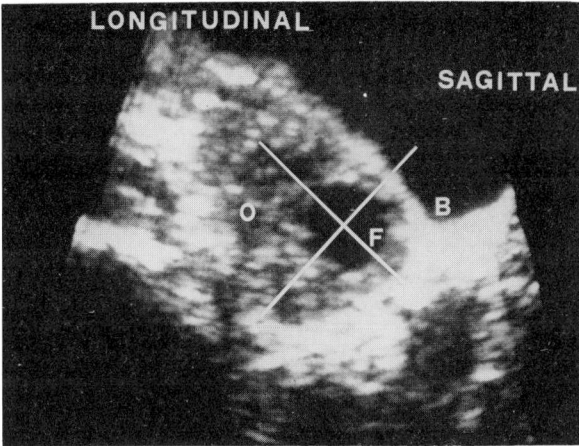

Fig. 7. Longitudinal and sagittal plane of the follicle (F)
O=Ovary   B=Urine bladder

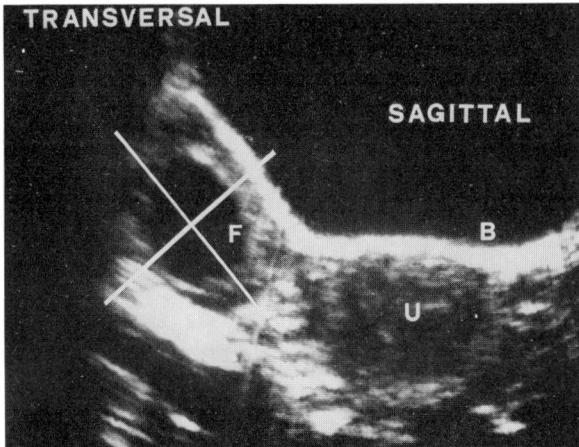

Fig. 8. Transversal and sagittal plane of the follicle

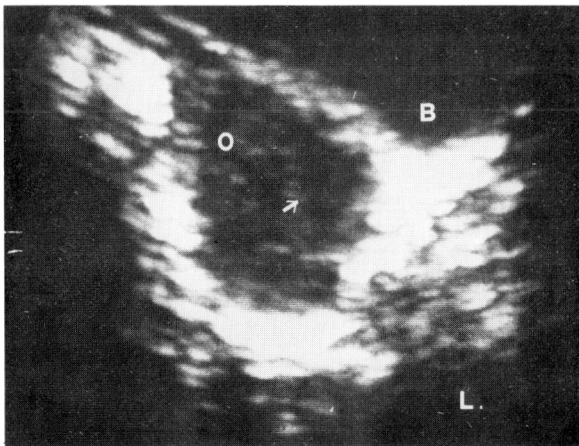

Fig. 9. Ovary (O) shortly after ovulation, residual loosening after
collapse of the follicle. L = Longitudinal scan

Mean Values of Follicular Size, Plasma 17ß-Estradiol, and Plasma Progesterone on the Day prior to Ovulation in Stimulated Ovulatory Cycles.

Kind of Stimulation	No. of treated cycles	Follicular Size mm $\bar{x} \pm$ SEM	17ß-Estradiol pg/ml $\bar{x} \pm$ SEM	Progesterone ng/ml $\bar{x} \pm$ SEM
Epimestrol	10	20.2± 0.8	198.0+20.9	0.84+0.14
Clomiphene I. unifollicular cycles	16	22.6± 0.7	283.9±17.6	1.85±0.32
II. multifollicular cycles	4	22.1± 1.7	570.0±120.7	337±1.18
Gonadotrophin I. unifollicular cycles	13	22.0± 0.7	320.4±32.6	1.42±0.24
II. multifollicular cycles	11	22.2± 0.5	972.9±110.4	4.24±1.25
Bromocryptine	2	21.0 ∅	215.0 ∅	0.7 ∅

Table 1

Mean plasma progesterone values on the day before ovulatory changes were detected tanged from 0.84 ng/ml (SEM ± 0.14) in the epimestrol to 1.85 ng/ml (SEM ± 0.32) in the clomiphene treated group (Tab. 1), when only unifollicular cycles were considered. When multifollicular development occurred, however, the mean plasma progesterone concentration exceeded the limit of 2 ng/ml described for spontaneous ovulatory cycles (2) on the day prior to ovulation (Tab. 1), thus demonstrating that more than one follicle was the source of progesterone excretion at this time. In half of the multifollicular cases treated with gonadotrophin the high progesterone concentration preovulatorily was accompanied by a BBT elevation and a decrease in the cervical score.

SUMMARY

It is well known that hormonal monitoring of the menstrual cycle fails to elucidate actual functional changes in the ovary and is not able to provide an exact parameter for follicular maturation. The described results show that follicular size measured by ultrasound is a dependable parameter for ovarian reaction regardless of the kind of stimulatin therapy and independent of uni- or multifollicular development, whereas 17ß-estradiol and progesterone concentrations in these cases differ significantly. For routineclinical practice, especially in gonadotrophin therapy, regular ultrasonic observation in thus the most reliable method in monitoring those patients. In addition this method makes it possible to induce ovulation even when high 17ß-estradiol values are found in multifollicular reaction, provided that only one or two predominant follicles are found and cervical mucus shows no progesterone influence.

Ultrasound Monitoring of Follicular Size as an Aid in In Vitro Fertilization and Transfer of Human Oocytes.

P.- H. Persson

In vitro fertilization and transfer of human oocytes is a technique under rapid development. To achieve fertilization in vitro it is important to obtain preo-ovulatory "eggs" as close to the normal time for ovulation as possible. To find the optimum time for collection is difficult; the parameters used are basal body temperature, serum progesterone and serum oestradiol. Hackelöer and others suggested monitoring of the follicular maturation by ultrasound.

To evaluate the usefulness of ultrasound monitoring of follicular growth before aspiration of follicles and in vitro fertilization, 57 women were examined by ultrasound two hours before laparotomy or laparoscopy. Fourty-seven of the women underwent operation due to either primary or secundary sterility. To secure ovulation these women were treated with clomiphene 50 mg daily for 5 days with the beginning on the 5th day of the cycle. 9.000 IU HCG (Gonadex[R]) were given 34 hours before the operation. The remaining 10 women were sterilized through laparotomy. Operation was planned to the 14th day of the cycle. These 10 women were only given 9.000 IU HCG 34 hours before operation. Ultrasound examination was performed with 400 ml of saline in the bladder. Only largest follicular diameter was measured.

At laparotomy or laparoscopy the visible follicles were aspirated with the aid of a neddle with 1 mm diameter connected to a vacuum pump with 200 mm Hg pressure. The follicular fluid was aspirated, its volume measured and the presence of oocytes immedaitely examined. Oocytes were classified as pre-ovulatory in the presence of a first polar body and a sticky, loose mass of cumulus cells. The oocyte was incubated with a sperm suspension in Tyrode's medium at 37°C and 5 % CO_2 pressure in an incubator for 24 hours, whereafter the egg was trans-

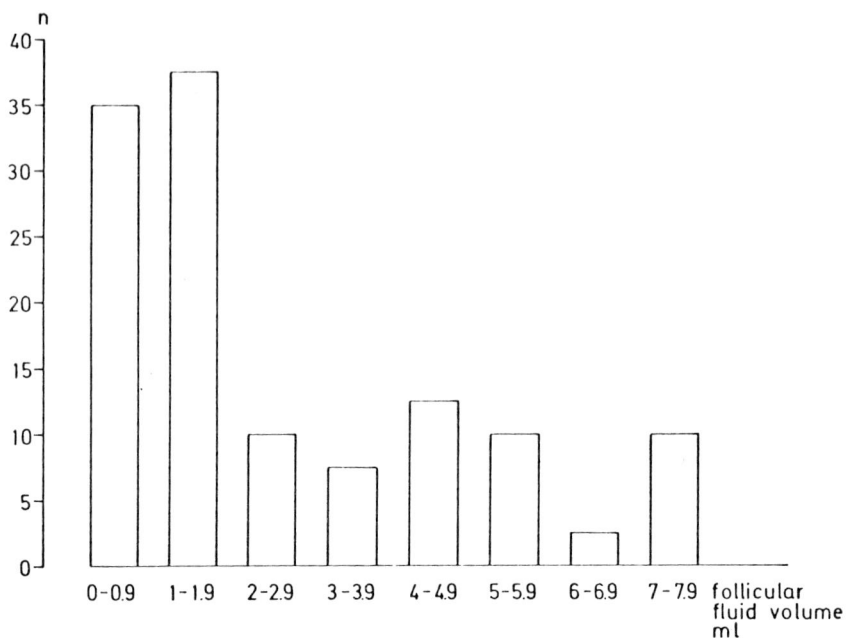

Fig. 10. Number of follicles and the follicular fluid volume from which preovulatory eggs could be obtained.

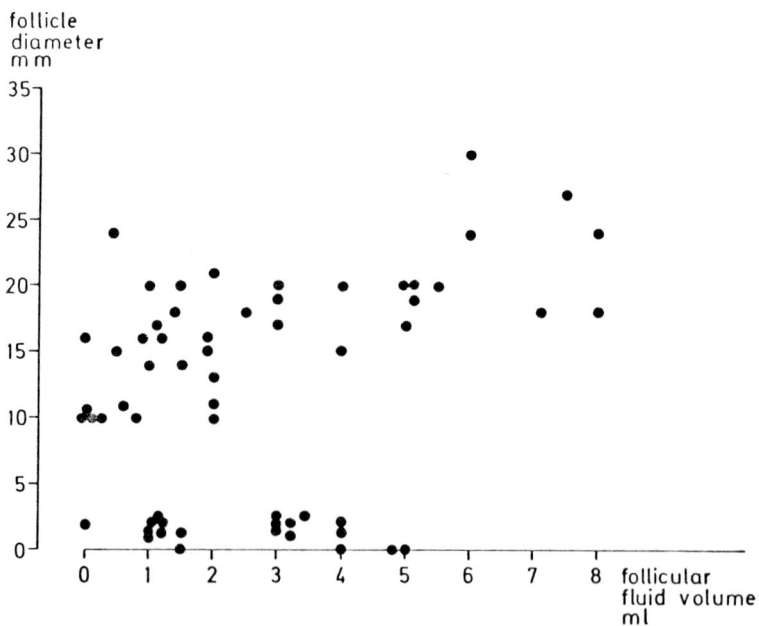

Fig. 11. Correlations between the diameter of the largest follicle measured by ultrasound and the volume of the follicular fluid obtained by aspiration at laparotomy or laparoscopy.

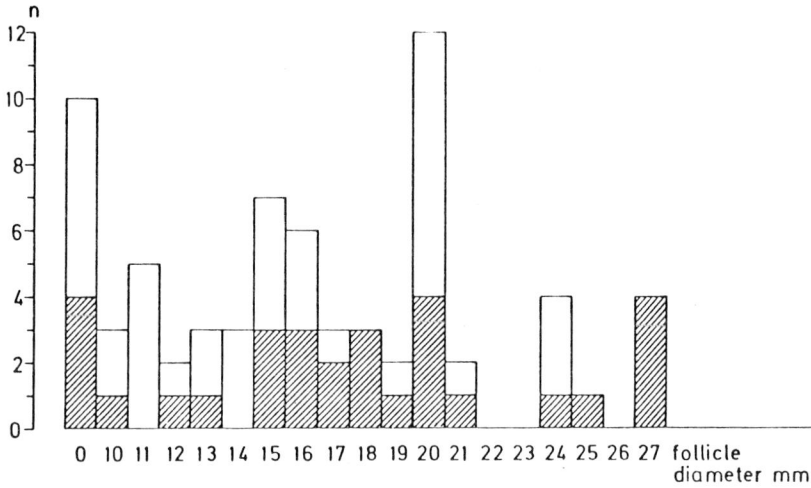

Fig. 12. Histogram of the follicular diameter measured by ultrasound. The shaded area depicts the proportion of the follicles from which preovulatory eggs could be obtained. In 10 cases ultrasound was unable to demonstrate follicles (0 mm). Four of these had large follicles at operation and preovulatory eggs could be obtained. These are regarded as false negative ultrasonic measurements.

ferred into Ham's medium for further development.
Cleaved oocytes were regarded as fertilized.

RESULTS

Pre-ovulatory eggs could be obtained from follicles at
almost any aspirated volume (Fig.10). There was no correlation between the largest obtained diameter of a follicle measured by ultrasound and the aspirated volume
(r = 0.36) (Fig.11). However, 30 women had follicles
with an aspirated volume of 2.0 ml or more. In 26 of
these women, ultrasound showed a follicular diameter
of 15 mm or more. In the remaining 4 women, who had
large follicles with pre-ovulatory eggs at laparotomy,
ultrasound was negative. The relation between the ultrasound estimated follicular diameter and the subsequent
finding of a pre-ovulatory oocyte is given in Fig. 12.

The method used for estimation of the volume of follicular fluid is inaccurate. By aspiration considerable
amounts of follicular fluid may be lost and/or incomplete emptying of the follicle may occur. Pre-ovulatory
oocytes could be obtained at almost any volume beyond
8 ml. The accuracy of the ultrasonic estimates of follicular diameter could thus not be verified by measurements of the follicular fluid volume. In four women
(13 %), pre-ovulatory oocytes could be obtained from
follicles with large volumes, which were not visualized
on the ultrasonic screen. These must be considered as
false negative ultrasonic results. The chance of obtaining a pre-ovulatory oocyte was 52 % if the follicular diameter obtained by ultrasound exceeded 14 mm.
With a diameter of 14 mm or less the chance of obtaining pre-ovulatory oocytes was 14 % if the false negative results are excluded.

THE ASSESSMENT OF OVULATION BY ULTRASOUND AND PLASMA
ESTRADIOL DETERMINATION.

R.H. Picker, R.D. Robertson, P.C. Wilson, D.M. Saunders,
Department of Obstetrics and Gynaecology and Ultrasound,
Royal North Shore Hospital of Sydney.
Sydney, Australia.

Presented to the 2nd World Federation of Ultrasound in
Medicine (Miyazaki, 1979).

In recent years, artificial insemination with donor
semen (A.I.D.) has become an accepted method of management for couples in whom the male partner is infertile.
The probable timing of ovulation and thus insemination

has been inferred by conventional means from Basal Body
Temperature (B.B.T.) and clinical assessment of changes
in cervical mucus. However, the reliability of the B.B.
T. and the accuracy of cervical mucus to pinpoint the
day of ovulation have been questioned. Limited supplies
of donor semen remain a major problem in most A.I.D.
programs. This study was designed to more accurately
assess the timing of ovulation in order to minimise
semen wastage.
The timing of ovulation was studied daily around the
peri-ovular period in 45 women attending an artificial
insemination clinic during 74 menstrual cycles by B-mode
ultrasound examination and plasma estradiol (E2) determination. Ultrasonic visualisation of the ovaries has
been previously reported and techniques for monitoring
follicular development under hormonal stimulus for ovulation induction have also been reported. In this series
using a Diasonograph NE 4200 machine equipped with a
3.5 mHz frequency transducer focused at 7-9 cm and using
an extremely full bladder as an ultrasonic window,
transverse echograms were taken at 1/2 cm intervals
cephalad from the pubis symphysis. Appropriate cephalad
or caudad angulation of the transducer was performed
according to the orientation of the anatomy scanned. The
echograms were recorded on multi-format x-ray film using
a Dunn camera with a 9 frame format. Ovarian follicle
size was measured and ultrasound patterns following ovulation were determined. The examinations were performed
on Day 6 of the cycle, Day 1 being the first day of menstrual bleeding and repeated every 3 days until evidence of follicular development was observed.(Figs. 13-17).
Ultrasonic examination then was performed on a daily
basis until changes associated with ovulation occurred.
Plasma E2 levels were determined also during this period
and the 2 parameters were compared with the probable
timing of ovulation as inferred by conventional means
from B.B.T. and clinical assessment of changes in cervical mucus. The day of ovulation assessed in this manner
was designated Day 0. Of the 45 women studied, 3 were
lost to ultrasound follow-up around the periovular
period and in another 2 the ultrasound findings were
incorrectly interpreted. Of the remaining 40 patients,
35 were normal and 5 patients were on treatment with
clomiphenecitrate for induction of ovulation. In all
normal cycles studied the maximum diameters of the follicles and the peak E2 determinations occurred within
2 days prior to and including the day of presumed ovulation. The follicle diameter increase was linear with
the mean maximum follicle diameter on Day minus 1 of
2.5 cm. The average of the values at this time for peak
E2 determination was 1660 pmol/l. The 5 clomiphene patients demonstrated varied results with multiple follicles varying in size from 2.5 to 3.5 cm diameter and E2

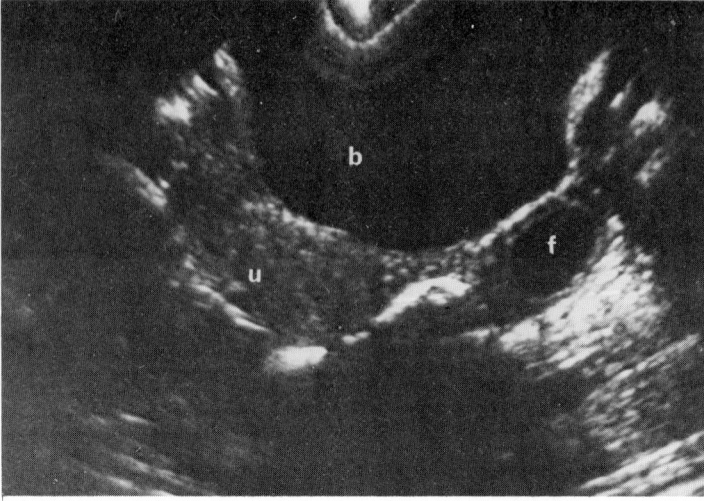

Fig. 13 **represents a transverse contact echogram through the full bladder demonstrating bladder (b), uterus (u) and left Graafian follicle (F).**

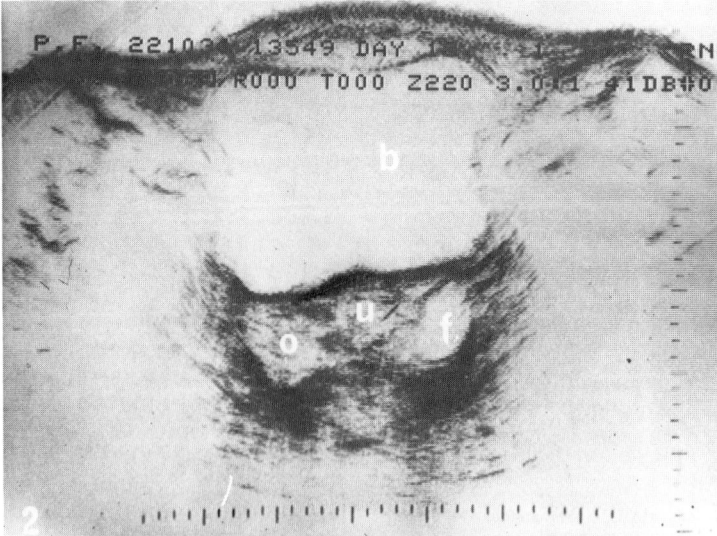

Fig. 14 **represents a transverse echogram using an Octoson demonstrating a full bladder (b), uterus (u), right ovary (o) and left Graafian follicle (f).**

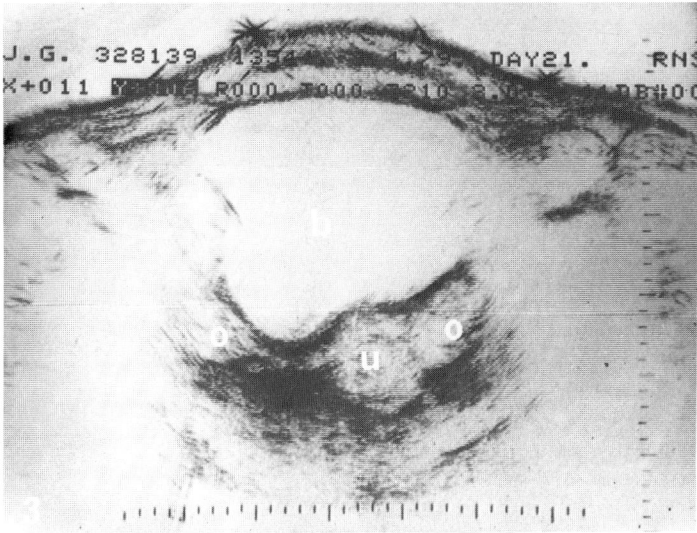

Fig. 15 represents a transverse echogram using an Octoson demonstrating a full bladder (b), uterus (u), right and left ovaries (o).

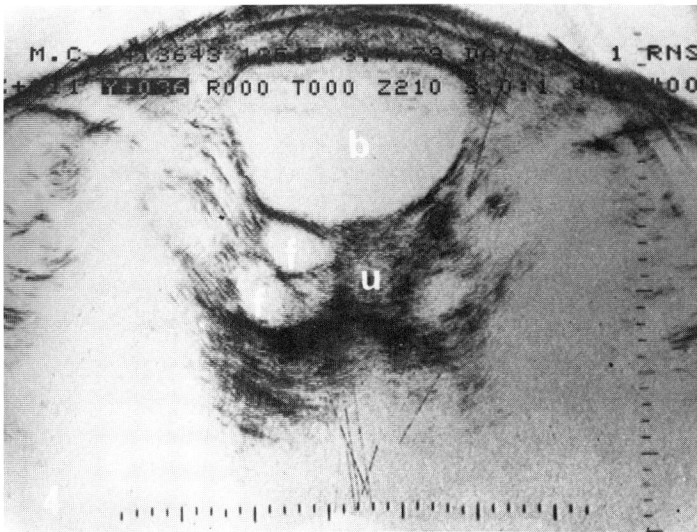

Fig. 16 represents a transverse echogram using an Octoson demonstrating a full bladder (b), uterus (u), and multiple right-sided follicles (f) in a stimulated patient.

407

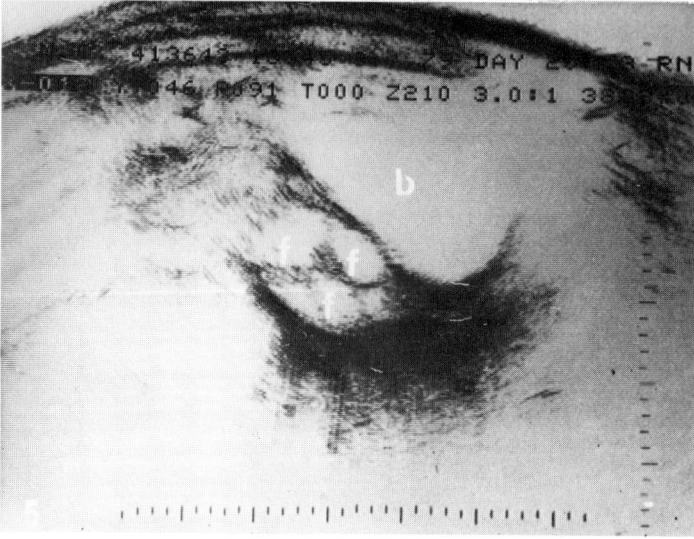

Fig. 17 represents a longitudinal echogram to the right of the midline using an Octoson demonstrating a full bladder (b), and multiple follicles in the right ovary (f).

levels varying from 2258 to 3846 pmol/l. Two definitive ultrasonic patterns were seen following ovulation. In 60 of the 74 normal cycles studied, follicular disappearance was noted. In the remaining 14 cycles, partial collapse of the follicle was noted with the appearance of internal echoes. The first pattern was taken to represent ovulation with collapse of the follicle and the subsequent development of a solid corpus luteum, and the second pattern was considered to represent ovulation followed by haemorrhage into the follicle which then underwent organisation. The authors believe the method is a simple, safe, clinically reliable means of determining the time of ovulation in women undergoing arteficial insemination and it is now used as a routine clinical tool in our A.I.D. program. Since this trial was performed ultrasonic evaluation of ovarian function is now undertaken in all AID patients to assess ovulation and in all patients undergoing ovarian stimulation for the production of ovulation. Other equipment employed has been a Picker 80 l grey scale unit and an Octoson water delay machine.

Monitoring of human ovulation by ultrasound compared to biochemical and clinical findings.

R. Terinde
Universitäts-Frauenklinik, Düsseldorf

Contribution to the Round Table "Ultrasound monitoring of ovarian stimulation" on the International Symposion on recent advances in ultrasound diagnosis (3), 1st - 5th October 1979.

This investigation is based on 535 ultrasound determinations of follicular development from -10 days to the day of ovulation or stop of hormonal therapy. 131 cycles in 65 patients with HMG/HCG-stimulation were controlled by ultrasound, clinical findings (cervical score, basal temperature) and determination of serum progesterone to confirm the day of ovulation.
In 104 of 131 cycles ovulation could be confirmed. In 18 cycles treatment was stopped because the ovaries developed multiple follicles within the meaning of policystic ovaries. In 4 cycles the ovaries showed no response to stimulation, in 5 cycles follicles between 1.9 and 2.5 were documented but no ovulation occured after HCG stimulation.
Figure 18 showes how the ovulation was verified in 104 cycles. Ultrasound monitoring was not involved in 21 cycles, that means 20 %. Lack of clinical findings was found in 25 cycles (24 %) and no progesterone determina-

tion in 30 cycles (29 %). These datas don't prove the value of each of these methods but the importance we express to them in clinical management of HMG/HCG therapy. Ovulation monitored by ultrasound was estimated when follicles of 1.9 cm or more were registrated or/and a corpus luteum occured.
In 25 of 83 cycles monitored by ultrasound the documentation of a corpus luteum proved the ovulation. This was found in the 4 cycles when no other method was used to confirm ovulation.
In discussion of missing ovulation monitored by ultrasound in 21 cycles (20 %) we had to notice several in part silly reasons (Figure 19). There is no doubt that ultrasound is totally wrong in some cases but looking at this figure one can hardly find out in which case ultrasound has made a mistake.

Looking at ovarian reaction to HMG/HCG stimulation we found out that in 40 % both ovaries developed follicles, in 53 % only one of the ovaries (Figure 20). No reaction was seen in 3 %. Follicular growth couldn't be monitored in one case, but seeing a corpus luteum it was suggested, that ovulation took place. Extreme obesity inhibited in three patients ultrasound monitoring of the ovaries. When only one of the ovaries was stimulated (Figure 21) in 60 % also one follicle could be seen at the time of ovulation, in 30 % two follicles and in 7 % three follicles. When both ovaries showed a reaction to HMG/HCG stimulation in 36 cycles (67.9 %) policystic ovaries occured. When only one ovary was stimulated a policystic development was registrated only in two cases (2.9 %).

There are different reasons why ovaries could not be visualized. Out of 476 determinations both ovaries could not be seen in 28 cases, one ovary in 50 cases. Listing up the reasons why failure in imaging the ovary occured most often a not satisfieing filled urinary bladder and extremely adiposity was found. In 27 determinations no explanation could be found why one ovary could not be seen, while the other one was easily visible.
Nevertheless these datas show that monitoring follicular growth is possible concerning the accuracy of this scanning method.

104 HMG-INDUCED CYCLES WITH OVULATION PROVED BY ULTRASOUND,
BASAL TEMPERATURE OR CERVICAL INDEX, OR PROGESTERON LEVEL.

	NO. OF CYCLES	(%)
ULTRASOUND, CLINICAL FINDINGS, PROGESTERON	46	(44,2)
ULTRASOUND, CLINICAL FINDINGS	16	(15,4)
ULTRASOUND PROGESTERON	17	(16,4)
CLINICAL FINDINGS, PROGESTERON	7	(6,8)
ULTRASOUND	4	(3,8)
CLINICAL FINDINGS	10	(9,6)
PROGESTERON	4	(3,8)

Figure 18.

21 HMG/HCG - CYCLES IN WHICH OVULATION COULD NOT BE VERI-
FIED BY ULTRASOUND

	NO. OF CYCLES
NO FOLLICULAR DEVELOPMENT MONITORED	2
OVARIES NOT VISIBLE IN CASES OF ADIPOSITY, DEFECT OF EQUIPMENT A, S, O,	7
FOLLICLES BELOW 1.9 CM IN DIAMETER AT THE TIME OF HCG - APPLICATION	4
AFTER INITIAL FOLLICULAR GROWTH NO MORE CYSTIC STRUCTURES	2
SPONTANOUS OVULATION WITHOUT HCG-APPLICATION	3
NO ORDER FOR ULTRASOUND AT WEEKEND	3

Figure 19.

OVARIAN REACTION TO HMG/HCG STIMULATION

	CYCLES	%
STIMULATION OF BOTH OVARIES	53	40,4
STIMULATION OF ONE OVARY ONLY	70	53,4
NO REACTION IN ANY OVARY	4	3,1
SPECIAL CASES	4	3,1
TOTAL	131	100

Figure 20.

NUMBER OF FOLLICLES WHEN ONLY ONE OVARY WAS STIMULATED

STIMULATION OF ONE OVARY (TOTAL)	ONE FOLICLE	TWO FOLLICLES	THREE FOLLICLES	POLY-CYSTIC OVARIES
70	42	21	5	2
	60%	30%	7,1%	2,9%

Figure 21.

<u>Discussion</u> by B.J. Hackelöer

Following the presented papers it seems obvious that
ultrasound offers new possibilities in the demonstration of follicular development. It represents a new aid
for the investigation and treatment of infertility i.e.
multiple pregnancies and hyperstimulations can be avoided (S.Nitschke, R.Terinde), ovulation could be induced
despite "too high" hormone levels (B.Funduk-Kurjak,
A. Christie), pregnancy rate was doubled (R. Picker),
and follicular fluid and ova could be collected after
volume estimation (H. Persson).
But there are still differences in follicular size measurements (range of 10-20 %) and difficulties even in
demonstrating the ovary. Therefore a reference plane
would be helpful.
Very often an image of two parallel lines outlining
lengthwise an echofree area was observed and followed
into the ovary.
This structure seems to be an ovarian vascular structure. The ovarian vessels reach the ovary through the
infundibulopelvic ligament and the mesovarium and give
rise to numerous spiral structures. The ovarian artery
seems to extend in accomodation to follicular development and may reach 3-10 mm in diameter and therefore
the visualization of this structure by ultrasound must
be possible. Since we observed this vessel-like structure and since we were sure about its importance we use
it as an indicator and guideline for ovarian imaging.
Another similar structure can sometimes be visualized
as well and can be identified as iliac vessel. It is
lying underneath the ovary but cannot be used as a good
guideline because of its instable relation to the ovary.

The ovarian vessels within the infundibulopelvic ligament have a stable relation to the ovary and therefore
we propose to use it as reference plane for ovarian
imaging. (see Figs. 22-25).

Two other questions were also discussed
1. The value of this non-invasive technique in comparison to another non invasive method the BBT. We found
   out that the follicular demonstration by ultrasound
   in order to prove ovulation was superior to the basal body temperature chart. BBT was unable to demonstrate ovulation in 15 % of our cases but Ultrasound
   had no false negative results.
2. Using modern digitalized compound-scanners it seems
   possible to differentiate much better than now
   between preovulatory follicles and the intrafollicu-
   lar changes occuring immediately after ovulation
   which means that the use of computersmay help in the
   demonstration of the corpus luteum.

Conclusion

Ultrasound monitoring of growing follicles was used over the last two years from different groups over the world. The result ist that this method is practicable reproducible and successful as a help in the treatment of ovarian stimulation and the investigation of infertility. There are still measurement difficulties but new technical development will offer new facilities.

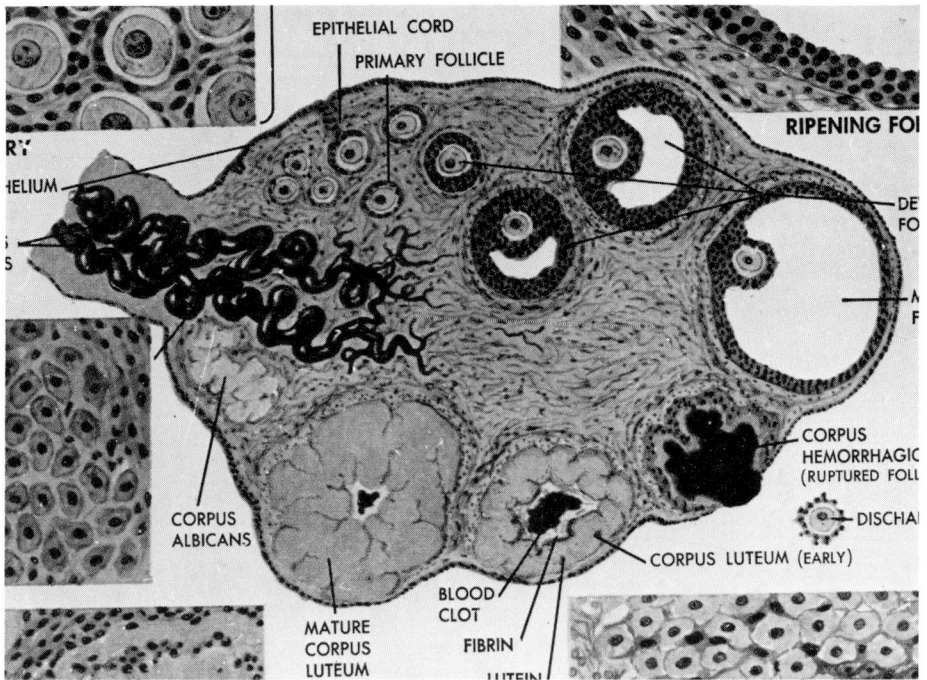

Figure 22. Ovarian vessels, anatomical situation

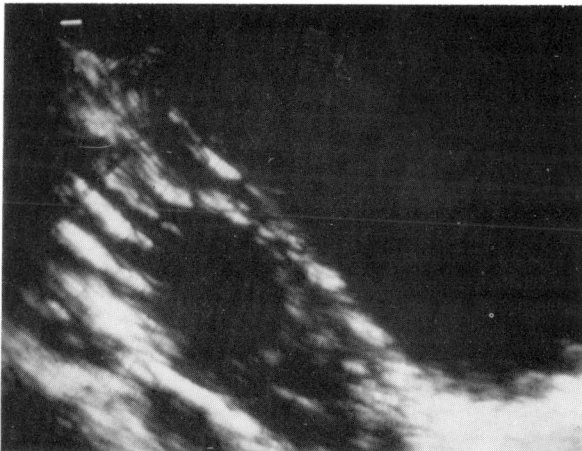

Figure 23. Demonstration of ovarian vessels (left)

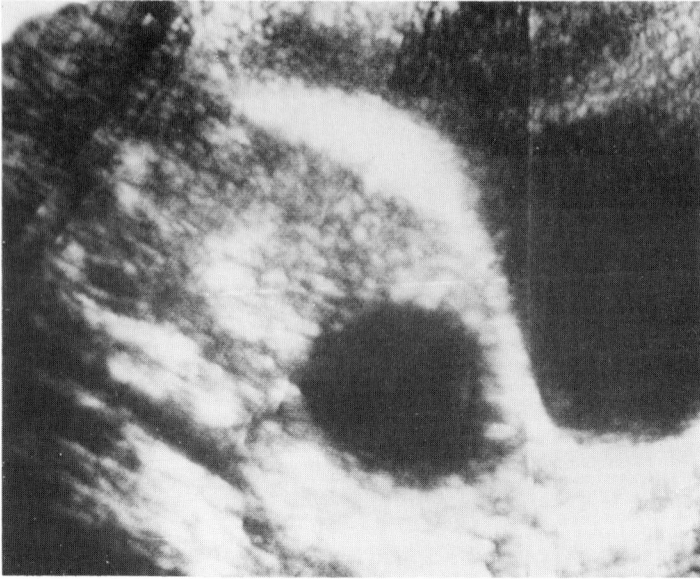

Figure 24. Ovary, follicle and ovarian vessel (left)

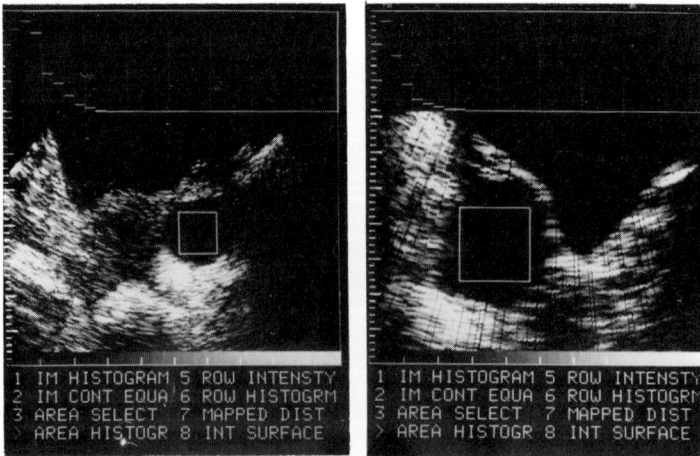

Figure 25. "Post-Processing" of a follicle structure
(right), so called "Area Histogram"

References:

1. Hackelöer, B.J., S. Nitschke, E. Daume, G. Sturm, R. Buchholz:
Ultraschalldarstellung von Ovarveränderungen bei Gonadotropinstimulierung.
Geburtsh. u. Frauenheilk. 37 (1977) 138

2. Hackelöer, B.J.:
The Ultrasonic Demonstration of Follicular Development during the Normal Menstrual Cycle and after Hormone Stimulation.
Proc. Int. Symp. on Recent Advances in Ultrasound Diagnosis, Dubrovnik, 1977

3. Hackelöer, B.J., S. Nitschke:
Ovarian imaging by ultrasound: An attempt to define a reference plane.
J.C.U., submitted for publication

4. Hackelöer, B.J., R. Fleming, H.P. Robinson, H. Adam, J.R.P. Coutts:
Correlation of ultrasonic and endocrinological assessment of human follicular development.
Am. J. Obstet. Gynec. 135 (1979) 120

5. Hackelöer, B.J., M. Hansmann:
Ultraschalldiagnostik in der Frühschwangerschaft.
Gynäkologe 9 (1976) 108

6. Funduk-Kurjak, B., Kurjak, A.:
Grey-scale ultrasound in monitoring ovarian stimulation.
Proceedings of the 59th Congress of Italian Gynecologists, pp. 280, 1978 a.

7. Funduk-Kurjak, B., Kurjak, A.:
Ultrasonic assessment of the growing ovarian follicle during the normal physiologic menstrual cycle.
Medicina 15 (1978) 132 (in Croatian)

8. Funduk-Kurjak, B., A. Kurjak:
Ultrasonic monitoring of follicular growth during the normal menstrual cycle and after stimulation.
Book of Abstracts, 3rd World Congress of Ultrasound, Myasaka, 22. - 27. July 1979 a.

9. Funduk-Kurjak, B., A. Kurjak, I. Puharic, I. Olajos:
Ultrasonic assessment of early pregnancy after stimulation of ovulation.
Perinatalni dani 1979, in print (In Croatian).

10. Abraham,G.E., Odell, W.D., Swerdloff, R.S., K. Hopper:
Simultaneous radioimmunoassay of plasma FSH, LH, progesterone, 17-hydroxyprogesterone and estradiol-17ß during the menstrual cycle.
J.Clin. Endocrinol. Metab. 34 (1972) 312-318

11. Johansson, E.D.B., J.D. Neill, E. Knobil:
Periovulatory levels of plasma progesterone and luteinizing hormone in woman.
Acta Endocrinol. 62 (1969) 82-88

12. Nitschke-Dabelstein, S., G. Sturm, E. Daume:
Neue Aspekte in der Beurteilung des Follikelwachstums unter besonderer Berücksichtigung medikamentöser Ovarstimulierung.
Arch. of Gynecol. 228 (1979) 42. Gynäkologen-

13. Nitschke-Dabelstein, S., B.J. Hackelöer, G. Sturm:
Ovulation and corpus luteum formation in ultrasonography.
Ultrasound Med. Biol. (submitted for publication)

14. Nitschke-Dabelstein, S., G. Sturm, B.J. Hackelöer, E. Daume, R. Buchholz:
Der Wert der Ultraschallüberwachung gonadotropin-stimulierter Patientinnen - ein Vergleich zwischen ultrasonographischen und endocrinologischen Parameter.
Geburtsh. und Frauenheilk. (submitted for publication).

12. ULTRASOUND AND THE RADIOLOGIST

H. B. Meire, Chairman

ULTRASOUND AND THE RADIOLOGIST

Hylton B. Meire.

Clinical Research Centre, Harrow, Middx, U.K.

INTRODUCTION

Since the introduction of grey scale display diagnostic ultrasound has been applied to an ever increasing range of organs and diagnostic problems. Whilst the art and science of ultrasound are still evolving the technique has already gained widespread acceptance in certain clinical situations. The purpose of this paper is to highlight those areas where ultrasound contributes most to patient management, or has permitted a reduction in conventional radiological techniques.

Kidney

The role of ultrasound in the detection and differential diagnosis of renal masses has been recognised for many years (6). In most institutions where ultrasound is now available all renal masses detected on IVU receive an ultrasound examination as their next investigation. In those patients where the lesion is clearly cystic needle puncture and diagnostic or therapeutic aspiration can be undertaken and arteriography avoided. In those patients with a complex or clearly solid lesion (Figure 1), many centres now also perform diagnostic aspiration of these. When the lesion is small ultrasound can be used to guide the biopsy needle.

Ultrasound also has a role in the further investigation of the non functioning kidney detected on IVU. Hydronephrosis can be excluded with 100% certainty and rarely a renal tumour may be detected. It is difficult to be certain of the diagnosis of unilateral renal agenesis but in the majority of patients the ultrasound findings will obviate the need for further radiological procedures. Ultrasound is also valuable for assessment of the response of hydronephrosis to treatment. This is particularly relevant in children undergoing ureteric re-implantation where serial radiographs may be undesirable. We have also used ultrasound to monitor patients with calculous renal disease where serial radiography is undesirable due either to age or abnormal sensitivity to radiographic contrast media.

We must balance against these potential reductions in radiography the occasional intravenous urogram which has to be performed to further evaluate a solid mass detected within the

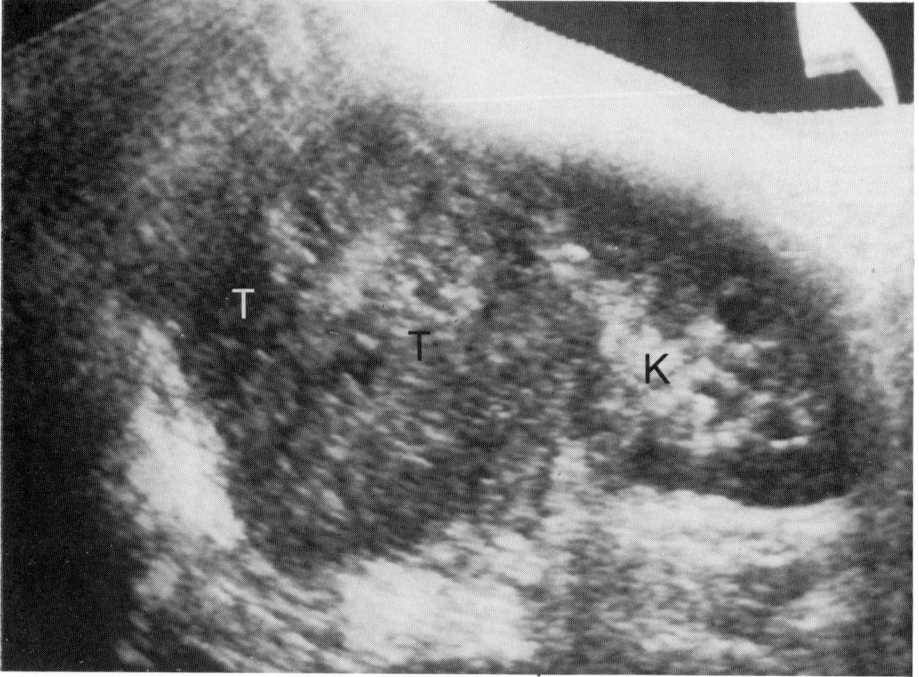

Figure 1 - Longitudinal posterior scan of kidney (K). There is a solid tumour (T) at the upper pole.

kidney as an incidental finding when examiningadjacent abdominal organs. In our department this occurs several times each year and not infrequently small solid renal masses clearly shown on ultrasound cannot be detected on conventional IVU's performed after the ultrasound examination.

Bladder

Ultrasound can be used for the assessment of bladder volume and is particularly valuable for the measurement of residual urine volume after micturition in children (3). In the adult both the diagnosis and staging of bladder tumours is feasible with ultrasound and patients treated with conservative surgery or drug treatment can have the progress of their disease monitored without recourse to repeated cystoscopies.

Liver

Ultrasound is pre-eminent for the diagnosis of liver metastases (Figure 2) and is used in our department for the routine screening of all patients with known primary malignant disease.

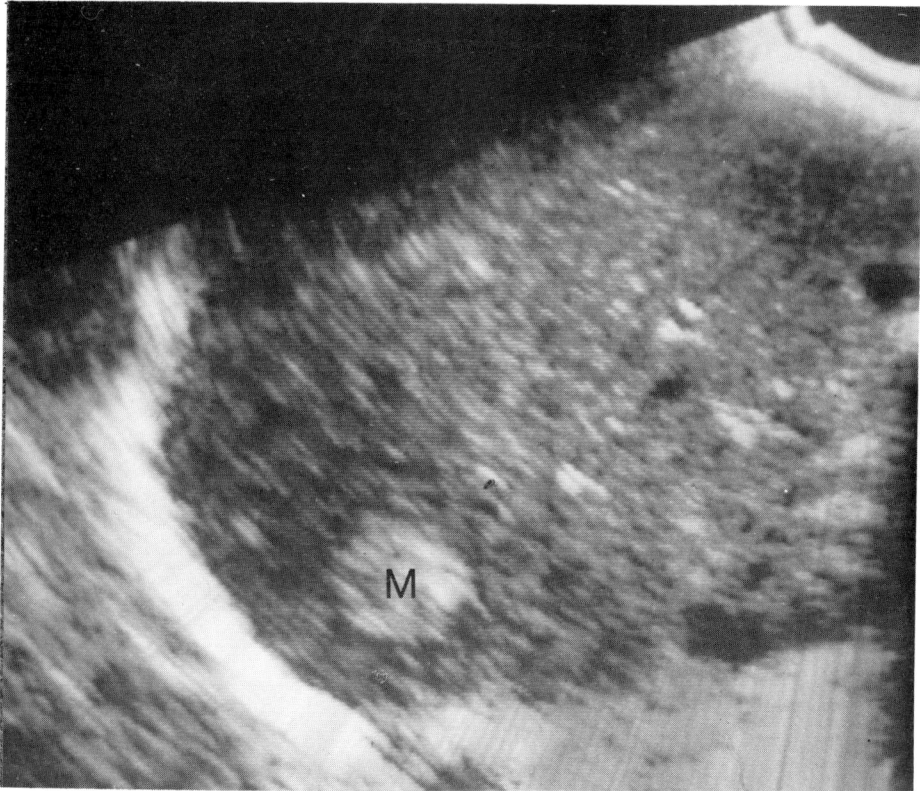

Figure 2 - Longitudinal scan of right lobe of liver. There is an echogenic metastases (M) posteriorly.

This not only permits a reduction in the number of radio nuclide scans performed but also helps the surgeon to plan his approach. In many patients unwarranted radical surgery has been avoided when unsuspected liver metastases have been detected.

Liver abscesses are also readily detected by ultrasound (Figure 3) and, as with lesions elsewhere, ultrasound is very valuable for directing the aspirating needle and for monitoring

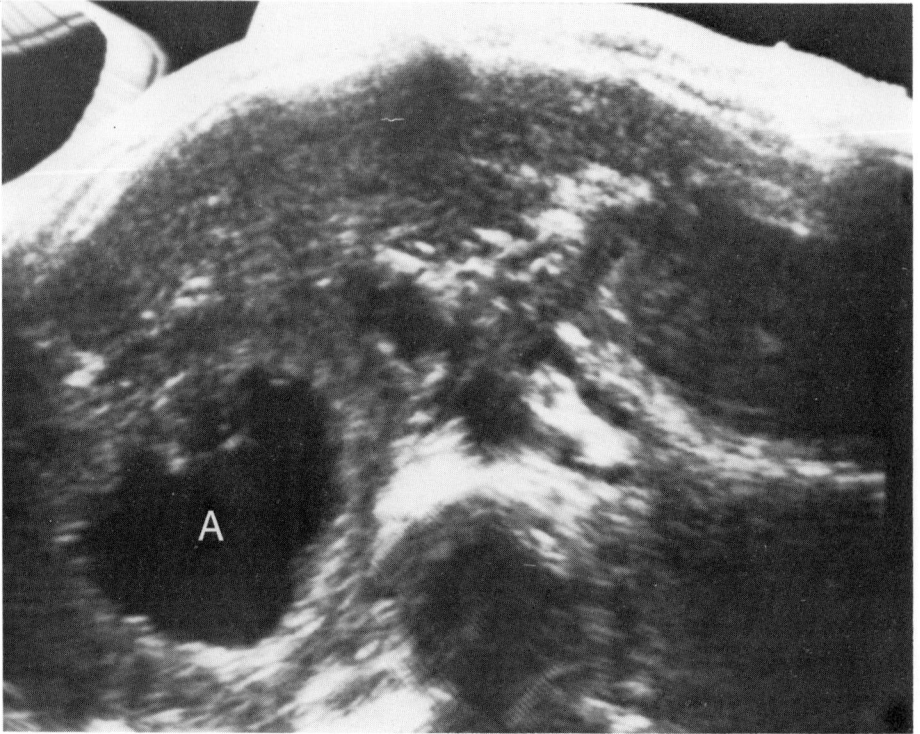

Figure 3 – Transverse scan of liver. There is a partially fluid abscess (A) posteriorly in the right lobe.

the response to treatment. The monitoring of liver abscesses by conventional radiographic techniques has proved unsatisfactory and ultrasound has made a substantial contribution to the management of this unpleasant disorder.

Jaundice

In a significant minority of patients with jaundice the clinical and biochemical findings fail to reliably differentiate medical from surgical causes. In this group of patients ultrasound can achieve differentiation with an accuracy approaching 100% (5). This is possible by detection of the dilated bile ducts (Figure 4) and many workers have found that in patients shown to have obstructive jaundice the level of obstruction can be ascertained in

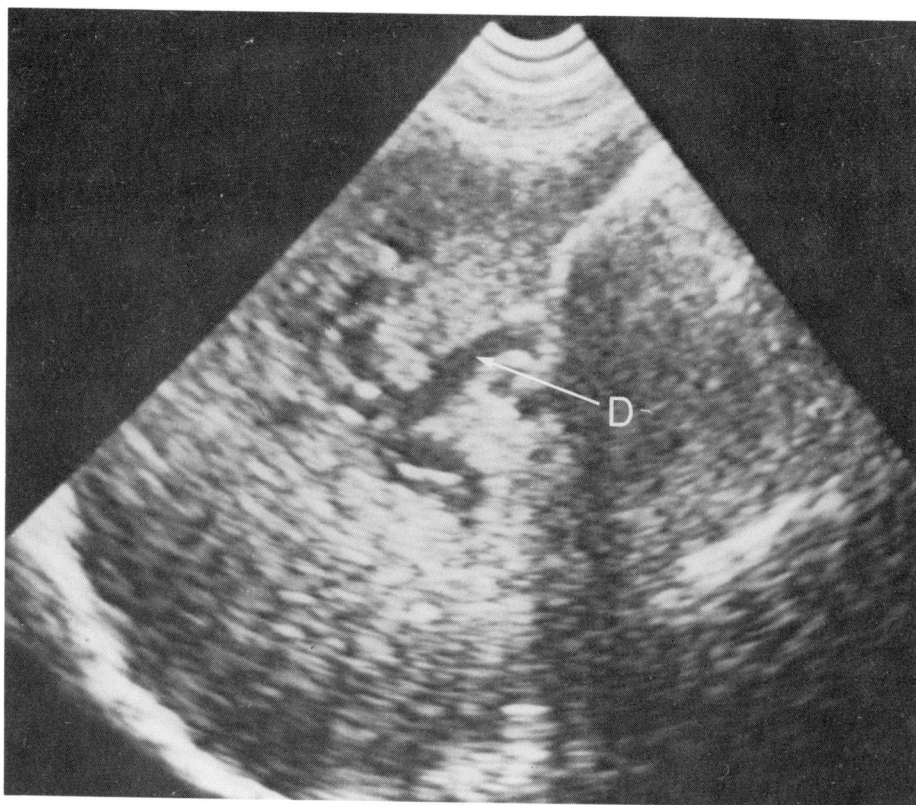

Figure 4 - Single frame from a rotating probe real time scan (EMI) showing a mildly dilated common hepatic duct (D).

over 70% of patients and the actual cause of obstruction may be clear in over half. The management of jaundice has thus been radically altered by the introduction of ultrasound scanning and the need for percutaneous transhepatic cholangiography, intra venous cholangiography, endoscopic retrograde cholangiopancreato-graphy etc. has been drastically reduced. In our institution patients with obstructive jaundice and a confident ultrasound diagnosis of the level and cause now receive no other investigations before being submitted for surgery.

Gall Bladder

The role of ultrasound diagnosis of gall bladder disease is under re-evaluation in many centres throughout the world at the

present time. Exponents of gall bladder ultrasound are now
suggesting that ultrasound examination should be the initial
diagnostic procedure for the diagnosis or exclusion of biliary
calculi and many workers claim success rates of well over 90% for
this procedure (1). Our own experience tends to support their
claims and thus a moderately expensive and time consuming
conventional cholec.ystogram can be replaced by a cheaper and
quicker ultrasound examination. Radiographic procedures can be
retained for the small percentage of patients in whom ultrasound is
unsatisfactory.

Pancreas

This is another organ in which the role of ultrasound imaging
is still under evaluation. With improved techniques and equipment
it is now possible to identify the head and body of the pancreas in
over 90% of patients (Figure 5) (2) and the advent of high
resolution real-time scanners should permit detection of the
majority of the pancreas in almost all patients. In a recent study
in our department we were able to show that a confident ultrasound
diagnosis of a normal pancreas was correct in over 85% of cases
whereas a computed tomographic diagnosis of normal pancreas was
correct in 72% of cases. CT however was more satisfactory than
ultrasound when pathological changes were present in the pancreas.
These results indicate that ultrasound examination of the pancreas
should be performed early in the investigation of this organ and
when a satisfactory examination reveals a normal pancreas there is
no need to continue with other more invasive and expensive
investigations in the majority of patients.

Thyroid

Ultrasound is invaluable for the assessment of localised masses
within the thyroid gland. As at other sites in the body solid
masses can be differentiated from simple cysts and the aspirating
needle can be accurately guided into the lesion. If therapeutic
aspiration of cystic masses is performed then ultrasound offers a
very satisfactory technique for the follow up of these patients. The
anatomical information obtained from an ultrasound scan.is almost
invariably more accurate than that obtained from isotope imaging
techniques, but the latter of course gives functional information
which is not available to the ultrasonologist. These two
procedures may therefore be complimentary but ultrasound can be the
first and only investigation in the management of patients with
solitary thyroid masses.

Abdominal Aorta

The abdominal aorta can be visualised by ultrasound in all
patients except those with gross obesity or excessive bowel gas. In
our experience abdominal aortic ultrasound is most frequently
requested in very thin elderly patients in whom there is a clinical
suspicion of a pulsatile abdominal mass. The aorta is invariably
detectable in these patients and its size and shape can be

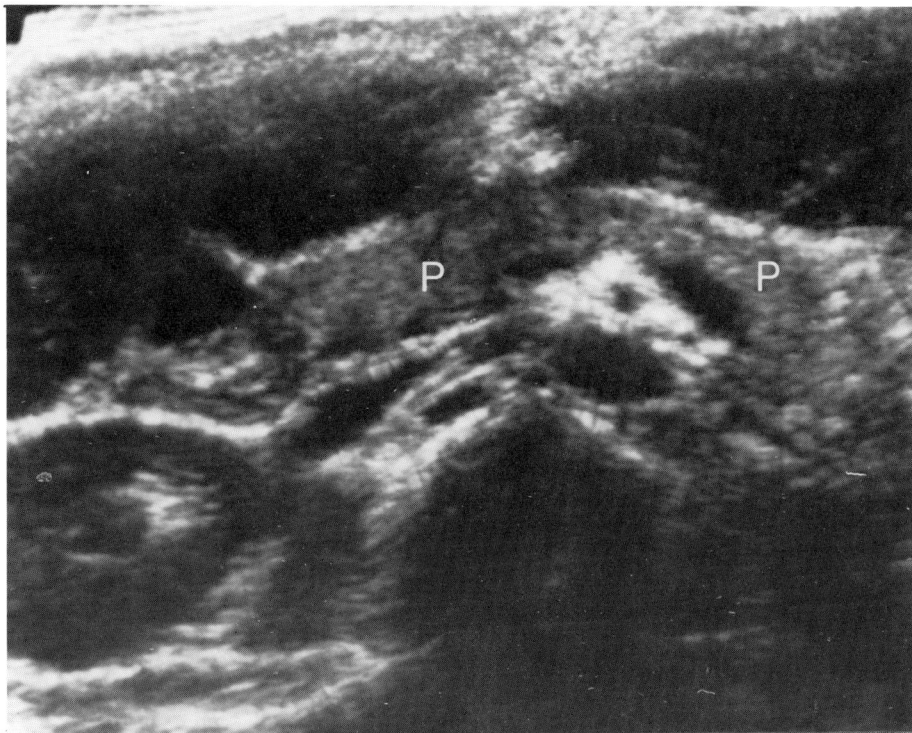

Figure 5 - Transverse scan of a normal pancres (P).

accurately measured and the clinical diagnosis of aortic aneurysm is generally disproven in our experience. The availability of ultrasound permits a small but highly significant reduction in the number of aortograms which would otherwise be performed. In those patients where ultrasound confirms the presence of asymptomatic aortic aneurysm the progress of the lesion can be readily monitored and further investigation instigated only if the aneurysm can be shown to be expanding detectably over a period of a few weeks.

Peripheral Vessels

The newly available pulsed doppler ultrasound vessel imaging systems now permit the non invasive imaging of the major superficial arteries and veins of the body. This form

of investigation is proving invaluable for the assessment of
patients with transient cerebral ischaemia and limb ischaemia. The
carotid and vertebral arterial systems can be reliably detected
(Figures 6 and 7) and those patients with significant extra cranial
disease can be referred for further investigation and possible

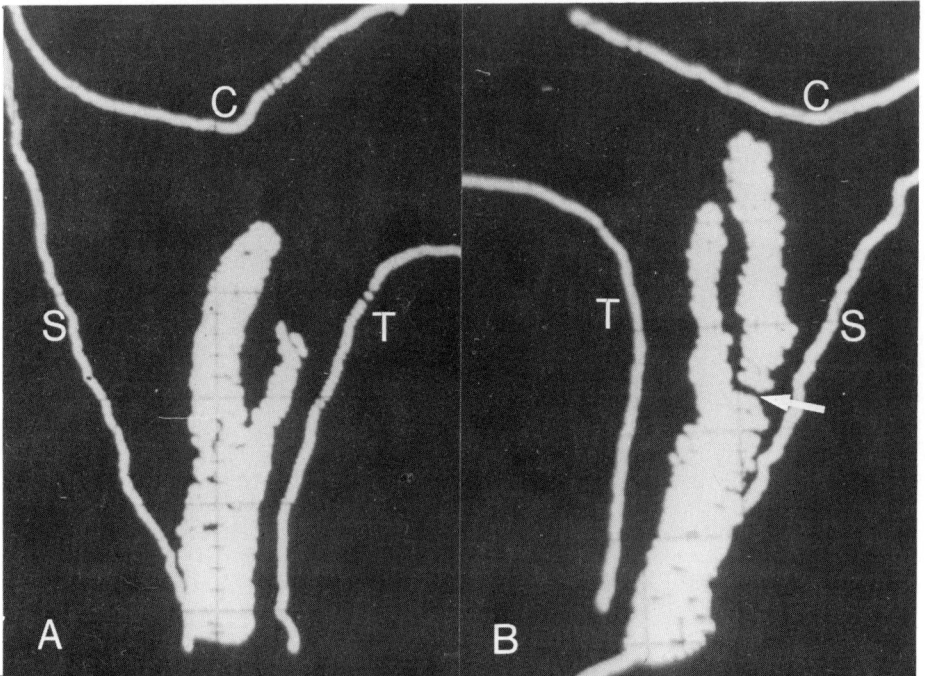

Figure 6(a) – Anterior MAVIS scan of normal right carotid
bifurcation. Chin (C), Sterno mastoid (S), Thyroid cartilage (T).
     (b) – Same patient's left carotid artery. There is a tight
stenosis (arrow) at the origin of the internal carotid.

surgery. Patients in whom the extra cranial vessels can be
confidently shown to be normal can be spared the trauma of an arch
aortogram and four vessel study.

     Patients with leg ischaemia can also be reliably assessed
before angiography and surgery (Figure 8). In addition the results
of surgery can be non invasively monitored and the efficacy of non-
invasive vascular dilatation techniques (e.g. the Dotter procedure)
can be assessed and the progress of the lesion monitored.

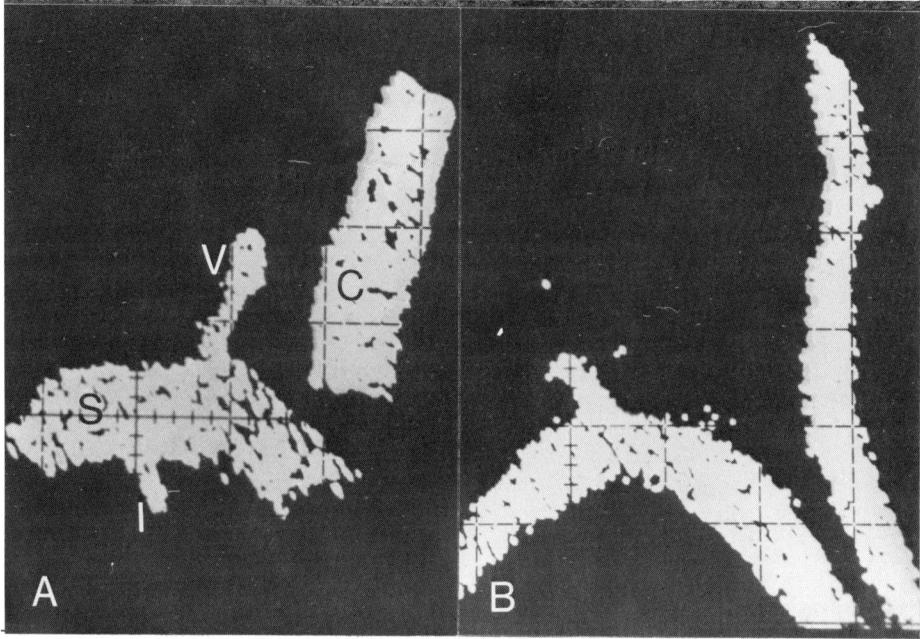

Figure 7(a) - Anterior MAVIS scan of normal right vertebral artery (V) Subclavian artery (S), Common carotid (C), Internal mammary (I).
    (b) - Anterior scan of patient with obstructed vertebral artery.

The deep veins of the leg can also be detected with a pulsed doppler vessel imaging system and a preliminary study in our department indicates that there is a close correlation between venography and ultrasound studies for the diagnosis or exclusion of deep vein thrombosis.

Obstetrics

Whilst much of the information obtained from an obstetric ultrasound examination early in pregnancy cannot be obtained at that time from radiographic techniques, the additional information made available to the obstetrician should permit him to rely less heavily upon obstetric radiography in late pregnancy. We have tested this hypothesis in our own institution and have noted that in 1974

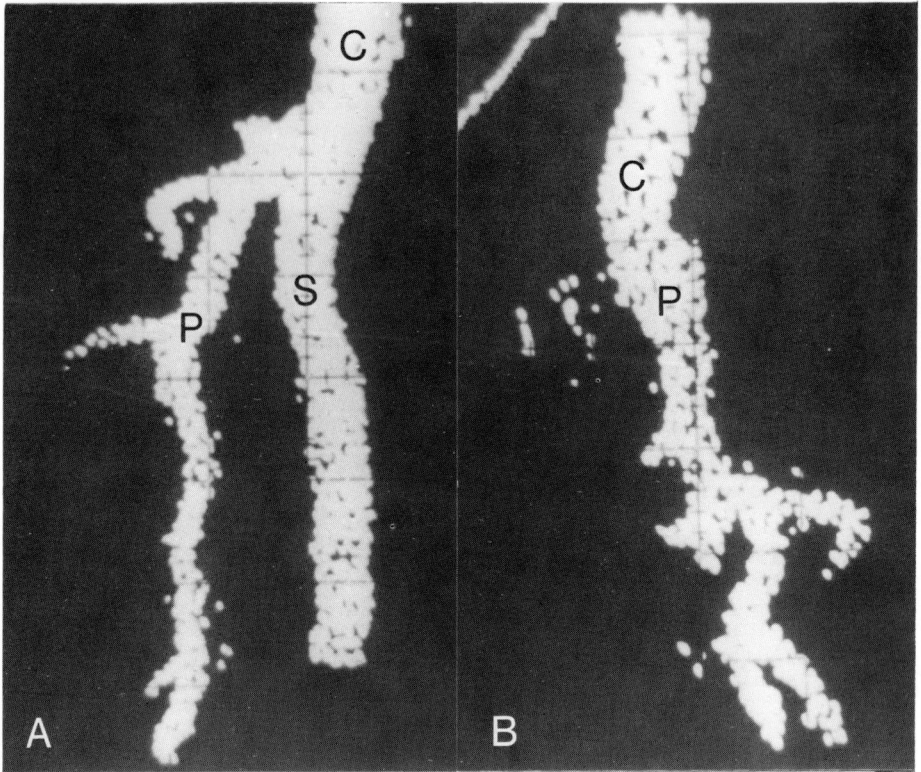

Figure 8(a) – Anterior MAVIS scan of normal right femoral artery.
Common femoral (C), Superficial femoral (S), Profunda femoris (P).
        (b) – Anterior scan of same patient's left femoral artery.
The superficial artery is blocked and the profunda hypertrophied.

(prior to initiation of the ultrasound service) 26.6% of all
pregnancies were subjected to radiography. Over the ensuing years
the number of ultrasound examinations has rapidly increased and by
1976 the obstetric radiography rate had been reduced to 12% (4). We
have recently examined the figures for 1977, 1978 and 1979 and note
that the reduction in radiographic procedures continues,
approximately 3% of patients being radiographed in 1979.

CONCLUSION

        In this brief review I have been able to show that not only has
patient management been improved by the availability of ultrasound
imaging techniques but that some reduction in alternative imaging
techniques has also been made possible.

It is impossible to assess the exact cost effectiveness of ultrasound in the different clinical situations indicated but since ultrasound is generally quicker and cheaper than all the special radiographic procedures discussed above it seems very likely that we should have little difficulty in persuading our hospital financiers that ultrasound is a good investment. Indeed, perhaps we should ask ourselves "However did we manage without it?".

REFERENCES

1. Anderson, J.C. and Harned R.K. (1977)
    Am. J. Roentgenol. 129; 975-7

2. Haber, K., Freimanis, A.K. and Asher, W.M. (1976)
    Am. J. Roentgenol. 126; 624-8.

3. Harrison, N.W., Parks, C. and Sherwood, T. (1976)
    Brit. J. Urol. 47; 805-814.

4. Meire, H. B., Farrant, P., and Wilkins, R.A. (1978)
    Brit. Med. J. 1; 882-3.

5. Sample, W.F., Sarti, D.A., Goldstein, L.I., Weiner, M. and
    Kadell, B.M. (1978)
    Radiology 128; 719-725.

6. Sherwood T. (1975)
    Brit. Med. J. 4; 682-3

THE VALUE OF THE ECHO PATTERN IN DIFFUSE LIVER DISEASE

K.C. Dewbury

Radiology Department, Southampton General Hospital,
Southhampton, United Kingdom

INTRODUCTION

The value of ultrasound in the detection of focal abnormalities of the liver is well established. In this respect, ultrasound is a sensitive diagnostic tool able, under
ideal circumstances, to detect focal lesions of as small as
½ cm. As well as demonstrating focal lesions within the liver, ultrasound is able in many instances to characterize
the lesions demonstrated. It is possible to recognize several different types of metastases, for example, echo-poor
metastases and the characteristic echogenic metastases. Echogenic metastases are characteristically associated with
colo-rectal primaries, but may also be seen with other GI
tract primary neoplasm (1). An example of echogenic metastases is shown in Fig. 1. In many instances, ultrasound is a-
ble to distinguish malignant focal disease from benign focal disease, such as vascular malformations, abscesses and
simple hepatic cysts. An example of the typical hepatic
cyst is shown in Fig. 2.

More recently, we have established an equally valuable
role for ultrasound, both in the detection and follow-up of
a group of diffuse liver diseases, which includes cirrhosis,
fatty infiltraion and hepatitis. These may all be recognized by a characteristic brightly reflective echo pattern.
The significance of this will be discussed.

GENERALIZED LIVER ECHO PATTERNS

Ultrasound imaging is essentially the mapping of tissue
elasticity gradients within an organ (2). All organs have a
characteristic textural pattern which corresponds in part to
the collagen skeleton of that organ. This characteristic
echo pattern may be defined by the size, distribution and
density of echoes within the organ, and is dependent upon
many factors, including the frequency of the transducer, the
signal processing of the system and the individual characteristics and build of the patient.

Four generalized liver echo patterns may be recognized:
a) Normal. The normal liver has a mid-grey reflectivity which
is interspersed with the vascular structures within the liver, the portal venous radicles being surrounded by a bright

432

cuff of echoes and the hepatic venous radicles appearing to have no wall echoes(1). The diaphragm and skin echoes stand out brightly in comparison to the normal liver parenchyma. The renal cortex has an echo amplitude slightly less than that of the normal liver, the renal collecting system standing out brightly within the centre of the kidney. An example of this normal pattern is shown in Fig.3.

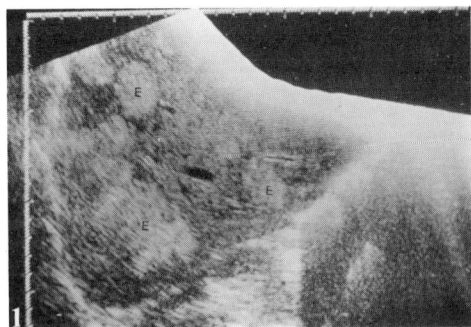

Fig. 1. A longitudinal scan showing echogenic metastases (E).

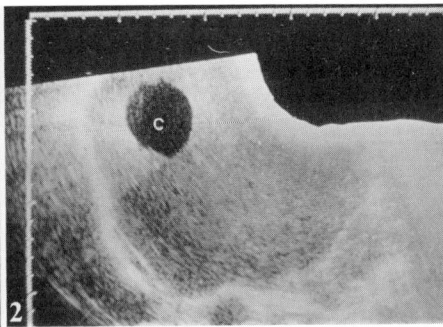

Fig. 2. A 3cm congenital cyst (C) in the right lobe of the liver.

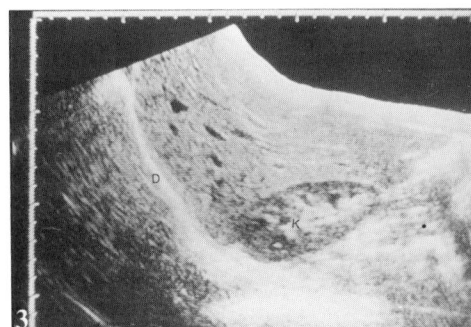

Fig. 3. A normal right lobe of liver and right kidney.

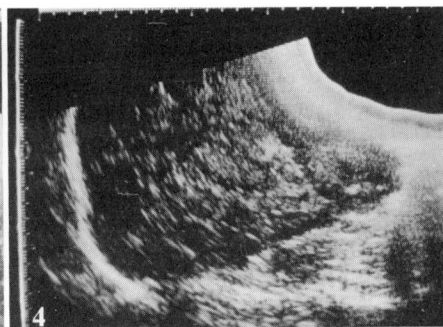

Fig. 4. Diffuse infiltration of the liver with metastases from carcinoma of breast.

b) <u>Disruptive</u>. The disruptive liver echo pattern may also be described as the replacement pattern, and is seen in conditions where almost the entire normal hepatic parenchyma is replaced. This situation may be seen in extensive metastatic replacement of the liver, an example is shown in Fig. 4. A disruptive echo pattern may also be seen in extensive polycystic disease of the liver where the liver is almost totally replaced by varying sized cysts and little normal hepatic parenchyma is visible. An example of this is shown in Fig. 5.
c). <u>Echo-poor</u>. The echo-poor liver is difficult to recog-

nize. Its recognition is markedly dependent on accurate swept gain and overall gain settings on the equipment. It has been described in severe cases of acute hepatitis and also in other acute infections of the liver, such as brucellosis.

d) Bright. The brightly reflective liver echo pattern is readily recognized at standard instrument settings, and is characteristically seen in a group of diffuse liver diseases which include cirrhosis, fatty infiltration and severe hepatitis (3).

CHARACTERISTICS OF THE BRIGHT LIVER ECHO PATTERNS

High amplitude echoes are returned from the liver parenchyma. These are recognized at standard instrument settings. Characteristically this produces disparity between the liver parenchyma and the cortex of the right kidney, which, in this instance, appears abnormally dark in comparison to the liver. The high amplitude echoes within the liver parenchyma produce a uniform mesh appearance, making the liver appear rather featureless(3). There is loss of visualization of the normal bright walls of the portal vein and decreased visualization of the smaller peripheral vessels (4). Distal attenuation of the beam may occur, but this is rather a subjective and variable feature. An example of a typical bright liver echo pattern is shown in Fig.6. Note the presence of the characteristic features described above. The A-scan from this patient is shown in Fig. 7. If this is compared with the A-scan taken from a normal patient shown in Fig. 8, it can be seen that the parenchymal echoes in the bright liver are a half to three quarters the size of the diagphragmatic echo, whereas in the normal A-scan the parenchymal echoes are a quarter to a third the size of the diagphragmatic echo. At liver biopsy, the patient shown in Fig. 6 had diffuse fatty infiltration of the liver with no

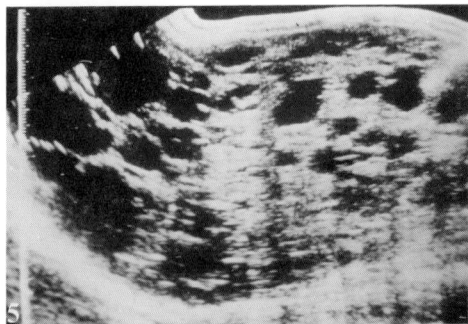

Fig. 5. Diffuse replacement of liver with multiple varying sized cysts in adult polycystic disease.

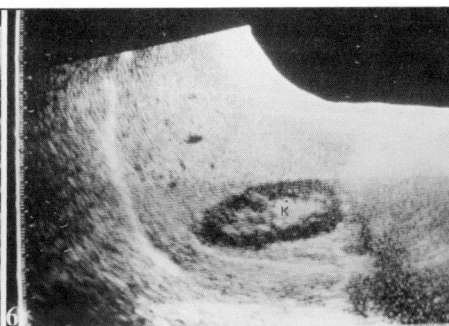

Fig.6. Brightly reflective echo pattern in a patient with fatty infiltration of the liver.

evidence of cirrhotic change. Fig. 9 is another typical example of a brightly reflective echo pattern, showing similar
features to those shown in Fig. 6. However, the biopsy report on this patient revealed evidence of micro-nodular cirrhosis with only a minimal fatty change within the liver.
Two strikingly different pathologies have produced remarkably similar ultrasound images. Fig. 10 is a further example of a typical brightly reflective liver echo pattern,
this taken from a patient with severe Hepatitis B and evidence of a minor degree of fatty infiltration in the liver
at the time of biopsy. Again, it can be seen that the appearances on the ultrasound image are similar to the two
previous examples. This important point, that differing
liver pathologies can give very similar bright liver echo
patterns, is summarized in Fig. 11, which shows longitudinal scans taken in the mid clavicular line from four different patients. The three brightly reflective scans are
taken from a patient with diffuse fatty infilitration, a
patient with cirrhosis and a patient with severe hepatitis.
A normal liver scan is shown for comparison purposes.

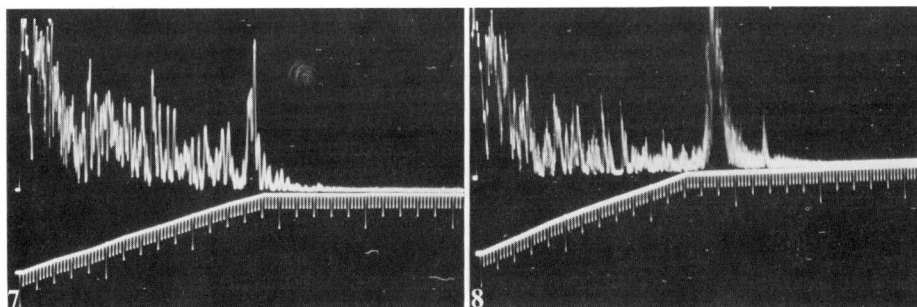

Fig. 7. A-scan from the patient shown in Fig. 6.

Fig. 8. A-scan taken from a normal patient. Compare with Fig.7.

ANALYSIS OF ULTRASOUND FINDINGS

Three separate, but related, studies have been carried
out to investigate the significance of the bright liver echo
pattern and its value in the detection of diffuse liver diseases. In the first study, over a ten-month period, a consecutive series of 60 patients was seen with a bright liver
echo pattern on the ultrasound images(3). In no case was the
histological diagnosis known at the time of the examination,
and follow-up was by analysis of the patients' records. A
subsequent biopsy was available on 47 of the patients and
these results are summarized in Table 1. There were no
false positives in this series. The finding, therefore, of
a bright liver echo pattern on ultrasound was considered
highly significant. It can be seen that this finding corresponds to one of a small group of liver pathologies. The

majority of patients were shown to have cirrhosis and the next largest group of patients were shown to have fatty infiltration and portal fibrosis. In this study, it was found that correlation with the severity of pathological change was poor. Both very early cirrhosis and minor degrees of fatty infiltration were detected and did not appear significantly different from more gross pathological changes of the same conditions. It became apparent during the study that several patients with established cirrhosis had normal liver ultrasound examinations. It was therefore apparent that ultrasound was not a reliable screening procedure for detection of cirrhosis, and that the histopathological reason for the bright liver echo pattern was more complex than simply the presence of fibrous tissue within the liver.

TABLE 1.   ULTRASOUND FINDING OF A BRIGHT LIVER

	HISTOLOGY	BRIGHT LIVER
1.	Cirrhosis	27
2.	Portal fibrosis/Fatty infiltration	16
3.	Severe hepatitis	2
4.	Cardiac cirrhosis	2
	TOTAL	47 patients

A separate study was therefore undertaken to establish the reliability with which ultrasound will detect cirrhosis (5). A group of 66 patients was collected who had had an ultrasound examination and liver biopsy within three months of one another and in whom the liver biopsy had shown cirrhosis of the liver. The patients were divided into two main groups depending on the type of echo pattern identified at the ultrasound examination. This is summarized below:

<u>BIOPSY PROVEN CIRRHOSIS</u>

66 patients

43 bright pattern   23 normal pattern

(50% other abnormalities)

In the first group of 43 patients a diagnosis of cirrhosis was strongly suggested by the recognition at ultrasound examination of a bright liver echo pattern. This confirms that ultrasound is not a reliable screening procedure for the detection of cirrhosis but that two out of three cases can be recognized. On a subjective basis, it is possible to subdivide the bright liver echo pattern into three types:
1. Marked fine bright pattern
2. Marked coarse bright pattern

3. Moderate bright pattern

Within all these three groups it is also possible to note the presence of significant distal attenuation of the sound beam. We have been unable to show any correlation between specific pathological findings and the subdivided ultrasound groups to suggest a tissue specificity for the findings. In this respect, our experience differs from that of other workers who have taken the two ends of the spectrum, the coarse bright liver with marked distal attenuation and the fine bright liver with no increase in attenuation, as being characteristic of cirrhosis and fatty infiltration respectively (6). In the second group of 23 patients with cirrhosis, the liver echo pattern was considered within normal limits. In spite of this, however, abnormalities were recorded in just over half the patients in this group, the most common abnormalities found being enomegaly, hepatomegaly, ascites, portal vein enlargement and portal vein fibrosis. In a clinical context these are all findings of relevance in a patient with cirrhosis. In the two groups, a careful analysis has been made of the full pathology reports and the findings of selected pathological features within the two groups are summarized in Table 2.

TABLE 2. COMPARISON OF PATHOLOGICAL FINDINGS

Selected features from biopsy reports	BRIGHT PATTERN (ultrasound group 1 --- 43 patients)	NORMAL PATTERN (ultrasound group 2 --- 23 patients)
Micronodular cirrhosis	50%	15%
Macronodular cirrhosis	10%	66%
Piecemeal necrosis	15%	50%
Fatty change	30%	15%

Comparison between the two main groups shows that there is a considerable amount of overlap, however a definite trend does become apparent. Micronodular cirrhosis, with or without fatty infiltration is more likely to yield a positive ultrasound result. In fact, if all the cases of micronodular cirrhosis are considered together, ultrasound will be positive in over 80% of cases. Macronodular cirrhosis, with or without piecemeal necrosis, is more likely to yield a negative result. Again, if these cases are considered as a group, ultrasound will be negative in approximately 80% of cases. Whilst this is only a trend, it is a substantial one in this series and may provide a clue as to the aetiology of the ultrasound appearances.

A further small study has been made of patients showing evidence of fatty infiltration of the liver but no evidence of cirrhosis. This is an uncommon condition, and so
this has been a rather small study. Twenty patients were
collected who had undergone ultrasound examination within
on month of their liver biopsy(7). In this series all the
ultrasound records were re-examined in random order, without prior knowledge of the patient's condition or of the
original ultrasound report. Twelve of the patients with a
fatty liver (60%) had a bright liver pattern. While only
three out of 10 patients with mild fatty infiltration had
a bright liver echo pattern, 9 of the 10 patients with histologically moderate or severe infiltration showed this pattern. It is clear that the sensitivity of detection of fatty infiltration by ultrasound is related to the severity of
pathological change. In this series overall 60% of patients
with fatty infiltration were detected, but in those patients
with moderate to severe changes the detection rate increased
to 90%.

The precise origin of bright echoes returned from the
liver remains unresolved. An increase in the fibrous tissue content of the liver has been shown to be the cause by
some workers (8). This does not seem surprising, as the
elastic modulus of collagen fibres is approximately a thou-
sand times greater than that of other soft tissues. This
produces large accoustic impedance mismatches, and therefore
strong echoes at collagen soft tissue interfaces. However,
in a comprehensive study of fatty tissue tumours, it has
been shown that fat is strongly echogenic(9). In our analysis of the bright liver echo pattern, we showed that fatty
livers with no evidence of fibrosis and cirrhotic livers
with no evidence of significant fatty infiltration may show
similar ultrasound appearances of bright echo patterns. The
precise reason why fatty tissue is echogenic is unclear. Experiments have shown that in vitro an emulsion of fat and
water is highly echogenic. This is probably because the ul-

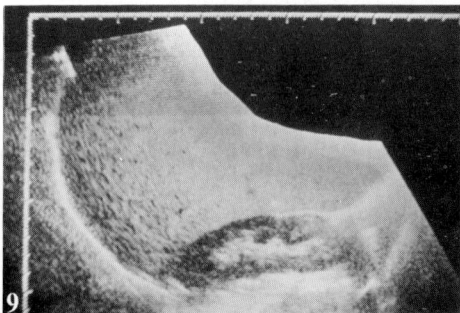

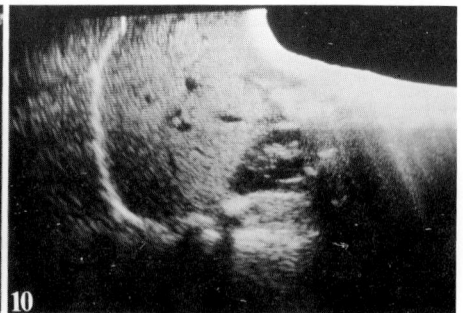

Fig. 9. An enlarged liver showing a brightly reflective echo
pattern. The patient had cirrhosis.

Fig.10. A brightly reflective
echo pattern seen in a patient with severe hepatitis.

trasonic velocity is reduced by about 10% in fat as compared with other soft tissues. This leads to relatively large accoustic impedence mismatches at soft tissue/fat interfaces. In fatty infiltration of the liver, the globular fat cells can be considered as an emulsion within the "water phase" of the surrounding soft tissues. It seems clear that there are two possible causes of brightly reflective echo patterns in the liver, fibrous tissue and fatty tissue.

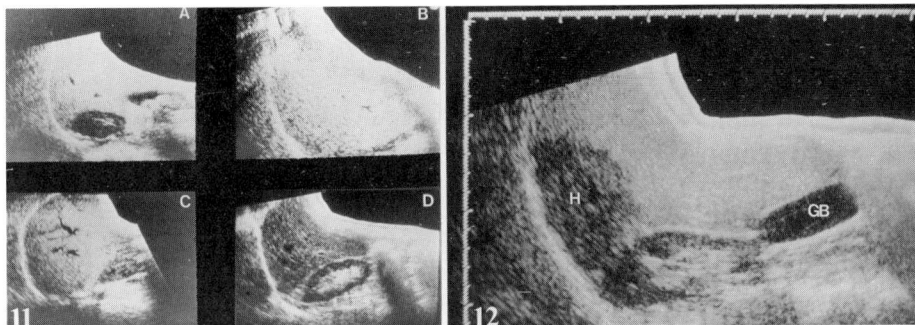

Fig. 11. The composite figure showing: a) fatty infiltration; b) cirrhosis; c) severe hepatitis; d) a normal liver. Note the similarity in appearance of the brightly reflective echo patterns.

Fig. 12. A brightly reflective liver echo pattern in patient with cirrhosis. A hepatoma (H) is seen posteriorly in the right lobe of liver.

SUMMARY

The finding of a brightly reflective liver echo pattern is highly significant. We have shown that there is a close correlation with cirrhosis and fatty infiltration. The false positive rate in our experience is extremely low, under 5%. Overall, about 65% of patients with either fatty infiltration or cirrhosis will be detected by ultrasound. However, if there is moderate to severe fatty change within the liver, ultrasound will detect 90% of these patients. If the patient has micronodular cirrhosis of the liver the pickup rate will be approximately 80%. These findings indicate that ultrasound is at least as valuable in the evaluation and detection of diffuse liver disease as in focal liver disease.

It should not be forgotten that focal liver disease and diffuse liver disease may coexist. The incidence of hepatocellular carcinoma is increased in patients with cirrhosis, and in Fig. 12 an example of a patient with cirrhosis of the liver is shown who has developed a hepatoma in the posterior part of the right lobe. Note the overall bright echo pattern of the liver which is disturbed in the region of the hepatoma which shows as a relatively echo-poor area.

439

1. Meire, H.B.(1979): British Journal of Radiology, <u>52</u>, 685-703.
2. Birnholz, J.(1979): In: Diagnostic Ultrasound in Gastro-Intestinal Disease, Churchill Livingstone, Chpt. 2.
3. Joseph, A.E., Dewbury, K.C. & McGuire, P.G. (1979): British Journal of Radiology, <u>52</u>, 184-188.
4. Gosing, B.B., Lemon, S.K., Scheible, W., Leopold, G.R. (1979): American Journal of Radiology, <u>133</u>, 19-23.
5. Dewbury, K.C. & Clark, B. (1979): British Journal of Radiology. (in press).
6. Taylor, K.J.W., Carpenter, D.A., Hill, C.R. & McReady, V.R. (1976): Radiology, <u>119</u>, 415-523.
7. Foster, K.J., Dewbury, K.C., Griffith, A.H. & Wright, R, (1979):British Journal of Radiology (in press).
8. Mcuntford, R.A. & Wells, P.T.N. (1972):Physics in Medicine and Biology, 17, 261-269.
9. Behan, M. & Kazam, E. (1978): Radiology, <u>129</u>, 143-151.

THE ROLE OF ULTRASOUND IN ACUTE POST TRANSPLANT RENAL FAILURE

H. Hricak, W.R. Eyler

Department of Diagnostic Radiology, Henry Ford Hospital, Detroit,
Michigan 48202

Diagnostic ultrasound is a reliable, noninvasive diagnostic procedure extensively used in the evaluation of patients with renal
transplants. Its application in the past has been in the diagnosis
of hydronephrosis and perirenal fluid collections. An increase in
renal volume and increased echogenicity of the kidney are reported
as diagnostic criteria of rejection. With the recent improvement in
ultrasound units, the renal anatomy can be well displayed and thus a
good analysis of the pathological changes within the kidney can be
achieved. We will discuss the sonographic parenchymal changes seen
during acute tubular necrosis and rejection.

MATERIALS

This presentation includes nine patients with rejection. The diagnosis was proven by clinical and laboratory data by radionuclide
studies, in two cases by arteriography and in two cases by nephrec-
tomy. There are six cases of acute tubular necrosis. Acute tubular
necrosis was proven by clinical and laboratory data, by radionuclide
studies and the most important by response to specific therapy.

METHODS

Within the first 24 to 48 hours after transplantation, control
studies should always be obtained to serve as a baseline for comparison with future scans. The patient is scanned in a supine position
using mineral oil as a coupling agent between transducer and skin.
Simple sector scans and linear scans are made parallel to and at
right angles to the longitudinal axis of the kidney.

We used commercially available gray scale units with 3.5 Mhz and
5 Mhz focused transducers. The scanning area includes the kidney
allograft with adjacent vasculature and perinephric tissue. Particular attention should be paid to the sensitivity (gain setting)
and the time gain compensation, (TGC). Too high a gain setting increases the tendency to record artifacts from echo-free structures,
while too low a gain setting prevents distinction between homogeneous solid structures and fluid collections. We used white
recording on a black background.

RESULTS

ACUTE TUBULAR NECROSIS

In our clinical experience, there are no sonographic changes seen
during acute tubular necrosis. The sonograms showed no alterations

throughout the course of ATN, (Fig.1). Significant kidney enlargement was not appreciated. The exact evaluation of the kidney enlargement in the immediate post transplantation period is difficult
since we do know that normal renal hypertrophy takes place at the
same time.

REJECTION

The previously reported increase in the renal volume was also seen
in our study. Increase in renal volume was not nearly as marked as
in the experimental studies, (3). The first sonographic change observed during acute rejection was enlargement of the medullary pyramids, (3,7), due to edema, (Fig.2). The cortex became either more
echogenic with the echoes being sparsely distributed or the cortical
echogenicity decreased, (2). Decreased echogenicity was either uniform or localized. The cortical medullary boundary became indistinct
in random locations, (3,7). A late sign of rejection was decrease
in the central sinus echoes, (7). In cases of renal rupture, secondary to rejection, perirenal fluid collections disappeared. Also,
crescent shaped fluid collections were seen without renal rupture
being present, (Fig.3).

DISCUSSION

Acute tubular necrosis and acute rejection are two major complications in the period after the transplantation. The therapy of the
two conditions is different making it very important to establish
the correct diagnosis. The therapy of acute tubular necrosis includes
only dieuretics and adequate hydration, while the dose of steroids
remains the same. In contrast, during acute rejection, the therapy
requires increases in the dosage of steroids. By clinical and laboratory parameters alone, the differentiation between the two conditions
cannot be achieved. Excretory urography, arteriography and retrograde pyelography do not provide critical information and may contribute to further renal damage. Furthermore, arteriography and
excretory urography are invasive procedures and as such should be
avoided where possible in every transplant patient. Radionuclide
studies are noninvasive procedures which provide us with functional
and anatomical information about the transplanted kidney. With
multiple radionuclide studies, the correct diagnosis can be suggested, but it should be emphasized that this cannot always be done
conclusively.

Sonographically, there are different patterns seen during rejection
as compared to ATN. While during the course of acute tubular necrosis, the sonograms show no alteration from the baseline study, there
are numerous findings seen during rejection. Some of the findings
of rejection are always present. The sonographic findings in rejection closely correspond to the pathological tissue changes and re-
membering that rejection is a dynamic process, the findings always
reflect the stage that the rejection process has reached.

SUMMARY

In acute post transplant renal failure, when the patient presents
with appropriate clinical and laboratory data and equivocal radionuclide studies, the differentiation between ATN and rejection can
be made by ultrasound.

REFERENCES

1. Conrad MR, et al: New Observations in Renal Transplants Using
    Ultrasound. Am J Roentgenol 131:851   1978
2. Hillman BJ, Birnholz JC, et al: Correlation of Echographic and
    Histologic Findings in Suspected Renal Allograft Rejection.
    Radiology 132 (3):673-676 Sep 1979
3. Hricak H, et al: The Role of Ultrasound in the Diagnosis of
    Kidney Allograft Rejection. Radiology 132 (3):667-672 Sep 1979
4. Hricak H, et al: Evaluation of Acute Post-Transplant Renal
    Failure by Ultrasound. Radiology Nov 1979
5. Hricak H, et al: Sonographic Findings Following Acute Renal
    Vein Thrombosis-Experimental Study. Presented AUR, May 1979
6. Hricak H, et al: Pitfalls in Hydronephrosis (In Preparation)
7. Maklad NF, Wright CH, et al: Gray Scale Ultrasonic Appearances
    of Renal Transplant Rejection. Radiology 131 (3):711-718
    Jun 1979

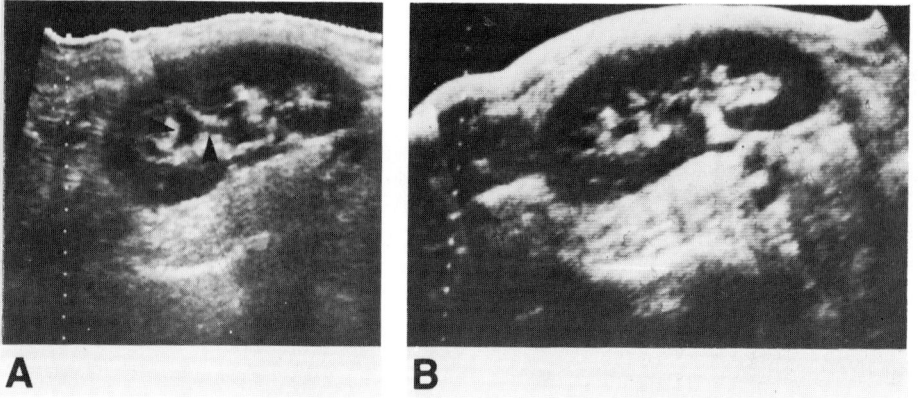

Fig. 1 ATN. a. Longitudinal scan 24 hours following surgery.
There is mild hydronephrosis. In the immediate post transplant
period, this is of no clinical significance. Dilated calyx (arrow)
and infundibulum (arrowhead). b. Seven days later. The serum
creatinine is 4 mg/dl. Hydronephrosis is no longer evident. The
renal parenchyma shows no change from the baseline study.

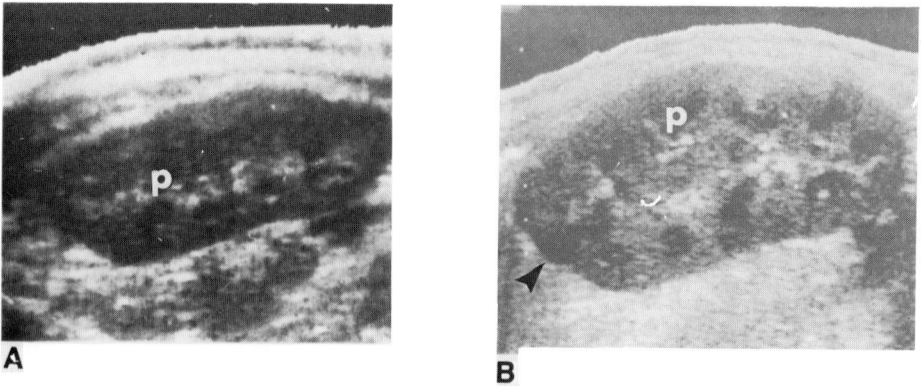

Fig. 2 Rejection. a. Longitudinal sonogram 48 hours after surgery.
Normal renal transplant. Normal renal pyramids (P). b. 10 days
later. The serum creatinine is 3 mg/dl. The kidney is enlarged and
the medullary pyramids (P) are now swollen and prominent. There is
also an anechoic area (arrow) along the cranial pole of the kidney
representing an area of hemorrhage or infarction.

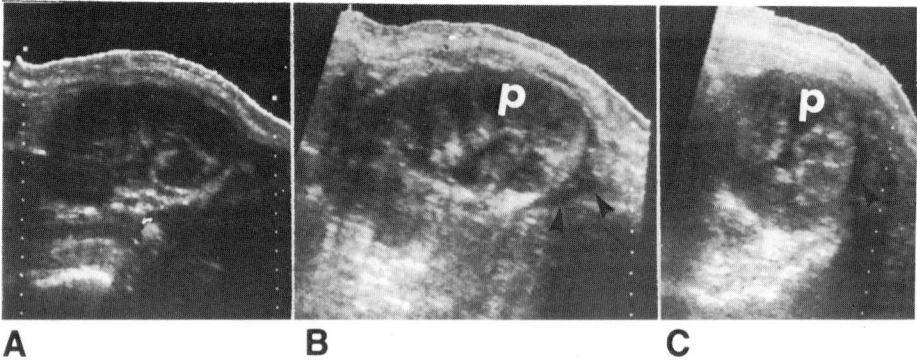

Fig. 3 Rejection. a. Normal renal transplant 24 hours following surgery. b. Eight days later. The serum creatinine is 3 mg/dl. Prominent renal pyramids (P). There is a crescent collection of fluid on the caudal pole of the kidney (arrow). c. Transverse scan taken at the same time as 3a shows prominent pyramids (P) and crescent collection of fluid (arrow).

13. INVITED REVIEWS

PULSATIONS OF INTRACRANIAL ECHOES IN RANGE: A MEANS OF MEASURING
PULSATILE FLOW THROUGH THE AQUEDUCT OF SYLVIUS IN MAN AND VARIATIONS
IN THIS FLOW WITH INCREASED INTRACRANIAL PRESSURE AND HYPERCAPNOEA

D.N. White

Queens University, Kingston, Canada.

INTRODUCTION

   Pulsations of echoes from interfaces in the brain both in amplitude and range have been observed since the earliest days of echoencephalography (1). Initially it was hoped that their measurement
might give information of clinical value especially in cases of cerebrovascular disease. These hopes have not been realised and, at the
present moment, little work is being carried out in this field.
This disillusionment results from similar factors that have led to
the decline in interest in echoencephalography. The technique has
marked limitations.
   We have described previously the measurement of intracranial
echo pulsations (2) and the reasons that recording the pulsations in
amplitude are less valuable than recording the pulsations in range
(3). Pulsations in amplitude are susceptible to artifact due to movement. This results either from movement of the transducer with respect to the skull or, more usually, from movement of the brain causing the interface to move out of the range gate or other interfaces
moving into the gate. Recording pulsations in range are subject to
the same artifacts but these are easier to identify (4). The use of
a tracking gate reduces these limitations for both types of recording.
Recording the pulsations in range is more informative than recording
pulsations in amplitude. Their magnitude can be measured in absolute
units and this magnitude is proportional to the pressure differential
across the interface that causes its motion. This is not the case
with variations in amplitude which depends on more complex factors.
Moreover a change in range indicates the direction of motion while
an increase or decrease in amplitude has no such significance.
   It is more difficult to circumvent the limitations resulting from
the marked and irregular scattering of the beam by the skull (5, 6
and 7). As a result, the interfaces from which recordings are made,
may be quite variously positioned with respect to the physical axis
of the beam and these positions cannot be determined. Moreover, this
pattern of irregular scattering varies markedly with any movement of
the beam with respect to the skull and it is never possible to remove
and replace the transducer so that the same pattern of scattering
recurs (8). This means that it is not possible to be certain of
recording either the movement or the amplitude of the pulsations from
any single interface in the same individual on separate occasions.
It is even less possible to record the pulsations from the same
cerebral interface in different individuals. It is for this reason
that we were able to show (9) that recording of the shape of the curve

449

of the pulsations in range is of little value. There is too great a variation between individuals and in recordings made from different interfaces in the same individual.

Within these limitations it is nevertheless possible to obtain information of value from recording the pulsations in range. By making continuous recordings from the same cerebral interface, while intracranial pressure was raised and lowered, we showed that the increase in the magnitude of range pulsations that occur as intracranial pressure rises are not the result of decreased damping as had previously been thought (10, 11 and 12) but rather as a result of redistribution of the cerebral circulation (13). With this technique we were also able for the first time to record modulation resembling Traube-Hering waves from the healthy human brain (14 and 15). We also recorded the marked ballistic movements in the ventricular walls and septum pellucidum in certain cases of hydrocephalus (16). It was this latter observation that suggested to us that pulsatile stress and strain at the interface between the brain and the ventricles might be more important as a cause of hydrocephalus than obstruction to the circulation of C.S.F. As a consequence we have proposed a new hypothesis to explain the aetiology of hydrocephalus (17) which may result in better prevention and treatment of this condition. We now report the ultrasonic observations which contributed to this new hypothesis.

METHOD

The multi-gated range and amplitude recording device that we developed for studying pulsations in range and amplitude has been previously described (3). It is able to record variations in range as small as 10 μm and, with the addition of a tracking system (4) as large as 7 mm. It is thus superior in its range to other range recorders such as that developed by Freund and Kapp (18) which is able to measure only the larger movements. It was for this reason that Freund (19) only recorded the larger range variations arising from the cerebral arteries and did not realise that the brain interfaces also moved in a pulsatile fashion but to a much smaller degree.

This system measures only the variations in range of those echoes within its gates in the vector of motion which is radial to the generator-receiver.

Despite the restrictions described above and this further restriction, information can be obtained from such recordings if an assumption is made. This assumption is that, in any one region of the brain, all the interfaces move in almost exactly the same direction and by almost exactly the same amount with each systolic pulsation. This assumption appears reasonable from an understanding of the effects of pressure or volume changes upon the semi-fluid contents of a largely closed system such as the cranium. It also seems reasonable since the propagation of the arterial pulse through the brain does not result in physical disruption of the cellular structure of the brain. Thus, if recordings are made from one region of the brain with the physical axis of the generator-receiver variously orientated with respect to this region, the maximal pulsatile variations in range recorded will represent both the true magnitude of motion and the vector of this motion for all the interfaces in this region.

450

It is not however possible to record the pulsatile motions of cerebral interfaces from any region of the brain from all possible orientations of the transducer. This results from the shape of the skull and the necessity for the transducer face to be placed flat on the scalp and for the generated beam to be normal to the underlying skull (21 and 5). The region of our particular interest, was that of the third ventricle and the anterior portion of the body of the lateral ventricle. It is possible to insonate this region along the three Cartesian axes with the transducer placed in the mid-frontal, vertical and supra-pinnal regions of the scalp.

RESULTS

By recording the magnitude of the systolic changes in range of a large number of interfaces along these three Cartesian axes in a large number of normal persons it is possible to see (Figs. 1 and 2) that systolic motion becomes maximal as this central region of interest, comprising the lateral and third ventricles, is approached. This increasing motion indicates that the brain itself increases in volume during systole. The vector of these increasing motions is largely inward and downward. Such an observation shows that, as a result of the increase in volume of the brain, the brain moves inward towards the lateral and third ventricles and downward towards the venous and C.S.F. pressure sinks in the posterior fossa and foramen magnum. This downward motion of all the intracranial contents no doubt compresses the basal cisterns of the C.S.F. and the basal venous sinuses. It is presumably restricted by the tentorium cerebelli. On the other hand, the magnitude of the systolic motions inward towards the ventricles (Fig. 2) decrease after the boundaries of these ventricles are reached. This observation demonstrated that there is compression of the lateral and third ventricles as has been shown to occur during pneumoencephalography by duBoulay (20) and in the intact human by ourselves (14 and 3). The incompressible C.S.F. within these ventricles must, as a result, be displaced in the only possible direction, downwards through the aqueduct of Sylvius towards the foramen magnum and the volume sink of the compliant spinal subarachnoid space.

It should be noted that occasional interfaces show magnitudes of motion considerably in excess of the envelopes we have drawn for the majority of the measurements we made. We believe these large movements are those from the regions of the cerebral arteries as recorded by Freund and Kapp's (18) system. Such movements are as large as a millimetre or more. That we did not display them as such large movements was due to the absence of the tracking facility at the time these measurements were made so that 0.2 mm was the largest motion we could then display.

These observations were novel and showed that the hypothesis previously proposed by Bering (22) that the arterial pressure wave was generated by the choroid plexus, was not tenable. The well-known observation that, at operation, the exposed brain moves outwards with each systolic pulsation is misleading and results from the fact that the cranium is no longer a closed system during a craniotomy.

These are qualitative observations. In our studies of the cause of hydrocephalus (17) we wished to have a quantitative estimate of the volume decrease of the C.S.F. within the third and lateral

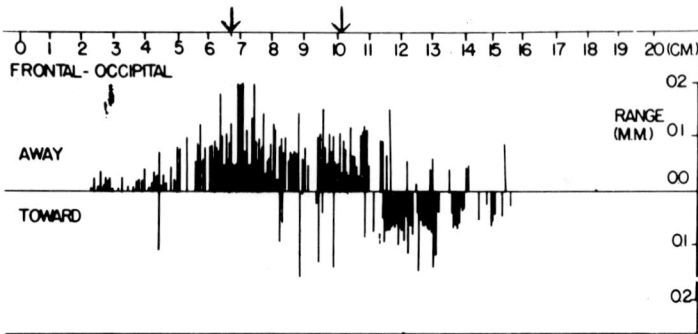

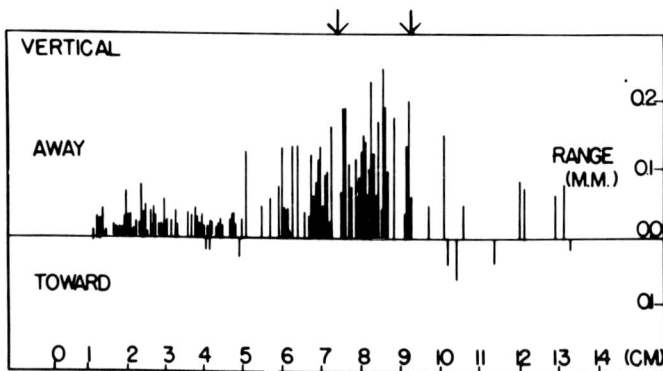

Fig. 1. The magnitudes of the systolic motion of a large number of cerebral interfaces at varying ranges along the fronto-occipital axis (upper) and vertical axis (lower). The arrows indicate the approximate position along both axes of the III ventricle. By comparison with Figure 2 showing the magnitudes of such systolic motion measured in the transtemporal axis, it will be noticed that the greatest movements of the brain in the vertical axis resulting from the propagation of the arterial pressure pulse are in a downward direction. These increase in magnitude as the III ventricle is approached showing that the brain above the ventricle is expanding: they decrease in magnitude at depths corresponding to the posterior fossa where measurements were difficult to make, presumably due to their restraint by the tentorium cerebelli. In the fronto-occipital axis the magnitude of the motions recorded also increase as the ventricular system is approached both anteriorly and posteriorly again showing that the brain is expanding in these regions. Note that the direction of movement from the cerebral expansion is always inwards towards the ventricles which are thus compressed.

452

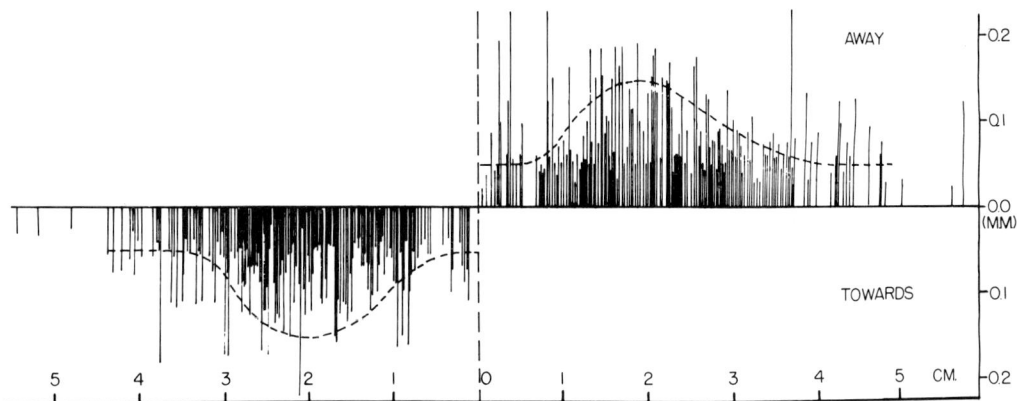

Fig. 2. The magnitude of the systolic movements in range of a large number of cerebral interfaces at varying distances from the cerebral midline in the transtemporal axis. The dotted lines correspond to the envelopes of the mean of all the motions measured. The magnitude of the motion increases up to a distance of 2 cms from the midline corresponding to the margins of the anterior portions of the bodies of the lateral ventricles. The brain is thus expanding lateral to this region. Medial to this region the magnitudes of the motions decrease showing the ventricles are being compressed. A few milli-metres to either side of the midline, corresponding to the position of the III ventricles, the interfaces are moving in opposite direc-tions as the two walls of the III ventricles are compressed.

ventricles resulting from the expansion of the brain caused by the arterial pulse so that we could calculate the rates of flow in the aqueduct of Sylvius during systole. If, with each systolic volume expansion of the brain, C.S.F. is displaced downwards from the lateral and third ventricles towards the compliant spinal subarach-noid space, we became interested in the limitations that might be imposed upon this venting pathway. Systole approximates 300 ms in duration during which period the appropriate volume of C.S.F. must be displaced downwards through the aqueduct of Sylvius, fourth ventricle and cisterna magna into the spinal subarachnoid space. It seemed obvious that the greatest difficulty in accommodating such flow would lie in the aqueduct of Sylvius because it is narrower than any other part of this pathway.

Calculation of the pressure-flow relationship that might be ex-pected in cylindrical tubes approximating the aqueduct in both length and diameter (dashed lines in Fig. 3) show that this is linear at lower rates of flow which are laminar. However above a certain rate, marked by the vertical bars, flow becomes disturbed and increasingly turbulent so that the relationship increasingly becomes quadratic. The question obviously arises whether such flows can be achieved with the pressure differential that is available across the two ends of the aqueduct of Sylvius.

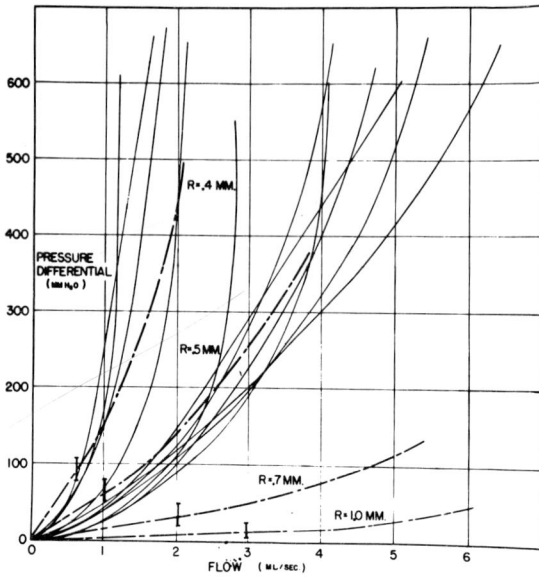

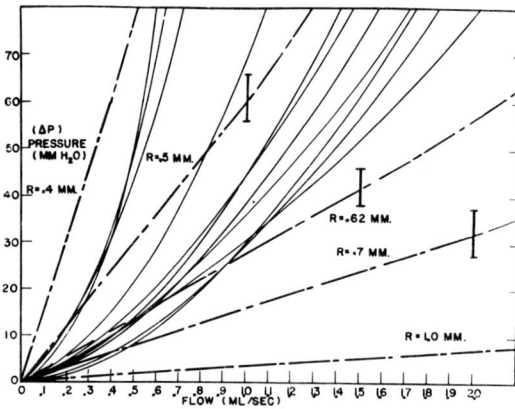

Fig. 3. The pressure-flow curves (dashed lines) calculated for water in cylindrical tubes 1.5 cm in length and with the varying radii indicated. The lower graph is an enlargement of the low flow and pressure region shown at the lower left of the upper graph. The vertical bars represent the transition points between laminar and turbulent flow.

The solid curves represent the pressure flow curves measured through the aqueducts of 12 normal human brain stems fixed in formalin.

However the aqueduct of Sylvius is not a regular cylindrical tube and it seemed more realistic to determine the pressure-flow relationship that can occur through it by experiment rather than by calculation. The solid lines in Figure 3 show the pressure-flow curves obtained by experiment through the aqueducts of twelve normal human brains fixed in formalin. There is very little experimental evidence of the pressure differential that occurs across the aqueduct in intact humans during systole. Bering (22) however recorded simultaneously the pressures in the lateral ventricles and cisterna magna of an 11 year old boy and found a differential between them of 13 mm H_2O. For methodological reasons this may be lower than the true differential pressure. However it will be appreciated that, with such pressures, flow through the cadaver aqueducts would amount to 0.25-0.85 ml s or 0.08-0.28 ml during the 300 m s of systole.

The question arises whether such volumes do in fact represent the quantity of C.S.F. displaced from the lateral and third ventricles with each heart beat. If there have been few measurements of intraventricular pressures in the intact human being, there have been none made of the volume of C.S.F. displaced by the systolic expansion of the brain. It was in making such measurements that the ultrasonic technique provided an unique tool.

In order to convert the varying centripetal motions we had measured into volume displacement of the C.S.F. from the lateral ventricles, it was necessary to determine the size of the lateral ventricles at the different regions in the transtemporal axis where the motion curves showed that compressive motion of varying degrees was occurring. We sectioned three normal fixed brains in the sagittal plane at approximately 5 mm intervals. One of these brains was chosen as having ventricles at the upper limit of normal size. We measured the surface area of the lateral ventricle in each section and plotted these areas against range in the transtemporal axis to either side of the cerebral midline (Fig. 4). By summing these areas we calculated that the two lateral ventricles of our three specimens had volumes of 43, 22 and 14 ml which corresponds with the volumes measured by Last and Tompsett (23) who found that the volume of the whole ventricular system averaged 22 ml with extremes of 7 and 57 ml. From the areas of the lateral ventricles at these varying ranges from the cerebral midline by means of the slopes representing systolic centripetal motion at corresponding ranges, it was possible to state that such motion would compress the lateral ventricles and reduce their volume by 0.07 or 0.10 ml for the two smaller ventricles and 0.08 ml for the larger ventricles. Similar volumes were obtained whether the slope of the curve of peak or average systolic motion of the cerebral interfaces was used. It will be noted that no increased volume of C.S.F. is vented from the brain with larger ventricles. This is due, of course, to the fact that the volume of C.S.F. vented from the lateral ventricles depends upon the volume increase in the brain and is independent of the volume of fluid contained in the ventricular system, only a small fraction of which is displaced with each systole.

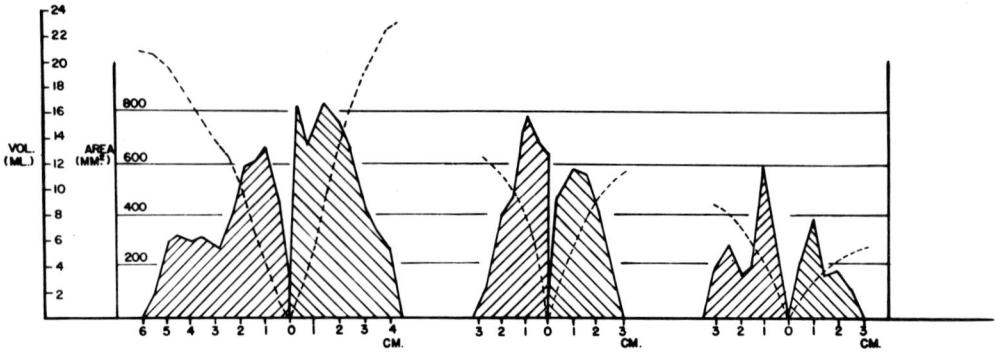

Fig. 4. The surface area of the lateral ventricles was measured in
three normal human brains from sections in the fronto-occipital plane
made at 0.5 cm intervals (cross-hatched areas). The volume of the
ventricles was then calculated at increasing distances from the midline (dotted lines). From these measurements it was possible, from
the slope of the envelope of the motions measured in Figure 2, to
calculate the volume reduction that such compressive motion at varying
distances from the midline would represent and hence the total reduction in volume of the ventricles as a result of such motion.

Within a few millimetres to either side of the midline, corresponding to the position of the walls of the third ventricle, the
interfaces are moving in opposing directions by approximately 0.05
mm. If the third ventricle is considered as a hemi-disc with an average diameter of 4.4 cms (24) the surface area of each of its lateral
walls will be approximately 7.5 cm^2. If the lateral walls each
moved inwards 0.005 cms, then the volume of the ventricle will be decreased 0.07 ml.
    It would appear therefore that from both lateral ventricles
and the third ventricle a total of about 0.27-0.20 ml of C.S.F. is
displaced downwards through the aqueduct during each period of cardiac systole. These volumes are slightly greater than those calculated from the pressure available across the aqueduct and quoted
above. For a number of reasons however we believe these results
are not incompatible (17).
    We were also interested in determining what factors might in-
fluence the volume of C.S.F. displaced from the lateral and third
ventricles through the aqueduct of Sylvius with each cardiac cycle.
We were especially interested in those factors which might increase
this volume to a quantity which could no longer be accommodated,
with the pressure available, by the narrow aqueduct. As was mentioned in the Introduction, it is not possible to make comparative
measurements of the systolic motion of cerebral interfaces from
different individuals such as two groups of patients with and without
raised intracranial pressure. Nor is it possible to make comparable
measurements from the same individual on separate occasions such
as in a patient with raised intracranial pressure which subsequently
becomes normal or vice versa. Comparable measurements must be made

456

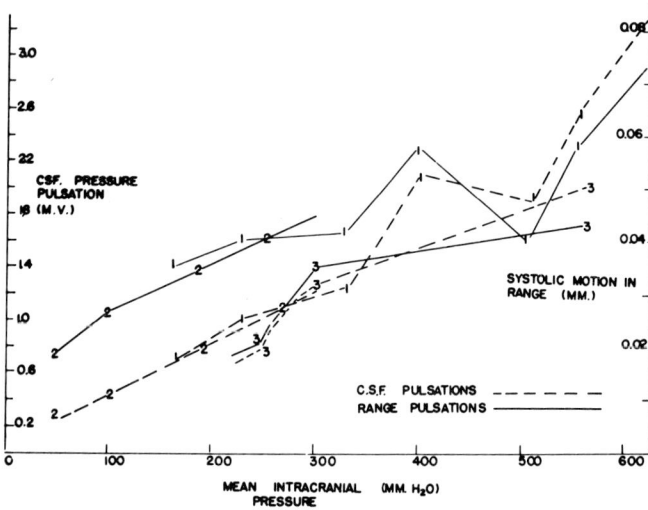

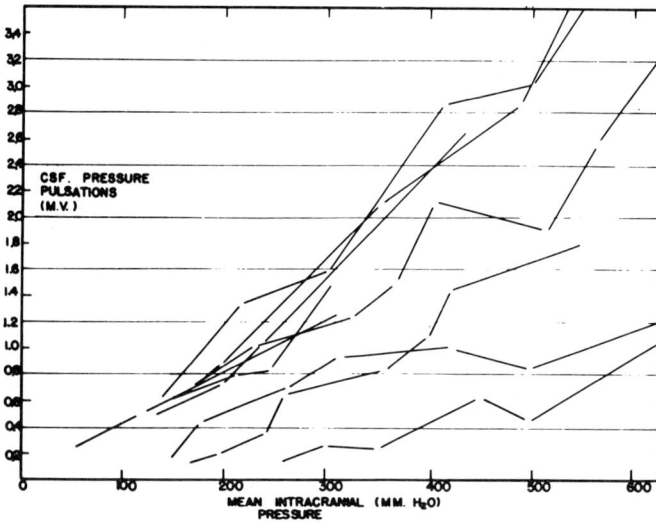

Fig. 5. Top. A comparison of C.S.F. pressure pulsations measured by means of changes in voltages developed by a strain gauge (dotted lines) and by changes in the magnitude of the systolic motion of cerebral interfaces (continuous lines) as mean intracranial pressure is increased by saline infusion into the lumbar subarachnoid space in 3 normal human subjects.

It should be emphasised that variations in motion in range are only proportional to differential pressures across the interface being imaged when they are all made from the same series of measurements from a single interface (3). Thus each of the three sets of measurements illustrated here should have an appropriate but different scale for the motion measured. Under these circumstances each of the three pairs of curves would coincide more closely than in this illustrations where, for convenience, one motion scale has been used for all three sets of measurements.

Bottom. Increases in the magnitude of the systolic pressure pulsations measured by a strain gauge as mean intracranial pressure is raised by saline infusion into the lumbar subarachnoid space of 9 human subjects.

457

on a single patient during a single recording session in which the transducer remains rigidly positioned with respect to the skull so that all measurements are made from the same interface.

With recordings made in this way we raised the intracranial pressure in 9 patients by infusions of saline into the lumbar subarachnoid space. We showed (Fig. 5 top) that the magnitude of the systolic motions we measured were proportional to the pressure pulsations. We then showed that (Fig. 5 bottom) the magnitude of the systolic pressure pulsations as recorded by a conventional strain gauge increases linearly with the intracranial pressure. However, when intracranial pressure was raised secondarily by means of increasing the alveolar pCO_2 in eleven patients (Fig. 6) the increase in the magnitude of the systolic motion of intracranial interfaces show an exponential rise. There is thus a fundamental difference in the increased pulsatile pressure or motions that result from primary increases in raised intracranial pressure and secondary increases that result from cerebral swelling due to vasodilatation (Fig. 7).

The reason for this difference is of some importance in the understanding of different causes of raised intracranial pressure. In the normal brain the pulsatile motions that we record are the result of pulsatile increases in intracranial pressure and volume due to the propagation of the arterial pulse through the cerebral vasculature. As the arterial pressure pulse propagates it expands and increases the volume of the blood vessels and hence of the surrounding brain as a whole. Normally this pressure pulse is wholly attenuated in the arteriolar system so that the pressure and volume increase results from the pulsatile distension of the cerebral arteries and, more particularly, the arterioles. When primarily vasodilatation occurs, as in hypercapnoea, the arterial pressure pulse is less attenuated and can propagate into the compliant capillary and venous systems. Thus the pulsatile pressure and motions initially increase markedly and only later become less marked as the capillary and venous resistance increases due to the secondary increase in intracranial pressure that results from the cerebral swelling. When the increase in intracranial pressure is primary, as occurs in brain oedema, the increased tissue pressure compresses the compliant veins and capillaries and thus increases vascular resistance. As a result, secondary arteriolar vasodilatation occurs in order to maintain cerebral blood flow by reducing arteriolar resistance. Since, with moderate increases in intracranial pressure, cerebral blood flow is maintained at a constant level, the total resistance of the cerebral vasculature also remains unchanged. However the arteriolar vasodilatation reduces arteriolar resistance while compression of the compliant capillary and venous systems by the surrounding tissue increases their resistance so that there is a progressive displacement of the site of maximal vascular resistance from the cerebral arterioles towards the compliant capillary and venous system. This effect had been previously observed using other techniques (25, 26 and 27). It also accounted for the observations of Jenkins and White (13) quoted in the Introduction, who showed that increases in intracranial pressure had no effect on the rise times or shape of the curves of the pulsations in range. As a result of these factors the pulsatile pressures and the movements of the cerebral interfaces

458

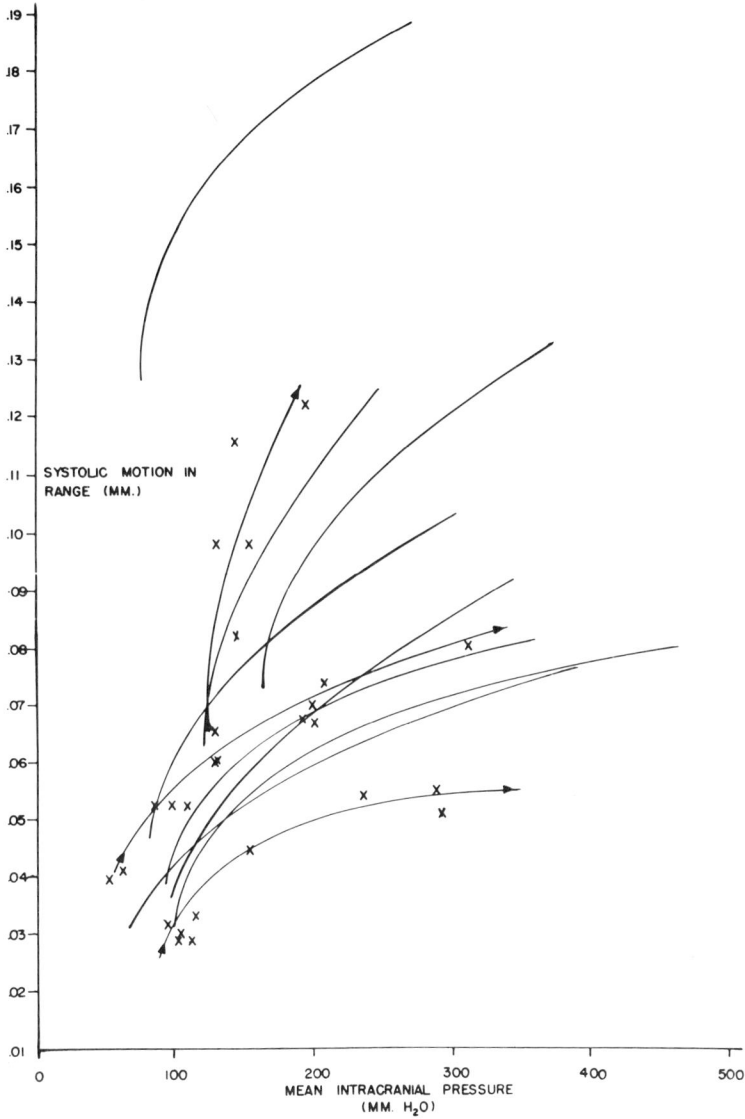

Fig. 6. Increases in the magnitude of the systolic pulsations in range as mean intracranial pressure rises due to increases in alveolar pCO_2 in eleven human subjects. Compare with Figure 5 (bottom).

459

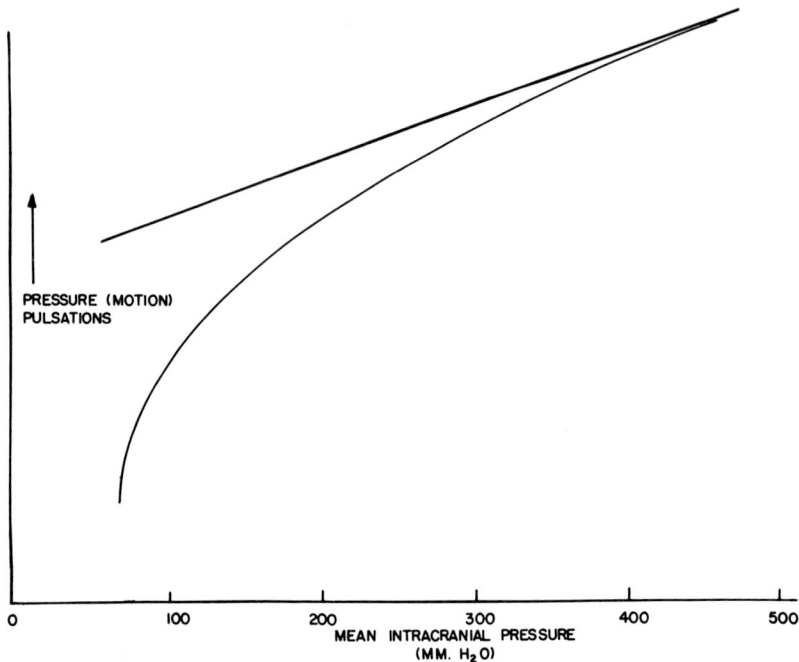

Fig. 7. Comparison of the rate of increase in cerebral pulsatile pressure resulting from primary arteriolar vasodilatation (curved line) and primary increased mean intracranial pressure (straight line). Because measurements of the systolic motion of cerebral interfaces are relative, the position of the two plots relative to each other is not significant, their curvature is significant.

thus caused, show a progressive and linear increase as mean intra-cranial pressure rises (Fig. 5). This observation is in contrast to the marked initial increase in pulsatile motion of cerebral inter-faces that results from primary cerebral vasodilatation (Fig. 6) when the flow of the arterial pressure pulse into the compliant capillary and venous systems is not initially damped by an increase in the surrounding tissue pressure.

   We believe that this difference between the rate with which mean intracranial pressure increases as a result of primary or secondary cerebral vasodilatation accounts for the well known clinical differ-ence in the onset of cerebral confusion and obtundity. Diseases that cause primary cerebral vasodilatation such as CO_2 narcosis, keto-acidosis, uraemia and metabolic encephalopathies cause confusion early in their course; diseases that cause secondary cerebral vasodilatation such as cerebral tumours or cerebral oedema due to trauma and other causes (excluding the initial concussive phase) produce cerebral confusion and reduced consciousness later in their development.

460

DISCUSSION

In the Introduction we emphasised the limitations to which the technique of recording intracranial echo pulsations is subject. While these are less serious if only pulsations in range are recorded, they do make it impossible to make comparative measurements on separate individuals or, on the same individual on separate occasions.

The two examples described in this paper show how these limitations can be circumvented. If it is desired to make absolute measurements such as the magnitude and direction of the movement imposed upon the brain by the arterial pressure pulse then a large number of measurements must be made in a large number of different individuals. Moreover, these measurements should be made from different directions so that the true magnitude and vector of motion can be estimated. In this way it is possible to average out the effects of the random scattering of the beam by the skull which result in uncertainty of the position, relative to the transducer axis, of any single interface the motion of which is being recorded. When motion of a large number of interfaces is measured the majority of these interfaces will be close to the transducer axis. When the motion of a large number of interfaces is recorded from all possible directions then the largest movement measured and its direction represents the true magnitude and direction of motion of that region of the brain.

If it is desired to make relative measurements such as the effects of increased intracranial pressure upon the systolic motion of the brain then these measurements must be made at a single recording session upon the same subject without moving the transducer. During this recording session the parameter being studied must be varied and the effect of these variations upon the systolic motions measured.

It is for these reasons that we find it difficult to envisage that this technique will be of value as a diagnostic tool in clinical medicine. Such diagnostic tools require that measurements made from persons suspected of disease be easily made and significantly different from those made on healthy persons. Measurements made from individual interfaces are subject to too great variations for such differences to be reliable. Recordings can obviously not be made from a large number of interfaces in sick persons. Finally, it is not possible, with available techniques, to make recordings continuously from the same interface over the days and weeks of a patient's illness in order to monitor variations in intracranial pulsatile movements.

REFERENCES.
Braak, J.W.G. ter, Greeze, P., Grandia, W.A.M. and deVlieger, M. (1961). The significance of some pulsations in echoencephalography. Acta Neurochir. 9:382-397.

2. Campbell, J.K., Clark, J.M., White, D.N. and Jenkins, C.O. (1970). Pulsatile echoencephalography. Acta Neurol. Scand. 46 Suppl. 45:1-57.

3. Clark, J.M., White, D.N., Curry, G.R., Stevenson, R.J., Campbell, J.K. and Jenkins, C.O. (1971). The measurement of intracranial echo pulsations. Med. Biol. Engng. 9:263-287.

4. White, D.N. and Stevenson, R.J. (1976). Transient variations in the systolic pulsations in amplitude of intracranial echoes: their artifactual origin. Neurology 26:683-689.

5. White, D.N. (1976). Ultrasonic Encephalography II. Ultramedison, Kingston, Ontario. pp. 251-269.

6. White, D.N., Clark, J.M., Curry, G.R. and Stevenson, R.J. (1976). The Effects of the Skull upon the Spatial and Temporal Distribution of a Generated and Reflected Ultrasonic Beam. Ultramedison, Kingston, Ontario.

7. White, D.N., Curry, G.R. and Stevenson, R.J. (1979b). The acoustic characteristics of the skull. Ultrasound Med. Biol. 4: 225-252.

8. White, D.N., Clark, J.M., White, D.A.W., Campbell, J.K., Bahuleyan, K., Kraus, A.S. and Brinker, R.A. (1971). The deformation of the ultrasonic field in passage across the living and cadaver head. Ultrasonographia Medica 1. (Edited by J. Bock and K. Ossoinig). Verlag der Wiener Med. Akad. p. 179-186.

9. Jenkins, C.O., Campbell, J.K., White, D.N. and Clark, J.M. (1971). Ultrasonic echo pulsations in range. A study of rise times and delay times. Acta Neurochir. 24:1-10.

10. Davson, H. (1956). Physiology of the Ocular and Cerebrospinal Fluid. Churchill, London. pp. 305-308 and 349-350.

11. Jeppsson, S. (1964). A method for recording the intracranial pressure with the aid of the echoencephalographic technique. Acta Chir. Scand. 128:218-224.

12. Jeppsson, S. (1967). A method for recording the intracranial pressure with the aid of the echoencephalographic technique. Proceedings in Echoencephalography. Springer-Verlag, Berlin. pp. 186-189.

13. Jenkins, C.O. and White, D.N. (1972). The rise time of intracranial echo pulsations and intracranial pressure. Acta Neurol. Scand. 48:115-123.

14. White, D.N., Jenkins, C.O. and Campbell, J.K. (1970). The compensatory mechanisms for volume changes in the brain. Proc. 23rd Conf. Engng. Med. Biol. p. 104.

15. Jenkins, C.O., Campbell, J.K. and White, D.N. (1971). Modulation resembling Traube-Hering waves recorded in the human brain. Europ. Neurol. 5:1-6.

16. White, D.N.,and Jenkins, C.O. (1971). Some observations on the fluttering midline echo in echoencephalography - a ballistocardiac effect and suggested cause of rupture of the septum pellucidum. Jo. Neurol. Neurosurg. Psychiat. 34:289-296.

462

17. White, D.N., Wilson, K.C., Curry, G.R. and Stevenson, R.J. (1979a). The limitations of pulsatile flow through the aqueduct of Sylvius as a cause of hydrocephalus. Jo. Neurol. Sci. 42:11-51.

18. Freund, H.J. and Kapp, H. (1966). Eine methode zur Registrierung arterieller Pulsationen mittels Ultraschall. Pflugers Archiv. 291:268-276.

19. Freund, H.J. (1966). Ultraschalldiagnostic cerebraler Gefassverschlusse. Verhand. d. Deutsch. Gesellschaft f. Innere Med. 72:653-656.

20. Boulay, G.H. de (1966). Pulsatile movements in the C.S.F. pathways. Br. J. Radiol. 39:255-262.

21. White, D.N. (1960). The six "laws" of echoencephalography. Neurology 20:435-444.

22. Bering, E.A. (1962). Circulation of the cerebrospinal fluid. J. Neurosurg. 19:405-413.

23. Last, R.J. and Tompsett, D.H. (1953). Casts of the cerebral ventricles. Br. J. Surg. 40:525-543.

24. Epstein, B.S. (1950). A pneumoencephalographic study of the normal third and fourth cerebral ventricles and aqueduct of Sylvius. Am. J. Roentgenol. Rad. Therap. 63:204-209.

25. Greenfield, J.C. and Tindall, G.T. (1965). Effect of acute increase in intracranial pressure on blood flow in the internal carotid artery of man. J. Clin. Invest. 44:1343-1351.

26. Shulman, K. and Verdier, G.R. (1967). Cerebral vascular resistance changes in response to cerebrospinal fluid pressure. Amer. J. Physiol. 213:1084-1088.

27. Lowell, H.M. and Bloor, B.M. (1971). The effect of increased intracranial pressure on cerebrovascular hemodynamics. J. Neurosurg. 34:760-769.

NEUROSONOLOGY: A CRITICAL SURVEY AND A PROPOSAL

Carlo Alvisi

Neurosurgical Institute, University of Bologna, Italy

Neurosonology is a new word created to define the field of application of ultrasound in detecting alterations of intracranial nervous structures and diagnosing brain diseases in particular.

During the last thirty years, the attempt to use ultrasound in neurology, neurosurgery and other related specialities has been made by many researchers and a great number of techniques and devices have been applied to obtain the major amount of information through exploring brain structures and intracranial and extracranial vessels. However, a large shadow covers this field of ultrasonology.

I believe that this uncertainty is due to many factors that are not easy to list. One of them, the most important in my opinion, is the ignorance of the possibilities of this technique: even now Oldendorf (1), in a very good article quotes "echoencephalography" as a means of checking only the "midline-echo". Another very important factor is the lack of information on the versatility of ultrasonic technology. The third one is the difficulty to realise that, by using ultrasound, it is now possible to check the morphology of the brain and the anatomical and functional state of the cerebral and extracerebral vessels.

The ultrasonographer and the neurologist must know how to interrogate the object under their examination and to adapt the means at their disposal in order to obtain precise data.

The purpose of this paper is to define the number of parameters explored by different ultrasonic methods, showing how useful they will be if integrated in an ideal future programme.

One of the most serious obstacles is the reliability of the data obtained and their meaningfulness. I know that no method exists without errors; however, I am aware that is possible to examine many different sources of data, compare these data and then integrate them so that a maximum definition can be reached.

In the following paragraphs, I have collected the parameters obtained by the methods and the techniques used or proposed for checking the morphology and/or the function of the intracranial and/or extracranial structures in order to detect the pathological changes that form the basis for diagnosis.

THE PARAMETERS AND THE METHODS FOR THEIR DETECTION

Dimension, site and shape of the ventricular complex (lateral ventricles, third and fourth ventricles) and the Sylvius acqueduct are detected by A-mode echoencephalography (2-5), by B-scan echoencephalotomography (6-10) and by real-time scansion (11-13).

Cranial theca is well measured by A-mode echography(14). Brain mantle thickness and external atrophy can be evaluated in A-mode echoencephalography (15-17) and in B-scan echoencephalotomography (11-13).

Pulsatility of the walls of the ventricles, of the surface of the insula, pulsations of the intracranial arteries, anterior cerebral artery, middle cerebral artery, intracranial portion of the internal carotid artery, basilar artery are recorded with T-motion technique, with the registration of the variations in amplitude and in range of the reflected echoes and with the real-time scansion(18-21).

Changes of the physical characteristics of the nervous tissue and patholgoical tissues are detected by means of the A-mode echoencephalography and B-scan echoencephalotomography (22).

The Doppler techniques are adopted for detecting the velocity of the blood and the direction of the flow inside the extracranial arteries, common carotid artery and its bifurcation, internal carotid artery, external carotid artery and its branches, vertebral artery, internal jugular vein (23-27).

The combination of the Doppler techniques with the A-mode or B-scan detection of the diameter of the above mentioned vessels can give the measurement of the blood flow and detect the changes of the lumen due to the aterosclerotic plaques or thrombosis (28).

The dimension of pons and cisterna pontis, the ponto-cerebellar angles are explored by B-scan echoencephalotomography (6,8).

MEANINGFULNESS OF PARAMETERS IN DIAGNOSTICS

The increased dimension of the entire cerebral ventricular complex as isolated data can be a sign of hydrocephalus. The degree of the pulsatility of the ventricular walls and the surface of the insula can indicate the participation of the vascular system or the intensity of the intracranial pressure. Further information is obtainable by checking the pulsations of the intracranial vessels and the characteristics of the circulation in the extracranial vessels. By means of the parameters - velocity, direction and blood flow - in the afferent vessels, it is possible to take into account the impairment of the intra and extracranial circulation. The characteristics of the velocity curves in the extracranial arteries and the comparison with the same data obtained from the internal jugular veins allow the detection of changes in the intracranial circulation.

To distinguish between the reduction of the vascular bed and the increased intracranial pressure the abovementioned morphological data can be used. The same parameters plus the ventricular complex shift or deformation co-operate in diagnosing tumours or other expansive processes. The presence of pathological echoes, detectable with a careful study and adapted equipment, enhances the possibility of the correct diagnosis of expansive processes.

CONCLUSIONS

Many ultrasonologists are quoted in this paper and perhaps they will be surprised by this collection of their data without any hint as to the reliability of the results of their research. The connotation of this paper cannot allow the complete exposition of "false positive" or "false negative".

The ultrasonologists or the neurologists or neurosurgeons or radiologists can argue against the attempt to summarize in an arbitrary synthesis the latest advances in the field of ultrasound applied to the diagnosis of nervous diseases.

However, I believe that while taking into account the correct criticism or every author, a new starting point is necessary for ultrasound in neurology before judging its usefulness.

We all want to obtain 100% correct results: this is the right attitude for a scientist, but nobody, as far as I know, has tried to collect all the data possible to obtain to give weight to each singly nor even to consider the real value of the combination of them all.

REFERENCES

1. Oldendorf, W.H. (1978): Neurology, 28, 517.
2. Kazner, E. and Hopman, H. (1973): Ultrasound in Med. & Biol., 1, 1.
3. Uematsu, S. and Walker, A.E. (1971): A manual of echo-encephalography, p. 54. The Williams and Wilkins Co., Baltimore.
4. Mikschiczek, D. (1977): Fortschr. Neurol. Psychiat., 45, 508.
5. Krogness, K.G. (1975): J. Neurosurg., 42, 508.
6. Alvisi, C., Cacciari, A. and Cavedoni, J. (1975): In: Ultrasound in Medicine, p. 839. Editors: D. White and R.E. Brown, Plenum Press, New York-London.
7. Alvisi, C and Cavedoni, J. (1975): Proc. Symposium Actualitatis Tomographiae, p. 106. Excerpta Medica International Congress Series n° 392, Amsterdam.
8. Valkeakari, T. (1975): In: Ultrasound in Medicine, p. 853. Editors: D. White and R.E. Brown, Plenum Press, New York - London.
9. Garrett, W.J., Warren, P.S. and Kossoff, G. (1979): In: Abstract, p. 98, 2nd Meeting of WFUMB, Miyazaki,

Japan. SCIMED Publ. Inc., Tokio.

10. Alvisi, C. (1979): In: Proc. 2nd Meeting of WFUMB, Miyazaki, Japan. Excerpta Medica, Amsterdam (in press).
11. Notermans, S.L.H. and Kamphuisen, H.A.C. (1977): Ned. T. Geneesk., 121, 1710.
12. Skolnick, M.L., Rosenbaum, A.E., Matzuk, T., Guthkelch, N. and Heinz, E.R. (1979): Radiology, 131, 447.
13. Fry, F.J., Barger, J.E., et.al. (1979): In: Abstract p. 40, 2nd Meeting of WFUMB, Miyazaki, Japan. SCIMED Publ. Inc., Tokio.
14. Nalin, A., Della Giustina, E., Ferrari, F. and Alvisi, C. (1978): J. Nucl. Med. All. Sc., 22, 21.
15. Alvisi, C., Mordini, B., Nalin, A. and Olivi, O. (1978): J. Nucl. Med. All. Sc., 22, 25.
16. Schiefer, W., Kazner, E. and Kunze, St. (1968): Clinical Echoencephalography, Springer Verlag, Heidelberg.
17. Alvisi, C., Cavedoni, J., Gnudi, S., Masiello, O. and Palmirani, R. (1978): J. Nucl. Med. All. Sc., 22, 67.
18. Smith, S.W., von Ramm, O.T., Kisslo, J.A. and Thurstone, F.L. (1978): Stroke, 9, 117.
19. Narikawa, H., Takahashi, L., Takase, S., Sato, G. and Itahara, K. (1979): In: Abstract, p. 151. 2nd Meeting of WFUMB, Miyazaki, Japan, SCIMED Publ. Inc., Tokio.
20. de Vlieger, M. (1979): In: Abstract, p. 41. 2nd Meeting of WFUMB, Miyazaki, Japan. SCIMED Publ. Inc., Tokio.
21. Uematsu, S. (1979): In: Abstract, p. 38. 2nd Meeting of WFUMB, Miyazaki, Japan. SCIMED Publ. Inc., Tokio.
22. van Venrooij, G.E.P.M., Boone, R.M. and Denier van der Gon, J.J. (1979): Acta Neurochirurgica, 49, 1.
23. Pourcelot, L. (1979): In: Abstract. p. 1. 2nd Meeting of WFUMB, Miyazaki, Japan. SCIMED Publ. Inc., Tokio.
24. Kaneko, J., Shiraishi, J., Inaoka, H., Okuda, J. and Sekiyama, M. (1979): In: Abstract, p. 37. 2nd Meeting of WFUMB, Miyazaki, Japan. SCIMED Publ. Inc., Tokio.
25. Reid, J.M. and Spencer, M.P. (1979): In: Abstract, p. 140. 2nd Meeting of WFUMB, Miyazaki, Japan, SCIMED Publ. Inc., Tokio.
26. Vogel, S., Pardemann, G. and Magnus, S. (1978): In: Abstract, p. 519. 3rd European Congr. "On Ultrasonics in Medicine", Bologna, Italy, Edizioni Centro Minerva Medica, Roma.
27. Jonkman, E.J., Tans, J.T.J. and Mosmans, P.C.M. (1978): Neurology, 218, 157.
28. White, D. and Curry, G.R. (1979): In: Abstract, p. 139. 2nd Meeting of WFUMB, Miyazaki, Japan. SCIMED Publ. Inc., Tokio.

CURRENT STATUS OF DIAGNOSTIC ULTRASOUND IN BREAST DISEASE

Kobayashi,T.

DEpartment of Central Clinical Laboratory,SChool of
Medicine, University of Occupational & Environmental
Health, Kitakyushu City, Japan 807

For the clinical management of breast cancer,there
is no doubt that the early detection is mandatory and
correct differential diagnosis is an important determina-
nt of prognosis.

Ultrasonography has been widely used for good modality to visualise soft tissue pathologies in many organs.
Breast echography has been highly appraised in the view
point of its high diagnostic accuracy,no physical hazard
like radiological approach and non-invasive technique.

The breast itself is soft and superficial organ,
therefore, it is ideal to use water coupling approaches
such as water tank immersion or water bag technique for
clinical purpose (Fig. 1).

Fig. 1

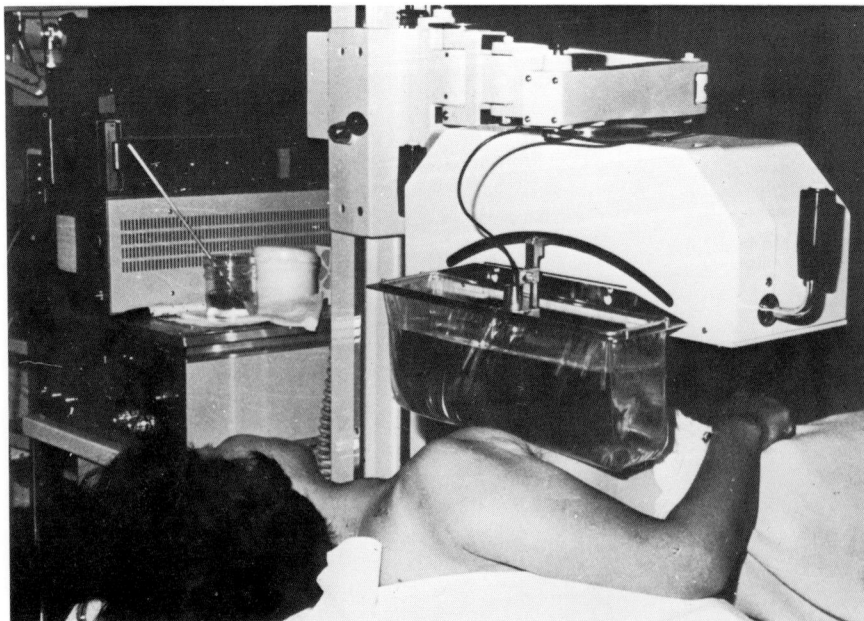

Current status of water coupling approaches in breast echography is summarized in Table I. Five equipments, that is,two in water tank scanning,and three in water bag scanning, are commercially available at the present.

As to the clinical applicability,water tank technique is rather good for large dense breast,whereas water bag technique seems to be good for small fibrous atrophic breast. For the water tank scanning,the prone position is used in hanging both breast down into tank,whereas the supine position is used in water bag scanning in placing its bag with degassed water upon the overlying skin of the target mass in one breast. Both scanning techniques can be used for the screening purpose of the breast,and also provides good gray scale image(Table I).

Table I

CURRENT STATUS OF THE ECHOGRAPHIC
APPROACHES TO BREAST CANCER

* Water Coupling Technique *

	Scanning in water-bath	Scanning in water-bag
Equipment available	i).U.I.Octoson (Australia) ii).Life Instrument (U.S.A.) Breast Scanner	i).Toshiba Sonolayergraph (Japan) ii).Hitachi EUB (Japan) iii).Aloka SSD (Japan)
Clinical Applicability	good for large dense breast	small & fibrous atrophic breast
Position in Examination	prone	supine
Applicability to screening	(+)	(+)
Display Quality	gray scale image	gray scale image
Diagnostic Accuracy Rate	good (over 85%)	good (over 85%)
Diagnostic Points	Boundary echo - Internal echo - Posterior echo	
Diagnostic Superiority	Scirrhous carcinoma-Papillary carcinoma-Medullary carcinoma	

As to the diagnostic criteria, three points can be used,that is,the boundary echo,internal echoes and posterior shadowing. The upper and lower figures show the echo signs suggestive for benign disease and amlignant disease respectively. Differential points can be divided into three categories; the boundary echo and shape shown in the left column, internal echoes shown in the middle column and the retromammary shadowing in the right column. As to the boundary echo and shape, it is regular and smooth,round,oval or hemioval in benign disease,whereas it is irregular and jagged,crab-like or polymorphous in malignant disease. As to internal echoes, it is homogeneous, uniform-sized or echo-free or anechoic in benign disease,whereas it is non-uniform-sized or heterogeneous in breast cancer. As to the posterior shadowing or retromammary shadowing, the tadpole-tail sign, the lateral shadow sign and accentuation of the posterior echo may appear in the benign disease,whereas the acoustic middle shadow sign and attenuation of posterior echo may appear in breast cancer.(Fig. 2).

Fig. 2

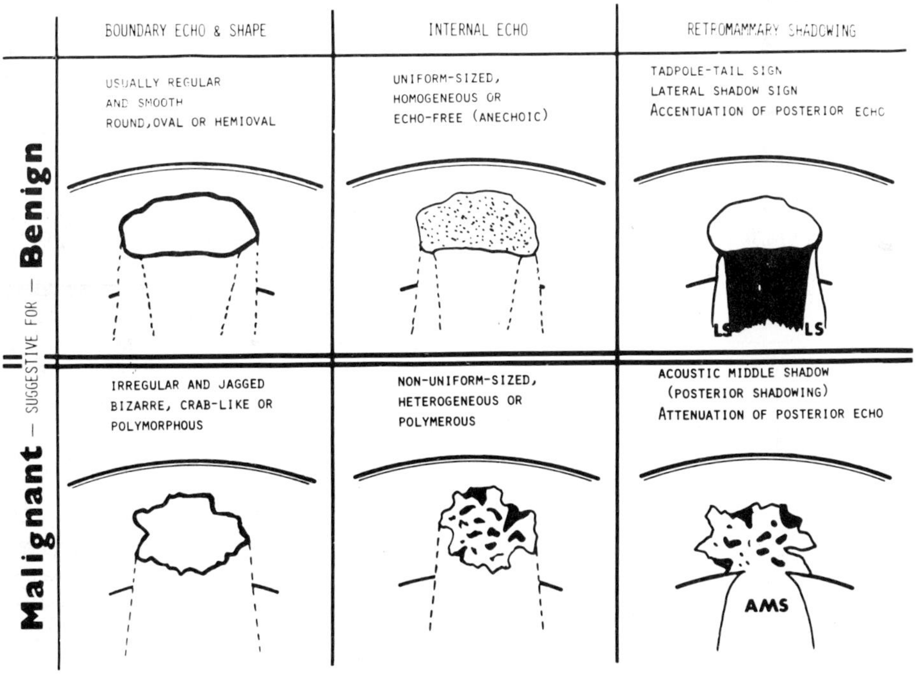

	BOUNDARY ECHO & SHAPE	INTERNAL ECHO	RETROMAMMARY SHADOWING
Benign	USUALLY REGULAR AND SMOOTH ROUND,OVAL OR HEMIOVAL	UNIFORM-SIZED, HOMOGENEOUS OR ECHO-FREE (ANECHOIC)	TADPOLE-TAIL SIGN LATERAL SHADOW SIGN ACCENTUATION OF POSTERIOR ECHO
Malignant	IRREGULAR AND JAGGED BIZARRE, CRAB-LIKE OR POLYMORPHOUS	NON-UNIFORM-SIZED, HETEROGENEOUS OR POLYMEROUS	ACOUSTIC MIDDLE SHADOW (POSTERIOR SHADOWING) ATTENUATION OF POSTERIOR ECHO

Figure 3 shows the typical echo gram of large benign cyst demonstrating regular smooth boundary with no echo rising from the inside of the cyst.

Figure 4 shows the gray scale echogram of small cyst and the lower echogram is expanded echogram

Figure 5 shows typical echograms of breast cancer, demonstrating irregular boundary with heterogenous internal echoes in varying size, and less attenuation of posterior shadowing, and this kind of echogram is often seen in the case of medullary carcinoma.

Figure 6 shows also typical echograms of breast cancer demonstrating strong attenuation of posterior shadowing, and often seen in the case of scirrhous carcinoma, the upper is taken by arc scanner and the lower one is recorded by linear scanner on the same patient,illustrating strong attenuation of posterior shadowing.

Fig. 3

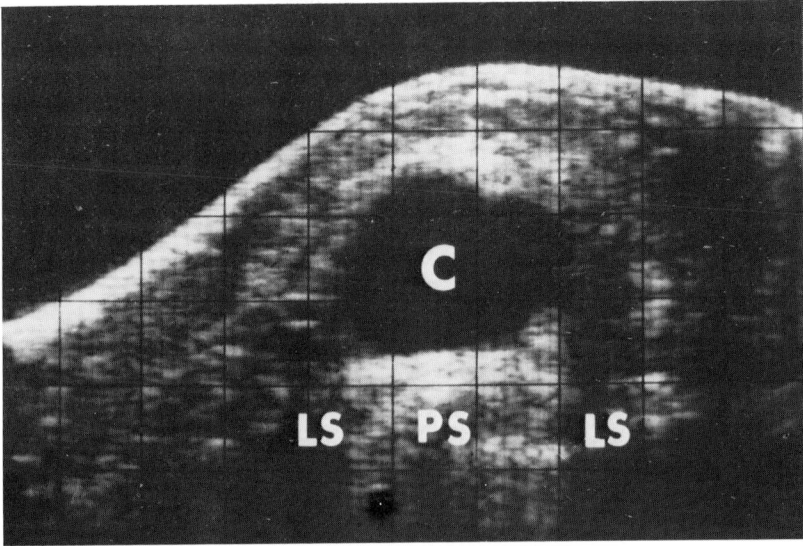

Fig. 4

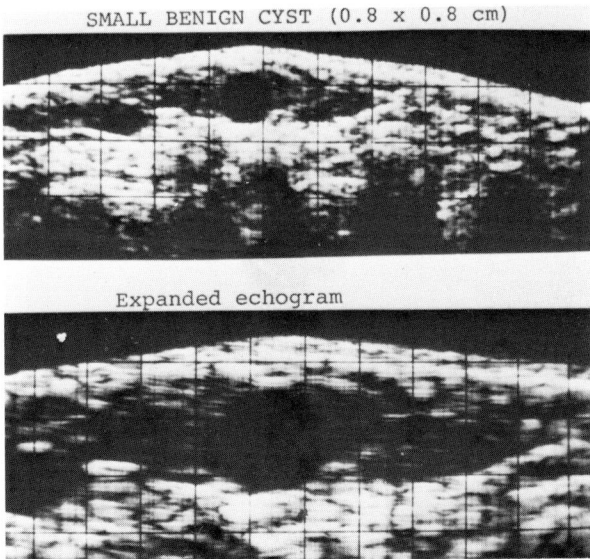

Fig. 5

MEDULLARY CARCINOMA (T 1)

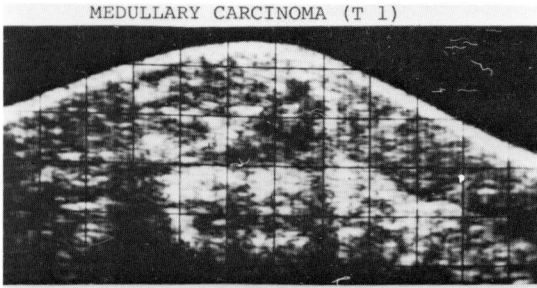

Expanded Echogram (Magnified)

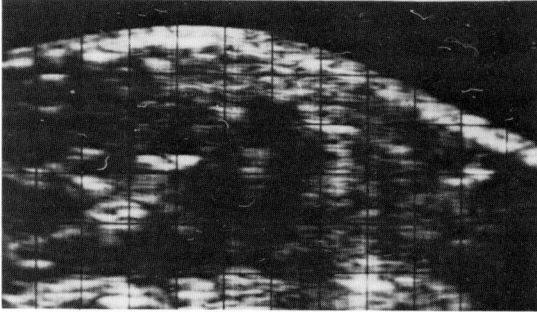

Fig. 6

SCIRRHOUS CARCINOMA (arc-scan)

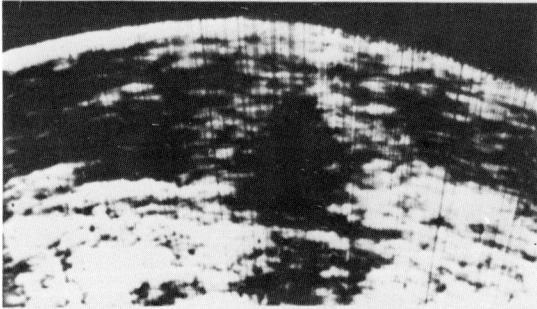

Same case (linear-scan)

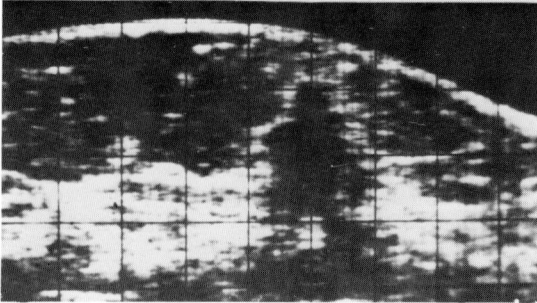

Diagnostic accuracy rates according to the tumor size;TNM classification and histological type are shown in comparison of the rates achieved by mammography, respectively in Tables II and III.

Table II. DIAGNOSTIC ACCURACY RATES
BY ULTRASOUND & MAMMOGRAPHY
ACCORDING TO T N M CLASSIFICATION

T N M	ULTRASOUND	%	MAMMOGRAPHY	%
T 1	31/40	78	28/37	76
T 2	52/58	90	49/56	88
T 3	13/14	93	12/14	86
Total	112 cases		107 cases	

Table III. DIAGNOSTIC ACCURACY RATES
BY ULTRASOUND & MAMMOGRAPHY
ACCORDING TO HISTOLOGICAL TYPE

Histological type	ULTRASOUND	%	MAMMOGRAPHY	%
SCIRRHOUS CARCINOMA	32/35	91	30/33	91
PAPILLARY CARCINOMA	26/31	84	25/32	78
MEDULLARY CARCINOMA	33/42	79	26/40	65
Total	108 cases		105 cases	

Ultrasonic tissue characterization study was carried out in analysing echo signs in routine clinical echograms and relevant microscopic specimen,especially collagen fiber content or connective tissue content in tumor mass of breast cancer. As illustrated in the table of diagnostic criteria, the retromammary shadowing or posterior shadowing is the important diagnostic information in breast cancer,that is, the acoustic middle shadow sign. It was my clinical impression that this sign might be closely related to the genetic bio-acoustic mechanism of ultrasonic attenuation, therefore, the investigation was carried out to check the histological specimens of the cases which showed strong posterior shadowing,especially the amount of connective tissue content or collagen fiber content in breast cancer, then it was found that the cases which showed collagen fiber content over 75% in 12 serially sliced specimens in given tumor mass demonstrating strong posterior shadowing or ultrasonic attenuation echographically,whereas less attenuation in cases showing collagen fiber content less than 25%.

This correlation was shown in Fig. 7.

Fig. 7

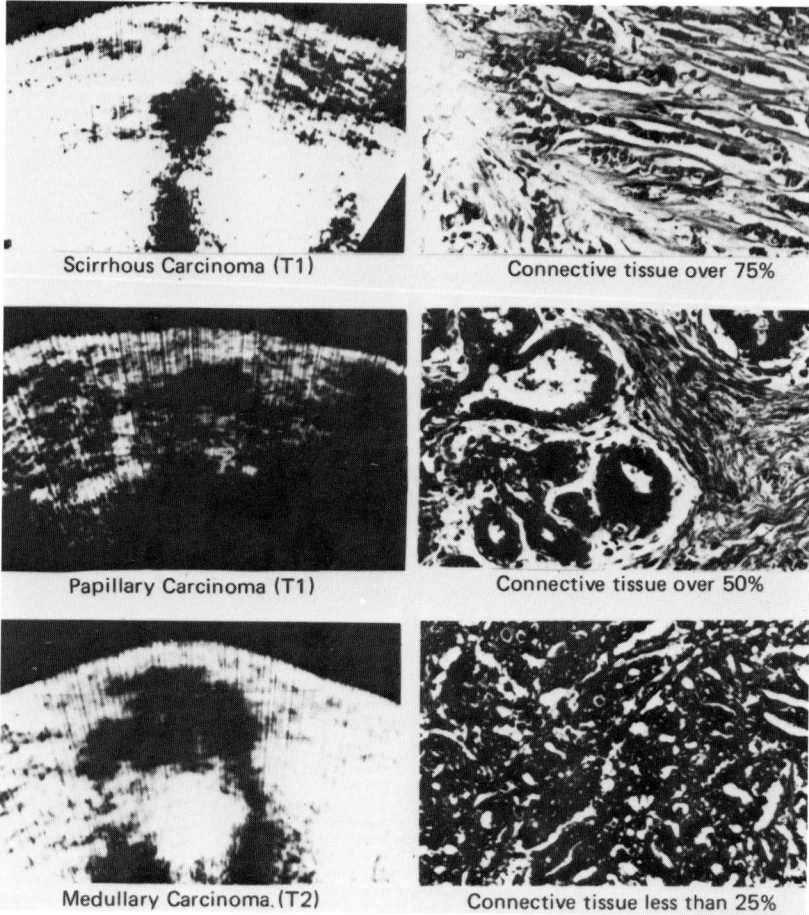

Scirrhous Carcinoma (T1)

Connective tissue over 75%

Papillary Carcinoma (T1)

Connective tissue over 50%

Medullary Carcinoma.(T2)

Connective tissue less than 25%

Ultrasonic tissue characterization speculated from clinical routine echograms are summarized in Tables IV and V.

Scirrhous carcinoma and cuctal carcinoma may tend to show strong attenuation,that is, strong retromammary or posterior shadowing just underneath the tumor mass echo, whereas any carcinoma in less collagen fiber content such as medullary carcinoma or mucous carcinoma may show less attenuation or on the contrary rather increased accentuation or intermediate in attenuation.

Difference in the nature of collagen fiber itself may play the role in producing the ultrasonic attenuation in breast cancer and fibroadenoma showing rather ultrasonic accentuation,and its speculation is shown in Table VI. The histo-chemical analysis is needed as to this problem

474

as further investigation.

In conclusion, connective tissue content or collagen fiber content may play important role to produce ultrasonic attenuation in routine clinical echogram.

ULTRASONIC TISSUE CHARACTERIZATION

CORRELATION BETWEEN ECHO-SIGNS IN CLINICAL ECHOGRAM ESPECIALLY
RETROMAMMARY OR POSTERIOR SHADOWING AND ACOUSTIC MECHANISM

1).Tadpole-tail sign
   (Arc-scanning)

2).Posterior strong echo
   (Linear scanning)

3).Lateral shadow sign
   (Arc & linear scanning)

1).Acoustic middle shadow sign
   (Arc & linear scanning)

2).Complete disappearance of
   bottom echo
   (Arc & linear scanning)

CLINICAL DIAGNOSIS

BENIGN TUMORS

Benign cyst

Fibrocystic disease

Fibroadenoma & others

INTERMEDIATE: Medullary Ca. & Mucous Ca.

MALIGNANT TUMOR

Scirrohous carcinoma

Ductal carcinoma

Papillary carcinoma

ULTRASONIC ACCENTUATION

TP
LS   LS   LS PSE LS

ULTRASONIC ATTENUATION

AMSS   AMSS

Table IV

DIFFERENCE IN CONNECTIVE FIBROUS TISSUE (COLLAGEN FIBER)

Ultrasonic ACCENTUATION

FIBROCYSTIC DISEASE
BENIGN CYST
FIBROADENOMA

COLLAGEN in product of

tissue-repairing process

PROBABLY DIFFERENCE IN HYDROXYPROLINE
ACTIVITY

Ultrasonic ATTENUATION

BREAST CARCINOMA

(Scirrhous type)

COLLAGEN in by-product of

cancer cell proliferation and

degenerative process

Table V

475

REFERENCES

1).Kobayashi,T.: Ultrasonic tissue characterization:
   Correlation of attenuation and echo-pattern
   Recent Advances in Ultrasound Diagnosis,edited by
   A.Kurjak, pp.28,Excerpta Medica,Amsterdam,1978

2).Kobayashi,T.: Clinical Ultrasound of the Breast
   Plenum Publishing Corporation,New York,1978

3).Fields,S. and Dunn,F.: Correlation of echographic
   visualization with biological composition and
   physiological state
   J.Acoust.Soc.Am. 54:809,1973

4).Calderon,G.,Vilkomerson,D.,Mezrich,R.,Etzold,K.F.,
   Kingsley,B.,and Haskin,M.: Differences in the attenuation of ultrasound by normal,benign, and malignant
   breast tissue
   J.Clin.Ultrasound 4:249,1976

5).Jellins,J.,Kossoff,G.,and Barraclough,B.H.: Comparative study of breast imaging by echography and xerography
   Recent Advances in Ultrasound Diagnosis,edited by
   Kurjak,pp.299,Excerpta Medica,Amsterdam,1979

6).Reeve,T.S.,Jellins,J.,Kossoff,G.,and Barraclough,B.H.:
   Ultrasonic visualization of breast cancer
   Aust.N.Z.J.Surg. 48:278,1978

ULTRASONOGRAPHY IN GYNECOLOGY: A 10 YEAR EVALUATION

S. Levi and H. Messai

Department of Obstetrics and Gynecology, Hopital Universitaire Brugmann, Brussels, Belgium

Shortly after its development by several pioneers such as Dussik(1942), Wild and Reid(1951), Howry et al(1955),Kikuchi et al(1957), Effert et al(1957), Donald et al(1958), practical use of ultrasonography (USG) grew rapidly. This diagnostic technique is widely available and is now applied for clinical investigations in any part of the human body.

The two-dimensional methods gave the powerful drive to the widespread use of USG and particularly in gynecology and obstetrics. The purely gynecological indications of USG remained, for a long time, restricted to the visualization of large abdominal or pelvic masses, and therefore its applications were few. Did not Donald et al(1958) comment on the interest of USG in gynecology through their experience of a hundred ultrasonically examined patients in these terms "...Our findings are still of more academic interest than practical importance, and we do not feel that our clinical judgement should be influenced by our ultrasonic findings... Preoprative diagnosis of histological structure...is an exciting prospect....Encourage great efforts to refine our technique".

Let us remember that at the beginning of the USG, the principal preoccupation was to affirm the presence or absence of an abdominal or pelvic tumour. Thereafter attempts to differentiate the solid tumours from the liquid one's were made particularly from the observation of differences in sound propagation in the tumour, in its surroundings or beyond this. Sunden (1964), Donald(1965), Kratochwil(1968), recommended to observe the modifications due to frequency changes as a tool for tissue characterization. Ultrasonic intensity alterations have also been used as an aid for the differential diagnosis of liquid and cystic tumours (Thompson et al 1967).

One of the earliest clinical evaluation of the interest of USG for gynecology was published by Thompson et al. (1967): after surgery in 82 patients,out of 100 ultrasonically examined patients, the ultrasonic results were classified in "good, fair or poor", which is in fact a very elementary way to appreciate the effectiveness: "No attempt was made to show the percentage of correct or incorrect diagnosis by the ultrasonic technique". The conclusion was that the gynecological USG could be useful: indeed, in 89% of the cases, the results were classified as good or fair. In another statistical work, Holländer(1968) evaluated the rate of correct diagnosis of tumors, using USG. He showed that, in a series of 93 patients with abdominal pelvis masses, 88% of the tumours were visualized. No tumour was described in 21 normal patients. These two papers related the reliability of extremely simple"diagnosis" made using the restricted possibilities of existing equipment. During the 10 years following the publications of these first numerical evaluations, statistical works on the USG and results of gynecological USG have been seldom: Levi(1971), Cochrane and Thomas(1974), Queenan' et al.(1975), Concordilas et al(1976), Schillinger et al(1976), Levi and Delval(1976).

Over these evaluations covering the entire gynecologi-.cal practice, we have to quote other reports on the value of USG in more restricted fields. These shown the possible spreading of indications: Zacutti and Brugnoli(1970) on ectopic pregnancies, Kratochwil et al.(1974) on recurrence of pelvic cancer, Janssens et al (1973)on the IUD, Calvo and Pacheco(1976) on endometrium, Ulrich and Sanders(1976) on pelvic inflammatory masses, Hackeloer et al(1977) on ovarian changes under gonadotropins influence, Exalto et al (1978) on the uterine congenital malformations, etc... All these very specialized investigations enter now in USG general practise, the accuracy of results is getting higher and as we shall see als further on in the light of our own results, the indications are thus more diversified in gynecology and the high disparity of the variety of USG indications is on the way to be reduced between obstetrics and gynecology.

Technical improvements have largely contributed to this evolution:with the A-scan, it was only possible to determine the size and the cystic or solid nature of a mass(Fig.1) which first was to be localized by manual palpation(Krato-

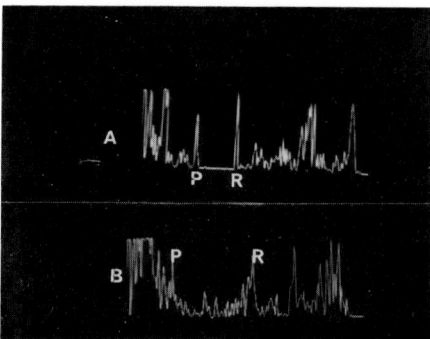

Fig.1. A-scan mode displays cystic & solid tumor echo pattern.A=cystic mass; B= solid mass; P=proximal echo and R=rear echo of masses (Kontron Abdoscan)

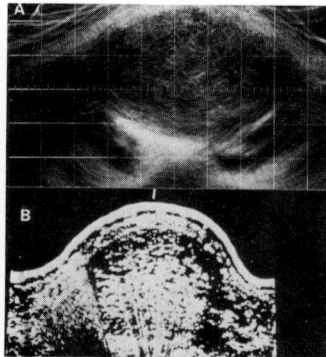

Fig.2. B-scan mode:A=manual compound scan with brightness mode (hydatidiform mole) and B=manual single scan with bistable mode(necrotic fibroid)(Aloka SSD 60)

chwil,1968). With the aid of the B-scan, linear or compound,
manual or automatic, it was possible to detect and to estimate the structure of masses with more or less luck depending upon whether the system was working in brightness-mode
or bistable-mode (Fig.2)(Levi,1972). New techniques have permitted to refine this diagnosis through a more detailed description of tissue structures. The grey-scale technique,
where the grey tones translate the echoes amplitudes are
among those. Originally, the processing of signals was only made analogically but now more and more digital processing is made (Fig.3). This should lead to computerized analysis. This last evolution allows us to anticipate, in a
near future, a very fine analysis of signals leading to
tissue characterization (Levi et al.1978). The parallel evolution of "slow" (differed time images) and "fast" techniques, (real-time images) (Fig.4), did not bring spectacular
improvements in gynecological as it did in obstetrical USG.
Nevertheless the use of real-time technique in gynecology,
as a step before the more classical and informative examination in differed-time, allows to save an appreciable amount
of time, to the benefit of more complicated cases when a
long-time examination is needed to resolve difficult echo-
patterns.

REPORT ON CLINICAL ACTIVITY OF OUR UNIVERSITY DEPARTMENT OF
GYNECOLOGICAL AND OBSTETRICAL USG

The first USG examination at the Clinque Obstetricale
et Gynécologique de l'Hopital Universitaire Brugmann in
Brussels was performed during February 1966. Only the A-
scan mode was used at the beginning and, in 1967, a B-scan
mode, manual-compound -scanner was at our disposal. At the
end of 1978, 23,395 patients had been investigated, which
corresponds to 42,077 examinations (Fig.5).

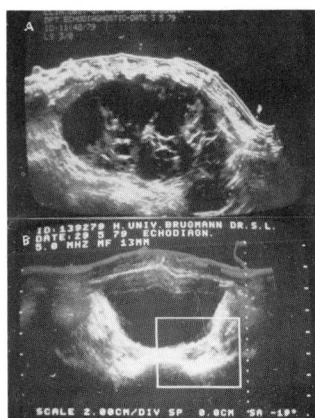

Fig. 3. A manual scan, grey-tone analog signals(complex ovarian tumor=cystad no-carcinoma)(Kretz Combison II). B=manual
scan, grey-tone digital signals. Left ovary is surrounded by
a frame used before zooming of this area, one of post-processing capabilities of this system(Unirad EDP 1000).

A. Evolution of the proportions between gynecological and obstetrical USG examinations . The need for a visual and innocuous technique was peremptorily demonstrated by the sudden interest shown for the USG and rapid progression of demands for obstetrical USG. In gynecology, the progression was slower; indeed several clinical and technical means to appreciate the anatomy and to make a diagnosis were already available for a long time. Furthermore the relative lack of precision of the early ultrasonography explains that the gynecological indications and the number of echographied patients were only few. The proportion of gynecological patients regularly grew from 1966 to 1978, moving up from 0% to 30% (Fig.6). The increasing precision and the larger diversity of gynecological USG indications are explanations of that growth.

B. Evolution of gynecological indications in USG . The Figure 7 shows the incidence variations of some 20 USG indications in gynecology. In 1970, 6 indications went over the frequency of 5%: uterine fibroid(23%), differential diagnosis of pelvis mass(21%) or of adnexial mass(8%) or be-

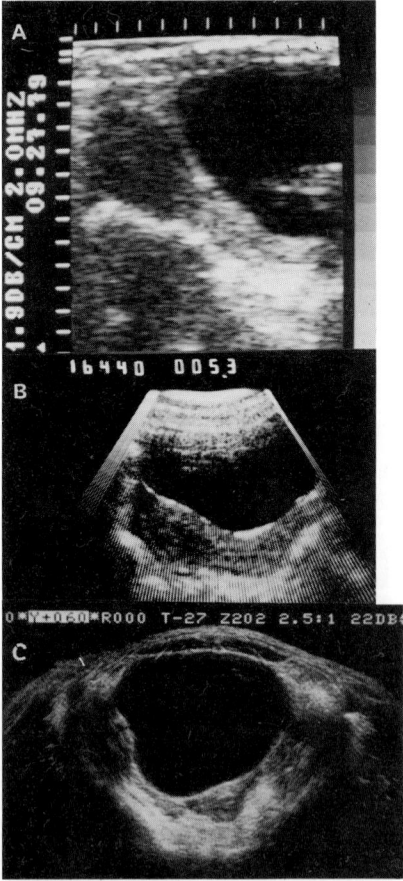

Fig. 4. A) automatic linear scanning, real-time,grey tones, 2 MHz: Normal uterus (Krontron Abdoscan)B) Automatic sector scanning, real-time, grey tones, 3.5 MHz: Normal uterus (Kretz Combison 100). C) Automatic compound scanning, grey-tones = one pelvis section displayed within a 2 sec/scan(Ausonics Octoson)

tween cystic and solid mass(17%), pain and mass(8%), hemor-
rhage(8%). In 1974, 2 and in 1978, 4 more indications were
above the 5% limit. The additional indications were respec-
tively:pain as single symptom(5 then 10%), pelvic status
(5 then 10%) mass and hemorrhage &7 then 11%), uterine size
(5 then 7%). Indications never mentioned before 1970 (less
than 0.5%) and well thereafter, are in 1978: monitoring of
previously diagnosed mass(4%), tubal pathology (ectopic
pregnancy excluded)(4%), ovarian size (2%), IUD (2%), follicle size (1%). This evolution will carry on, sustained
by the technical evolution and the improvement of observation qualities.

Dpt Echodiagnostic (Clin.Ob-Gyn.) Hop.Brugmann

REPARTITION ACTIVITE de 1966 à 1978

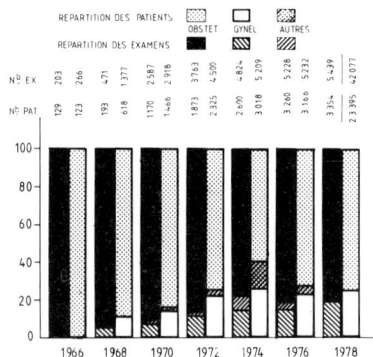

INCIDENCE OF USG GYNECOLOGICAL PATIENTS

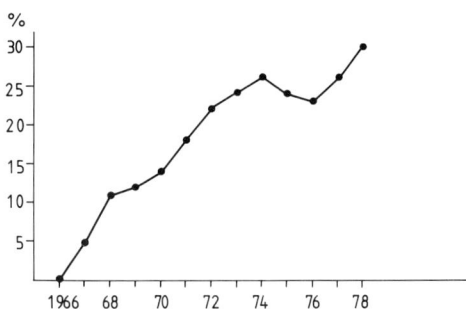

Fig. 5. Total number of patients and examinations performed in Diagnostic Ultrasound Dept. performed each
year since 1966 and distribution of these cases be-
tween obstetrics, gynecology and other indications
(even years only).

Fig. 6. Percentage of gynecological indications between all
ultrasonically examined patients.
(The absolute number of patients,
from 1966, are 0,6,21,74,164,
272,422,570,696,754,778,861,
1046, and total = 5664)

C. Value of USG in gynecology: comparison between the echographic and operative descriptions. Out of 5664 USG pelvic
examinations, 956 operative controls were available to appreciate the validity of the sonographic information. The
information brought by the USG was divided into 4 groups
(Fig. 8).
1. Exact information: means that the pathology was correctly localized (uterus, ovaries, tubes or other) and that the
pathology type was defined with a minimum of details (solid,
liquid or complex tumour, one or more masses, necrotic zones)
2. Useful information: means that the USG information was
correct but not specific enough, e.g. the interpretation of
USG revealed an adnexial solid tumour while an ovarian tumour or pedonculated myoma was found during the operation;
USG diagnosis of cystic para-uterine tumour while ovarian
cyst or an hydrosalpinx was found.

481

3. <u>Missing information</u>: means that a lesion was not observed
with USG when the surgical finding was positive. About 90%
of that situation occurred in cases where two different abnormalities were coexistent: e.g. fibroma and ovarian cyst,
but ovarian cyst was not described by USG.
4. <u>False information</u>:means that the anomaly was erroneously
diagnosed. e.g. ovarian cyst for uterine myoma; hydrosalpinx for normal tubes; uterine fibroma for solid ovarian
tumor.

EVOLUTION OF THE USG INDICATIONS

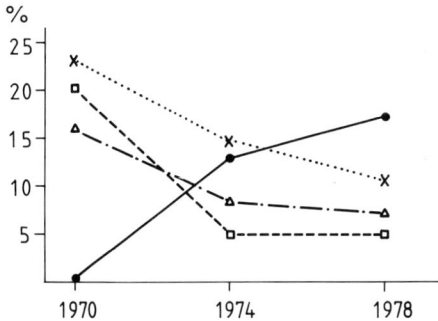

Echodiagnostic unit of Ob-Gyn. Dpt. Univ.
Brugmann Hosp. Brussels

**EVALUATION of INFORMATIONS
OBTAINED FROM U.S.G.**

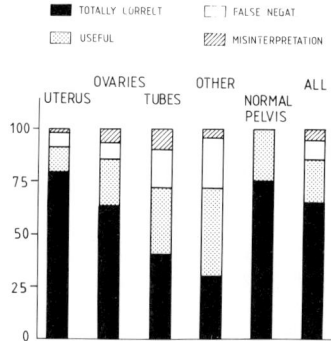

Fig. 7. Evolution of the percentage of some examples of
ultrasound examinations.
X....X = uterine fibroid?
  - - = pelvic mass:differ-
         ential diagnosis?
  - - = ovarian mass:solid
         cystic?
_____ = USG for indications
         never mentioned be-
         fore 1970.

Fig. 8. Results of 956 USG
examinations, all controlled
by surgery.

    In the rubric "normal pelvis", the USG <u>exact informa-
tion</u> means that a normal pelvis, as described by laparoscopy or laparotomy, was also described as normal by USG; <u>use-
ful information</u> means that minor anomalies were described
but not after surgery when the pelvis was succintly expressed as "normal" (e.g. USG description of the somewhat irregular outlines of the uterus, retroversion...).
    The USG information appears to be precise or useful in
more than 86% of the cases, inexact in 14% (false negatives:
9% and erroneously interpreted anomalies: 5%). These rates
are to be compared with the increasing incidence of impre-
cise clinical indications for USG examinations. The rate
of correct USG information is increasing only slowly but
one should take into account an important factor which is
the evolution of the selection of cases referred to USG.

As the ratio USG examination surgical indication shows it, in the first five years, more than 70% of pelvic USG examinations were followed by operation; for the last five years the rate was less than 15%.

The gynecological USG seems to evoluate to a more extended conception: a method for screening pelvic anomalies.

CONCLUSION

The contribution of the USG in gynecology is incontestably positive. The traditional gynecological examination requires a visual and innocuous complement, simple and without disagreement for the patient and inexpensive. This complement is brought by the USG with reliability in a non-invasive way such as no other exploration can do it. Numerous expected improvements should give more complete information; these are connected to the technological development and the introduction of computer with their large spectrum of possibilities.

REFERENCES

1. Calvo Ch.C, Pacheco L.A.(1976): Acta Gin 27, 157-170.
2. Cochrane W.J., Thomas M.A.(1974): Radiology, 110, 649-654.
3. Corcondilas E., Calfopoulos P., Michalas S., Kaskarelis D.(1976): Vie Med Canada, 5, 938-939.
4. Donald I, McVicar J., Brown T.G. (1958): Lancet, 1, 1188-1194.
5. Donald I, (1965): J Obstet Gynaec Br Commonw, 72,907-929.
6. Dussik K (1942): Z Ges Neurol Psychiat, 174, 153.
7. Effert S., Erkens H., Grosse-Brockhoff F.(1957): Dtsch Med Wschr, 82, 1253.
8. Exalto N., Eskes T.K., Hein P.R.(1978): Europ J Obstet Gynec VIII, 369-375.
9. Hackeloer B.J., Nitschke S. et al.(1977): Geburtsch Frauenheilk, 37, 187-190.
10. Hollander H.J.(1968): Med Klin, 63, 1175-1180.
11. Howry D.H., Holmes J.H., Cushman C.R., Posakony G.J. (1952): Geriatrics, 10, 123-128.
12. Janssens D. et al. (1973): Contraception, 8, 485-495.
13. Kikuchi Y. et al. (1957): J Acoust Soc Amer, 29, 824.
14. Kratochwil A (1968): Ultraschalldiagnostik in Geburthilfe und Gynäkologie. Stuttgart, G. Thieme.
15. Kratochwil A. et al.(1974): Geburt.Frauenh. 34,742-752.
16. Levi,S (1971): Schweiz Z Gyn Geburtsh, 2, 11-24.
17. Levi,S (1972): Diagnostic par ultrasons en gyn-obstetrique.
18. Levi, S & Delval R.(1976): Acta Obstet Gynec scand,55,261-266.
19. Levi, S et al(1978): In: Recent advances in ultrasound. p.36.
20. Queenan JT(1975): Amer J Obstet Gynecol., 123, 453-465.
21. Schillinger H, et al(1972): Geburtsh Frauenh., 36,976-982.
22. Sunden B(1964): Acta Obstet Gynec Scand, 43, supple 6.
23. Thompson HE et al(1967): J Obstet Gynecol, 98,472-481.
24. Ulrich PC, Sanders RC(1976): J Clin Ultr. 4,199-204.
25. Wild JJ, Reid JM(1952): Amer J Path, 28, 839.
26. Zacutti A, Brugnoli C.A.(1970): Acta Eur Fertil,2 ,445-468.

TWO METHODS FOR QUANTIFIED ULTRASONIC TISSUE CHARACTERIZATION

Kjell Lindström and Nils-Gunnar Holmer

Department of Biomedical Engineering, University Hospital, Malmö Allmänna Sjukhus, Malmö, Sweden.

The importance of ultrasonic echography has increased greatly during the last few years, and its impact on health care now exceeds all early expectations. It´s non-invasive and non-destructive properties further enhance the usefulness in clinical medicine. However, further evolution is restricted by the subjective interpretation of clinical ultrasound data. The talent and skill of the operator is still the prime factor for validity, reliability and reproducibility of the diagnostic results.

The ability of ultrasonic echography to visualize directly soft tissue structure is dependent upon partial reflection of acoustic energy at interfaces of juxtaposed tissues exhibiting different acoustic impedance. The limited dynamic range of most standard ultrasonic pulse echo equipment do often restrict the visual display to specular (mirror-like) reflections from large vessels, tense connective tissues such as present in organ capsules etc. The diagnosis is then performed on an "anatomical map" made from shape, size and position of structures delineated by the echoes from their boundaries.

Because no soft tissue is completely homogeneous, reflections - very variable in amplitude but detectable nevertheless - can be recorded from every region of an organ being scanned. Echoes from internal structures are often two to three orders of magnitude smaller than obtained from large interfaces at normal incidence. The recent use of so called grey-scale echography permits simultaneous display of normal specular reflections as well as these internal echoes which considerably increases the reliability of portrayal of soft tissue organs. Their signature; i.e. size, pattern and distribution of internal echoes is dependent on the structural organisation and architecture of examined tissues and may be used to classify various types of soft tissue.

It is essential that the different organs can be portrayed with representative magnitude of echoes. Many physical factors affect the propagation of ultrasound through tissue, and the wide dynamic range of grey-scale echography further accentuates artifacts due to beamwidth, beam side lobes and multiple reflections within the examined structure.

The purpose of this paper is twofold:

1) To discuss the physical parameters that influence on the ultrasound echosignal returning from various

normal and abnormal tissues.

2)   To devise methods for quantitative tissue characterization (including automatic setting-up of the
ultrasound scanner) to reduce the uncertainty resulting from subjective interpretation.

PHYSICAL FACTORS AFFECTING MAGNITUDE OF ECHO-SIGNALS

When an ultrasound wave propagates through a medium,
its intensity is reduced as a function of distance. As the
main objective of echography is to portray the magnitude of
echoes, it´s appropriate to analyze the different factors
which affect the magnitude of echoes.
By working out special compensation criteria for each
of the factors and control the receiver gain so as to counteract the losses, it should be possible to compensate for
the attenuation. Some of the major factors affecting the
attenuation are briefly discussed below.

a)   Diffraction

The ultrasound beam can be analyzed by applying
Huygen´s Principle on the transducer surface. This surface
is considered to be an array of separate elements, each ra-
diating spherical waves in the forward direction. Under
steady state conditions the elements move in synchrony with
equal amplitudes. Then the spherical waves from each very
small element interfere constructively to reinforce each
other in some points and destructively in other. The result
is a tendency to form maxima and minima of intensity in the
transmitted sound waves. As a consequence of this the ultrasound is concentrated within a beam. Further, the ultrasound beam becomes more uniform with increasing

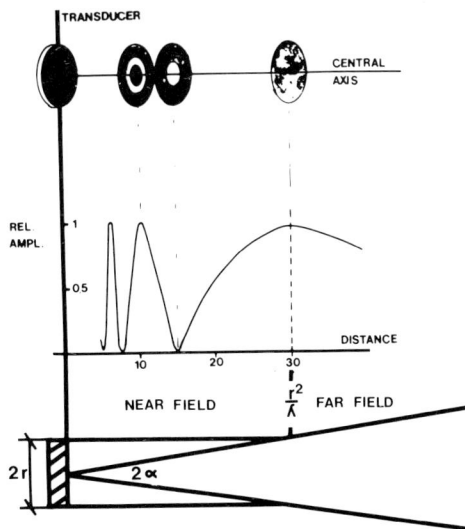

Figure   1

485

distance from the source.

It can be shown that in a practical situation ($r \gg \lambda$) the near field extends out to a distance that is approximatively equal to ($r\uparrow 2/\lambda$), where r is the radius of the circular disc transducer and λ the wavelength of the ultrasound.

Beyond the limit of the near field there is no longer any possibility of complete reinforcement of the spherical waves from each small element at the transducer surface. The radiation can therefore be assumed to travel outward in the form of a cone whose apex is at the crystal, as illustrated in Fig. 1. The beam is roughly cylindrical in the near field but diverges at angles $\pm\alpha$ (i.e. half the angle formed by the apex of the cone) in the far field. The angle of divergence, α, can be derived from

$$\sin \alpha \simeq 0.6 \, \lambda/r$$

Consequently, the shape of the ultrasound field depends upon the radius, r, of the transducer and the wavelength, λ, of the ultrasound. Thus, if the wavelength is decreased in relation to the radius of the transducer, the sound beam will spread less and become more defined and intense.

For any specific ultrasound transducer, it is possible to calculate or preferably measure the losses due to diffraction for subsequent compensation.

b)   Absorption by tissue

There is often a state of confusion concerning the meaning of absorption versus attenuation. As pointed out by Wells (1), absorption refers to the conversion of ultrasound to thermal energy (mechanical losses), attenuation refers to the total propagation losses, including absorption. The absorption mechanism in biological materials is dependent on many different factors. At Megahertz frequencies, the relaxation mechanism is the one most commonly observed.

In order to compensate for absorption, the intensity losses as function of depth penetration is calculated. Where absorption is uniform the losses are proportional to the ultrasound intensity I. Thus for a plane wave propagating in the X-direction, we have

$$(dI/I) = - k \, x$$

where k is the absorption coefficient. By integrating this equation and applying the boundary condition: $I = I_0$ for $x = 0$, one obtains the equation for the intensity at the depth $I(x)$

$$I(x) = I_0 \, e^{-kx}$$

For normal soft tissue it is found that the absorption

coefficient is proportional to the frequency, f, of the
ultrasound. The equation can thus be written as

$$I(x) = I_0 \, e^{-\alpha f x}$$

where $\alpha = k/f$. The losses for soft tissue are often given
as an average rate of 0.5 dB/cm, MHz.

Most electronic circuits used for time-gain-compensa-
tion (TGC) of the ultrasound echo-signals are designed out
of the assumption that the general form

$$I(x) = I_0 \, e^{-kx}$$

can be used for the total attenuation as well. To include
the various forms af attenuation, k is then assigned a
rather complex frequency dependence. As the ultrasound
pulse traverses through many different structures of diversified form and size, this assumption is invalid in clinical use and the resulting TGC-function is consequently often unsufficient.

The characteristic of an adequate TGC-circuit, correc-
ting for absorption and diffraction is shown in Fig. 2.

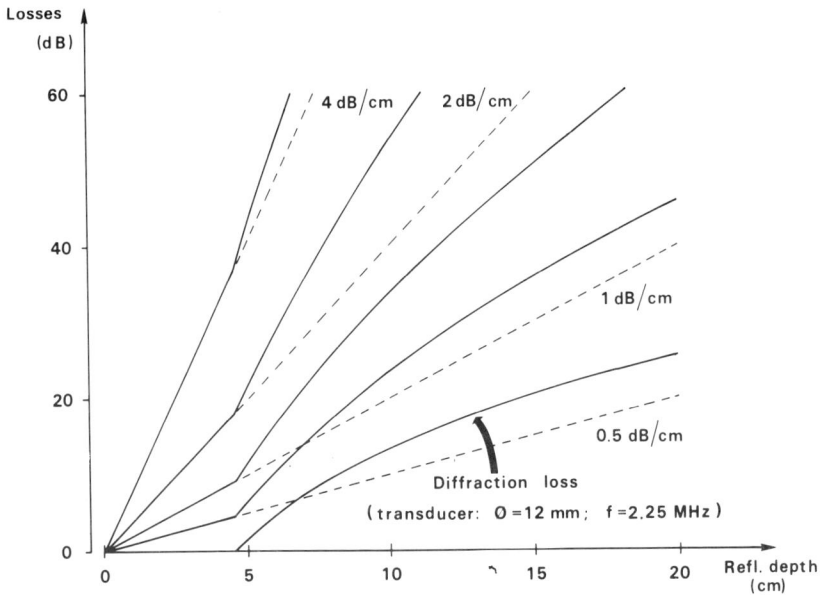

Figure   2

c)   Reflection

So far consideration has been restricted to ultrasound propagation through homogeneous media. From acoustic
point of view, a medium is homogeneous if both density and

487

sound velocity are constant throughout the region of the medium disturbed by the ultrasound wave. The effect of in-homogeneities on the sound wave depend on their intrinsic properties and their geometries. The simplest type of in-homogeneity is a plane interface between two different ho-mogeneous media having characteristic impedances, Z_1 and Z_2, respectively.

In general, part of the incident sound energy is re-flected back into medium (1) and the remainder transmitted into medium (2). The pressure reflection coefficient, (R), i.e. the ratio of the amplitude of the reflected wave to that of the incident wave, depend upon the characteristic impedances of the two media and on the angle of incidence of the incident wave.

For normal incidence, formula and resulting reflection are given in Fig. 3. As can be seen, there is a linear re-lation between the pressure reflection coefficient (R) and changes in the acoustic impedance ($\Delta Z/Z_1$) up to about 0.1 (5% error). Most biological soft tissue interfaces falls into this category.

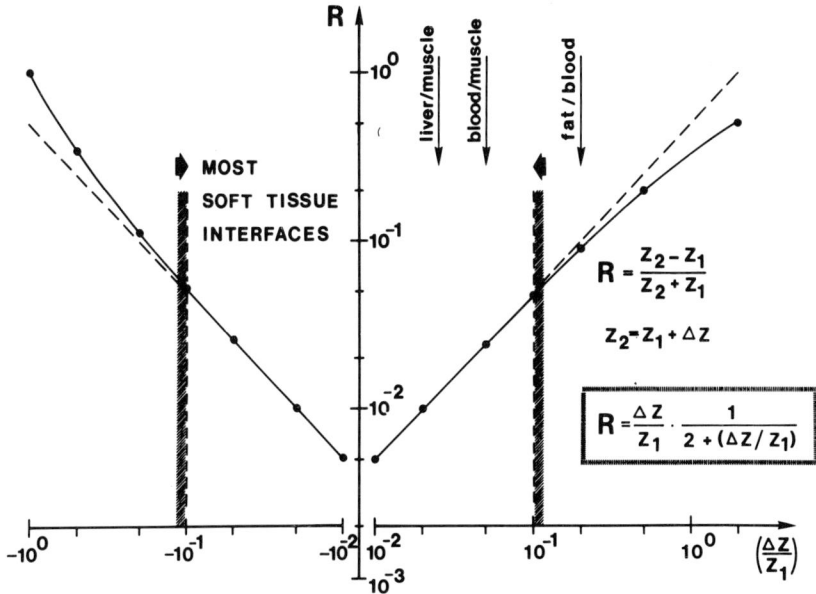

Figure 3

If the sound wave is transmitted through a number of different media, partial reflection may occur at each in-terface. Even if each of the reflections is quite small, the resulting attenuation can be quite prominent with in-creasing number of interfaces, as shown in Fig. 4. This is one of the reasons for the occurence of so called shadowing behind dense structures, often used as a clinical sign for

488

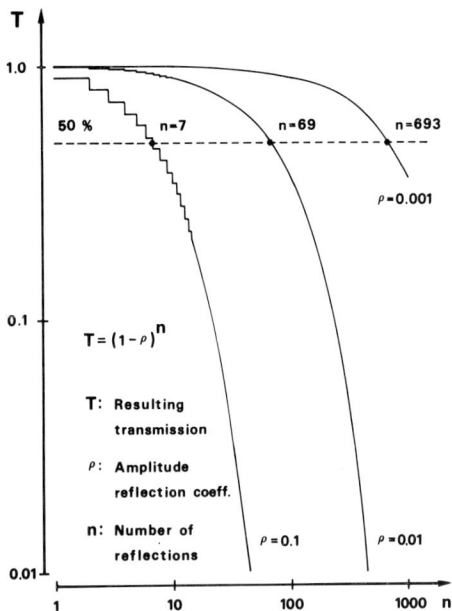

Figure 4

the existence of for example a solid tumour.

The losses calculated in Fig. 4 assume independent reflections. If the intermediate medium, Z_2, between two media, Z_1 and Z_3, is sufficiently thin little losses will take place and the resulting sound transmission coefficient will be the same as for a wave moving directly from medium (1) to medium (3).

Multiple reflections can sometimes cause serious artifacts by displaying echoes in positions where no interface really exists. When they occur, initially echoes are obtained from all the genuine interfaces. In addition, a set of "new" echoes are produced as a result of multiple reflections between the different interfaces. Such multiple reflections can be of the axial type, produced by a pulse reflected backwards and forwards more than once along the line of sight, or of the unaxial type owing to reflection from any other discontinuity out of the line of sight. These echoes occur particularly when a highly reflecting surface is located near the transducer. It is very difficult to eliminate such artifacts in an automatic mode, but with experience they can often be recognized as the small genuine internal echoes have a distribution pattern which differs from that obtained from multiple reflections. It is of cause unsuitable to make use of areas containing such "false" multiple reflections for tissue characterization.

Reflection of sound waves will always take place when there is a discontinuity in the characteristic impedance. At a plane boundary having dimensions large compared with

489

the wavelength, specular (mirror-like) reflection will take place. Where, however, the boundary has dimensions which are comparable with or less than one wavelength, scattering will take place, i.e. the beam is reflected in all directions.

Scattering may also be caused by the presence of a large number of small acoustic inhomogeneities distributed in the tissue. This is the way internal echoes are generated in for example the liver, solid tumours and even some fluid filled structures like cysts.

By scattering, energy is diverted from the main sound beam and the observed attenuation is directly proportional to the volume of the scattered object and also to the fourth power of the frequency. As compared to specular reflection, the scattered reflections exhibit smaller variation in echo amplitude with changing angle of incidence. This can be taken advantage of to display the position of an organ even when it is not possible to show the echoes from the boundaries due to their inclination to the beam.

d)   Angle of incidence and aperture

The reflectivities of various soft tissue interfaces are normally given for the rather idealized case of normal incidence on a perfectly flat boundary. The magnitude of echoes from large interfaces is large when the interface is normal to the beam, but is critically dependent on inclination. Organs and major structures are not completely smooth, but exhibit surface irregularities. As the ultrasound frequency is increased, the surface seems to become "rougher" as the wavelength decreases and becomes comparable with the irregularities. Simultaneously, the surface

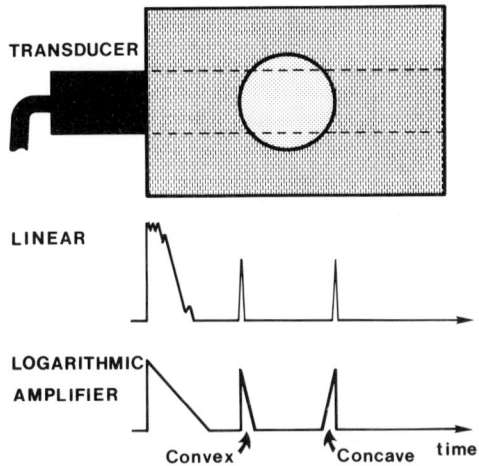

Figure 5

exhibits smaller variation in echo amplitude with changing angle of incidence.

The form of the echo envelope obtained can sometimes give additional information about geometry of the echoproducing interface. The use of logarithmic amplifiers seems to be especially useful in this aspect. As seen in Fig. 5, convex and concave interfaces can easily be discriminated between, dependent upon if the triangular echo envelope has a steep or slow front.

The use of a transducer with very good lateral resolution is not sufficient to produce accurate ultrasound pictures. Image distorsion due to limited numerical aperture, a disadvantage with most of the present scanning systems, is shown in Fig. 6. The limitation is illustrated on a highly reflecting surface, angulated against the ultrasound beam, using a) an ultrasound system with high lateral resolution but small numerical aperture, and b) an ultrasound system with high lateral resolution and large numerical aperture.

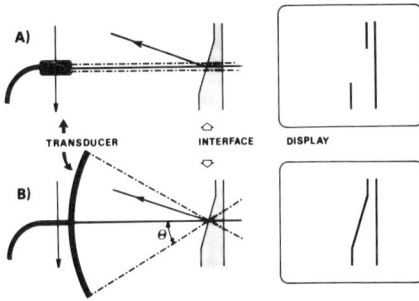

A)

TRANSDUCER   INTERFACE   DISPLAY

B)

θ

Figure 6

e)   Propagation velocity

Normally, echography equipment are constructed out of a presumption that the velocity of ultrasound in human tissues has a single value, often given as 1540 m/sec. As the ultrasound velocity for soft tissue can differ between 1470 - 1640 m/sec, the absolute accuracy of the method is limited and geometrical forms may be displayed distorted. This limitation might be the ultimate barrier in the work to improve resolution and fidelity in ultrasound pictures.

When an ultrasound wave meets the large interface between two media with different velocity of sound, a reflected wave returns in medium (1) at the velocity, c_1, as that with which it approached the interface. The transmitted wave continues into medium (2) beyond the interface at a velocity, c_2, corresponding to propagation in medium (2). Just as in optics, the well-known laws of reflection and

refraction of plane waves apply, i.e. the angle of incidence is equal to the angle of reflection, and Snell's law,

$$\frac{\sin \theta_1}{\sin \theta_2} = \frac{c_1}{c_2}$$

regulates the angle of transmission.

Significant differences between sound velocities in
different areas under investigation result in registration
errors in the B-mode display. Further, it must be remem-
bered that the ultrasound beam is widened or narrowed upon
oblique transmission into a second medium, thereby changing
the actual intensity in the sound beam.

If $c_1 < c_2$, then for some critical angle of incidence,
the refracted ray makes an angle of 90° with the normal to
the interface. If the angle of incidence is equal to or
greater than the critical angle, no acoustic energy is
transmitted into the second medium.

METHODS FOR TISSUE CHARACTERIZATION

All echography systems are capable of displaying two
acoustic parameters of tissue, namely the amplitude of the
acoustic echo and its site of origin. Different display
methods emphasize one type of information to the exclusion
of the other. In the A-mode type of presentation there is
good visual representation of the amplitude data. However,
A-mode suffers from the fact that there is a complete loss
of anatomical orientation, so that one does not know the
precise lateral relationship of one echo to another. Anatomical orientation is essential for correct interpretation
of the amplitude data, because the amplitude of the echo is
in large measure determined by the angle of incidence of
the incident sound beam and the absorption of overlaying
tissues. B-mode, on the other hand, provides excellent orientation and anatomical information, but the contrast gradient of the B-mode echograms is so low that it is difficult to distinguish amplitude differences with the naked
eye with this type of presentation.

Optimum differential diagnosis demands that both amplitude and anatomical data be simultaneously evaluated in
reading a diagnosis. Scanned deflection modulation (2) displays both the source of the echo and its relative amplitude, thus retaining the best features of both the A- and
the B-modes.

For the tissue characterization methods described below, it is necessary to utilize even more accurate information. Ultrasound scanners with display line selector,
similar to the TD-recorder (3), are therefore normally utilized providing simultaneously excellent spatial orientation and accurate A-mode presentation from any part of the
display.

Combining all the factors affecting the magnitude of ultrasound echoes, it should be obvious that current available TGC-circuits are inadequate to compensate for total attenuation. In fact, it is often seen how picture information can be degraded due to misuse of the TGC-circuit.
There are two possibilities to improve the situation:

a)   The "large dynamic range"-approach, where the echography system is designed with a dynamic range, sufficient to record all returning information for further processing and calculation without any previous adjustment.

b)   The "reflection correction"-approach, where all known losses are compensated for as far as possible, and in an automatic way to reduce subjective interpretation.

"LARGE DYNAMIC RANGE"-METHOD

The aim to eliminate correction for losses from echography equipment has required development of novel instrumentation for amplification and signalprocessing. We have designed a new amplifier-detector-combination, which can compress an input signal of 100 dB dynamic range to an output signal range of 30 dB. Such an amplifier makes TGC unnecessary and enables to some extent direct observation on the A-mode display of the attenuation of the ultrasound pulse in the tissue.

a)   Quasi-logarithmic amplifier-detector

It is possible to construct logarithmic amplifiers in many different ways, most of which result in systems with

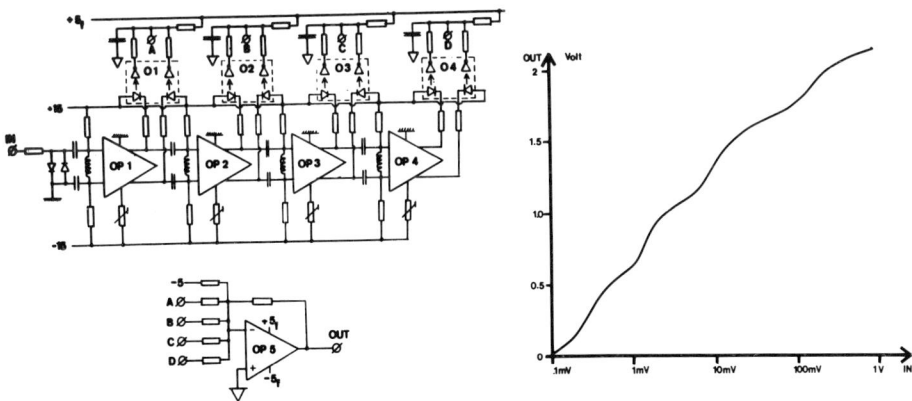

Figure   7a   7b

493

poor frequency response. However, using so called piece-
wise linear approach, wide-range quasi-logarithmic amplifiers can be designed with frequency response sufficient
also for echography. By summing the outputs of cascaded
limiting amplifiers, isolated and demodulated through opto-
couplers, the resulting output signal can be made proportional to the logarithm of the input signal.

A block diagram for a 4-stage cascade amplifier (using opto-couplers at each stage) is illustrated in Fig. 7a.
The output signals from each opto-coupler are added by
OP-5. For a given input signal, the two last amplifiers
OP-3 and OP-4 might be saturated, whereas OP-1 and OP-2 are
not. The dynamic range of the cascaded amplifier-detector-
combination is thus much larger than the range of each
single stage of the amplifier. The gain-transfer characteristic for the four cascaded stage design is shown in
Fig. 7b. The dynamic range and amplification can be fixed
upon by the number of cascaded stages used. If large dynamic range and amplification is desired, the signal-to-noise
ratio can be improved if a low-noise pre-amplifier precede
the cascaded stages.

Compared to an ordinary linear amplifier, the dynamic
range of the present amplifier is about 500 times larger.
This quality is displayed in Fig. 8, where the A-mode of a
reflectoscope showing several echoes of decreasing ampli-

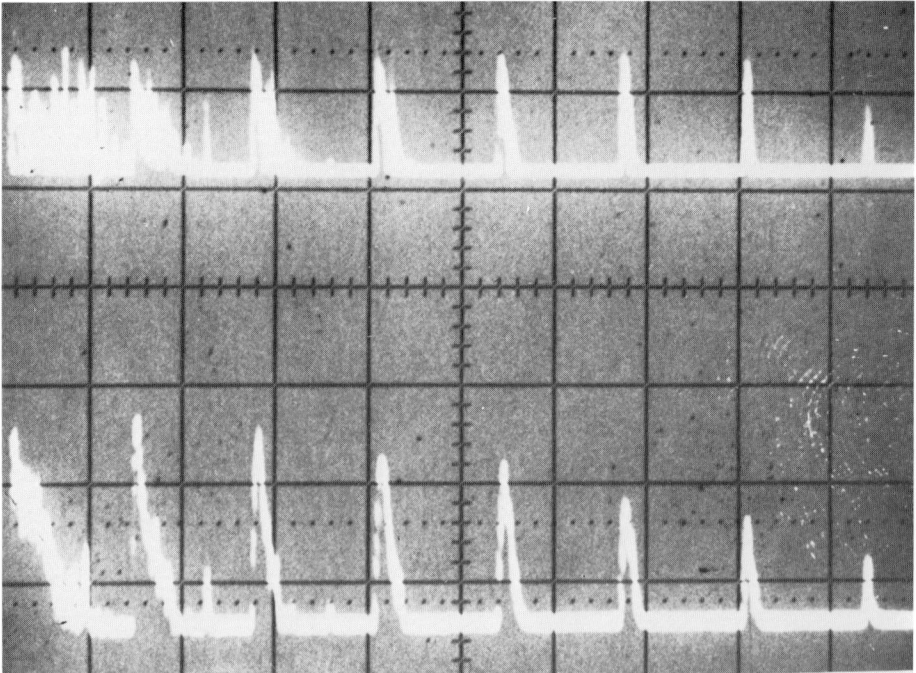

Figure 8

494

tude is amplified by a conventional (linear) reflectoscope amplifier (upper trace) and the present amplifier (lower trace). From the figure it is obvious that the conventional amplifier saturates for all echoes except the last one, while the logarithmic amplifier shows the decreasing amplitude of the echoes. Further, it should be observed that the decrease of the transducer oscillations caused by the transmitter pulse can be observed with the new amplifier.

The quasi-logarithmic amplifier has proved to perform very well and it can be widely spread because of its simplicity both in technical design and use. Its enormous dynamic range makes it particularly suitable to process signals when the received echoes show a large dynamic range.

b) Attenuation measurement

The quasi-logarithmic amplifier with its large dynamic range is well suited for attenuation measurements. A simplified block diagram of an apparatus, designed to measure total echo attenuation as a function of distance, is shown in Fig. 9. It is possible to connect this apparatus to most different kinds of ultrasound scanners.

Assuming equal reflection coefficients and perpendicular reflection surfaces the amplitude of the reflected echoes can be described by the equation

$$A(x) = A_0 \cdot e^{-k' x}$$

At the distance x_1 we measure

$$\log(A(x_1)) = \log A_0 - k' x_1$$

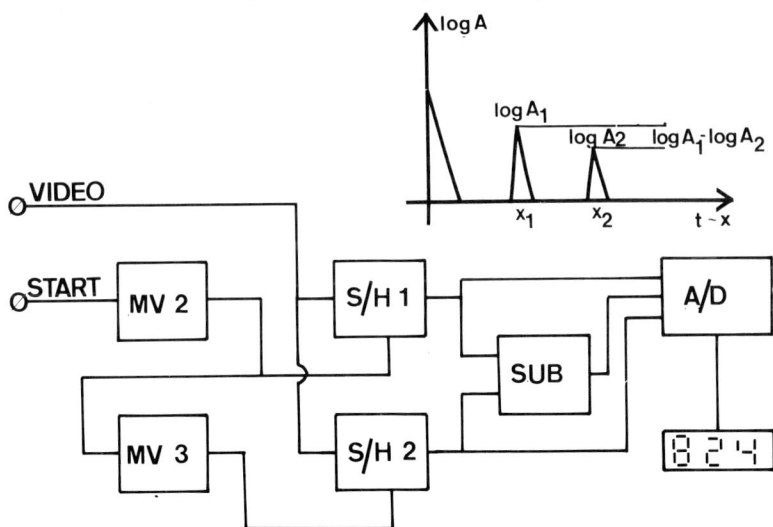

Figure 9

495

A similar relation holds for x_2. The difference between these two measurements

$$\log(A(x_1)) - \log(A(x_2)) = k' \ (x_2 - x_1)$$

which can be easily measured electronically with sample-and-hold circuits (S/H) sampling $\log(A(x_1))$ and $\log(A(x_2))$ and a difference amplifier subtracting the values. The result is displayed via an A/D-converter. By this technique the attenuation factor k is calculated

$$k' \ = \ \frac{\log(A(x_1)) - \log(A(x_2))}{x_2 - x_1}$$

During in vitro tests in our laboratory, we found it necessary to compensate for beam divergence before absorption value could be calculated. However, with such compensation, the measurements for pure absorption became accurate and reproducable. In clinical investigations, however, some problems were revealed depending on moving structures, angled surfaces etc.

A newly designed equipment shown in Fig. 10, using a fast 8-bit A/D-converter and a memory which can be examined by a μ-computer, is presently built to circumvent these problems.

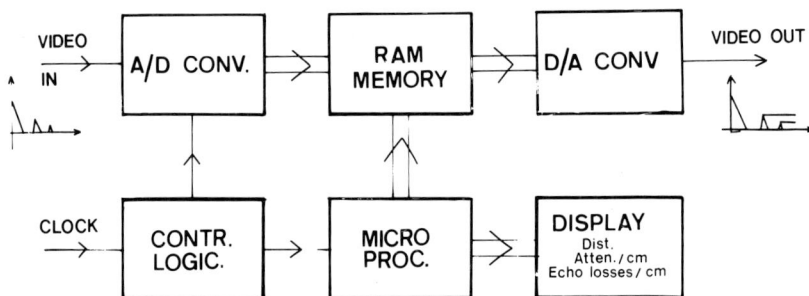

Figure   10

"REFLECTION CORRECTION"-METHOD

In diagnostic ultrasound, the amplitude of received echoes shows a large variation with time due to various physical factors. The conventional correction method, the TGC, is often found to be inadequate to display all echoes well.

In some cases, like one-dimensional echocardiography, TGC can produce adequate echoes when the examination depth is divided into separately controllable segments. Unfortu-

nately, this type of compensation is not possible for compound or real-time scanners, since in this case, the TGC
should be adjusted to match the individual attenuation and
reflection of the ultrasound beam for each scan line. There
is consequently a strong need for better TGC-methods.

a)   Normal TGC-compensation

The attenuation of an ultrasoundwave, as it progresses
through homogeneous soft tissue, is often approximated to
an exponential decrease. If the TGC-circuit in the echoscope is used to increase the receiving gain exponentially
with time, echo amplitudes can be made the same for occasional similar boundaries at different distances. The effect
of the TGC-circuit is schematically illustrated in Fig. 11.

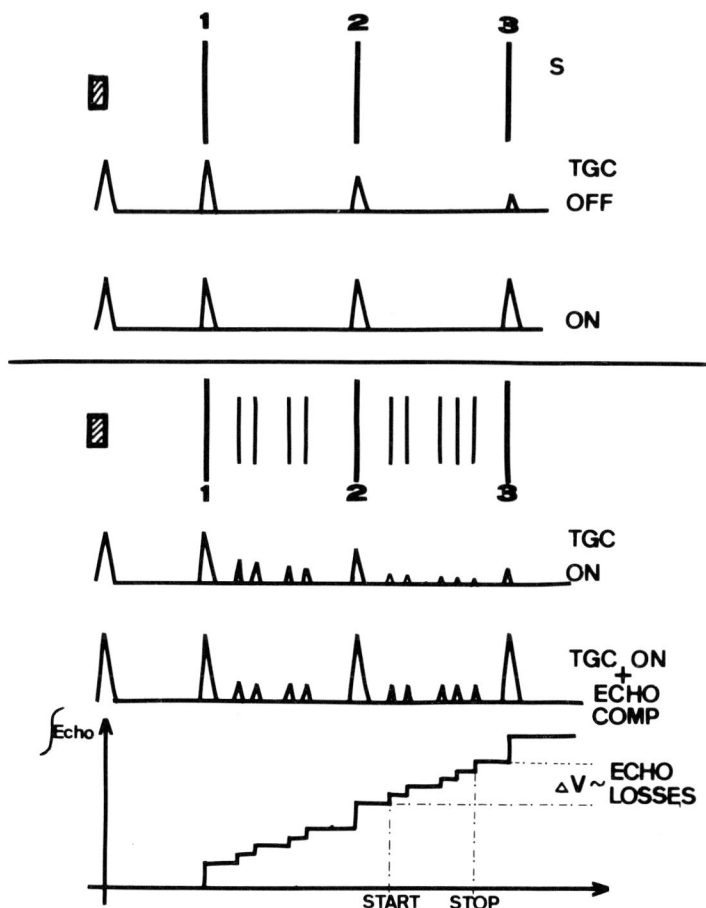

Figure   11

This simple model is not applicable in clinical echography, owing to additional echo-losses. If many reflecting boundaries are traversed quite large losses can result, as discussed above. The TGC-circuit, designed for absorption in soft tissue only, must be adjusted in such a way, that it will give an acceptable average compensation for both absorption and reflection losses. As a result, large variations in echocompensation might appear in different parts of produced ultrasound pictures (fig. 11, middle).

b)   Automatic TGC

This difficulty can be circumvented by the use of automatic reflection correction(4). If the detected echo signals are integrated during each sweep, a voltage proportional to attenuation due to reflections only will result. This signal can be used as additional control voltage for the TGC-circuit, whereby normal tissue absorption as well as the reflection losses can be compensated for. The function of this automatic TGC is schematically illustrated in Fig. 11 (bottom).

c)   Tissue characterization

The integrated echo signal from each sweep contains information of the spatial echo losses. By measuring the difference voltage on the integrated echo signal from two predetermined positions along the ultrasound beam, an estimation of the echo reflection losses in the tissues in the corresponding part of the tissue can be made (5),(6). Thus, the echo losses in different tissues can be measured, which may give valuable information about the tissue in question

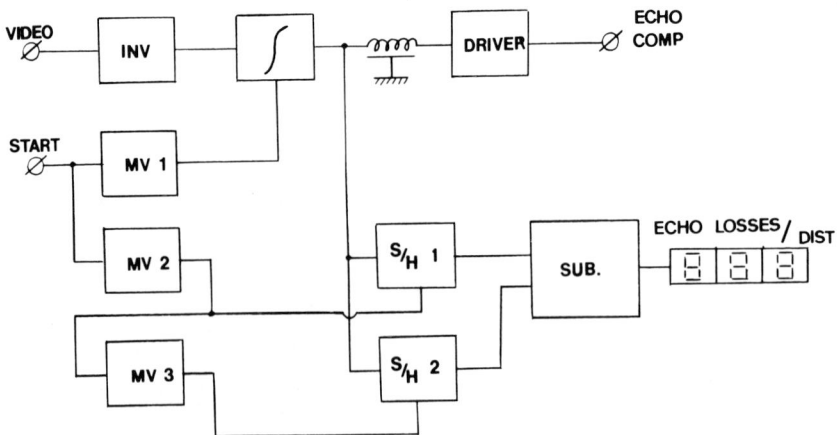

Figure   12

(systic-solid, or classification of solid tumours). A circuit for this measurement is shown in Fig. 12. The starting
point for the region of measurement is determined by an adjustable delay (MV 2) and the end point by an additional
adjustable delay (MV 3). The sample-and-hold circuit (S/H 1)
holds the integrated value at the starting point while a
second circuit (S/H 2) keeps the end point value. These two
voltages are subtracted and the difference voltage is displayed on a digital voltmeter.

This equipment can be connected to the video signal
output of almost any echoscope, and makes it possible to
classify different kinds of tissue due to reflection losses.

d)   Calibration

For clinical use, it is important to set up the ultrasound scanner properly. The TGC shall compensate for the
basic soft tissue absorption and the loop-gain of the echo
compensation must be adjusted for adequate compensation of
reflection losses. This can be performed by means of a
special test object, shown in Fig. 13(left).

The upper part of the test object is constructed from
two tissue equivalent materials, with a slight difference
in acoustic impedance. If no attenuation takes place between the two boundaries, reflection of equal amplitude would
result. If the TGC-circuit is designed so that dB/cm-cor-
rection is adjustable, this parameter is adjusted until the
two echoes have equal amplitude, as shown in Fig. 13(right).
The TGC is now calibrated.

In the lower part of the test object, a simulated tumour is added to the middle section. Such a "tumour" can
be constructed from a natural sponge filled with gelatin
containing "scatterers"(7). When the transducer is placed
in the echocompensation position, the echo from the right

Tissue Equivalent Test Object for Calibration

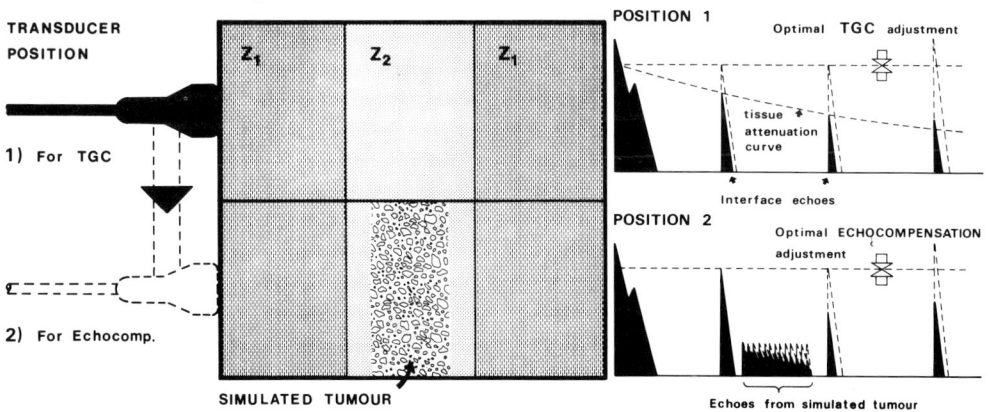

Figure   13

boundary will again be small as a result of reflection losses in the "tumour". By adjusting the loop-gain, so as to restall its amplitude, the gain of the echo-compensation circuit corresponds to the reflection losses and the tissue characterization device is calibrated for clinical work.

e)   Limitations

Transducer beam pattern: As shown above, large additional signal losses can result when measuring in the far zone of the transducer. However, by the use of calibrated transducers, these losses can be compensated for in the echocompensation circuit.

Scattering, angle of incidence: If the aperture of the transducer is insufficient (as is often the case) the actual reflection losses can be much greater than received reflections indicate. This effect is to same extent compensated for when calibrating the system in the test object. However, even when the compensation is insufficient, the resulting compensation is reproducable.

Selection of measurement area: By proper selection of measurement area, the influence of various artifacts can be reduced to a minimum. By comparing measurements from different parts of the organ structure under investigation a good estimate of the reliability of the measurement can be obtained. Finally, comparison of reflection losses in a selected area to that of a known structure in the body, such as muscle, can further increase the accuracy of the method.

Measurement length: The present technical solution of the echocompensation circuit includes a delay of about 2 μsec to avoid so called hunting. This corresponds to a tissue layer 1.5 mm thich, why echolosses always should be averaged over a length of at least 5 mm.

CONCLUSION

Much work is presently going on around the world to find methods and devices for ultrasonic tissue characterization. In spite of relatively complex scanning- and signal processing techniques, few clinically useful in vivo-methods have so far been deviced.

We have described two simple methods, intended for clinical use. Both are combined in one apparatus, to enable measurement of echo-losses as function of distance as well as the total echo attenuation. A simplified block diagram of the apparatus is shown in Fig. 14. It is possible to

500

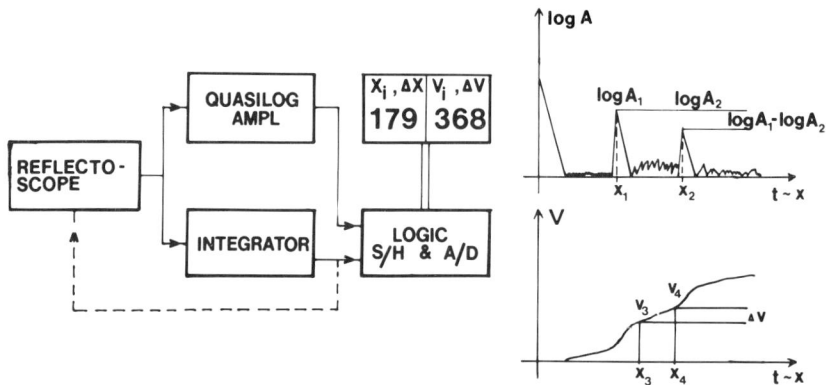

Figure 14

connect different types of ultrasound scanners to the apparatus.

a)   The "large dynamic range"-method makes use of a newly
developed quasilogarithmic amplifier for absolute attenuation measurement in different organs. The method has proved
to work well in vitro, whereas the accuracy is decreased
due to transducer movement artifacts in vivo. A new micro-
processor controlled version is under construction and will
hopefully improve its usefulness into the clinic.
     The new quasilogarithmic amplifier has already proved
its great value for investigations where the range of echoes
is very large. A specialized version of the logarithmic
amplifier, without one single external control, is already
in clinical use at our hospital for ultrasound investigation of sinusitis.

b)   The "reflection correction"-method has shown encouraging results in in vitro tests and is now under clinical
tests. An extra bonus with the echocompensation-technique
is the improved quality of the processed ultrasound pictures. A switch is included to turn-off the echocompensation
and restore the normal TGC-function, to retain the well-
known clinical signs from normal ultrasound scanning (echo-
shadows etc).
     Preliminary clinical results, achieved in collabora-
tion with Dr P.-H. Persson, has shown that it is possible
to differentiate between healthy and retarded foetuses due
to tissue characterization. The integral of back-scattered
echoes from the fetal liver was measured between the echoes
of the foetal abdominal wall and foetus venosus. The result shows significant changes for the fetal liver of growth
retarded infants. These results will be published elsewhere.

REFERENCES

1. Wells, P.N.T.(1977): Biomedical ultrasonics. Academic
    Press, London.
2. Baum, G.(1971): In: Recent Advances in Diagnostic
    Ultrasound, p. 109. Editor: E. Rand. Charles C.
    Thomas Publisher, Springfield.
3. Lindström,K., Maršál,K., Gennser, G., Bengtsson, L.,
    Benthin, M. and Dahl, P. (1977): Ultrasound Med.Biol.,
    Vol. 3, 143.
4. Holmer, N.-G., Lindström, K. and Lilja, B.(1977): Nya
    aspekter på time gain control (TGC), Svensk förening
    för medicinsk ultraljuddiagnostik 1977-10-14,
    (In swedish).
5. Holmer, N.-G. and Lindström, K.(1978): New Methods in
    Medical Ultrasound, p. 278. LUTEDX/(TEEM-1001)/1-420/
    1978, Lund - Malmö.
6. Lindström, K. and Holmer, N.-G.(1978): Abstracts,
    Third International Symposium on Ultrasonic Imaging
    and Tissue Characterization, p. 124. Editor: M. Linzer,
    National Bureau of Standards, Gaithersburg.
7. Edmonds, P.D., Reyes, Z., Parkinsson, D.B., Filly,R.A.
    and Busey,H.(1979): In: Ultrasonic Tissue Character-
    ization II, p. 323. Editor: M. Linzer, National Bureau
    of Standards, Spec.Publ. 525, U.S.Government Printing
    Office, Washington.

14. FREE COMMUNICATIONS

THE ROLE OF ULTRASOUND IN THE DIAGNOSIS AND MANAGEMENT OF THE INCOMPETENT CERVIX

Maher Mahran

Ain Shams Ultrasound Unit, Ain Shams University, Cairo, Egypt

The diagnosis of the incompetent cervix depends upon the history, clinical examination and different methods of investigation. The history is very suggestive when abortions follow a difficult instrumental delivery or induced abortion. However congenital imcompetent cervix is well known when a normal non-instrumental delivery is followed by repeated abortions. Clinical examination cannot diagnose a patulous internal os. However it can diagnose associated defects which might play an important role such as cervical tears, very short cervix and partial or complete loss of the portio vaginalis.

Usually the diagnosis is not complete without testing or demonstrating the defect of the internal os. This is done either by passing Hegar's dilator or by hysterogram. An internal os which allows the passage of Hegar's dilator 6 mm diameter or more without resistance is incompetent. A hysterogram done by a special technique can demonstrate the degree of damage to this region. However none of these methods of investigation can be used during pregnancy. This difficulty arises when the patient is seen for the first time pregnant. The introduction of ultrasound made it possible for the first time to document the diagnosis and to measure the internal os during pregnancy. (Fig.1). In the non pregnant state ultrasound offers an easier, quicker and safer method of diagnosis.

MATERIAL

This study includes 92 pregnant women diagnosed clinically as cases of repeated abortions due to incompetent cervix. All were examined by ultrasound to confirm the diagnosis and to decide the line of treatment. The internal os was measured in 34 cases. Many patients had more than one measurement especially in the follow up. Twenty normal pregnant women were used as control. All had the anteroposterior diameter of the internal os measured.

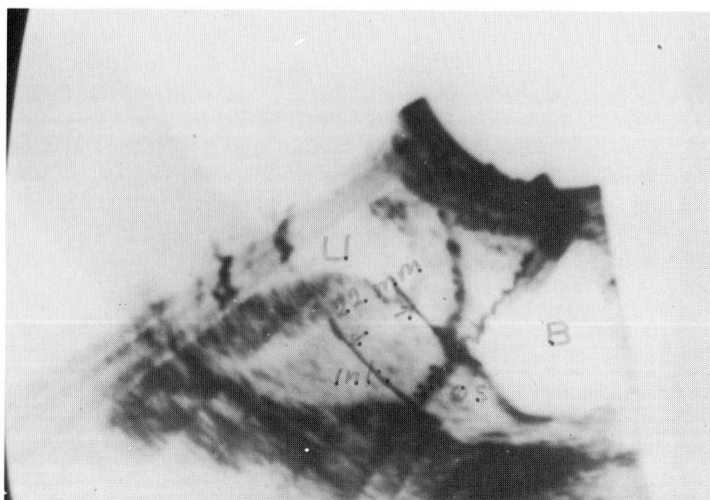

Figure 1. Longitudinal scan showing a patulous internal os measured by two electronic markers. (22 mm)

METHOD

The localization of the region of the internal os was done by longitudinal scan, using NE 4200. We use the angle between the bladder base and the vault as a marker at the level of the internal os. This was confirmed after inserting Foley's catheter in the uterus. The lower level of the ballon is at the level of the angle of the bladder. This proves the validity of our landmark to identify the region of the internal os. In order to check the validity of the measurement, the region of the internal os was measured in uteri submerged in water bath and in non pregnant women by ultrasound and Hegar's dilators in 10 women and in two uteri. The difference did not exceed 1-2 mm more in the ultrasound measurement. This could be partly explained by the thickness of the mucosal lining.

The patient is prepared as usual by the full bladder technique avoiding overdistension. The region of the internal os can be identified by the angle created by the reflection of the peritoneum from the supravinal cervix to the bladder. This angle can be easily demonstrated in the majority of cases.

It is important to remember the anatomy of the cervix which is formed of an outer fibromuscular layer lined by the cervical mucous membrane which rests immediately on the muscle layer and surrounds the cervical canal which usually contains some cervical secretion. Accordingly the following measurements could be identified:

1 - Outer muscular measurement between the outer surface
    of the fibromuscular layer.
2 - Inner muscular measurement between the inner surface
    of the fibromuscular layer.
3 - Inner mucosal measurement between the inner surface of
    the cervical mucose.

The last two measurements could be used to assess the
integrity of the internal os. However it is not always
easy to measure the inner mucosal diameter in contrast to
the inner muscular diameter where the muscle wall can be
clearly delineated.

The patient is prepared as usual by the full bladder
technique avoiding overdistension. It is important to
scan the cervical region longitudinally at very near distance i.e. every few mms until the widest diameter is available for measurement, otherwise the diagnosis can be easily
missed. Funneling of the cervical canal and failure to
demonstrate its integrity are bad prognostic signs.
(Fig. 2).

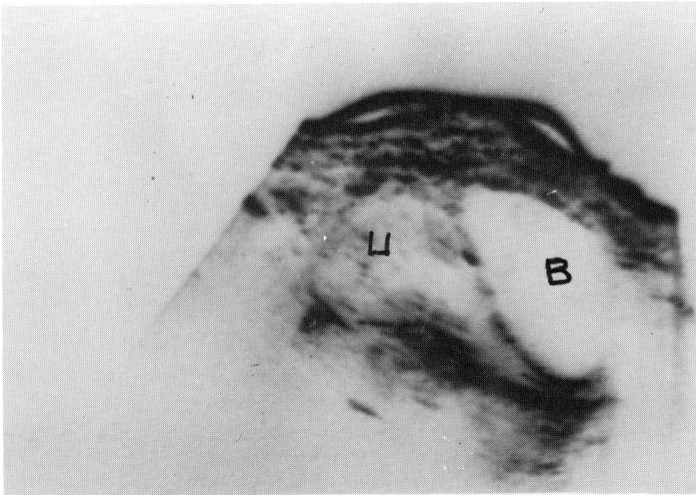

Figure 2. Longitudinal scan demonstrating funneling of
the internal os.

The measurement of the internal os was done in 34
cases of repeated abortions. The evaluation of the other
48 cases was done by descriptive terms, tight, dilated or
funneling of the internal os. (Fig. 3). The internal os
antero posterior diameter was measured in 20 normal pregnant women in the first and second trimester and the
results were compared.

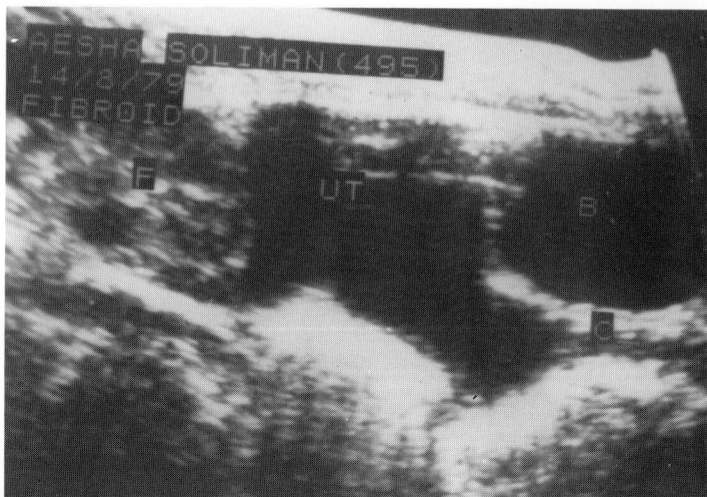

Figure 3. Longitudinal scan demonstrating a major degree of cervical imcompetence associated with submucous fibroid.

RESULTS

Ultrasound examination of 92 cases revealed that 4 patients were not pregnant and 4 patients had missed abortion and these 8 cases were excluded from the study. In the remaining 84 cases the cervix was not diluted in 9 cases. These 9 cases were treated medically. In the remaining 75 cases the os was dilated and they all had cerclage done, transvaginally in 65 cases and transabdominally in 10 cases. In the one case who underwent vaginal cerclage there was twin pregnancy.

The followup of the nine women who were treated medically revealed two cases of missed abortion who were evacuated. In two cases the internal os dilated progressively and both underwent vaginal cerclage.

The measurements of the anteroposterior diameter of the internal os in 20 normal pregnant women are listed in Table 1. The mean diameter during the first trimester is 9.5 mm. The mean diameter during the second trimester is 11.8 mm. The measurements of the internal os in 34 cases of repeated abortions are listed in Table 2. The mean diameter in the first trimester is 15.3 mm and in the second trimester 19.4 mm. (Table 3.) A statistically significant difference ($P < .01$) exist between the diameter of the internal os in normal pregnant women and in repeated aborters. (Fig. 4 and Fig. 5.)

508

TABLE 1. Measurement of internal os in 20 cases of normal pregnancy.

PREGNANCY DURATION	INTERNAL OS MM.	MEAN MM.
1ST TRIMESTER	16, 9, 6, 8, 9	
	10, 6, 10, 12, 11	9.5
2ND TRIMESTER	11, 13, 10, 9, 11	
	16, 14, 14, 9, 11	11.8

TABLE 2. Measurements of internal os in 34 cases of repeated abortions.

PREGNANCY WEEKS	INTERNAL OS MM.	MEAN MM.
→ 8	16, 14, 13	14.3
9, 10	19, 14, 18, 16, 5	
	21, 14, 20, 10, 9	15.6
11, 12	11, 9, 25, 20	16.4
13, 14	15, 29, 28, 10, 11, 32	20.8
15, 16	15, 23, 9, 33, 15, 19	19.0
17, 18	19, 20	19.5
19, 20	15, 30, 11	18.6

TABLE 3. A comparison between the mean internal os measurement in 20 normal pregnant women and in 34 women with history of repeated abortions.

	NORMAL PREGNANCY	REPEATED ABORTION
1ST TRIMESTER	9.5 MM	15.3 MM
2ND TRIMESTER	11.8 MM	19.4 MM

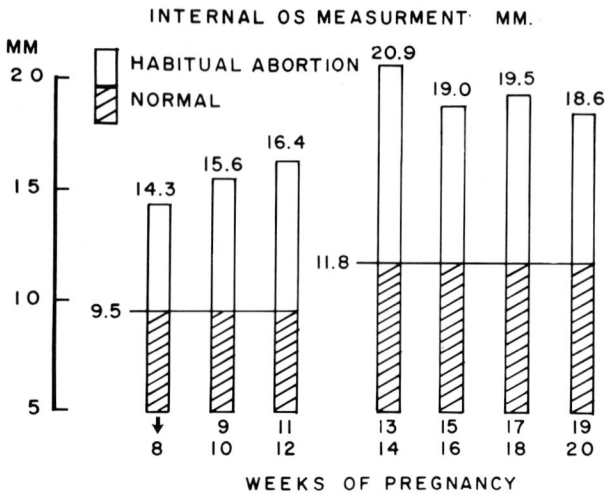

Figure 4. Internal os measurements in cases of repeated abortions compared to the mean diameter in normal pregnancy.

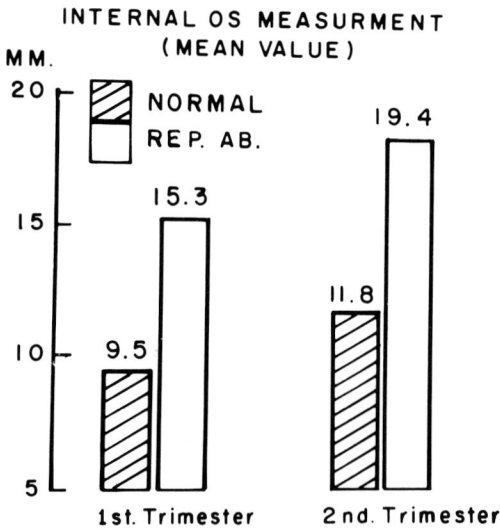

Figure 5. Internal os measurement (mean value) in cases of incompetent cervix compared with normal pregnancy.

DISCUSSION (Indication of Ultrasound)

I. Diagnosis

Ultrasound is the only method for investigation and confirmation of the diagnosis of the patulous internal os during pregnancy. It is easy to diagnose a dilated or a patulous internal os the same as the condition is diagnosed

510

by hyterosalpingography in the non-pregnant state with the exception that in ultrasound we are scanning and measuring the anteroposterior diameter of the cervical canal while in the latter the transverse diameter is visualized. There are many degrees of weakness, and measurement of the region of the internal os is important. Until a normal background is established for different durations of pregnancy and for different parities, measurements could only be used for comparative reasons in the follow up of the same patient. It is important in the process of ultrasound scan that other contributing factors to the process of abortion be looked for such as associated uterine anomalies or uterine fibroids, (Fig. 3).

Our results indicate a significant difference in the diameter of the internal os between normal cases and cases of repeated abortions diagnosed clinically as patulous internal os. A measurement of 15 mm or more during first trimester or 20 mm or more during second trimester should be considered as a diagnostic parameter of incompetent cervix and should be taken with other criteria as an indication for cerclage. In a recent study the diagnosis of patulous internal os is documented when a pear shaped distortion of the isthmus is seen on a median longitudinal scan and when the anteroposterior diameter is above or equal to 20 mm, (Irondelle et al. 1978).

II. Planning of treatment

There is no doubt that the availability of ultrasound examination is of great help especially in borderline cases. Taken into consideration with the clinical history a decision is taken whether to operate or to start a conservative treatment with sonographic follow up.

III. Preoperative evaluation

The role of ultrasound is very important in cases where the operation of cerclage is decided upon especially for the following points:
1.To confirm the diagnosis of pregnancy.
Ultrasound examination confirms the pregnant state. Pregnancy tests have false positive results. Clinical examination is risky and might cause abortion. It is well known that cases were operated upon who were discovered to be non-pregnant later on. Once the diagnosis is confirmed the operation could be done if it is indicated. In our series 4 patients turned to be non-pregnant.
2.To establish the diagnosis of fetal life.
It is important before operating to establish fetal life. This cannot be done at such an early period of pregnancy without the help of ultrasound. Cases are known where cerclage was done on a uterus containing a dead fetus or a missed abortion. Real time scan establish the presence of fetal life and assess fetal well being. In

our series 4 cases proved to have missed abortion.

3.To exclude fetal abnormality or disease.

The common neural tube defects can be diagnosed at early months of pregnancy. These must be excluded especially if there is a history of abnormalities before operating. Another important condition is vesicular mole. Cases are known who where operated upon by vaginal cerclage for a uterus with molar pregnancy.

4.To exclude twin pregnancy.

Twin pregnancy does not contraindicate cervical cerclage. However its presence indicates the need for extra care and other lines of treatment beside the operative intervention. It might indicate the modified technique at double cerclage and necessitate a very careful follow up.

5.To exclude placenta praevia.

Early in the second trimester the placenta can be easily located and a placenta praevia of the serious type can be diagnosed. This has to be taken into consideration regarding whether to operate or not and when to operate. Our policy is that if we do not operate, we carry on the expectant treatment with ultrasound follow up. If placental migration is established we operate.

During the first trimester, the chorionic tissue is localized occasionally in the lower part of the uterus near the internal os. Although this might not identify the future placental site yet we tend to postpone the operation under these circumstances and follow the patient up.

IV. Follow up

1.Follow up of expectant treatment

Expectant treatment is indicated in mild or borderline cases of patulous internal os. The essence of the treatment is rest: physical, mental and sexual. Tokolytic drugs and psychotherapy are important additions. In the past once expectant treatment was decided upon it was implemented to end whether success or failure. Now with ultrasound available the region of the internal os can be monitored every two weeks or even every week or whenever new symptoms arise such as lower abdominal pain or excessive vaginal discharge. Progressive dilation indicates impending abortion or premature labour and is an indication for operative intervention. In our series two cases out of six undergoing expectant treatment were operated according to these criteria and successfully continued pregnancy to full term.

2.Follow up after vaginal cerclage

Every patient who underwent vaginal cerclage should be followed up by ultrasound. The first postoperative scan and measurement will evaluate the operative success. Further scans will ensure the maintenance of operative success. If the internal os starts to dilate, there is an

512

indication to reoperate. Fetal well being is also continuously assessed during these examinations.

3.Follow up after transabdominal cerclage

Severe cases of patulous internal os are treated by
transabdominal cerclage, (Mahran, 1978). These cases are
monitored regularly after the operation. The aim is to
evaluate the success of the operation and to monitor the
fetus and its intrauterine growth. (Fig. 6). In all these
patients pregnancy is terminated by abdominal section at
term. If the patient becomes pregnant again the condition
of the internal os has to be evaluated by ultrasound. If
the internal os measurement is satisfactory the patient is
allowed to continue pregnancy with operative intervention.
If the os is dilated the operation has to be repeated.

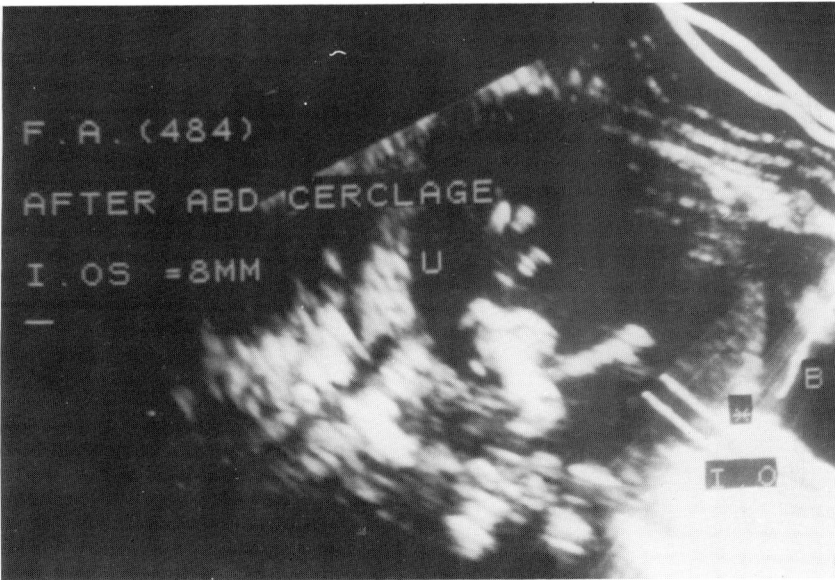

Figure 6. Measurement of the internal os after transabdominal cerclage (8 mm).

There is no doubt that ultrasound plays an important
role in the clinical management of the problem of repeated
abortions due to cervical incompetence.

ACKNOWLEDGEMENT

I would like to acknowledge the real help and enthusiasm of my assistants Dr. Said El Tohamy, Dr. Amira Saleh
and Dr. Aida Megahed in the preparation of this work.

REFERENCES

1.   Irondelle, D., Seneze, J. and Bourbigot, Y. (1978):
     Rev. Fr. Gynecol. Obstet. 73, 531
2.   Mahran, Maher. (1978) Obstet. Gynecol. 52, 502

APEX ORBITAE - A SPECIAL PROBLEM IN ULTRASOUND DIAGNOSIS

Bozidar Ilic and Ilija Nagulic

Eye University Hospital and Neurosurgical University
Hospital, Beograd, Yugoslavia

The diagnostic and surgical problems concerning the
deep portion of the orbit are still waiting to be solved.
In this particular anatomical area the bony walls are superimposed with soft tissues and all important structures
from the functional point of view are concentrated on the
region of the optic canal and superior orbital fissure. For
that reason the apex of the orbit has attracted steady attention among contigious specialities: ophthalmology, neurosurgery, otolaryngology and maxillofacial surgery.

The anatomical apex of the orbit is formed by the optic foramen, which is limited by two roots of lesser wing
and by the body of the sphenoid. This anatomical notion
was enlarged to include the superior orbital fissure and its
content, as a result of attempts to divide the orbital space
into different layers and zones. Benedict (1949) distinguished 3 layers and 3 zones of the orbital cavity. The subject of our consideration will be the third zone of Benedict.

The border between the second and apical Benedict's zone
is a virtual frontal plane crossing the entrance of the central retinal artery to the optic nerve, at about 10mm behind the eyeball.

According to Mennig (1970) this border is placed more
behind, to be 10mm in front of the optic canal. Apex of
the orbit is of special diagnostic and surgical interest for
Mennig. Nevertheless in this small region important diagnostic and surgical problems are encountered because:
1. It is a very small space--about 2 cm in diameter.
2. An almost closed place -- surrounded by orbital bones on
   all sides, except forward, where it is hidden by the
   eyeball.
3. Very dense and crowded area with nerves, vessels and
   muscles.
4. The surfaces of normal structures are oriented almost
   parallel to the sound beam, which results many times in
   a repeated total reflexion, interference of echoes and
   an increased noise level. These anatomical properties
   make it difficult to distinguish between the normal and
   pathological structures.
5. Relatively large acoustic shadow of strong reflecting
   normal structures, such as lens and sclera, observed

especially in B-mode ultrasonography.
6. In the neighbourhood of the intracranial cavity and the possibility of spreading pathological processes in both directions (meningiomas, astrocytomas, infections). Impossibility to detect by ultrasound the bone infiltrations and bone defects in this region.
7. Difficult to differentiate tissue because of necessity of applying the lower frequency of ultrasound.
8. Sometimes it is almost impossible to confirm our preliminary diagnosis by operative and histological findings because of the very difficult surgical approach to this region.

The list of problems we discussed here seems to not yet be exhausted.

To illustrate these problems, we present here some of our cases.

The first figure shows negative ultrasonography in a case of massive invasion of orbital apex with destruction of sphenoidal wings, involving the temporal muscles. Histologically it was a fibroma chondromixoides.

The ultrasonograms of the astrocytomas are typical and usually do not cause difficulties for an experienced examiner. The echograms and CT scans of 2 cases of astrocytomas are presented on Figures 2,3,4.

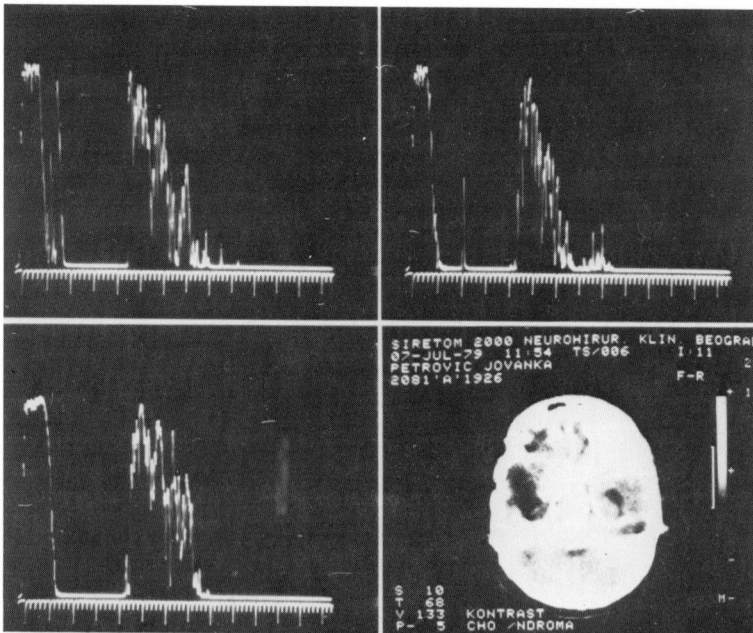

Fig. 1. Negative ultrasonography in case of massive invasion of the orbital apex with destruction of sphenoidal wings. Histological findings: Fibroma chondromixoides

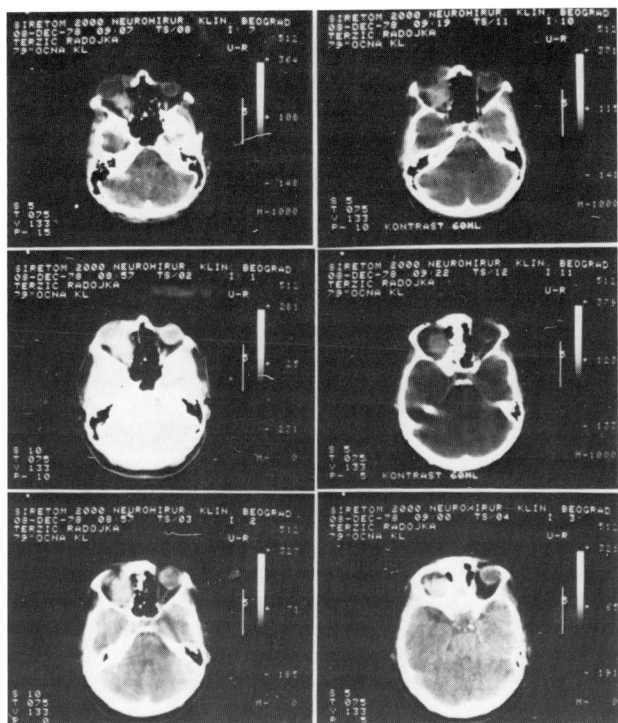

Fig. 2. CT scans of an astrocytoma of the apical region.

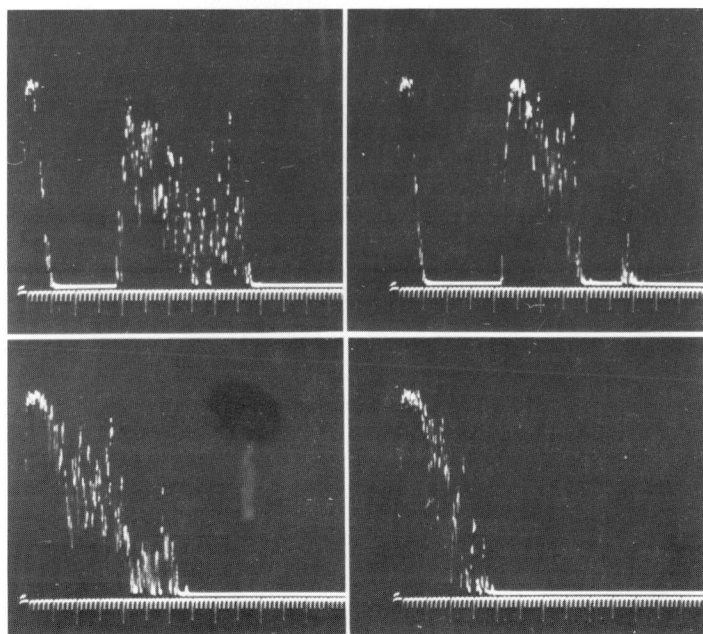

Fig. 3. Ultrasonograms of the case shown in Fig. 2. Typical finding with clearly seen septal echoes.

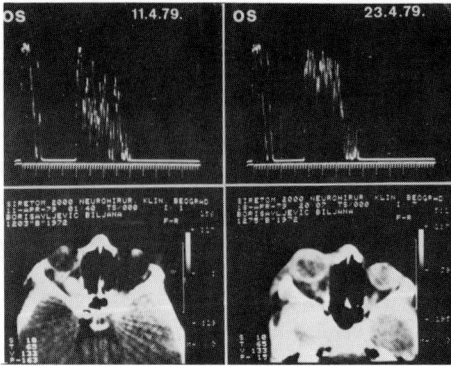

Fig. 4. Ultrasonograms and CT scans of an astroctyoma of the apical region before and after operation.

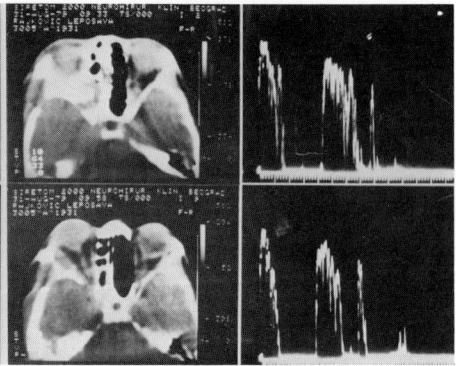

Fig. 5. A great tumoral invasion of orbit and the middle fossa with poor ultrasonic finding.

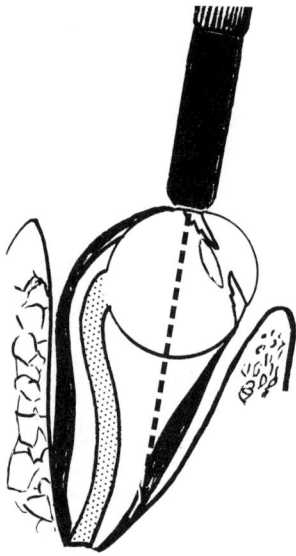

Fig. 6. In extreme abduction of eyeball, the retrobulbar space becomes more approachable to ultrasonic investigation.

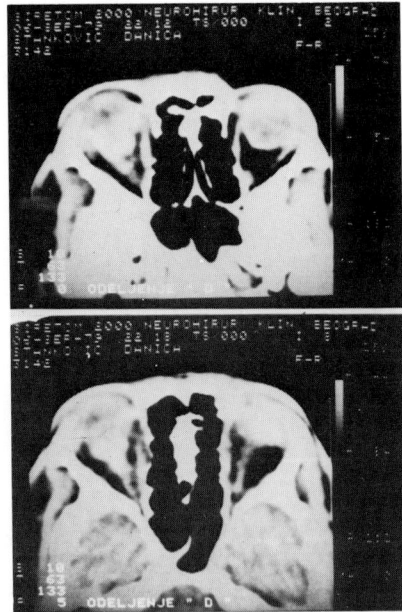

Fig. 7. CT scan of an intraconic tumor.

On Figure 5 we demonstrate a great tumor invasion of the orbit and the middle fossa with poor ultrasonic finding.

Applying the proble in the habitual position against the cornea in order to investigate the retrobulbar intraconic and apical space, we often are not able to detect a

small, even large, tumors of this region. We explain this
by the difficulties listed above. We have tried to investigate the whole retrobulbar space, especially the apex, using the transducer in vertical position, when the eyeball
is in extreme abduction. In that position of the eyeball
the optic nerve is dislocated close to the ethmoidal wall
and the lental atenuation is avoided. Even small tumors
become clearly visible in this position (Figs. 6,7,8).

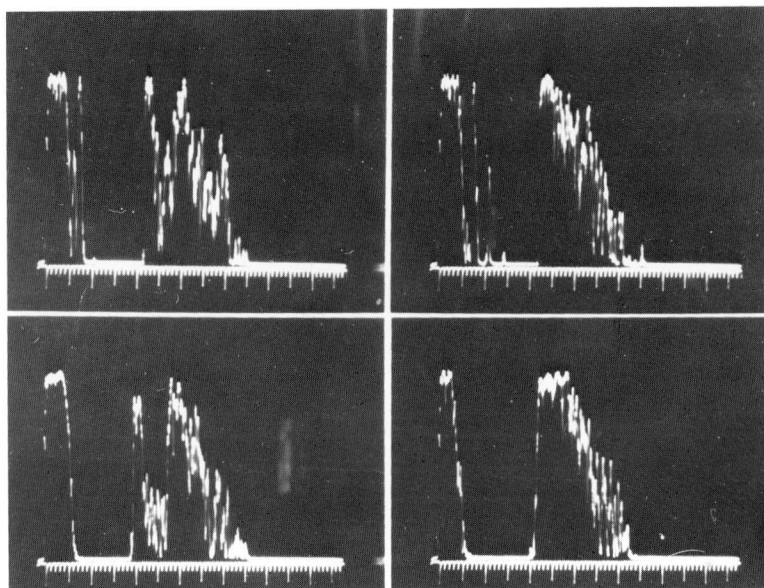

Fig. 8. Ultrasonograms of case in Fig. 7. Upper: Transcor-
neal echogram with lental echo and poor presentation of the
tumor. Lower: The same in abduction of the eyeball, with no
lental echo. Tumor becomes clearly visible and tissue differentiation possible. The echogram of normal opposite eye
is shown on right side.

CONCLUSIONS

The difficulties of ultrasonic diagnosis of the apical
region of the orbit are due to many particular reasons, such
as small size of well hidden space, dense crowded important
normal structures (nerves, vessels and muscles), acoustic
shadows, total reflexion and interference of echoes.

To avoid some of these difficulties we use vertical
position of the transducer in extreme abduction of the eyeball. Using this technique we are able to detect and differentiate even small tumors.

COMPARATIVE STUDY OF ULTRASONOGRAPHY AND COMPUTERIZED
TOMOGRAPHY IN DIAGNOSIS OF SPACE-OCCUPYING LESIONS OF
THE ORBIT

Ilija Nagulic, Bozidar Ilic, Petar Dimitrijevic

Neurosurgical University Hospital, Beograd Eye University
Hospital, Beograd, Yugoslavia

The diagnostic evidence of orbital lesions has greatly
improved with echography and computerized tomography. Computerized tomography has been until now one of the most important methods for identification of space-occupying lesions of the orbit. This method is non aggressive, rapid,
painless and certain. However, it can not substitute all
of the other investigative methods for orbital pathology.
Orbital diagnoses remain a serious problem requiring all
available equipment.

We shall try to analyze some diagnostic complications
we were faced with this last year during joint investigations
held at the Service for CT Scanning of the Neurosurgical University Hospital and at the Service for Ultrasonography of
the Eye University Hospital in Beograd. Our services possess a tomograph Siretom 2000 and a Kretz 7200 MA apparatus
for ultrasonography.

The results of this parallel investigation using two
methods on 29 patients are presented. Twenty-three patients
underwent surgery and the preoperative diagnosis obtained
by both methods was histologically controlled.

In the first group of 18 patients, findings obtained
with ultrasonography and computerized tomography were in
full agreement with the operative findings (Table 1). An
example from this group is demonstrated in Figure 1, showing a choroidal melanoma penetrating the orbit and the max-
illar sinus. Although infiltration of the sinus was not
found by standard cross-section tomography, it was proved
by conventional roentgenography of paranasal sinuses.

Another interesting case from this group is one with
polymorphism of cavernous haemangioma (Figure 2).

In two cases from the second group, the ultrasonic findings were precise and were confirmed by surgery. Computerized tomography gave false-positive results (Table 2 and
Figure 3).

The case of myositis is shown in Figure 3. This patient underwent surgery twice. The echography was always
negative. The biopsy of the muscle proved the diagnosis of
myositis.

In a case of fibroma chondromixoides the ultrasonography was false-negative, while CT presented a large tumoral
mass in the orbit and middle fossa.

The ultrasonography was also negative in a case of arteriovenous malformation, where the CT scans revealed the presence of a flebolyth (Figure 4). We were able to prove the presence of foreign bodies--clipses, during the control ultrasonography after surgery(Figure 5).

TABLE 1. FINDINGS OF ULTRASONOGRAPHY, CT AND SURGERY

Meningioma	4
Astrocytoma	4
Cavernous haemangioma	3
Malignant melanoma of choroid spreading into orbit	2
Lymphoblastoma metastaticum	1
Cyst	1
Mikulitz's disease	1
No histology	1
	18

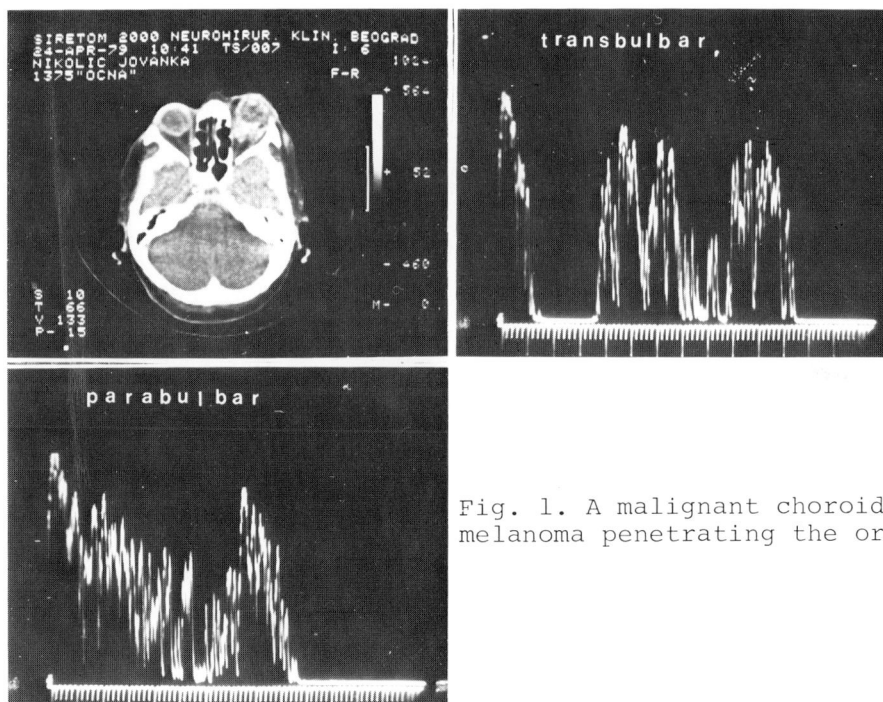

Fig. 1. A malignant choroidal melanoma penetrating the orbit.

The last group includes 7 cases, 6 of them did not have surgery. In one case the operative findings were negative (Table 3). The case of negative operative findings is presented in Figures 6,7,8.

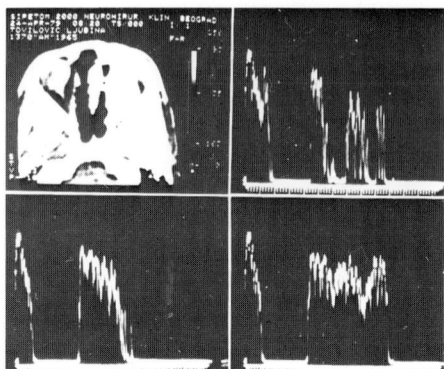

Fig. 2. A great cavernous haemangioma. Polymorphism of ultrasonic image;cystic form of one portion of tumoral mass is shown on echogram above.

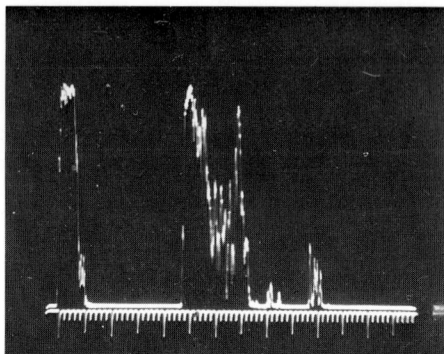

Fig.3. The echographic presentation of hypertrophic extraocular muscle.

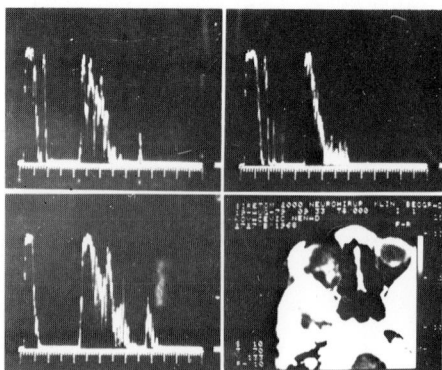

Fig. 4. An arteriovenous malformation with negative ultrasonic finding.

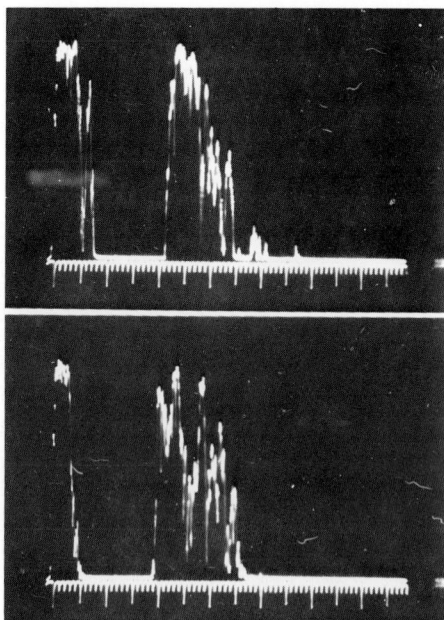

Fig. 5. The case from Fig. 4 postoperatively. The echoes of of clipses.

The case of congenital glaucoma-buphthalmus of the right is extremely interesting (Figure 9). A real diagnostic dilemma has developed. Is it a classic case of pseudo-proptosis caused by the different sized eyeballs, or a pseudo-pseudoproptosis with a tumor of the optic nerve behind the hydrophthalmic eyeball? The child has not yet been operated on. From April to September 1979, there were no changes in the clinical findings. Our decision has been to wait and watch.

TABLE 2. CT, ECHOGRAPHIC AND SURGICAL FINDINGS

	CT - Incorrect
	Echography - Corresponding operative findings
1	- Myositis
2	- Scleritis pseudotumorosa

TABLE 3 ECHOGRAPHIC AND CT AGREEMENT

No surgery		6
Negative operative findings		1
No surgery:		
Meningioma	1	
Congenital glaucoma	1	
Myositis	1	
Osteoma	1	
Grave's disease	1	
Without final diagnosis	1	
Total	6	

In a great majority of our cases the two methods described were sufficient to make a correct diagnosis of orbital lesions. This means to detect, localize and to determine the nature of the tumor.

In the group of 29 patients analyzed, a correct pre-operative diagnosis was made by both methods in 25 of the cases. In 4 cases the localization of the lesion was established by one of the two methods.

If ultrasonography and computerized tomography do not reveal the lesion in the presence of positive clinical signs of orbital disease, two positions can be taken.
1. to wait and repeat the investigations after 1 month or later, or
2. to use all other diagnostic methods trying to find the cause of proptosis.

The decision depends on the attitude of the clinician and on his experience. Orbital lesions have to be investigated by a highly specialized team of experts.

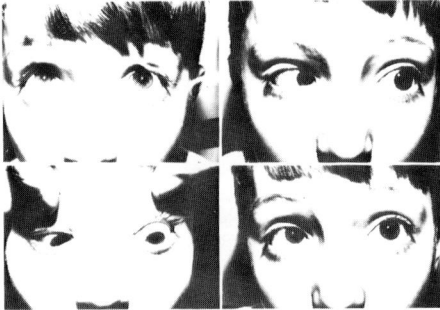

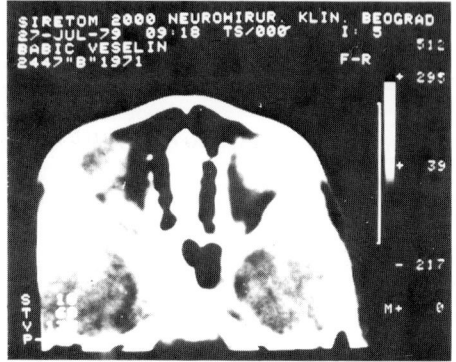

Fig. 6. Positive clinical finding-discrete proptosis of left eye with paralysis of VI nerve.

Fig.7. CT scan of child from Fig.6 shows a well limited mass in the apical region of the left orbit.

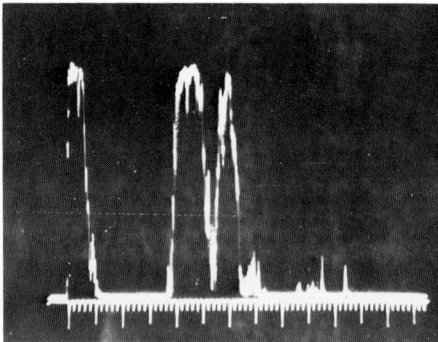

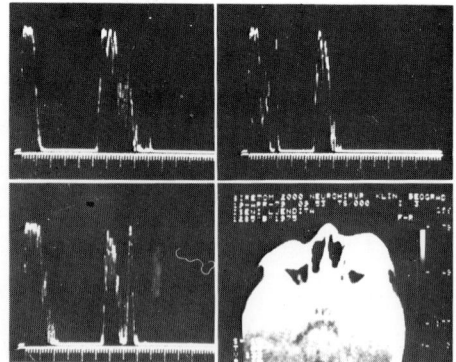

Fig. 8.Ultrasonogram of case shown of Fig. 6 and 7 is also positive. Operative finding was negative.

Fig. 9. Case of congenital glaucoma-hydrophthalmus. An enlarged optic nerve on the echogram?

MINIATURIZED ULTRASONIC REAL-TIME SCANNER AS CLINICAL AID IN ACUTE GYNECOLOGICAL SITUATION

K. Maršál and P.-H. Persson

Department of Obstetrics and Gynecology, University of Lund, Malmö, Sweden.

Diagnostic ultrasound equipments have been improved and their operation has been considerably simplified in recent years. In obstetrics and gynecology, the ultrasonic real-time method has offered new possibilities to monitor the intrauterine condition of the fetus and to visualize the organs within the female pelvis. In 1978, a miniaturized hand-held linear array equipment was presented (1). The small size of the equipment might slightly impair the image presentation, but in return it offers obvious advantages. It was therefore considered worthwhile to evaluate the equipment in clinical practice. We used the hand-held scanner as a bedside tool in a specific and relatively common situation at the gynecological emergency wards.

MATERIAL AND METHODS

For two weeks, all women attending the Department of Gynecology at the University Hospital of Malmö for vaginal bleeding after an amenorrheal period of six or more weeks were examined by the miniaturized hand-held ultrasound scanner*. The results of the ultrasonic examination were not available to the clinician at the gynecological examination and thus did not influence the management. The women were also examined by a conventional ultrasound compound B-scanner by an experienced operator. The full-bladder technique was always used. The presence of a gestational sac in utero and/or fetal heart activity was especially sought.

RESULTS

The study group consisted of 20 women aged 18-41 years (Table I). The duration of amenorrhea was 6-16 weeks, mean 9.4 weeks. Eleven women appeared to have an intrauterine pregnancy, gestational age 7-16 weeks. In all of them, the hand-held scanner identified the intrauterine amniotic sac (Table II). Eight of the 11 pregnancies demonstrated fetal heart activity; in one woman as early as in the 8th week. In three women (two in the 7th and one in

---

*Minivisor[R], Organon Teknika, Oss, The Netherlands

the 8th gestational week), fetal heart activity was not seen. Conventional B-scan examination failed to identify fetal heart activity in one of the 7-week pregnancies but succeeded in all other instances. The subsequent course was favorable in all pregnancies except one, which ended in spontaneous abortion nine weeks after the examination (41 years old multiparous woman with multiple intrauterine myomas). Two women with 9 and 10 weeks' amenorrhea and no demonstrable amniotic sac or fetal heart activity were found to have had spontaneous abortion proved at curettage and at subsequent histological examination. Three women, amenorrheal for 7, 8, and 10 weeks, had ectopic pregnancy proved at laparotomy. In two of them, no gestational sac was found by ultrasound; in one, a gestational sac was seen but no fetal heart activity. The repeated examination 2 days later failed to reproduce the finding, and a negative result was verified by conventional B-scan examination. In none of these women could adnexal masses be seen by the hand-held scanner or by the compound scanner. In four women with amenorrhea of 6-13 weeks, no pregnancy could be proved clinically or biochemically. All had a normal sized uterus, as shown both by the hand-held scanner and by the conventional B-scanner.

DISCUSSION

The clinical usefulness of the miniaturized real-time scanner in the diagnosis of threatening abortion was greater than expected. The gestational sac was positively identified in all pregnancies with normal subsequent course; fetal heart activity could be detected as early as in the 8th week and in all cases from the 10th week. This result is comparable with other studies performed by conventional scanners (2). In this context, it is important that we did not get false negative results, which could wrongly influence the clinical management. The investigation confirmed the known difficulties of diagnosing ectopic pregnancy by ultrasound.

The small size and the comparatively low cost of the hand-held scanner recommend it as a good complement to clinical examination in the gynecological emergency ward. Furthermore, the hand-held scanner can obviously be useful in the delivery ward for estimates of the fetal position, fetal viability, and placental site. The measuring capacity of the equipment is insufficient for precise fetometry.

Careful use of the device with appreciation of its limitations makes it a helpful bedside facility. Experience of full-size ultrasound imaging seems to be a prerequisite for the proper use of the miniaturized real-time scanner.

526

REFERENCES

1. Ligtvoet, C., Rijsterborgh, H., Kappen, L. and Bom, N. (1978): Ultrasound in Med. & Biol., 4, 91.
2. Jouppila, P. (1976): Acta Obstet. Gynecol. Scand., 55, 131.

TABLE I. Clinical findings in 20 women with amenorrhea

Clinical diagnosis	Duration of amenorrhea		Total	HCG test positive
	6-10 wks	11-16 wks		
Intrauterine viable pregnancy	7	4	11	11
Incomplete abortion	0	2	2	2
Ectopic pregnancy	2	1	3	1
Non-pregnant	2	2	4	1*
Total	11	9	20	15

*False positive finding

TABLE II. Ultrasonic findings in 20 women with amenorrhea

Clinical diagnosis	Presence of gest. sac			Fetal heart action		
	Amenorrhea			Amenorrhea		
	≤10 wks	>10 wks	Total	≤10 wks	>10 wks	Total
Intrauterine viable pregnancy	7	4	11	4	4	8
Incomplete abortion	0	0	0	0	0	0
Ectopic pregnancy	1*	0	1	0	0	0
Non-pregnant	1*	0	1	0	0	0
Total	9	4	13	4	4	8

*False positive finding

BLIGHTED OVUM (HYDROVUM) - ULTRASONIC, CLINICAL AND CYTOGENETICAL ASPECT

Bulić M., Singer Z.

From the Department of Gynecology and Obstetrics,
Clinical Hospital "Dr O. Novosel" Zagreb, Yugoslavia

Cases of disturbed or failed early pregnancy have clinically been classified into diagnostic categories such as abortus imminens, incipiens, in tractu, incomplete or missed abortion. These are, however, only descriptive stages of a process which may result in either complete abortion or further pregnancy development.

Inmmost cases such dilemmas are resolved by ultrasonic examination (U.S.). It enables us to develop new categories (7) based on findings of the gestation sac, the embryo and its movements. One of these categories is Blighted ovum (B.O.).

The cause of spontaneous abortion may be a genetic disease, at the chromosomal or genic level, or enviromental factors. Investigation of couples with repeated abortions has shown that one of the partners is the carrier of balanced chromosomal translocations, the incidence being cca 5% (5). Cytogenetic investigation of aborted tissues would yield more reliable results in this respect (4).

We have cytogenetically investigated samples of aborted tissues previusly determined by U.S. as B.O. The purpose of the investigation was to determine wheder more significant chromosomal aberations are present and, if so, which of them are responsible for B.O. Should genetic disease be found to predominate in such cases, couples affected by conceptus maldevelopment are at high risk for repetition in subsequent pregnancies.

MATERIAL AND METHODS

Out of more than 6000 U.S. examinatins (1976-1979), 94 typical B.O. typical B.O. findings have been established (incidence 1:63.8). Pregnancy was terminated in the ward and macro- and microscopic confirmation of ultrasonic findings was possible in 78 cases (82.97%). Cytogenetic investigation was performed in 21 cases (22.33%). The diagnosis is based on criteria established by Donald et al.(3) on the gestation sac finding without an embryonic echo (Fig.1), with growth retardation of the gestation sac, expressed as the area of gestation sac, even a reduced rate between two measurements (2).

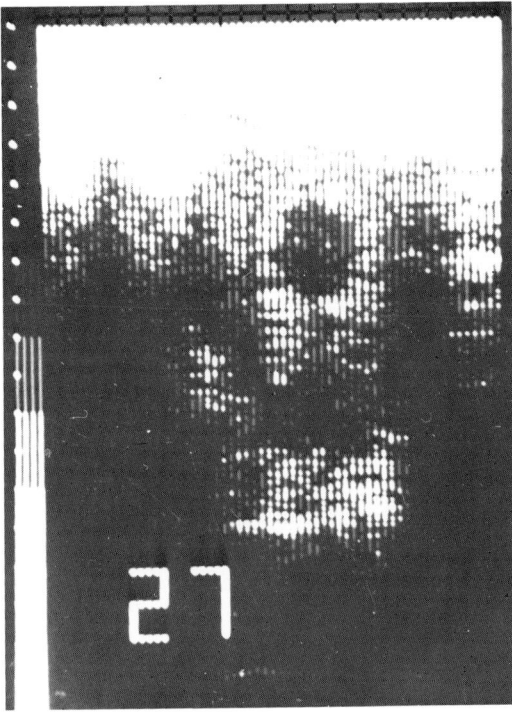

Fig. 1

Fourteen-week pregnancy. Well-outlined gestation sac, (area 5.7 cmm^2, mean diameter 2.7 cm, corresponding eight weeks of pregnancy), without fetal echo, Transversal section; Real-time technique.

Material for cytogenetic investigation was sampled immediately after evacuation, in sterile conditiones, and transported to the cyto- genetic laboratory right away. Small parts of tissue (2 sq.mm) were prepared, by mechanical maceration, for the X and Y test, and for cultivation by the Cover Slip technique. The nutrient was the Minimum Essential Medium /MEM/ according to Eagle, and 25% of Fetal Calf Serum /FCS/. Chromosomes were identified by the Quinacrine fluore- scent technique and the tripsin Giemsa banding (G) mathod (6,1,8).

RESULTS

Clinical results are based on a retrospective study of data rela-- ted to the 94 B.O. cases determined by ultrasonic examination.

Table 1
Age of pregnant women with B.O. finding

Y	e	a	r	s			
Less than or	20	21–25	26–30	31–35	36–40	More than 40	Total
	11	23	21	23	11	4	94

The age of 38 women (40.42%) was more than 30 years, which is significantly higher than the figure for our general population.

Table 2.
Fertility

No pregnancy	32	51 (54.26%)
No delivery	19	
One or more deliveries		43 (45.75%)
One or more spontaneous abortions		51 (54.26%)

The incidence of spontaneous abortions is significant.

Table 3
Gestation age of B.O. at the first examination

w	e	e	k	s		
Less than 10	10–11	12–14	15–17	17–20	More than 20	Total
	4	24	37	15	9	5	94

Most of the cases were in the second trimester of pregnancy. The size of conceptus was small, by ultrasonic criteria, the difference between gestation age and the ultrasonic measurement being 3–10 weeks.

The clinical course was asimptomatic in 24.47% of cases; 63.80% of cases had less pronounced, shorter or longer-term bleeding. Gestagen therapy was applied in 31% of cases.

Macroscopically detritic embryos were found in 2 out of 78 cases. Microscopic findings most often involve hydropic villi and abnormal vascularisation (57 cases or 73.00%). In these 57 cases trophoblast swelling was found in 11 cases, and a microscopically determined hydatic mole in 2 cases.

The results of cytogenetic investigation, which were of the highest interest, are presented in Table 4.

Table 4
Results of cytogenetic investigation

Karyotype	N	X test	Y test	Remarks
46,XX	4	+	–	Two cases of Herpes V.vag.
46,XY	4	–	+	M.Hunter, one case
47,XXY	1	+	+	Klinefelter sy.
47,XXX	1	++	–	Triple X
45,X	3	–	–	Turner sy.
47,XXE18+	1	+	–	Edwards sy. female
47,XYE18+	1	–	+	" male
69,XXY	1	+	+	Triploidy
69,XYY	1	–	++	"
		–	+	Now growing in vitro
∅	4	–	+	(Two cases of neg.immuno-
		+	–	biological pregnancy test)
		–	+	

In 4 cases cultivation failed (two of these had negative immuno-biological pregnancy test). The X and Y test could be determined in all cases, and the karyotype in the remaing 17 cases (8o.95%)(Fig.2). Normal male or female karyotypes were found in eight cases. One of them related to a couple with X linked mucopolysaccharidosis (M.Hunter) in male offspring, and we concluded that genopathy was the cause of B.O.

Two cases were interesting becouse the finding indicated Herpes virus vaginitis; we bel ieve that the viral environmental factor may be the reason for the teratogenic effect.

Gonosomal numerical aberrations were found in 5 of 17 investigated cases. Autosomal numerical aberrations were found in 2, and polyploidy (triploidy) also in 2 cases.

The potential cause inderlying disturbed development (B.O.) could be established in 12 aut of 17 cases (70.59%) out of which 9 (52.90%) karyotypic abnormalities.

CONCLUSIONS

1. Typical ultrasonic B.O. findings make their corelation with clinical, pathohistological and cytogenetic findings possible.
2. We are suggesting a new name for this entity, i.e., Hydrovum, becouse it describes the fluid content of gestation sac and hydropic changes in the chorionic villi. We would consider it useful for

international use, particulary in countries using Latine terminology in medical diagnosis, by analogy with terms such as Hydrocephalus, Hydramnion etc.

3. Couples with detected and confirmed Hydrovum pregnancy belong to the high risk group in relation to the repetition of the genetic diseases in subsequent pregnancy. Accordingly, we suggest genetic counselling and an early detection of the genetic disease by early amniocentesis.

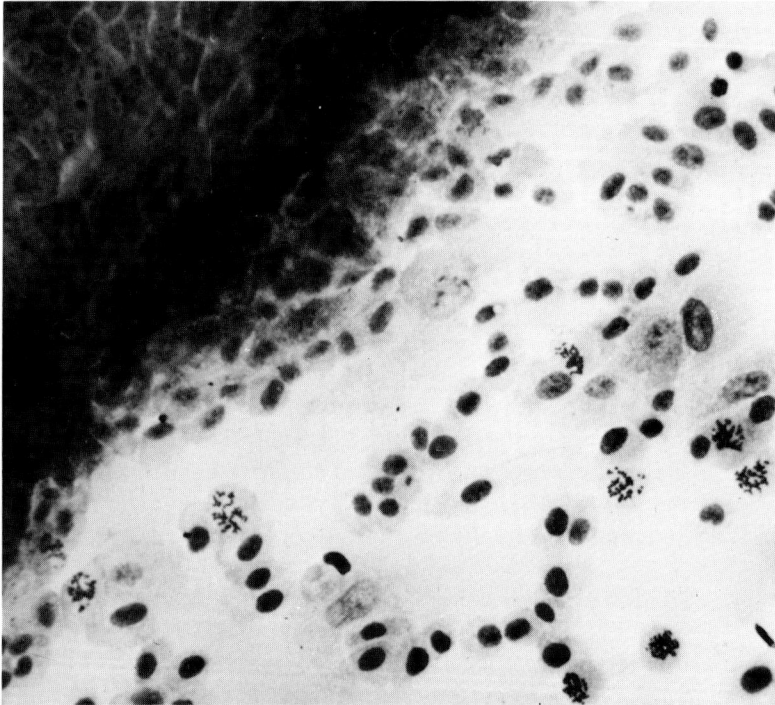

Fig. 2
Growing tissue from the gestation sac explant after 14 days in culture. Cover slip technique. The margin of the explant is seen in the top left-hand corner (darker area) and dividing cells with many metaphases.

REFERENCES

1. Beck,M., Singer,Z., Uroić,M.(1974): Works of Immunological Institute Zagreb, 17,37.

2. Bulić,M., Vrtar,M. (1976): In White a. Brown: Ultrasound in Medicine, Vol. 3A, Plenum Press, New York a. London, p. 6o3.

3. Donald,I., Morley,P., Barnett,E.(1972): Journal of Obstetrics and Gynaecoly of the British Commonwealth, 79, 3044.

4. Hamerton,J.L. (1971): Human cytogenetic, Vol.II, Academia Press, New York a. London, p. 379.

5. Heritage,D.W., English, S.C., Young, R.B., Chen, A.T.L.(1978): Fertility and Sterility, 29, 414.

6. Paul, J.(1972): Cell and tissue culture. 14th edition, Churchil Livingstone, Edinbourg a. London, p. 172.

7. Robinson,H.P. (1975): British Journal of Obstetrics and Gynaecology, 82, 849,

8. Schmid,W.(1976): Acta Paediatrica Scandinavica, Suppl. 259, 57.

FETAL BREATHING MOVEMENTS IN LABOUR UNDER EPIDURAL ANALGESIA

Marko Križ and Višnja Latin

Department of Obstetrics and Gynecology, University of
Zagreb, Zagreb, Yugoslavia

Although reports about fetal breathing movements(FBM)
and whole body movements (WBM) in pregnancy are well documented (1,2), there are just a few reports on this phenomenon during labour. Studies about FBM and WBM under obstetric analgesia are even less common. The purpose of the
present study was to examine the influence of continuous
epidural analgesia with low Xylocaine (Lignocaine)doses on
FBM and WBM in well established labour.

MATERIALS AND METHODS

The material consisted of ten healthy parturients in
well established labour with regular and painful contractions and a cervix opened 3-4 cm. The purpose of the investigation was explained to the patients and an informal
consent was obtained. Their age, parity and gestational
age are shown in Table 1.
Nine of them had singleton pregnancies and one had triplets. Thirty minutes before application of the epidural
block the incidence of FBM and WBM was investigated by ADR
real-time machine. The investigation was undertaken at the
15 degrees left lateral position which was achieved by a
supporting pillow placed under the right hip. After that
the epidural catheter was inserted and the test dose of 100
mg of 2% Xylocaine was injected. The technique of FBM
observations, as well as the method of epidural block in
labour, has been previously described by the authors (4,5).
After waiting for ten minutes for the epidural block
to take, which was confirmed by the pin-prick test and
questioning the parturient, we waited another ten minutes
because it has been previously demonstrated(6), that the
fetal concentration of the local anesthetic reaches its
peak 10-30 minutes after epidural administration. The real-
time assessment of fetal activity was then repeated for another thirty minutes. During the investigation period, as
well as during labour, the infusion of Ringer solution was
running into one of the forearm veins of the examinees. Glucose was neither given i.v. nor was it ingested.

RESULTS

All labours were uneventful. The analgesia was good or

excellent in all cases. There was no hypertension or any
other side effects. The incidence of WBM and FBM before
and after analgesia as well as the birth weight and Apgar
scores are shown in Table 2.

TABLE 1. AGE, PARITY AND GESTATIONAL AGE OF EXAMINES

	AGE (years)	PARITY	GESTATIONAL AGE (weeks)
MEAN	27.7	1.6	39.1
RANGE	21-33	1-3	33.3-40.4

TABLE 2. THE INCIDENCE OF FETAL MOVEMENTS BEFORE AND AFTER
EPIDURAL ANALGESIA, BIRTH WEIGHTS AND APGAR SCORES

	WBM		FBM		Birth weight	Apgar	
	Before	After	Before	After		1	5
1.	0	3x	0	0	3980	6	8
2.	0	0	0	0	3910	6	9
3.	0	0	0	0	3620	10	10
4.	0	0	0	0	3710	9	10
5.	1x	0	0	0	3000	10	10
6.	3x	0	0	0	1900	9	10
7.	3x	3x	0	0	3930	10	10
8.	3x	1x	0	0	4160	10	10
9.	0	0	0	0	3550	10	10
10.	0	0	0	0	1690	8	9
	0	0	0	0	1970	8	9
	0	0	0	0	1870	6	6

DISCUSSION AND CONCLUSION

The method of obstetric analgesia should never in any
case impair fetal well being. It has been shown earlier
that epidural analgesia has no adverse effects on the placental blood flow (7). It has been also demonstrated that
maternal smoking (8) or the administration of drugs such as
pethidine or pentobarbitone(9) could have some influence on
FBM. Although the incidence of FBM and WBM is reduced in
labour, in comparision to the antenatal period, it could be
potentially used as a useful indicator of fetal well being
in normal and high risk labour. Our first results show that
from this aspect the use of Xylocaine for the epidural
block in labour is a safe and good obstetric analgetic method.

REFERENCES

1. Marsal, K. (1977): Ultrasonic assessments of fetal breathing movements in man. Thesis, Malmo, pp. 1-49.
2. Gennser, G. (1978): In: Recent advances in ultrasound diagnosis. (ed. A. Kurjak). Excerpta Medica, Amsterdam-Oxford, pp. 187-188.
3. Wittmann, B.K., Davison, B.M., Lyons, E., Frolich, J. and Toweel, M.E. (1979): Brit. J. Obstet. Gynecol. 86, 278.
4. Kurjak, A., Latin, Visnja and Czajkowski, Z. (1978): In: Fifth Conference on Fetal breathing. pp. 95-105, Nijmegen.
5. Kriz, M. and Kurjak, A. (1977): Jugoslav. ginek. opstet. 17, 381.
6. Belfrage, P., Raabe, N., Thalme, B. and Berlin, A. (1975): Am. J. Obstet. Gynecol., 121, 360.
7. Jouppila, R., Jouppila, P., Hollmen, A. and Kuikka, J. (1978): Br. J. Anaesth., 50, 563.
8. Gennser, G., Marsal, K. and Brantmark, B. (1975): Am. J. Obstet., Gynecol., 123, 861.
9. Boddy, K., Dawes, G.S., Fisher, R.L., Pinter, S. and Robinson, J.S., (1976): Br. J. Pharmac., 57, 311.

FUNCTIONAL EVALUATION OF FETAL MOVEMENTS BY REAL-TIME

A. Ianniruberto and E. Tajani

Department of Obstetrics and Gynecology, City Hospital
'M. Sarcone', 70038 Terlizzi (Bari), Italy.

Quantitative evaluation of fetal movements is nowadays accepted as a reliable index of fetal vitality and general well-being (4,7,8,9,10), but when the purpose is to investigate specific neuromotor competence and development of motricity, the qualitative analysis (or motoscopic examination), made possible by real-time ultrasound scanning, is required.

MATERIAL AND METHODS

We have studied 1500 pregnancies between the 7th and the 42nd week by using a real-time gray scale ultrasound apparatus and a linear array multicrystal transducer of 2.5 MHz (Aloka Echo Camer SSD-202) .

Fetal movements have been studied during a period of 5-20 minutes and the examinations have been performed at morning after breakfast and before administering medications.

Gestational age was determined by knowing the last menstrual period or by performing measurements of the CRL or the BPD.

Of the 1500 pregnancies, 820 have been followed at weekly intervals, in order to detect the development of new motor features. The fetal motor behaviour patterns have been classified according to the gestational age, in which they have started to be recognized. Some movements eventually disappeared and others continued to be present up to the term of pregnancy.

The material has been analyzed according the same criteria used in neurological examination of the newborns, with the collaboration of a team of neuropediatricians guided by Prof. A. Milani Comparetti.

RESULTS

The numerous significant patterns of motor behaviour observed have been ordered according to the week of pregnancy when they start to be recognized and to the period of their persistence, as following (the numbers refer repectively to the gestational week of beginning and ending

+ Aloka Comp. Ltd., Tokyo, Japan

of each motor pattern):
(1) Rapid, vermicular and weak movements involving all
body of the embryo: 7-10; (2) rapid movements with extension and flexion of all body: 9-20; (3) extension movements
of the head, trunk, lower limbs with various postures or
downwards extension of the upper limbs: 10-20; (4) extension movements of the head, trunk and lower limbs: 11-40;
(5) the fetus pushes its feet against the uterine wall,
extending the lower limbs and trunk and pushes with its
head against the opposite wall: 14-40; (6) changes in lying posture: jumping, creeping, climbing: 11-40; (7) rotation of the head: 12-40; (8) isolated and/or independent
movements of the limbs and head: 11-40; (9) hands are
brought into contact with the head, face and mouth: 12-40;
(10) total response to mechanical stimuli: 12-25; (11) motory response only in directly concerned parts: 20-40:
(12) mouth opening with tounge protrusion: 14-40; (13) extension and crossing of the lower limbs: 14-26; (14) sucking, swallowing, breathing: 14-40; (15) sudden and vigor-
ous movements of the diaphragm: hiccups: 24-40; (16) body
and breathing movements more frequent after maternal meals:
26-40; (17) the hands clasp together, they grasp the umbilical cord and move it: 22-40; (18) motory response to
sound stimuli: 28-40.

DISCUSSION

The study of the fetal movements by using a real-time
ultrasound apparatus seems to be a useful parameter for the
evaluation of fetal well-being. Reinold, for the first
time, has noted that in cases of fetal compromission the
spontaneous fetal movements are absent, infrequent or
sluggish. The quantitive analysis has been attempted also
by other authors, either by ultrasonography or by clinical
evaluation (2, 7, 8, 9, 10, 11). It has been reported a
definite correlation between the number and amplitude of
the fetal movements and the fetal conditions.
Our contribution to the study of the fetal movements
has been a pattern analysis of the motoscopic findings
recorded at different stages of pregnancy. The challenge
is not to list more and more items for the performance
expected at each weekly developmental step, but instead to
detect the functional appointments.
Our method is based on the principle that a recognizable motor pattern is a modulating function available in
the process of motor programming and of motor development.
The stock of patterns available contains the primary authomatisms belonging to the genetic endowment characteristic
of the species and the secondary authomatisms acquired by
learning.
Patterns seen in the fetus are primary authomatisms
appearing in a fixed sequence and interacting among each
other in a condition, like the intrauterine set, where the
influence of epigenetic factors on the developmental pro-

cess can be considered relatively scarce.

Some of these primary authomatisms can be easily recognized as related to functional competence of the fetus and appear in the neonate as the so called 'primative reflexes' which will disappear in the following weeks. Some are already emerging motor behaviours organizing permanent functions for extrauterine life.

Milani Comparetti had already put forward the hypothesis based on retrospective interpretation of neonatal motor behaviour that certain so called primitive reflexes were in fact remains of fetal functional competences.

Some belong to the fetal competence of being born such as the 'locomotion for presentation' (creeping, placing and 'walking' in the newborn) such as the 'propulsion needed for the fetal collaboration in labour ('supporting reflex' in the newborn), such as the startle pattern (Moro reflex used for the first inspiration).

Ecoscopic examination of fetal patterns has completely confirmed this hypothesis.

From among the numerous patterns observed only those have been selected which seemed functionally meaningful and of which we were able to define functional correlations. We have recognized the following fuctional patterns: (1) Sharp, sudden jerks with flexion and extension, which are symmetrical, involving the whole body, and result in jumps, which then allow the fetus to change its lying position (we have interpreted them as an antigravity function); (2) creeping and climbing (interpreted as locomotion); (3) propulsion, with the same pattern that is eventually used by the fetus to cooperate during delivery; (4) smooth, isolated movements of the head and of individual limbs; (5) rotation of the head, sucking, swallowing, breathing; (6) early 'startle' responses, responses to mechanical and auditory stimuli.

We have noted that in the event of acute anoxia the fetus shows a phase of hyperkinesia then a phase of akinesia followed, if it survives, by the recovery of motricity but sometimes with patterns of earlier stages of motor development. The regression of fetal motor behaviour, interpreted as signs of brain disorder, is also noted in cases of severe chronic fetal hypoxia or lesions of the CNS.

The suggestion is made that the regression observed during fetal life can be also recognizable in neurological conditions in later life. In fact, the abnormal patterns domineering in certain forms of cerebral palsy are identical to some of those seen in the early stages of normal fetal development.

In each regression syndrome the 'tyranny' of two fetal patterns can be recognized as overpowering all others and producing the typical poverty of movement (lack of freedom of movement); for this reason we have called the condition 'diarchy' (tyranny of two). Diarchies recognizable in cerebral palsy are two with the dominance of

two couples of patterns. The first regression syndrome
(I Diarchy) reproduces (a) the pattern of the earliest
antigravitary function in the fetus when by jerks in flexion and in extension it jumps up and floats down again
continuously until the lying down body surface has changed
(13th week of gestational age), and (b) the pattern of leg
scissoring and arm flexion.

The second regression syndrome (II Diarchy) reproduces (a) the pattern of extension with arms pushind downwards and (b) the aspecific startle pattern which can be
seen in the fetus from the 13th week of gestational age
and is a permanent feature throughout life used functionally as a Moro reflex at birth for the first inspiration.

The two regression syndromes seen in case of a brain
lesion constitute a clinical entity of their own.

In conclusion, our motoscopic findings in the fetus
allow: (1) To see that these match retrospective interpretation of findings in the newborn, thus confirming the
validity of the theoretical model; (2) to put forward
pattern analysis as an effective method for developmental
diagnosis and prognosis; (3) to demonstrate regression to
earlier patterns of motor behaviour when fetal suffering
has occurred; (4) to demonstrate that types of individual
fetal behaviour persist during the first weeks or months
of extrauterine life.

REFERENCES

1. Birnholz, J.C., Stephens, J.C. and Faria, M. (1978):
    Fetal Movement Patterns: a Possible Means of Defining
    Neurologic Developmental Milestones in Utero. Am J
    Roentgenol, 130, 537.
2. Henner, H., Haller, U., Wolf-Zimper, O. et al. (1975):
    Quanitification of Fetal Movements in Normal and Path-
    ological Pregnancies. Proc., Second European Congress
    Ultrasonic in Medicine, Munich, May 12-16, 1975, 316,
    E. Kazner Ed., Excerpta Medica, Amsterdam.
3. Humphrey, T., (1970): Funciton of the Nervous System
    during Prenatal Life; in Stave, U: Physiology of the
    Perinatal Period. Appleton Century Crofts, New York.
4. Ianniruberto, A., (1977): Human Fetal Movements in
    Normal and Pathologic Pregnancies; in Poor Intra-
    uterine Fetal Growth, B. Salvadori and A. Bacchi Eds.
    Edizioni Centro Minerva Medica, 257.
5. Ianniruberto, A., Iaccarino, M. and Tajani, E., (1978):
    Lo studio del feto con gli ultrasuoni a tempo reale;
    in Medicina Fetale, Simposio Internazionale, Gorizia
    8-10 giugno, Monduzzi Edizioni, Bologna, 117.
6. Milani Comparetti, A. and Gidoni, E.A., (1978): Inter-
    pretazione funzionale della motricità fetale; in
    Medizina Fetale, Simposio Internazionale, Gorizia 8-10
    giugno, Moduzzi Edizioni, Bologna, 69.
7. Pearson, J.F. and Weaver, J.B., (1976): Fetal Activity
    and Fetal Wellbeing In:Evaluation.Brit Med. J., 1: 1305

8.   Reinold, E. (1973): Clinical Vaule of Fetal Spontan-
     eous Movements in Early Pregnancy, J. Perinatol Med 1:
     65.

9.   Reinold, E. (1976): Ultrasonic in Early Pregnancy.
     Diagnostic Scanning and Fetal Motor Activity. Series
     Editor Keller, P.J., Karger, S., Basel.

10. Sadovsky E. and Polishuk, W.Z. (1977): Fetal Movements
     in Utero: Nature, Assesment, Prognostic Value, Timing
     of Delivery. Obstet Gynecol 50: 49.

11. Timor-Tritsh, I., Zador, I., Hertz, R.H. et al. (1976):
     Classification of Human Fetal Movements. Am. J Obstet
     Gynecol 126: 70.

ULTRASOUND-GUIDED FETOSCOPY USING REAL-TIME SCANNING

V. Jovanovic and R. Rauskolb

Universitäts-Frauenklinik, Giessen, West Germany

In the field of invasive diagnostic methods, the use
of sonar techniques in the form of ultrasound-guided puncture continues to gain in clinical importance (1-3). This
holds primarily for the introduction of instruments into
the amniotic cavity during pregnancy in cases where this is
necessary for clarifying specific diagnostic questions.

A generally low risk to the mother is always offset by
a much harder to calculate risk to the fetus during such
operations. Invasive methods such as amniocentesis or fetoscopy chiefly jeopardize a pregnancy by directly damaging
the fetus itself or by causing a lesion on the placenta
and/or the uterine wall. The question of how to avoid such
dangers to the fetus in the clinical application of a method
so vital for the prenatal diagnosis of congenital defects
stands rightly in the focus of current interest.

For the ultrasound-guided puncture, the use of a real-
time scanner is the obvious choice. After years of experience in amniocentesis using the Vidoson 635, it seemed
reasonable to assume that the same sort of penetration of
the amniotic cavity but with a slightly "thicker" endoscope
would be similarly safe and acceptable for mother and fetus.

TECHNIQUE - VIDOSON 635

The fetoscope is made up of a trocar sleeve and the
endoscope and has a maximum outside diameter of 3.2 mm. For
the fetoscopy the patient is positioned on a normal gynaecological chair. Following a thorough ultrasound diagnosis,
the patient is given a local anaesthetic and the trocar
sleeve introduced into the amniotic cavity. For this purpose the ultrasound transducer of the Vidoson is mechanical-
ly fixed longitudinally on the abdominal wall and above the
puncture area.

The selection of the best site for insertion depends
both on the localization of the placenta and on the position
of the fetus,in particular on the presentation of the fetal
region important for diagnosis. This is where the striking
and comparatively unfavourable dimensions of the Vidoson
transducer can in individual cases give rise to serious
problems, both in locating the optimal puncture area and in
fixing the transducer so as to allow for unimpeded insertion
The sites which regularly proved to be least problematical

for ultrasound-guided penetration using the Vidoson were the sectors of the supra-pubic puncture area lying immediately to the right and left of the median line.

The trocar's entry into the amniotic cavity can be followed in detail on the ultrasound monitor with a high degree of clarity. The removal of the trocar is usually accompanied by a gush of amniotic fluid.

TECHNIQUE - ADR-SCANNER (3,5 MHz)

For the past one and a half (1 1/2) years we have been able to work with an ADR-Scanner, which has a much smaller and more manageable transducer. Since then we have performed amniocentesis almost exclusively with this equipment, since it has in our view made the puncture procedure technically simpler and more acceptable for the patient. It thus seemed the obvious next step to use the new device for fetoscopy as well.

For fetoscopy with the ADR-Scanner, the patient is positioned on a normal examination table. The size and mobility of the ADR transucer mean that it can be placed in a position on the abdominal wall which allows for transabdominal penetration in practically any area between the Fundus uteri and the symphysis. However, for fixing this transducer in the chosen sector a second person experienced in work with the equipment is required. Besides fixing the transducer it is the assistant's job, by means of fine adjustments in the transducer's exact positioning during the insertion procedure, to make sure that the fetoscope is kept constantly within the path of the ultrasound waves and thus visible as it enters the amniotic cavity. If this is managed, it is equally possible by means of the ADR-Scanner to follow the introduction of the trocar sleeve in every detail.

Exact co-ordination of the tasks performed simultaneously by the operator and assistant is difficult to achieve and requires joint technical training. Both should have experience in fetoscopy and be interchangeable with regard to their respective tasks within the team. This technique has involved only minor alterations in the insertion procedure practised so far; time and work-effort are not affected.

TABLE 1. ULTRASOUND-GUIDED FETOSCOPY WITH REAL-TIME SCANNER

FETOSCOPIES	VIDOSON 635	ADR-3,5 MHz
	N	N
Prior to planned abortion (14 to 22 weeks)	73	25
Diagnostic cases	26	13
Total (137)	99	38

First practical experience with the ADR-Scanner was accumulated with the earlier equipment through fetoscopies carried out prior to planned abortions (Table 1). Meanwhile in 13 out of a total of 38 diagnostic cases we have succeeded in satisfactorily placing the trocar-sleeve intra-amniotically with the help of the ADR-Scanner. In the process, we have been struck by a comparatively strong reflexion coming from the surface of the trocar sleeve, which can occasionally give rise to difficulties in identifying the fetoscope as it enters the amniotic cavity.

Because of the ADR-transducer's favourable dimensions (Table 2), the trocar sleeve can be inserted at a steeper angle to the edge of the transducer, thus reducing the "traumatised distance". This applies particularly where insertion is directed transversely to the longitudinal axis of the transducer, although in such cases usually only part of the sleeve or indeed only its tip is visible on the monitor. On the other hand, a transducer positioned transversely is easier to fix on the slippery abdominal wall.

TABLE 2. REAL-TIME SCANNERS USED FOR ULTRASOUND-GUIDED FETOSCOPY

	Vidoson	ADR
Transducer dimensions	-	+
Variety of puncture area	-	+
Assistant	+	-
Traumatised distance	-	+
Sterility	-	+

+ Advantage
- Disadvantage

Similarly problematical with both types of equipment remains the question of local sterility. This problem seems to us to be easier to solve with the ADR or with other multi-element scanners. After disinfection of the skin, only sterile oil is used during the ultrasound diagnosis and the transducer itself is packed in a sterile plastic bag.

DISCUSSION

With regard to the possibility of direct injury to the fetus and/or of a lesion on the placenta, the insertion procedure constitutes the most critical phase in the course of a fetoscopy. Here the ultrasound-guided technique has proved itself beyond a doubt as the best method available; compared with a "blind puncture" it guarantees a high degree of safety (2,3). The two scanners discussed exhibit quite different advantages and disadvantages when comparing their potential but each has proved itself in its own way in clinical use.

REFERENCES

1.   Rauskolb,R.(1977): Dtsch. Med. Wschr., 102:1341.
2.   Rodeck,C.H.,Campbell,C.(1978): Lancet I, 1128.
3.   Jonatha, W.D.(1977): In:Gynäkologie und Geburtshilfe. Forschungen - Erkenntnisse. Egermann, Wien,Vol.II:657.

ALTERNATIVE METHOD FOR OBJECTIVE RECORDING OF FETAL MOVEMENTS IN THE THIRD TRIMESTER OF PREGNANCY

K. Maršál, K. Lindström and U. Ulmsten

Department of Obstetrics and Gynecology, University Hospital, Malmö, Sweden

Recent years have seen increasing evidence on the clinical usefulness of the monitoring of fetal body and limb movements (FM) when evaluating the well-being of the fetus in utero (1,2,3). It is desirable to perform such monitoring of FM by objective means, as the maternal subjective reporting of FM is impaired by considerable errors (4).

Real-time ultrasound technique is very useful for the observations of fetal motoric activity in the first and second trimester of pregnancy (1). Indeed, it became a method of choice for this purpose. However, during the last three months of pregnancy, only parts of the fetal trunk and extremities can be visualized by a real-time scanner (5,6). Furthermore, the real-time method gives no quantified signals of FM; continuous supervision by the observer is necessary. Therefore a new method for recording FM was designed; it can serve as an alternative or a complement to the ultrasound method.

Four piezo-electric crystals are used as transducers and are placed at the maternal abdomen. When the fetus moves, electric signals are obtained from the crystals. By processing the four signals, outsignals X and Y are produced (Fig. 1). They represent the vector indicating the centrum of the fetal activity in a co-ordinate system. A sum of all primary signals represents the total activity (outsignal Z). The momentary fetal motoric activity is presented at the oscilloscope screen. For each sequence of fetal movements, a new signal is displayed and the activity during a 5-minute period is summed by photographing the oscilloscope screen (Fig. 2). The outsignal Z is also recorded graphically and the incidence of FM signals is registered by an automatic counter.

The new method (called FM-detector) has so far been applied to 37 women with uncomplicated pregnancies during the last trimester. On average, the recording time was 30 min; the recorded incidence of FM was 17 % of time, and the number of movements ranged from 7 to 155 per 30 min. In ten women, FM were recorded subjectively by the mothers and simultaneously by the FM-recorder and real-time ultrasound scanner. In the real-time image, the following main types of FM were recognized:

1. Stretching movements of the fetal trunk;
2. Rolling movements of the whole fetal body;
3. Isolated movements of the fetal extremities or fetal head;
4. Hiccups — intense repetitive movements of short duration;
5. Fetal breathing movements — rhythmic retractive movements of the fetal thorax and simultaneous expansive movements of the fetal abdomen due to contractions of the fetal diaphragm.

Combinations of the different FM types occurred. In the display from the FM-detector, hiccups and isolated movements of the extremities could be recognized. More experience is probably necessary to identify the various movements of the fetal body. Fetal breathing movements were not detected by the FM-detector.

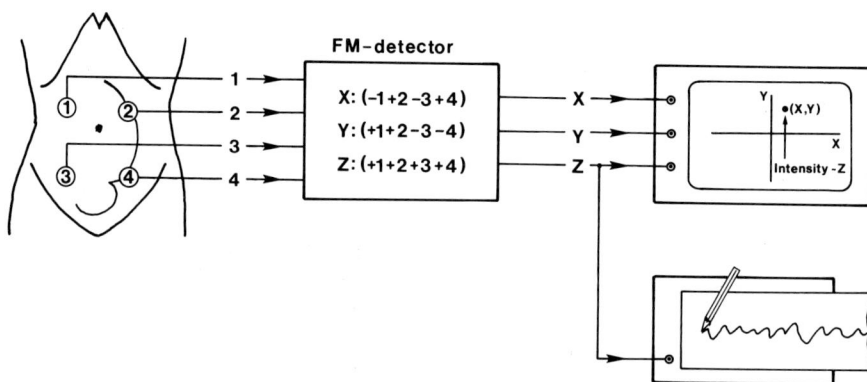

Figure 1. Fetal movements detector — schematic drawing of the set-up and principle.

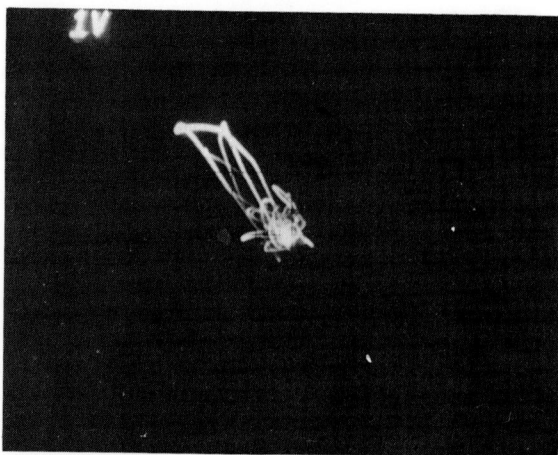

Figure 2. Oscilloscope display of the fetal movements recorded by the FM-detector during 5 min.

The three methods — one subjective and two objective — were evaluated concerning the agreement in detecting FM. Only 62 % of the FM registered by the FM detector and the real-time ultrasound method were also recognized subjectively by the mothers. The FM-detector and real-time method agreed in 92 % of the movements. Both methods missed approximately the same proportion of FM.

The new method for objective recording of FM is suitable for long-term registration of movements; it is non-invasive and causes no discomfort to the mother. It can be used simultaneously with real-time ultrasound technique for analysis of various FM patterns and also together with abdominal fetal ECG. Further studies will show whether the method is applicable as a clinical tool for monitoring the fetal condition in high-risk pregnancies.

REFERENCES

1. Reinold, E. (1976): In: Ultrasonics in early pregnancy. S. Karger, Basel.
2. Sadovsky, E., Yaffe, H. and Polishuk, W. (1974): Int. J. Gynaecol. Obstet., 12, 75.
3. Pearson, J.F. and Weaver, J.D. (1976): Br. Med. J., 1, 1305.
4. Wenderlein, J.M. (1975): Z. Geburtsh. Perinat., 179, 377.
5. Holländer, H.-J. (1978): In: Real-Time Ultrasound in Perinatal Medicine, p. 28. Editor: R. Chef. S. Karger, Basel.
6. Reinold, E. (1979): In: Proceedings IIIrd International Symposium on Recent Advances in Ultrasound Diagnosis. Editor: A. Kurjak. Excerpta Medica, Amsterdam. (In press.)

THE ASSESMENT OF FETAL MOVEMENTS IN EARLY PREGNANCY

B. Hodek

Department of Gynecology and Obstetrics, University Hospital "Dr. M. Stojanović", Zagreb, Yugoslavia

Before the ultrasound was used in obstetrics, the fetal life in utero could only be recognized after the 18th to 20th week of pregnancy by means of subjective data from the pregnant woman, feeling or not feeling fetal movements. This information was objectively confirmed by auscultation of the fetal heart. By ultrasound we can prove fetal life in utero by recording fetal heart beats or by evidence of fetal movements. Diagnostics is already possible from the 7th to 8th week of gestation, but the findings are positively certain from the 10th week (1, 3). Recording of fetal heart beats is performed by the compound scanner, using A- and B-scan, or by combining the B-scan and the Doppler device. Fetal movements are monitored by the compound scanner also using A- and B-scan. This method may consume a lot of time and is complicated especially for an unexperienced examiner.

Ultrasound "real time" technique made monitoring of fetal movements much simpler. This is a very rapid and relatively easy way to obtain results. It is important to mention that the whole fetus must be visualized in the scan plane. In very early pregnancy the fetal parts cannot be distinguished, but echoes which originate from the gestational sac are clearly visible.

Reinold was the first to report fetal movements in detail (4, 5,6,7). The floating movements in the amniotic cavity are due to specific fetal weight, which is slightly greater than the amniotic fluid, so that even a small impulse is enough to change its position, and make it float in the amniotic fluid (2). Another factor which enables this extraordinary motility is the fact that the volume of amniotic fluid is four times greater than the volume of the fetus in early pregnancy while at the end of the second half of pregnancy the volume of amniotic fluid is just one fourth of the fetal volume (8).

There are longer or shorter rest periods between movements which are presumably due to the sleeping fetus, intake of certain drugs by the mother, or lack of space within the amniotic cavity. The observation period is usually 3 to 5 minutes. If the observation period must be shortened for various reasons, or there are no spontaneous movements, the "motor provocation test" is applied. By palpating the abdomen or by vaginal examination the fetus is indirectly moved and in this way subsequent movements are induced. This test can be positive only from 10th week of pregnancy. If there are no spontaneous movements during

the observation period or the "motor provocation test" is negative
the fetal state is considered to be impaired and fetal death will
occur 12 to 24 hours after the last recording of movements. In this
period fetal heart beats are still present.

Method and results

"Real time" technique was used in the investigation of fetal movements by means of the "VidoSon 738" Siemens device. First we wanted
to establish the frequency of fetal movements according to gestational age in normal pregnancy and then to examine the movements in
threatened pregnancy.

The first group consisted of 45 gravidas with uncomplicated pregnancies in the 10th to 20th week of gestation. Five of them were excluded from the group because they lost the live fetus due to an incompetent cervix. Surgical treatment was not applied because of bad
finding on the cervix. Thus the group finally consisted of 40 gravidas.

The second group consisted of 18 gravidas. These were: 5 gravidas from
the first group, 13 gravidas with clinical signs of threatened pregnancy or ultrasonic examination movements demonstrating an impaired
fetus. The observation period was five minutes and a fixed scan plane
technique was applied. This technique is necessary because otherwise
we could be lead to erroneous counts of fetal movements. Examinations
were performed in weekly intervals. The pregnancy was followed for
four more weeks, e. g. till the 24th week of gestation, because with
analysis of fetal movements the prognosis of fetal well-being cannot
be given for a longer period of time due to the many negative factors
which can occur during the later period of pregnancy.

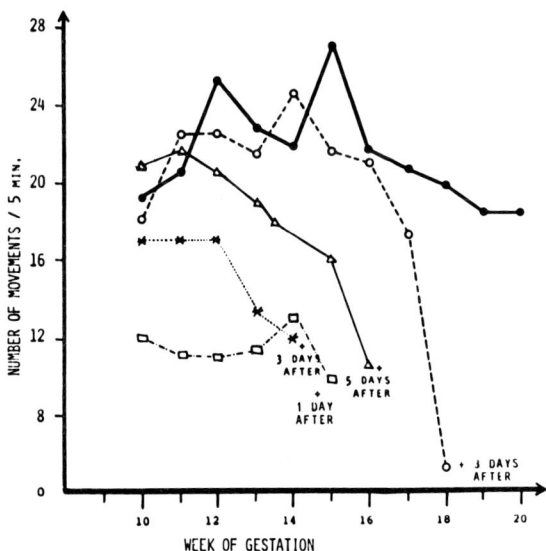

The fig. 1 shows the correlation between the number of movements in a 5 minute period and gestational age from the 10th to 20th week of pregnancy. The thick filled curve demonstrates the mean values of movements for each week of gestation. The number of movements increases from the 10th week and reaches its peak in the 15th week. A slight fall in frequency in the 13th and the 14th week is explained by a smaller number of samples, but tendency of increase is present from the 10th to 15th week. From the 15th week the frequency decreases so that by the 20th week the value is lower than in the 10th week. In all 40 gravidas the pregnancy developed normally until the 24th week.

In the second group consisting of 18 gravidas it is interesting to analyze the frequency of movements in four pregnancies during which fetal death occured. They are demonstrated by three discontinued curves and one thick filled curve. In three cases, the regular frequency of movements was present at the begining of the examination. In two of them, very early in the 11th and 12th week respectively, a progressive fall of frequency occured, while in the third the frequency followed a normal increase till the 14th week when the frequency fell suddenly and fetal death occured. In the fourth case a low frequency was already present in the 10th week. This state continued until the 14th week when the frequency dropped further and the fetus died 24 hours after this last examination. At the time of examination only two movements were registered and the "motor provocation test" was negative.

The frequency of fetal movements was constantly within normal values in the five cases where mothers lost their fetus due to an incompetent cervix. This can be understood because the cause of terminated pregnancy was not in the feto-placental unit so neuromuscular fetal activity was not impaired.

In the remaining nine cases the frequency was constantly near the normal values, altough intermittent signs of threatening abortion were present. In all of these cases the pregnancy progressed to the 24th week. In analyzing them it is evident that the fetus was not impaired in spite of clinical signs of threatened pregnancy, and vice versa.

Conclusion

Our own results, as well as the data from literature, confirmed that by monitoring fetal movements we obtained a valuable prognostical parameter of fetal well-being in utero. This parameter is only complementary, and must be used concurently with other methods of monitoring fetal intrauterine condition.

REFERENCES

(1) Bovicelli, L., Orsini, L.F., Rizzo, N., Coppola, P., Foschi, G., Montacuti, V., Pazzaglia, L., Calderoni, P., Stratico, G., Orlandi, C. (1978): Diagnostic and prognostic value of fetal heart activity in early abnormal pregnancy. IIIrd European congress on ultrasonics in medicine, Bologna Oct. 1.-5. X 78. Proceedings, p. 433.

(2) Hofman, D., Holländer, H.J. (1968): Uber den Nachweis fetalen Lebens und die Messung des kindlichen Schädels mittels des Zweidimensionalen Ultraschallechoverfahrens. Gynekologia 165, 60.

(3) Joupilla, P. (1976): Fetal movements diagnosed by ultrasound in early pregnancy. Acta Obstet. Gynec. Scand. 55, 131.

(4) Reinold, E. (1971): Beobachtung fetaller Aktivität in der ersten Hälfte der Gravidität mit dem Ultraschall. Pädiat. Pädol. 6, 274.

(5) Reinold, E. (1971): Fetale Bewegungen in der Frühgravidität. Z. Geburtshh. Gynäk. 174, 220.

(6) Reinold, E. (1972): Aussagekraff der durch Ultraschall beobachten Kindesbewegungen. 5. Dt. Kongr. Perinatale Medizin, Berlin 1972. Thieme, Stuttgart, p. 25.

(7) Reinold, E. (1973): Klinische Bedeutung der fetalen Spontanbewegungen in der Frühgravidität. J. Perinatal. Med. 1, 65.

(8) Reinold, E. (1976): Ultrasonics in early pregnancy. Karger, Basel 1976.

HUMAN FETAL STOMACH PROFILES

J.W. Wladimiroff, R. Leijs and B. Smit

Department of Obstetrics and Gynaecology, Academic
Hospital Rotterdam Dijkzigt, Erasmus University Rotterdam,
Rotterdam, The Netherlands

Following an explosion of studies on fetal respiratory, cardiac and urinary function and somatic activity, it is not surprising that one has also turned to the study of fetal stomach activity. It is only due to recently improved image resolution of real-time ultrasonic scanning equipment that detailed studies on fetal stomach filling and emptying patterns became possible. Vandenberghe (1,2) was the first to carry-out extensive studies in this particular field of fetal dynamics; his work is presented elsewhere in this book.

We were interested in fetal stomach profiles in normal pregnancy during the last trimester of pregnancy.

TECHNIQUE AND PATIENTS

The fetal stomach can be clearly visualized on a dynamically focussing linear array two-dimensional real-time scanner (3) (Fociscan, Organon Teknika). First an oblique cross-section of the upper-abdomen showing the largest saggital section of the stomach is obtained. The maximum longitudinal (diameter a) and transverse diameter (diameter b) can now be measured (Fig. 1). This is followed by a scan, which is at right angles to the saggital plane of the stomach allowing measurement of the largest antero-posterior diameter (diameter c).

Assuming the fetal stomach being of a prolate elipsoid shape, fetal stomach volume (FSV) can now be calculated:

$$FSV = \frac{4}{3} \times \pi \times \frac{Diam\ a}{2} \times \frac{Diam\ b}{2} \times \frac{Diam\ c}{2}$$

A total of 62 normal pregnancies between 30 and 41 weeks was studied. In each patient the following aspects of fetal stomach dynamics were studied over a period of one hour between 9.00 am and 9.00 pm.:

- The rate and pattern of fetal stomach filling and emptying.
- Maximum and minimum stomach volumes.
- Relationship to maternal meals and time of the day.

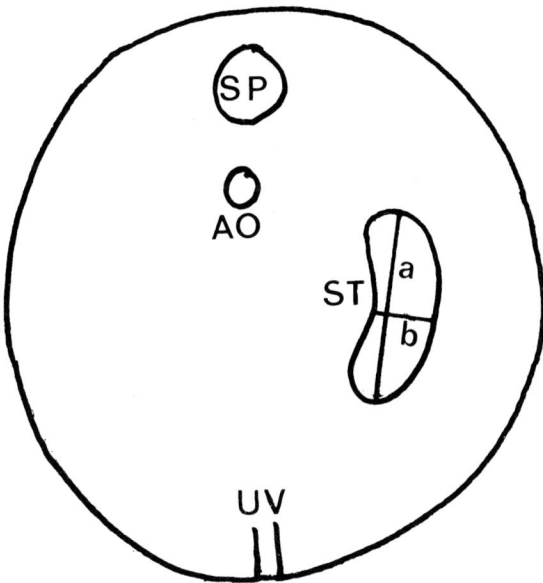

Figure 1. Schematic representation of an oblique cross-section of the fetal upper-abdomen demonstrating saggital section of the stomach. SP=spine; UV=section of umbilical vein; ST=stomach; a=largest longitudinal and b=largest transverse stomach diameter.

RESULTS

Fetal stomach filling is non-linear (Fig. 2), filling time usually ranges between 10 and 30 minutes (63%), but may take only a few minutes or as long as 45 minutes (Fig. 3). The process of fetal stomach emptying takes less than 5 minutes in the majority of cases (58%), but may last up to 30 minutes (Figs. 2 and 3). The process of fetal stomach filling and emptying seems to be accelerated following maternal meals. In a considerable number of patients (47%), no visable change in stomach volume over a period of more than 20 minutes is observed (Figs. 2 and 4). These so-called constant stomach volumes are usually found to be below the level of 4 ml (79%) and are nearly always seen during the pre-meal periods.

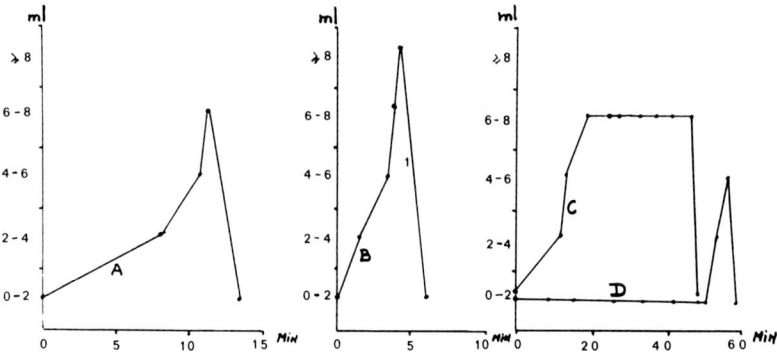

Figure 2. Examples of non-linear stomach filling, stomach emptying and constant stomach volumes.

Maximum stomach volumes are usually less than 2 ml in the study period between 30 and 33 weeks and less than 6 ml between 38 and 41 weeks (Fig. 5). Only during the latter part of pregnancy volumes of more than 8 ml can be demonstrated. Minimum stomach volumes are always less than 2 ml.

The incidence of fetal respiratory movements is significantly higher ($p < 0,001$) during fluid-filled fetal stomachs (mean 32.5%) as compared with empty stomaches (mean 19.6%) (Table I).

Peristaltic activity of the fetal stomach towards the pyloric exit is nearly always observed during the first hour following a maternal meal (Figs. 6a - 6d).

There is no difference in fetal stomach profile when comparing the 9.00 - 12.00 a.m., 12.00 - 3.00 p.m., 3.00 - 6.00 p.m. and 6.00 - 9.00 p.m. study period.

DISCUSSION

The finding of a non-linear stomach filling pattern is not surprising since this process is determined by the rate and quantity of liquor being swallowed over a particular period of time.

The maximum stomach volumes in our study are slightly lower than those measured by Vandenberghe (2), although the same formula was applied.

The presence of periods of relative stomach inactivity (constant volumes) are in keeping with fetal rest and activity states. A higher fetal stomach activity was observed following maternal meals, although no diurnal variation could be established.

The observation of peristaltic contraction waves in the fetal stomach underlines once more that vital

554

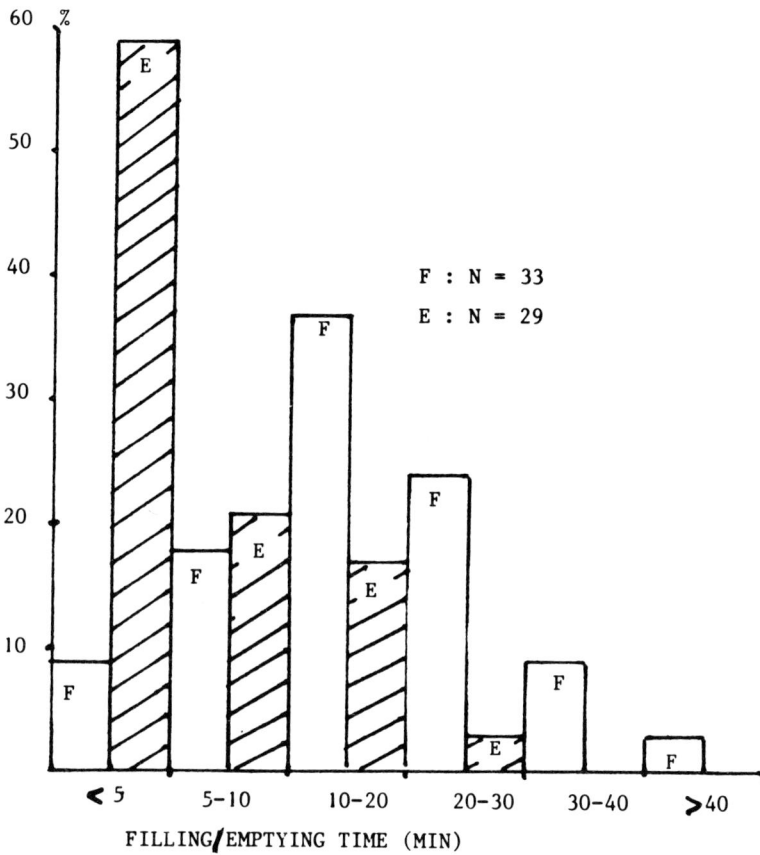

Figure 3. Stomach filling (F) and emptying (E) times.

functional processes are already well-established during
intra-uterine life.

The finding of significantly higher fetal respiratory
activity in the presence of a fluid-filled stomach as
compared with an empty stomach should instigate more
extensive studies on the interaction between fetal
respiratory, digestive and cardio-vascular activity in
order to deepen our insight in these still largely
unexplored fields of fetal dynamics.

Table I. Percentage incidence of fetal respiratory movements in fluid-filled and empty fetal stomachs.

FULL	EMPTY
37 %	17 %
22 %	25 %
54 %	16 %
42 %	22 %
19 %	24 %
25 %	17 %
24 %	10 %
32 %	26 %
42 %	14 %
28 %	25 %
X = 32.5 %	X = 19.6 %

(% incidence F.R.M.)

$p < 0.001$

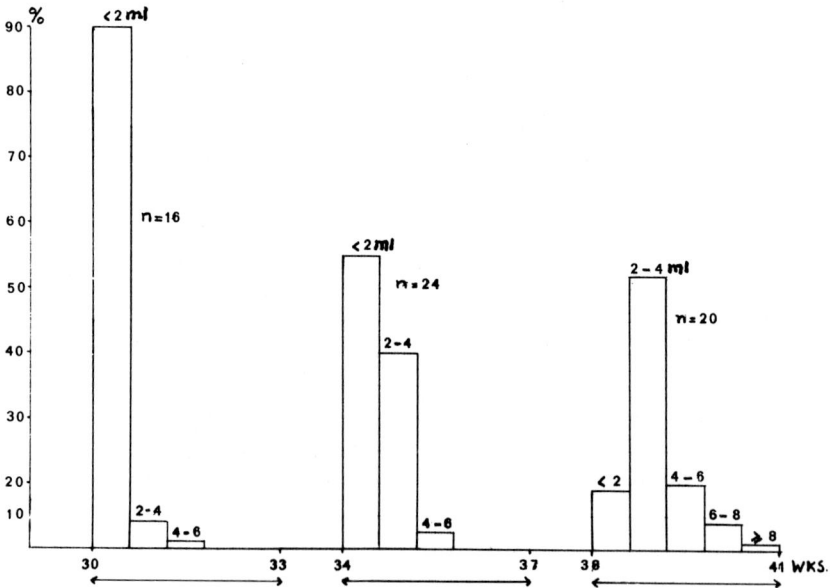

Figure 5. Maximum stomach volumes divided into groups of < 2, 2-4, 4-6, 6-8 and $\geq$ 8 ml between 30 and 41 weeks of gestation.

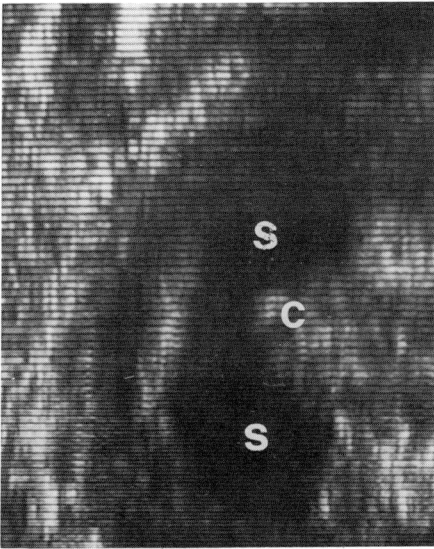

Figure 6a.

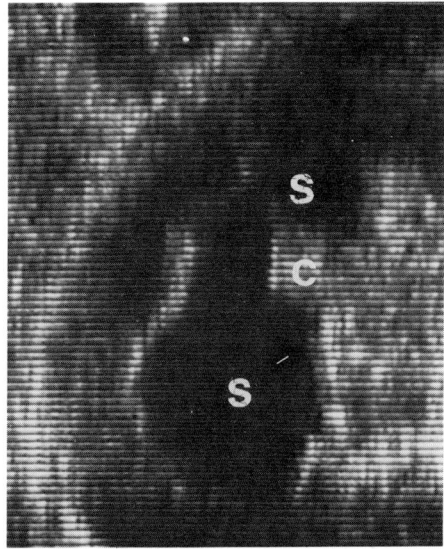

Figure 6b.

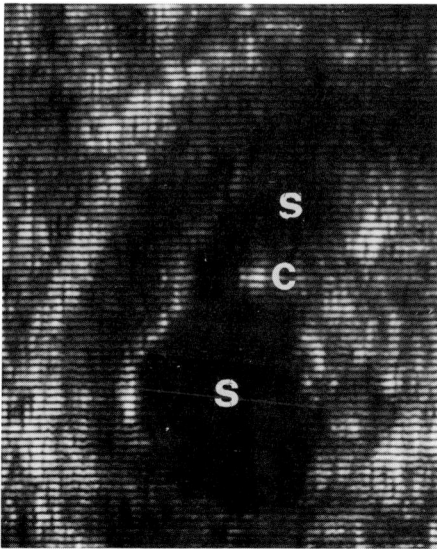

Figure 6c.

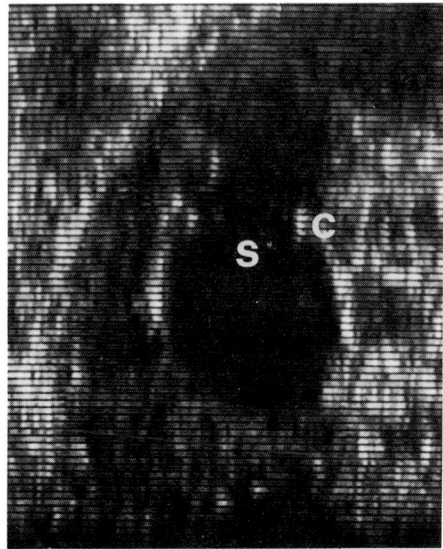

Figure 6d.

Figures 6a - 6d. Peristaltic activity (C) in fluid-filled fetal stomach (S).

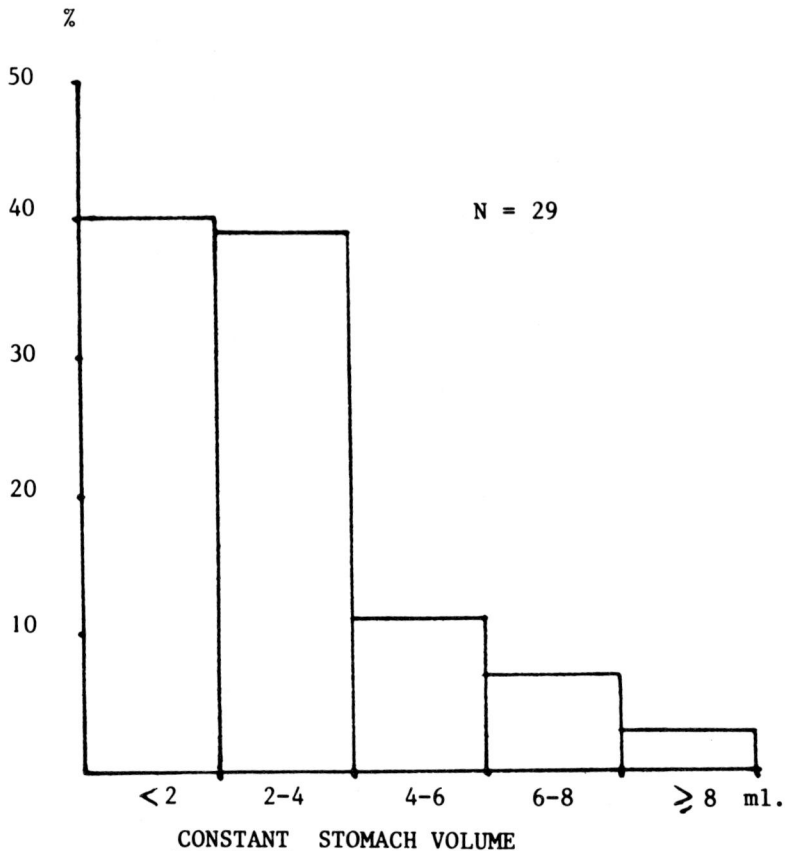

Figure 4. Constant stomach volumes, defined as no visable change in stomach volume over a period of more than 20 minutes.

REFERENCES

1. Vandenberghe, K. and De Wolf, F. (1978):
   In: Abstract Book 3rd European Congress on Ultrasonics in Medicine, pp. 417-418, Minerva Medica, Bologna, Italy.

2. Vandenberghe, K., and De Wolf, F. (1979):
   In: Abstract Book 4th World Congress on Ultrasonics in Medicine, p. 132, Miyazaki, Japan.

3. Ligtvoet, C.M., Ridder, J., Hagemeijer, F. and Wladimiroff, J.W. (1977):
   In: Ultrasonics International 1977, p. 111, Editor: Z. Novak, IPC Science and Technology Press, Guildford, England.

INDEX OF AUTHORS